Memory: Organization and Locus of Change

Memory: Organization and Locus of Change

Edited by

LARRY R. SQUIRE

NORMAN M. WEINBERGER

GARY LYNCH

JAMES L. McGAUGH

New York   Oxford
OXFORD UNIVERSITY PRESS
1991

Oxford University Press

Oxford New York Toronto
Delhi Bombay Calcutta Madras Karachi
Petaling Jaya Singapore Hong Kong Tokyo
Nairobi Dar es Salamm Cape Town
Melbourne Auckland

and associated companies in
Berlin Ibadan

Published by Oxford University Press, Inc.,
200 Madison Avenue, New York, New York 10016

Oxford is a registered trademark of Oxford University Press

Library of Congress Cataloging-in-Publication Data
Memory: organization and locus of change/
edited by Larry R. Squire ... [et al.].
p. cm. Includes bibliographical references and index.
ISBN 0-19-506921-8
1. Memory—Physiological aspects. 2. Neural plasticity.
I. Squire, Larry R.
QP406.M457 1991 612.8′2—dc20 91-16012

This work relates to Department of Navy Grant N00014-90-J-4008 issued by the Office of Naval Research.
The United States Government has a royalty-free license throughout the world in all copyrightable material
contained herein.

Research sponsored by the Air Force Office of Scientific Research, Air Force Systems Command, USAF,
under grant or cooperative agreement number, AFOSR 91-0105. The U.S. Government is authorized to
reproduce and distribute reprints for governmental purposes notwithstanding any copyright notation therein.
The views and conclusions contained in this document are those of the authors and should not be interpreted
as necessarily representing the official policies or endorsements, either express or implied, of the Air Force
Office of Scientific Research or the U.S. Government.

9 8 7 6 5 4 3 2 1

Printed in the United States of America
on acid-free paper

Preface

This book is the fourth in a series that began in 1984. Like the previous volumes in the series, *Neurobiology of Learning and Memory*, *Memory Systems of the Brain*, and *Brain Organization and Memory: Cells, Systems, and Circuits*, this book is the result of a conference organized by the Center for the Neurobiology of Learning and Memory of the University of California, Irvine. The Fourth Conference was held at Irvine on October 17–20, 1990. Contemporary work on memory is directed at several levels of analysis and draws on a number of different disciplines. In particular, questions about memory make use of the methods and approaches traditionally associated with both psychology and neuroscience. The contents of this volume reflect this diversity as well as the excitement of what has been for many years a highly productive area of research.

The book begins with an introductory chapter that considers the psychology of memory at the global, structural level. The remainder of the book is divided into three related parts. The first focuses on recent approaches, which are based in part on new technology, that aim to measure and describe activity in relatively large populations of neurons. The second focuses on memory at the level of brain systems. One major theme to emerge from work at this level is that memory is composed of multiple, separable components and that different components can be identified with specific anatomical structures and connections. The third part focuses on molecular and cellular studies of how individual neurons and their synapses show history-dependent behavior. This work concerns both short-lasting changes in synaptic plasticity as well as longer-lasting changes in connectivity that depend on altered gene expression and morphological growth and change. Altogether, the chapters provide a rich summary of the breadth and the excitement of contemporary research on the biology of memory.

The conference and the preparation of this book were generously supported by the Office of Naval Research, the Air Force Office of Scientific Research, the National Science Foundation, the UCI Office of Research and Graduate Studies, the Irvine Company, UCI Global Peace and Conflict Studies, G.D. Searle & Co., and Beckman Instruments, Inc.

We are especially grateful to Lynn Brown, Nan Collett, Lori LaSalle, Deanna Sanders, and Lillian Fontana for their sustained and superb assistance in all phases of this project.

L.R.S.
N.M.W.
G.L.
J.L.McG.

Irvine, California
May 1991

Contents

Contributors   xi

1. *Concepts of Human Memory*   3
   ENDEL TULVING

I Distribution of Learning-Induced Brain Activity

2. *Insights into Processes of Visual Perception from Studies in the Olfactory System*   35
   WALTER J. FREEMAN

3. *Optical Imaging of Architecture and Function in the Living Brain*   49
   AMIRAM GRINVALD
   TOBIAS BONHOEFFER
   DOV MALONEK
   DORON SHOHAM
   EYAL BARTFELD
   A. ARIELI
   RINA HILDESHEIM
   EUGENE RATZLAFF

4. *Modular Organization of Information Processing in the Normal Human Brain: Studies with Positron Emission Tomography*   86
   MARCUS E. RAICHLE

5. *Structures in the Human Brain Participating in Visual Learning, Tactile Learning, and Motor Learning*   95
   PER E. ROLAND
   BALÁZS GULYÁS
   RÜDIGER J. SEITZ

6. *Does Synaptic Selection Explain Auditory Imprinting?*   114
   HENNING SCHEICH
   E. WALLHÄUSSER-FRANKE
   K. BRAUN

II Functional Roles of Brain Systems

7. *Memory Representation in the Hippocampus: Functional Domain and Functional Organization* 163
   HOWARD EICHENBAUM
   NEAL J. COHEN
   TIM OTTO
   CYNTHIA WIBLE

8. *Systems and Synapses of Emotional Memory* 205
   JOSEPH E. LEDOUX

9. *Alterations of the Functional Organization of Primary Somatosensory Cortex Following Intracortical Microstimulation or Behavioral Training* 217
   GREGG H. RECANZONE
   MICHAEL M. MERZENICH

10. *Localization of Primal Long-Term Memory in the Primate Temporal Cortex* 239
    YASUSHI MIYASHITA
    KUNIYOSHI SAKAI
    SEI-ICHI HIGUCHI
    NAOHIKO MASUI

11. *Mnemonic Functions of the Cholinergic Septohippocampal System* 250
    DAVID S. OLTON
    BENNET S. GIVENS
    ALICJA L. MARKOWSKA
    MATTHEW SHAPIRO
    STEPHANIE GOLSKI

III Locus of Cellular Change

12. *The Anatomy of Long-Term Sensitization in Aplysia: Morphological Insights into Learning and Memory* 273
    CRAIG H. BAILEY
    MARY CHEN

13. *Activity-Dependent Neuronal Gene Expression: A Potential Memory Mechanism?* 301
    CHRISTINE M. GALL
    JULIE C. LAUTERBORN

14. *Variants of Synaptic Potentiation and Different Types of Memory Operations in Hippocampus and Related Structures*   330
GARY LYNCH
JOHN LARSON
URSULA STAUBLI
RICHARD GRANGER

15. *Local Plasticity in Neuronal Learning*   364
E.N. SOKOLOV

16. *What the Chick Can Tell Us About the Process and Structure of Memory*   392
STEVEN P.R. ROSE

Index   413

Contributors

A. ARIELI
Department of Neurobiology
Weizmann Institute of Science
Rehovet, 76100
Israel

CRAIG H. BAILEY
Center for Neurobiology and
  Behavior
College of Physicians and Surgeons
Columbia University
722 West 168th Street
New York, New York 10032

EYAL BARTFELD
Department of Neurobiology
Weizmann Institute of Science
Rehovet, 76100
Israel

TOBIAS BONHOEFFER
Max-Planck Institute for Brain
  Research
Deutschordenstrasse 46
D-6000 Frankfurt
Germany

K. BRAUN
Institute of Zoology
Technical University Darmstadt
Schnittspahnstrasse 3
D-6100 Darmstadt
Germany

MARY CHEN
Center for Neurobiology and
  Behavior
College of Physicians and Surgeons
Columbia University
722 West 168th Street
New York, New York 10032

NEAL J. COHEN
Amnesia Research Laboratory
Beckman Institute
Department of Psychology
University of Illinois at Urbana-
  Champaign
Urbana, Illinois 61801

HOWARD EICHENBAUM
Department of Psychology
University of North Carolina at
  Chapel Hill
CB# 3270, Davie Hall
Chapel Hill, North Carolina 27599

WALTER J. FREEMAN
Department of Molecular and
  Cellular Biology
Division of Neurobiology
University of California
Berkeley, California 94720

CHRISTINE M. GALL
Department of Anatomy and
  Neurobiology
University of California
Irvine, California 92717

BENNET S. GIVENS
Department of Psychology
Johns Hopkins University
Charles & 34th Streets
Baltimore, Maryland 21218

STEPHANIE GOLSKI
Department of Psychology
Johns Hopkins University
Charles & 34th Streets
Baltimore, Maryland 21218

RICHARD GRANGER
Center for the Neurobiology of
    Learning and Memory
University of California
Irvine, California 92717

AMIRAM GRINVALD
Laboratory of Neurobiology
Rockefeller University
1230 York Avenue, Box 138
New York, New York 10021
and
Department of Neurobiology
Weizmann Institute of Science
Rehovot, 76100
Israel

BALÁZS GULYAS
Division of Positron Emission
    Tomography
Department of Neurophysiology
Karolinska Institute and Karolinska
    Hospital
Box 60500, S-104 01 Stockholm
Sweden

SEI-ICHI HIGUCHI
Department of Physiology
University of Tokyo
School of Medicine
7-3-1 Hongo, Bunkyo-ku
Tokyo 113, Japan

RINA HILDESHEIM
Department of Neurobiology
Weizmann Institute of Science
Rehovot, 76100
Israel

JOHN LARSON
Center for the Neurobiology of
    Learning and Memory
University of California
Irvine, California 92717

JULIE C. LAUTERBORN
Department of Anatomy and
    Neurobiology
University of California
Irvine, California 92717

JOSEPH E. LEDOUX
Center for Neural Science
New York University
4 Washington Place
New York, New York 10003

GARY LYNCH
Center for the Neurobiology of
    Learning and Memory
University of California
Irvine, California 92717

DOV MALONEK
Department of Neurobiology
Weizmann Institute of Science
Rehovot, 76100
Israel

ALICJA L. MARKOWSKA
Department of Psychology
Johns Hopkins University
Charles & 34th Streets
Baltimore, Maryland 21218

NAOHIKO MASUI
Department of Physiology
University of Tokyo
School of Medicine
7-3-1 Hongo, Bunkyo-ku
Tokyo 113, Japan

JAMES L. MCGAUGH
Center for the Neurobiology of
  Learning and Memory
University of California
Irvine, California 92717

MICHAEL M. MERZENICH
Coleman Laboratory
Keck Center for Integrative
  Neuroscience
University of California
San Francisco, California 94143

YASUSHI MIYASHITA
Department of Physiology
University of Tokyo
School of Medicine
7-3-1 Hongo, Bunkyo-ku
Tokyo 113, Japan

DAVID S. OLTON
Department of Psychology
Johns Hopkins University
Charles & 34th Streets
Baltimore, Maryland 21218

TIM OTTO
Department of Psychology
University of North Carolina at
  Chapel Hill
Chapel Hill, North Carolina 27599

MARCUS E. RAICHLE
Division of Radiation Sciences
Washington University School of
  Medicine
501 S. Kingshighway, Box 8225
St. Louis, Missouri 63110

EUGENE RATZLAFF
IBM T.J. Watson Research Center
P.O. Box 218
Yorktown Heights, New York
  10598

GREGG H. RECANZONE
Laboratory of Sensorimotor
  Research
National Eye Institute
National Institutes of Health
Bethesda, Maryland 20892

PER E. ROLAND
Laboratory for Brain Research and
  PET
Nobel Institute of Neurophysiology
Karolinska Institute
Doktersringen 6F
S-104 01 Stockholm
Sweden

STEVEN P.R. ROSE
Brain and Behaviour Research
  Group
Open University
Milton Keynes MK7 6AA
United Kingdom

KUNIYOSHI SAKAI
Department of Physiology
University of Tokyo
School of Medicine
7-3-1 Hongo, Bunkyo-ku
Tokyo 113, Japan

HENNING SCHEICH
Institute of Zoology
Technical University Darmstadt
Schnittspahnstrasse 3
D-6100 Darmstadt
Germany

RÜDIGER J. SEITZ
Medizinische Einrichtungen
Der Universitat Dusseldorf
Neurologische Klinik
Moorenstr. 5
D-4000 Dusseldorf 1
Germany

MATTHEW SHAPIRO
Department of Psychology
McGill University
Montreal, Quebec
H3A 1B1, Canada

DORON SHOHAM
Department of Neurobiology
Weizmann Institute of Science
Rehovot, 76100
Israel

E.N. SOKOLOV
Department of Psychophysiology
Moscow State University
Marx Avenue 18
103009 Moscow
USSR

LARRY R. SQUIRE
Veterans Administration Medical
  Center (V-116A)
University of California, San Diego
3350 La Jolla Village Drive
San Diego, California 92161

URSULA STAUBLI
Department of Psychology
McGill University
Montreal, Quebec
H3A 1B1, Canada

ENDEL TULVING
Department of Psychology
University of Toronto
Toronto, Ontario
M5S 1A1, Canada

E. WALLHÄUSSER-FRANKE
Institute of Zoology
Technical University Darmstadt
Schnittspahnstrasse 3
D-6100 Darmstadt
Germany

NORMAN M. WEINBERGER
Center for the Neurobiology of
  Learning and Memory
University of California
Irvine, California 92717

CYNTHIA WIBLE
Brockton Veterans Administration
  Hospital
Psychiatry 116A
Brockton, Massachusetts 02401

Memory: Organization and Locus of Change

1

Concepts of Human Memory

ENDEL TULVING

Scientific study of human memory has been proceeding apace for over a hundred years. Original experiments on normal memory by Ebbinghaus, early clinical observations of pathological memory by Korsakoff, and pioneering studies of conditioning and learning in animals by Pavlov and Thorndike laid the foundations of a science of memory that has been expanding ever since and that now has branched out in many directions. Today, learning and memory are explored at several levels of analysis in different organisms from a number of complementary perspectives.

The first century of research on human memory has had two major effects: (a) it has produced a wealth of empirical data, and (b) it has forcefully demonstrated the enormous complexity of learning and memory. In so doing, it has also promised more of the same in the future—an ever-increasing number of detailed facts, and an even greater complexity. An individual practitioner can take defensive action against this dual onslaught in either of two ways: concentrate on some narrow corner of the domain and seek order and harmony locally, or ignore the minutiae and contemplate the broad outlines of the total scene. Although one's choice depends on temperament and previously reinforced behavior, observation suggests that one's selection of the strategy for minimizing perplexity also correlates with age. Young investigators like confrontations with specific problems; older ones prefer to look down on things from the stratosphere.

In this chapter I discuss some general ideas in the broad field of human memory. Ideas are the lifeblood of science. In the final analysis, the fortunes of any scientific discipline depend at least as much on the quality of its ideas as on the raw facts about Nature. It is easy to agree with Ernst Mayr when he says that "those are not far wrong who insist that the progress of science consists principally in the progress of scientific concepts" (Mayr, 1982, p. 24). The reason that, say, a telephone directory fails to pass muster as a scientific publication is that one cannot have any interesting ideas about its contents, although it qualifies splendidly on several other relevant criteria: it provides a large number of very tightly organized empirical facts, a large proportion of the information in it can be regarded as quantitative, and the number of accurate predictions even a small directory allows greatly exceeds the number of predictions possible on the basis of the best contemporary models and theories of memory.

I will refer to the ideas that I wish to discuss as "concepts" in order to convey the impression that they are not just fleeting thoughts anyone might have about the subject matter, but rather that they are products of careful thought, sometimes a great deal of hard thought. But it should be clear that, even under the cloak of the more respectable term, a concept is nothing more than an idea, a thought, or a hunch about something. As such, it can be powerful or impotent, brilliant or shallow, enduring or ephemeral. It can help or hinder, encourage or frustrate, inspire or stifle.

In other fields of scientific endeavor, concepts vary in the importance of the role they play. Some concepts are central, whereas others play secondary, tertiary, and further subsidiary roles. Central concepts of other sciences are universally known. They include things such as force and acceleration in classical mechanics, metabolism in understanding living matter, homeostasis in defining disease states, atmospheric pressure in the understanding of weather phenomena, and lithospheric plates in the science of plate tectonics. These concepts are central in that their absence would greatly hamper the exposition of theory in which they play a part, and in that the understanding of the target phenomena would be incomplete in their absence.

The concepts of human memory to be discussed in this chapter are not quite in the same class as the major concepts of more mature sciences, but they are broad and general, transcending individual phenomena and stretching across the boundaries of particular models and theories. In this sense they are central to the science of human memory. The concepts I discuss are well known to all practitioners inside the field, and familiar to many others. The justification for reviewing them on the present occasion lies in the fact that concepts have a habit of changing over time, and that sometimes these changes escape wider notice. Most of us practicing researchers exhibit a remarkable tendency to become imprinted on and remain attached to the initial formulation of a concept, despite changes, sometimes radical changes, that it undergoes as a result of further work and thought. A periodic reexamination of the status of ideas and concepts in a field need not be a total waste of time.

I classify the concepts to be discussed into two broad categories: processing concepts and classificatory concepts. Processing concepts have to do with processes that comprise individual acts of memory; classificatory concepts represent ideas about different kinds of learning and memory, or memory systems.

PROCESSES OF REMEMBERING

One of Ebbinghaus's numerous contributions was the adoption of the study/test paradigm for the study of memory. The paradigm has remained a successful standard ever since. In the study phase, experimental subjects are presented some information or learn a task; in the test phase, the retention of the information or the task-based skill is assessed. We take the study/test paradigm for granted and do not always realize its influence in shaping our approach to and thoughts about our subject matter. Memory is inextricably intertwined with other cognitive functions of the brain in the ceaseless flux of behavior and experience. The study/test paradigm allows the experimenter to create a multitude of laboratory analogues of single *acts* of memory that constitute the flux in real life, and makes the individual discrete acts the objects of observation and analysis. From this perspective, to study memory is to study acts of memory; to understand memory means to understand the mechanisms and component processes whose workings and interactions determine the course and outcome of an act of memory. The identity of and relations among the component processes demarcate the conceptual structure of an act of memory.

General Abstract Processing System

A conceptual structure of a single act of human memory, dubbed General Abstract Processing System (GAPS), is schematically represented in Figure 1.1 (Tulving, 1983). It depicts the stages of encoding, storage, and retrieval of an item of information, and interrelations among them, within the conventional study/test paradigm.

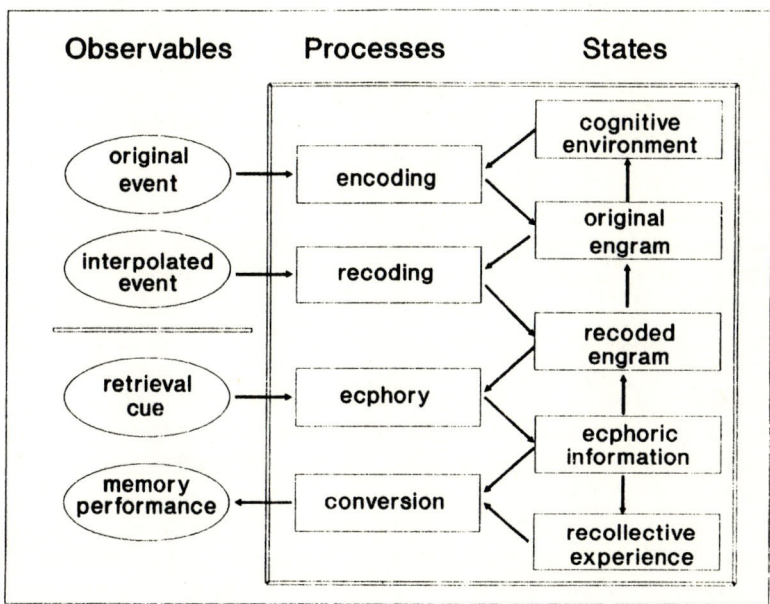

FIGURE 1.1. General Abstract Processing System (GAPS): A conceptual structure of component processes of an act of remembering. (From Tulving, 1983)

GAPS specifies three different kinds of concepts: observable components, hypothetical processes, and hypothetical states. States represent the end products of the processes. The arrows in the diagram represent the relations among the concepts; each arrow can be interpreted as "influences".

The central concepts of GAPS are *encoding, engram, ecphory,* and *ecphoric information.* Encoding is the process that converts the event information into an engram (memory trace or representation); ecphory is the process that combines the information in the engram and the retrieval cue into ecphoric information. Ecphoric information determines recollective experience, the end product of an act of cognitive memory.[1] Encoding and engram are the principal components of *storage* of information in memory; ecphory and ecphoric information are the principal components of *retrieval* of the stored information.

The act of remembering begins with the encoding of a perceptual or conceptual event within a given cognitive environment that represents all aspects of the state of the system that are relevant to the event and its encoding. It ends with the creation of a cognitive state referred to as ecphoric information. It is constructed on the basis of both the (usually recoded) engram and the retrieval cue. In episodic memory, ecphoric information determines the nature of recollective experience, the conscious re-experience of the original event. In semantic memory, the ecphoric information determines the contents of the retrieved bundle of knowledge. In laboratory studies, and frequently though not always in real life, the cognitive contents of recollective experience and retrieved knowledge are converted into overt behavior, usually in verbal or some other symbolic form. Such conversion is, strictly speaking, not a component of the act of remembering. A person's verbal description of the retrieved cognitive contents is a postecphoric, nonmemory process; its relation to ecphoric information and recollective experience can take any one of a number of different forms (cf. Buschke, 1987, Fig. 22–1).

The structure of GAPS is abstract. It does not constrain the treatment of the component processes that comprise the storage and retrieval of information about experienced events in formal modeling or their analysis at the physical and physiological levels. It neither prescribes nor proscribes the specific nature of component processes. It is compatible with many particular theoretical ideas or physiological characterizations of the underlying mechanisms and processes. GAPS does, however, make explicit the general categories of component processes of remembering. By postulating the existence of these processes, it points to the necessity of their analysis at *all levels.*

The outcome of any act of memory is generally useful to the individual to the extent that ecphoric information and recollective experience accurately reflect the original extent of or correspond to the originally stored fact. A great deal of evidence exists showing that the correspondence between the original event or fact and its ecphorized form may be highly variable, from near-perfect reproduction to glaring discrepancies. In cognitive psychology of memory this correspondence defines the dependent variables of primary interest.[2]

GAPS has been shaped by what is known about the factors and variables that determine remembering as it manifests itself at the level of cognition and behavior. The component processes of GAPS reveal the sources of multiple determinants of the nature and contents of recollective experience and its correspondence with the original event or comprehended fact. It explicates the variability of this correspondence, from highly accurate recreation of the original experience to remembering of events that in fact did not occur or retrieval of facts that are not true. It summarizes the types of experimental interventions that are not only possible in the study of memory but whose omission from the analysis would necessarily result in an incomplete understanding of memory.

Synergistic Ecphory

GAPS makes explicit the synergistic nature of retrieval. Retrieval in earlier times meant the "utilization" of traces, or stored information (Melton, 1963), or "the use of memory in neuronal and behavioral operations" (Dudai, 1989, p. 6). These definitions, widely accepted even today, embody the strong "storage bias" that characterized psychological thinking about memory for a long time, and still does so for most laypersons. The storage bias leads people to identify retrieval with the performance of what the individual has learned, or with the output from the memory system. In the traditional thought, performance is determined by past learning: the output from the memory system depends on the earlier inputs as represented by the informational contents of the engram. Even in early information-processing models of memory (Atkinson & Shiffrin, 1968; Waugh & Norman, 1965), one of the basic assumptions was that of a one-to-one relation between what had been stored and what could be recalled. Thus, retrieval was thought to provide a nondestructive test of what has been stored. In theoretical terms the concept of retrieval as performance was conceptualized as "activation" of the engram. GAPS suggests that the matter is more complex. The antidote to the storage bias is synergistic ecphory.

I use the term *synergistic ecphory* to express and emphasize the idea that the outcome of an act of memory depends critically not only on the information contained in the engram but also on the information provided by the retrieval environment, or retrieval cues. "Synergistic" serves to remind us that ecphory, the main component process of retrieval, is governed by these two sources of relevant information, one derived from the past, the other one representing the present. Thus, synergistic ecphory as a concept differs from and supersedes the historically earlier concept of activation of engram. It also accents the contrast between the storage-oriented study of memory and the orientation in which retrieval plays an equally decisive role.

For over three-quarters of a century after Ebbinghaus's ground-breaking work, strong storage bias prevailed. To study memory meant to study storage. In the associative orientation this meant the study of acquisition and loss, strengthening and weakening, transfer and interference of associations. Performance was little more than a device for measuring the changes in storage.

The thinking governed by the storage bias began to change in the 1960s, when storage and retrieval processes were analytically and experimentally separated and an explicit distinction drawn between *availability* and *accessibility* of stored information (Tulving & Pearlstone, 1966). Availability was determined by the same variables that determine storage; accessibility was a joint function of availability *and* retrieval cues. The distinction between availability and accessibility did not depart greatly from that between learning and performance, or between the engram and its activation, but it prepared the way for a more radical break with the past. This break came when it was discovered that different encoding operations performed on structurally fixed units of information could lead to large differences in the remembering of these units (e.g., Craik & Tulving, 1975; Hyde & Jenkins, 1969; Mathews, 1977), and that the effectiveness of structurally fixed retrieval cues could vary greatly with differences in these encoding operations (e.g., Barclay, Bransford, Franks, McCarrell, & Nitsch, 1974; Fisher & Craik, 1977; Thomson & Tulving, 1970; Tulving & Osler, 1968; Tulving & Thomson, 1973; Watkins & Tulving, 1975). The idea of performance as activation of engrams was superseded by the more advanced concepts of encoding specificity (Tulving & Thomson, 1973), transfer appropriate processing (Morris, Bransford, & Franks, 1977), and synergistic ecphory (Tulving, 1982). A more complete story of these developments, together with a survey of relevant experimental evidence, is presented elsewhere (Tulving, 1983).

Synergistic ecphory, the idea that remembering occurs as a result of *interaction* between storage and retrieval, or between engram and ecphory, implies that to understand memory means to understand this interaction. It implies that any specification of an engram *independently* of ecphory is necessarily incomplete, as is any specification of ecphory independently of the engram. The specification of the engram has to refer to ecphory, exactly as the specification of the ecphory must refer to the engram. Synergistic ecphory also implies that any physical determination of the properties of the engram independently of ecphory may turn out to be impossible, inasmuch as the engram does not exist in the absence of ecphory: it cannot be distinguished from the rest of the neural aftereffects of the encoding process. Such *physical indeterminancy* of the engram is to be contrasted with its *biological determinacy*, as reflected in the products of the interaction between storage and retrieval.

Initial attempts have been made to identify storage and retrieval processes, or the engram and ecphory, at the level of brain activity, with success that augurs well for the future. One example is provided by Neville, Kutas, Chesney, and Schmidt (1986) who studied event-related potentials (ERPs) during both encoding and subsequent recognition of words, and found that the amplitude of the late positive component (P650) recorded at encoding was different for words subsequently recognized and those not recognized. Another example of electrophysiological study of brain events correlated with memory processes is the study reported by Smith and Halgren (1989) who found rather large differences in the ERP patterns for words previously presented and recognized as such by the subjects and words not previously presented. They interpreted this "word-repetition" effect on ERPs as reflecting dynamic neurocognitive activity whereby the information provided by the retrieval cue (the test word) is brought into interaction with the information contained in the engram of the original presentation of the word—that is, synergistic ecphory. A third example, based on a different technique, is a preliminary study of regional cerebral blood flow that showed different patterns of cortical activation correlated with retrieval of episodic and semantic information (Tulving, 1989; Tulving, Risberg, & Ingvar, 1988).

CLASSIFICATION OF MEMORY

A relatively recently adopted new approach to the study of memory has to do with the classification of memory (Sherry & Schacter, 1987; Tulving, 1985c, 1986). The classification approach *complements* the process-oriented approach to memory; it is not an alternative to it. The general purpose of the classification enterprise is analysis and description of memory as a structured assembly of separable but normally closely interacting brain systems and subsystems whose collaborative functioning is expressed in behavior, cognition, and conscious awareness. A basic premise of classification research is that all nontrivial empirical generalizations about learning and memory necessarily hold only within certain boundaries. Classification research attempts to define these boundaries in terms of different memory systems and subsystems.

The objectives of classification research are threefold. Classifiers seek to construct a classificatory scheme that (a) identifies major systems and subsystems of memory, (b) specifies their properties and characteristics, and (c) delineates the nature of the relations among them. The pursuit of the classification enterprise also includes the search for the solutions of a variety of related methodological and pretheoretical problems. These include issues such as the rules and principles of classification research, the nature of relevant empirical evidence, the logic of acceptable inferences from the data, the relations between memory tasks and memory systems, and the creation and adoption of suitable terminology (Tulving, 1985c).

The Concept of "System"

What do we mean by "memory system"? The concept of "memory system" itself is still evolving, and undoubtedly will be modified, refined, and sharpened as classification research unfolds. In an early formulation (Tulving,

1984a), I tried to make explicit what I perceived as rather broadly held tacit assumptions as to what memory systems are and what they do, notions that I thought reflected the views on the issue by most researchers. As these general ideas about systems have not been substantially challenged or changed greatly in the intervening years, and as they are not widely known, they may be worth re-recording here:

> (1) Different systems serve separate, largely nonoverlapping behavioral and cognitive functions. They mediate the acquisition and retention of different kinds of information and knowledge. . . . (2) Different systems operate according to different laws and principles. Although all learning and memory systems share some features—they all enable the organism to make use of information acquired on an earlier occasion—all the processes of different systems need not be the same: what is true of one system is not *necessarily* true of another. (3) The behavioral and cognitive functions of different systems are represented in the brain by different neural structures, different neural mechanisms, or both. Each such structure or mechanism is specialized for a particular set of behavioral or experiential functions. It is sometimes possible for one neural learning and memory system to substitute for another, albeit at a less efficacious level; it is also possible for the activity of one of the neural systems to modulate that of another. (4) Different systems have developed at different stages in the phylogeny of the species, representing the responses of the species to changes in environmental demands for survival. Analogous changes may occur in the ontogeny of individual members of the species in some cases: depending upon the time course of the maturation of the brain, different kinds of learning and memory functions become possible at different ages of the developing individual. (5) Different systems differ from one another with respect to the format of representation of acquired information. . . . The after-effects of a behavioral event registered in a more primitive system may carry minimal information about the past event, although sufficient information to determine or modify future behavior or experience. On the other hand, representations (engrams, memory traces) laid down in a more advanced system may preserve a good deal of detailed information about the past event. (6) In the course of an organism's interaction with its environment, several systems may participate in the storing of information, use of information, or both, in a particular situation. The cooperation among the systems may be so smooth that casual observation of behavior creates the impression of a single system in action. (Tulving, 1984a, pp. 177–179)

In this formulation, a memory system is defined by its brain mechanisms, type of information it handles, and the principles of its operations, with a good deal of overlap in all three aspects envisaged among different systems. Sherry and Schacter (1987), in their discussion of the concept of memory system, endorse the ideas that different memory systems are characterized by different modes of operation and different brain structures. They also elaborate on the evolutionary rationale for the emergence of different memory systems, arguing that different systems evolve in response to the need for information storage and retrieval devices for specific purposes, under conditions where the needs satisfied by different systems are said to be *functionally incompatible*. But Sherry and Schacter (1987) reject the notion that the type of information is different in different systems (Tulving, 1984a). This kind of disagreement is a symptom of the developing understanding of classification; its resolution is one of the many tasks awaiting memory classifiers. One solution is to postulate that a given system may indeed process different kinds of information, but that each of its subsystems deal with only one type of information. An example of this idea is provided by the word-form and the structural description subsystems of the perceptual representation system (PRS) that has been postulated to mediate perceptual priming effects (Schacter, 1990; Tulving & Schacter, 1990). The mode and rules of operation of the two subsystems are assumed to be the same, but the types of information on which the two subsystems operate are diffeent, as are presumably their neural underpinnings.

The systems approach has been criticized in cognitive psychology, primarily because of perceived lack of evidential support and because the whole idea is thought to violate the principle of parsimony. Some cognitive psychologists indeed seem to be greatly alarmed at the prospects of what they view as "proliferation" of memory systems, such alarm being caused by as few as four systems (Zacks, 1984). One fear frequently expressed is that if postulation of different memory systems is accepted as a legitimate scientific practice, there is nothing to prevent any investigator, on finding a new dissociation, from declaring the existence of yet another system, or a pair of systems. The principle adopted by these believers in unitary memory is that the movement towards multiple memory systems has to be stopped before it is too late. Roediger (1990a) has compared the postulation of multiple systems with the listings of instincts and Gestalt "principles" of perception, and has predicted the same dire fate for memory systems that befell these other sorry scientific misadventures.

Five Memory Systems

A number of classificatory schemes of human memory have been described and discussed. Initially these took the form of various dichotomies, such as those between short-term and long-term memory (e.g., Shallice & Warrington, 1970; Warrington & Shallice, 1969), episodic and semantic memory (Kinsbourne & Wood, 1975; Tulving, 1972; Warrington, 1975), and procedural and declarative memory (Cohen, 1984; Cohen & Squire, 1980; Squire & Cohen, 1984). Now, however, more comprehensive structures have been proposed (e.g., Johnson, 1990; Squire, 1987; Tulving, 1983, 1987; Warrington, 1979; Weiskrantz, 1987, 1990).

One such tentative general classification scheme for human memory systems is presented in Table 1.1. It includes five major learning and memory systems: *procedural* memory, perceptual *priming*, *short-term* memory, *semantic* memory, and *episodic* memory. Each of the five systems is large

TABLE 1.1 Major Human Memory Systems—1990

1.	Procedural memory: Skills; simple conditioning
2.	Perceptual representation system: Perceptual priming of identification of objects
3.	Short-term memory: Highly accessible information from recent cognitive inputs
4.	Semantic memory: General knowledge of the world
5.	Episodic memory Conscious recollection of the personal past

and complex, comprising a number of subsystems for which evidence at the present stage of our knowledge is of variable quality.

The ordering of the major systems in the overall classification scheme corresponds roughly to their presumed developmental sequence, with the procedural system the earliest, and the episodic the latest. The ordering of the systems also reflects the conjectured relations among the systems: many operations of the higher ones depend on, and are supported by, the operations of the lower ones, whereas lower systems can operate essentially independently of the higher ones.

The scheme in Table 1.1 does not include primitive forms of learning, such as sensitization and habituation, because little work has been done with them in humans, and sensory (iconic and echoic) memory (Coltheart, 1983), because little is known about their relation to forms of memory other than short-term memory. Two entries in Table 1.1, semantic and episodic memory, are sometimes categorized together as *declarative* (Cohen, 1984; Cohen & Squire, 1980; Squire & Cohen, 1984) or *propositional* memory (Tulving, 1983), as they share a number of features. Another frequently used distinction is that between implicit and explicit memory (Graf & Schacter, 1985; Roediger, 1990b; Schacter, 1987b). Implicit memory designates the *expression* of stored information without awareness of its acquisition coordinates in space and time—that is, expression of what the individual *knows* without necessarily remembering how, when, or where the knowledge was acquired. Explicit memory, on the other hand, refers to the expression of short-term and episodic memory, expression of what the person consciously *remembers* as a personal experience. In Table 1.1, procedural, PRS, and semantic memory would be classified as implicit; short-term and episodic memory would be classified as explicit memory.

The procedural system is an *action* system; its operations are expressed in behavior, independently of any cognition. Skillful performance of perceptual-motor tasks and conditioning of simple stimulus–response connections are examples of tasks that depend heavily on the procedural memory system. The general model of procedural memory is provided by what Hirsh (1974) called "performance line storage," characterized by the kind of learning that is preserved after hippocampectomy, differentiating it from "contextual retrieval," which requires representational storage and depends on the integrity of the hippocampal system.

The other four are *cognitive* systems. They mediate changes in cognition, or thought. In the course of normal everyday activity, the computational outputs of the cognitive memory systems typically guide overt behavior, but such conversion of cognition into behavior, as we already noted about GAPS, is not an obligatory part of memory. Rather it is an optional postmemory, or postecphoric, process. Indeed, in the laboratory the products of cognitive memory systems are analyzed in the form of "pure" experience or thought, with behavioral responses serving merely as indicators of properties of cognitive processes.

Perceptual priming is a specific form of learning that is expressed in enhanced identification of objects as structured physical-perceptual entities. Perception of an object at Time 1 primes the perception of the same or a similar object at Time 2 in the sense that the identification of the object can require less stimulus information or less time than it does in the absence of priming.

Short-term memory, also referred to as *primary* memory (Waugh & Norman, 1965) or *working* memory (Baddeley, 1986; Baddeley & Hitch, 1974), registers and retains incoming information in a highly accessible form for a short period of time after the input. Short-term memory makes possible a lingering impression of the individual's present environment beyond the duration of the physical presence of the stimulus information emanating from the environment.

Semantic memory makes possible the acquisition and retention of factual information in the broadest sense; the structured representation of this information, semantic knowledge, models the world. Semantic knowledge provides the individual with the necessary material for thought—that is, for cognitive operations on the aspects of the world beyond the reach of immediate perception. An example of the capabilities of semantic memory is knowledge of location of objects in the nonperceived space; another is classification of objects, events, or situations—or symbolic descriptions of them—into higher-order conceptual categories depending on their functions and uses.

Episodic memory enables individuals to remember their personally experienced past—that is, to remember experienced events as embedded in a matrix of other personal happenings in subjective time. It depends on, but transcends, the range of the capabilities of semantic memory. The most distinctive aspect of episodic memory is the kind of conscious awareness that characterizes recollection of past happenings. This awareness is unique and unmistakably different from the kinds of awareness that accompany perceptual experiences, imagining, dreaming, solving of problems, and retrieval of semantic information. To distinguish the episodic-memory awareness from these other kinds, I have referred to it as autonoetic consciousness (Tulving, 1985b). It has been successfully brought under experimental scrutiny by Gardiner and his coworkers (e.g., Gardiner, 1988; Gardiner & Java, 1990; Gardiner & Parkin, 1990).

The evidence for the distinction between and among different forms of memory, and memory systems, are derived from *dissociations* between outcomes of tests that are known or can be assumed to rely differentially on different systems. Outcomes of tests are said to be dissociated if they differ as a function of an independent variable, or with subjects and their brain states. Evidence for separate or separable systems is provided by different *convergent* dissociations. Despite the fears and misgivings expressed by unitarians, it is unlikely that a competent classifier would propose a new memory system, or a new pair of systems, after observing a single novel dissociation. The logic of the dissociation methodology has been thoroughly discussed by Shallice (1988). The dissociation evidence that bears on the issues of classification of memory is growing by leaps and bounds. It has been reviewed by Richardson-Klavehn and Bjork (1988), Schacter (1987b), Shallice (1988) and Shimamura (1986).

Classification of memory requires a multilevel approach. Functional analysis of memory systems must necessarily be combined with neuroanatomical and neurophysiological analyses. Behavioral data on their own are seldom sufficiently compelling to allow preclusion of alternative interpretations. Differentiation of systems at the level of neural pathways and networks, and eventually perhaps even at the level of cellular and synaptic mechanisms, is an important part of the classification research. Although the available knowledge on neuroanatomical localization of function is still fragmentary, a good deal of progress has been made in recent decades in identifying the regions of the brain that are critical for the operations of different systems. Reviews of relevant evidence include those by Squire (1986, 1987) and Weiskrantz (1985, 1987).

In the remainder of this chapter, I will consider two issues that have emerged in classification research and that illustrate the role of concepts in the study of human memory. The first issue is the recently discovered phenomenon of perceptual priming and the perceptual representation system (PRS) that has been postulated as the system subserving such priming. Perceptual priming represents a relatively recent discovery; it is under vigorous investigation today, and it holds every promise of becoming an even more acute focus of study in the future. The second issue is the distinction between episodic and semantic memory. The current thinking about the nature of, and especially the relation between, these two forms of memory have changed since the introduction of the distinction some 20 years ago, and the reality of the distinction has been energetically denied by some. (For one set of objections, see Baddeley, 1984; McKoon, Ratcliff, & Dell, 1986; Ratcliff & McKoon, 1986; Roediger, 1984).

PERCEPTUAL PRIMING AND PRS

A perceptual representation system (PRS) is the latest addition to the developing list of memory systems (Schacter, 1990; Tulving & Schacter, 1990). It consists of several known and probable subsystems, which mediate perception of different objects as structural entities and facilitate such perception through priming. *Perceptual priming* was identified as a distinct form of memory only recently, although the basic phenomena have been known for some time. It differs from two other major forms of priming, *semantic* priming (Meyer & Schvaneveldt, 1971; Neely, 1977) and *conceptual* priming (Hamann, 1990; Roediger & Blaxton, 1987; Roediger, Weldon, & Challis, 1989; Srinivas & Roediger, 1990; Tulving & Schacter, 1990), in that perceptual priming operates on physical-perceptual *appearances* of objects, including words, and has little to do with their *meaning*, whereas both semantic and conceptual priming operate at the level of meaning, and have little to do with the perceptual appearance of the words.

The idea that priming might be subserved by a system other than those already known was suggested by Tulving, Schacter, and Stark (1982), at a time when the distinction between perceptual and conceptual priming was not yet appreciated. The tentative priming system was initially referred to as the QM (for "quasi-memory") system (Hayman & Tulving, 1989; Tulving, 1985a), to reflect the assumption that in some sense it seemed to belong somewhere "between" perception and memory. Kirsner and Dunn (1985) explicitly suggested that priming was a form of perceptual learning. The term PRS was adopted from the neuropsychological literature on disorders of reading and of object perception as historically prior, more comprehensive, and more appropriate (Schacter, 1990; Schacter & Tulving, 1990).

A prototypical perceptual priming experiment, consisting of two stages, resembles a prototypical explicit memory experiment. In the first (study) stage, the subject is presented with a stimulus object (target), such as a word, a face, a picture, or a line drawing of an object. In the second (test) stage, separated from the first by a shorter or longer interval, the subject is presented with a cue containing incomplete or impoverished *perceptual* information about one of the target objects. The subject's task is to identify the cued target, or to assign it to a larger category. Thus, for example, in the test stage, the subject might be given a graphemic *fragment* of a word, such as P – I – I – G, or — AG – EN –, and asked to name the word. Other kinds of perceptual cues that have been used include word *stems, n* initial letters of words (e.g., Warrington & Weiskrantz, 1970), incomplete line drawings of the target objects (e.g., Snodgrass & Feenan, 1990; Warrington & Weiskrantz, 1968), and tachistoscopic presentations of targets (e.g., Jacoby & Dallas, 1981; Musen & Treisman, 1990; Schacter, Cooper, & Delaney, 1990). It is the perceptual similarity between cue and target that defines the phenomenon as perceptual priming. In conceptual priming the relation between the cue and the target is specified in terms of their meaning. The subject's objective is always to identify the target.[3]

The *priming effect* is measured in terms of some function of the difference between the probabilities of identifying words encountered and words not encountered in the study stage of the experiment. The priming test differs from explicit memory tests in the question posed to the subject: "What is this word?" versus "What did you see in the study list?" Answers to both questions are influenced by the study episode, and in this sense represent aftereffects of the same original event, but the aftereffects are radically different, in a number of ways, and thus suggest they are expressions of different memory systems.

First, unlike the expression of other kinds of cognitive memory, priming is nonconscious. An individual perceiving an object more efficiently because of priming is not aware that the act of perception has benefited in any way from earlier exposures to the same or a similar object. In the laboratory, priming effects occur regardless of whether subjects know or do not know anything about the relation between the study and test stages of the experiment, or whether they know or do not know that their memory is being tested (Bowers & Schacter, 1990). Second, even when subjects are aware of the relation between the study and test stages, priming effects are as large for the stimulus items that they consciously remember having seen earlier as they are for the stimulus items that they do not remember (e.g., Jacoby & Witherspoon, 1982; Tulving et al., 1982). Third, unlike episodic and semantic memory, perceptual priming is sensitive to the compatibility between the perceptual format of the studied item and the test cue. Priming effects are considerably reduced or even absent if the priming test is given in a format different from the presentation format, as when auditory presentation is followed by a visual test (e.g., Jacoby & Dallas, 1981; Morton, 1979), when pictorial presentation is followed by a verbal test (e.g., Roediger et al., 1989), or when bilingual subjects are presented words for study in one of their languages and tested for corresponding translations in the other (e.g., Kirsner & Dunn, 1985; Roediger & Blaxton, 1987). Fourth, again unlike episodic and semantic memory, perceptual priming is little affected by variations in the semantic encoding operations performed on target items at study (e.g., Graf & Mandler, 1984; Jacoby & Dallas, 1981). Fifth, priming is preserved in anterograde amnesia, whereas episodic memory is not (e.g., Graf, Squire, & Mandler, 1984; Tulving, Hayman, & Macdonald, 1991; Warrington & Weiskrantz, 1970, 1974). The most natural interpretation of this fact is that priming does not require brain structures or mechanisms whose damage in amnesia results in a severe impairment in the patient's ability to consciously recollect recent happenings. Sixth, perceptual priming is largely invariant across developmental stages (young children to adults to elderly people), which are correlated with systematic differences in episodic memory performances (e.g., Light, Singh, & Capps, 1986; Mitchell, 1989; Naito, 1990; Parkin & Streete, 1988). These findings suggest that the neural pathways that subserve episodic remembering, maturing late in childhood and deteriorating early in old age, are not necessary for priming, and that their functioning does not contribute anything substantial to the operations of the priming system. Seventh, perceptual priming is less affected by alcohol and drug treatments than are other forms of cognitive memory (e.g., Hashtroudi, Parker, DeLisi, Wyatt, & Mutter, 1984; Nissen, Knopman, & Schacter, 1987), again suggesting differences in the brain mechanisms underlying the operations of the two forms of memory. Finally, although it has sometimes been asserted that priming effects are short-lived (e.g., Squire, 1986) at least some priming effects are long lasting. In one experiment it was found that a single presentation of a familiar word for a few seconds in a list of 100 other words produced priming effects that could be readily detected more than 16 months later (Sloman, Hayman, Ohta, Law, & Tulving, 1987). In another study it was found that the amnesic patient K.C., about whom more later in this chapter, exhibited virtually undiminished priming effects in fragment completion a year after repeated exposures to the target words. Thus, he could "read" fragments such as – – RCR – – T, – A – G – YL –, and – E – I – W, which can give difficulties to nonprimed normal readers, 12 months after having been repeatedly primed with the target words (Tulving et al., 1991).

There are other characteristics of perceptual priming that distinguish it from other forms of cognitive memory, but the given summary includes the major features and illustrates the overall nature of dissociation evidence that bears on the classification problem. The main point to be made is that the evidence (a) comes from a variety of sources, and (b) presents a complex picture, any component of which would have been difficult or impossible to predict, on the basis of what was known about other forms of memory, before the facts were discovered in the laboratory.

Some independent observers of classification research have expressed reservations about the force of dissociation evidence. Weinberger (1990), for instance, has suggested that dissociations could simply reflect differential thresholds of different behavioral manifestations of a single underlying process. He has also wondered about how one can go beyond the conclusion that a dissociation implies anything other than just lack of identity. These concerns may be reasonably raised in connection with any one single dissociation, but they lose their potential relevance when confronted with the totality of evidence. The idea of differential thresholds may account for, say, differential effects of drugs on explicit memory and priming, but it is directly at variance with the many findings of stochastic independence between explicit recognition and implicit priming (e.g., Jacoby & Witherspoon, 1982; Musen & Treisman, 1990; Schacter, Cooper, & Delaney, 1990; Tulving et al., 1982). As to the idea that dissociations point to lack of identity, there is no problem there. The concept of multiple systems includes, and transcends, the notion of lack of identity. It provides an explication of how the dissociated task performances are not identical, as well as how they are.

The multiple contrasts between priming and the phenomena of explicit memory, plus some others discussed elsewhere (Schacter, 1990; Tulving and Schacter, 1990), converge on the idea that perceptual priming is subserved by a distinct memory system, the PRS. The PRS integrates perceptual inputs into highly specific neurocognitive representations of objects to which, as a result of priming, access can be gained on the basis of diminished stimulus information. It can do so independently of episodic and semantic memory (Tulving et al., 1991) and probably independently of short-term memory, although, like all other memory systems, it normally interacts closely with other systems, receiving inputs from them and sending outputs to them. It reaches its optimal functional capability in development before other cognitive memory systems do. Finally, it consists of a number of subsystems. One such (word form system) mediates priming of visual words, another (structural description system) mediates priming of natural visual objects (Schacter, 1990).

Little is known about the neuroanatomical and neurophysiological correlates of PRS. Observations of preserved perceptual priming in amnesic patients suggest that priming is mediated by the brain structures outside the medial temporal and diencephalic regions that are damaged in amnesia. There is evidence that visual identification of words activates the extrastriate region of the occipital lobes bilaterally (Petersen, Fox, Posner, Mintum, & Raichle, 1988) and that object identification depends on the right posterior cortical region (Warrington & Taylor, 1978). It can be surmised that visual priming of words or objects also depends on these cortical areas.

EPISODIC AND SEMANTIC MEMORY

The distinction between personal and impersonal forms of memory has been around for some time, under different labels. More or less detailed characterizations of these two basic forms of memory had been provided by clinically oriented students of memory and memory pathology (e.g., Claparède, 1911; Nielsen, 1958; Reiff & Scheerer, 1959), as well as philosophers (e.g., Locke, 1972). In a report of his extensive clinical neurological investigations of memory and amnesia, Nielsen described the two forms as follows:

> A study of pathways of memory formation has revealed a basic fact not suspected when this study began—there are two separate pathways for two kinds of memories. The one is memories of life experiences centering around the person himself and basically involving the element of time. The other is memories of intellectually acquired knowledge not experienced but learned by study and not personal. (Nielsen, 1958, p. 25)

Corresponding to these two kinds of memories are two types of amnesia:

> Amnesia is of two types: (1) loss of memory for personal experiences (temporal amnesia), and (2) loss of memory for acquired facts (categorical amnesia). Either may be lost without the other. (Nielsen, 1958, p. 15)

In an essay that I wrote in 1972 I adopted the terms *episodic* and *semantic* as designations of the two forms. At the time, most of the evidence relevant to the distinction within cognitive psychology was anecdotal. Since 1972 the database relevant to the distinction has expanded greatly, much more directly relevant information has become available, and considerable progress has been made in the understanding of the properties of the two systems and their interrelation.

The initial distinction between episodic and semantic memory served a largely heuristic function, and the two concepts are often used in this atheoretical sense. "Episodic memory" defined in this heuristic or "processing" sense designates acquisition and retention of a particular type of information, in a particular type of situation. The information is what has been denoted as *declarative* or *propositional*; the situation is one in which retrieval is said to be *explicit*. The GAPS framework discussed earlier in this chapter holds for episodic memory (or declarative memory, or explicit memory) defined in this heuristic sense. "Semantic memory" defined in the same sense refers to the acquisition and retention of associative, imaginative, factual, and semantic information independently of the particular circumstances surrounding its acquisition. This information, too, can said to be declarative or propositional.

The second sense of "episodic memory" refers to a hypothetical neurocognitive system. It represents a more recent development, and it is in this "systems" sense that I discuss it here. The episodic system confers on its possessor the unique capability of storing information about personal happenings in subjective space and time (Tulving, 1983, 1984b). This stored episodic information serves as the basis for the conscious recollection of aspects of the original events, in a distinctive form of awareness that has been labeled autonoetic awareness (Tulving, 1985a, 1985b, 1987). Episodic memory system subserves remembering of the temporal order of past events (e.g., Hirst & Volpe, 1982; Milner, Petrides, & Smith, 1985; Shimamura, Janowsky, & Squire, 1990), as well as the setting, or context, within which events occur (e.g., Mayes, Meudell, & Pickering, 1985). Although, because of lack of a suitable language, it is difficult to study autonoetic awareness in lower animals, some features of episodic memory—information about temporal order and place of happenings—have been investigated, and evidence for memory capabilities analogous to episodic memory found (e.g., Hirsh, 1974; Kesner & DiMattia, 1984; Olton, 1984; Ruggiero & Flagg, 1976; Thomas, 1984).

The initial idea concerning the relation between episodic and semantic memory was that they represented two parallel subsystems of declarative memory (Tulving, 1983), and some writers have retained this idea (e.g., Squire, 1987). A more reasonable current hypothesis, however, is that the episodic system is a unique system embedded within and supported by semantic memory in some of its operations (Tulving, 1984b). A corollary hypothesis is that semantic memory precedes episodic memory in ontogenetic development and phylogenetic progression. Episodic memory has evolved from semantic memory to acquire functional capabilities not possessed by an unvarnished semantic system, but in some of its operations it has remained highly dependent on semantic memory (Tulving, 1984b, 1987). Thus, for instance, it looks as if no new information could be stored in episodic memory if semantic memory were totally dysfunctional (cf. DeRenzi, Liotti, & Nichelli, 1987), although new information could be stored in semantic memory in the absence of a functioning episodic system, as presumably happens in very young children and in lower animals without episodic memory.

Among other implications of these ideas about the relation between the two systems is the rejection of the popularly held assumption that information enters the semantic system *through* the episodic system, a sort of a "first episodic, then semantic" kind of a notion (e.g., Squire, 1987). New information enters semantic memory through the perceptual systems, not through episodic memory. The evidence for this hypothesis is derived from studies of amnesic patients.

Anterograde Amnesia and the Episodic/Semantic Distinction

The amnesic syndrome consists of a selective and severe impairment of certain forms of memory caused by lesions in the medial temporal lobe and midline diencephalic structures, as well as possibly other regions of the brain. (For reviews, see Markowitsch & Pritzel, 1985; Squire, 1986, 1987; Weiskrantz, 1985, 1987). The core of the syndrome is anterograde amnesia, characterized by highly deficient functioning of episodic memory. The amnesic patient is incapable of remembering any personal happenings and experiences beyond the period covered by short-term memory (Rozin, 1976). Yet amnesic patients typically are unimpaired on tasks that are heavily dependent on procedural memory, PRS, and short-term memory systems (Schacter, 1987a; Shimamura, 1986; Squire, 1987; Weiskrantz, 1987), and their other intellectual functions—perception, language, and thought—are completely or largely intact.

What is not yet clear is the relation between amnesia and semantic memory. Usually, although not always, an amnesic patient has retained much of the premorbidly acquired general knowledge, suggesting a dissociation between the preserved semantic memory and the impaired episodic memory (Cermak, 1984; Kinsbourne & Wood, 1975, 1982), but such comparisons are confounded, and therefore inconclusive. More revealing are studies in which experimentally controlled new semantic learning and episodic recollection of such learning are directly compared.

In a recently conducted extensive study of a densely amnesic patient, K.C., we obtained evidence of his ability to learn new semantic knowledge and to retain it, as far as we could tell, normally over a long interval of time. We also caught a glimpse of the reasons why such new semantic learning has been declared to be beyond the capabilities of amnesic patients in many previous studies (Tulving et al., 1991).

K.C., a 40-year-old man, suffered closed-head injury in a traffic accident in 1980, with extensive damage to several regions of the brain, especially in the left hemisphere (for further details, see Tulving et al., 1991). One consequence of this damage was extremely dense anterograde amnesia and a total absence of any autobiographical recollections from the time before his accident. Thus K.C. is one of the few amnesics described in the literature whose episodic memory is completely dysfunctional (Tulving, Schacter, McLachlan, & Moscovitch, 1988). In the study of his ability to learn new semantic information (Tulving et al., 1991), we taught him 64 three-word sentences (such as REPORTER SENT REVIEW, and STUDENT WITHDREW INNUENDO) over a number of widely distributed learning trials. At the time of subsequent retention tests, he was given the first two words of the sentence as a cue (e.g., STUDENT WITHDREW) and asked for the third word that would complete the sentence. At the end of the training, he was capable of producing 38 of the 64 target words. After a 12-month interval, during which K.C. was not exposed to any of the materials, this number had fallen to 25, still demonstrating considerable retention over such a long interval. Data from another experiment with K.C. (Hayman & Mcdonald, 1990) suggested that the success of K.C.'s semantic learning was at least partly attributable to the method we used. The tests administered to K.C. *during* the multiple distributed learning trials were such that they largely eliminated incorrect, potentially interfering responses to sentence frames, resulting in "errorless" learning. As normal subjects suffer less from interference than do memory-impaired individuals, these results suggest that normal subjects' intact episodic memory allows the learners to overcome interference and to correct errors in a fashion not possible for amnesic subjects. At any rate, minimization of interference seems to be an important determinant of semantic learning by amnesics. In one formal attempt to teach H.M. new vocabulary words (Gabrieli, Cohen, & Corkin, 1988) it was found that he was not capable of doing so. It is not inconceivable that this outcome, too, is at least partly attributable to rather large amounts of interference engendered by the method that these investigators used.

The fact that a densely amnesic subject such as K.C. can learn new semantic information illustrates the conclusions that Nielsen (1958) drew about two types of memory and two types of amnesia. But it may appear surprising in light of the widely held belief that amnesic patients are incapable of such learning (e.g., Rozin, 1976; Squire, 1987). Even if surprising, our findings do not stand alone. A number of other recent studies have demonstrated under controlled conditions that amnesic patients *can* learn new semantic information, even if slowly and laboriously in comparison with nonamnesic control subjects (e.g., Glisky & Schacter, 1988; Glisky, Schacter, & Tulving, 1986a, 1986b; Kovner, Mattis, & Goldmeier, 1983; Mattis & Kovner, 1984; McAndrews, Glisky, & Schacter, 1987; Schacter, Harbluk, & McLachlan, 1984; Shimamura & Squire, 1987, 1988). Thus, amnesic patients who cannot recollect the learning episode any more than they can recollect any other postmorbid personal happenings can nevertheless acquire new semantic knowledge. Our findings with K.C. fit well into this general pattern.

These facts contraindicate statements sometimes made to the effect that amnesia is a condition characterized by the impairment of "only one type of memory," declarative memory, which stores "facts and episodes" (Squire, Shimamura, & Amaral, 1989, pp. 212–213), and statements like "We favor the view that the defining feature of amnesia is an impairment in the ability to establish declarative memory, whereas the ability to establish procedural memory is preserved" (Shimamura & Squire, 1987, pp. 471–472). These statements reflect the fact that amnesics' performance on semantic learning tasks is decidedly subnormal: although they can learn new facts, they do so less effectively than do normal subjects. The inference drawn from this fact is that amnesics' semantic learning ability is subnormal, together with a further generalization that, as both semantic learning ability and the ability of episodic recollections are impaired in amnesics, amnesia consists of impairment of declarative memory.

Although these inferences appear to be quite straightforward and reasonable, they overlook the fact that semantic learning, even if slow in comparison with normal subjects, is possible in anterograde amnesia, whereas conscious recollection of any personal episodes, including the learning episodes, is not possible. The comparison between semantic learning and episodic recollection is one between some and none. What could such a dissociation—some versus none—mean? To pursue this matter, let us briefly examine two widely used concepts in neuropsychological studies of memory. One of these is "normal memory." The other one has no specific designation; for ease of reference I will label it as "codetermination of task performances by different systems," or simply "codetermination."

Normal Memory and Codetermination of Tasks

"Normal" memory in today's clinical neuropsychology is defined in terms of performance on a battery of psychometric tests or conventional laboratory experiments that conform to the study-test paradigm. Amnesic patients' performance on these measuring instruments is very poor in comparison with that of the normal standardization group, hence "subnormal." From the point of view of the systems approach, however, the concept of "normal" memory would be defined in terms of normal functioning of all memory systems and subsystems. The "normal memory" baseline of any brain-damaged person with impaired memory is defined by the same person's premorbid functioning. As this information is usually not available, "normal memory" usually refers to the levels of performance of people without brain damage who are comparable to the patient or patients in other intellectual respects. These "normal" subjects perform "normally" on memory tasks, because their various memory systems, some of which contribute to or codetermine such performance, are unimpaired.

One of the most fundamental assumptions of neuropsychology is that the carrying out of any cognitive task is complexly determined. In the systems orientation, the assumption is that any cognitive task is codetermined by the operations of a number of different systems and subsystems. Impaired performance on a task by a brain-damaged individual, under otherwise *optimal processing* conditions of encoding, storage, and retrieval (Buschke, 1987), implies dysfunctioning of one or more of the relevant systems or subsystems. If a system is damaged, the person's performances on memory tasks suffer, commensurately with the extent of the damage to the system and the extent that the system normally contributes to, or codetermines, the performances in question. I refer to these ideas collectively as the *concept of codetermination*.

Codetermination helps us to interpret properly various kinds of findings resulting from comparisons of brain-damaged patients and normal subjects. If we know that a patient is amnesic and that episodic memory is dysfunctional, and we observe that the patient's short-term and perceptual priming performances in various tasks are normal, we can draw *two* closely interrelated conclusions: (a) the brain pathways necessary for episodic memory are not necessary for short-term memory and perceptual priming (mediation of performances by different systems), and (b) the intact episodic system of the normal subjects does not codetermine short-term and perceptual priming performances (independence of short-term and perceptual priming systems from episodic memory).

On the other hand, consider a situation in which we have good reasons to assume that (or in which in fact) two systems, M1 and M2, do codetermine the performance on a task. That performance will then be impaired in a patient suffering from damage to, or loss of, one of the systems, M1, in comparison with "normal" performance, even if the patient's other system, M2, functions normally. As an example consider the situation in which M1 and M2 are episodic and semantic memory, respectively, and the task is learning a list of unrelated paired associates. Assume that an amnesic patient's episodic system is dysfunctional whereas the semantic memory system is intact. Assume further that the learning of new associations is codetermined by both systems. If these assumptions are granted, then it follows that the amnesic patient will exhibit subnormal learning of paired associates despite the fact that the patient's semantic learning ability is preserved.

The logic of codetermination is simple and noncontroversial; it has been used (e.g., Cermak, 1986; Milner, Corkin, & Teuber, 1968) and explicitly discussed (e.g., Schacter, 1985; Schacter, Delaney, & Merikle, 1990) often enough in interpretations of outcomes of experiments comparing patient and subject populations. Yet the full implications of codetermination have sometimes been overlooked.

The concept of codetermination, applied to the results that have been obtained in experiments comparing amnesics and normal subjects learning new semantic information, including our recent findings with K.C. (Tulving et al., 1991), allows us to draw the following inference. Learning of new semantic knowledge need not be impaired in amnesic patients even if their ability to acquire such knowledge appears to be subnormal; the superiority of normal subjects' performance on the semantic learning task may be partly or even wholly attributable to their intact episodic memory.

This conclusion or hypothesis, of course, is drastically different from the conclusion that amnesic semantic memory is impaired along with episodic memory, and that empirical facts from studies with amnesic patients do not throw any light on the distinction between episodic and semantic memory (e.g., Squire & Cohen, 1984; Squire, 1987; Squire et al., 1989). The hypothesis of partially or wholly preserved semantic memory in at least some amnesic patients may turn out to be wrong. It does, however, provide a viable logical alternative to the hypothesis that amnesia is an impairment of declarative memory, thus allowing comparative assessments of the validity of the two hypotheses in future research. It also provides an interesting demonstration of the close interaction between facts and ideas, a demonstration of how concepts must shape research in order to stay viable, and how they in turn must be shaped by the results of the research.

The hypothesis that semantic learning ability is preserved in some amnesics implies that these amnesics would perform normally in all semantic learning tasks in which normal subjects could not rely on their intact episodic memory. It is difficult to create such a situation. How can one make or instruct people not to remember something of which they are reminded by a cue? However, some indirectly relevant evidence has recently been reported by Dagenbach, Horst, and Carr (1990). These researchers found that previously unknown vocabulary words taught to university students showed no semantic priming effects when tested with very short intervals – stimulus onset asynchrony (short SOAs) – between primes and targets, although subjects were capable of fluently responding with the newly learned words to their synonyms as cues in paired-associate tests. Such semantic priming effects are simple to observe for pairs of words that are closely related in semantic memory (e.g., Meyer & Schvaneveldt, 1971; Neely, 1977), a finding once more confirmed by Dagenbach et al. (1990). The absence of similar effects with recently learned pairs of words therefore suggests that the integration of new associations between words into semantic memory requires many trials of practice even in normal subjects, and that the excellent recall of the associations in an explicit memory test may reflect the operations of the episodic memory system.

The matter will probably turn out to be more complex than the brief summary here suggests, but at least the hypothesis that the semantic memory system, in the absence of episodic memory, acquires information slowly is a novel one that is clearly worth pursuing. The clarification of the role that episodic and semantic systems play in learning of semantic information would add to our understanding of the nature of, and the relation between, the two systems.

CONCLUSION

I have examined and discussed some ideas and concepts that figure prominently in contemporary research and study of human memory. Among the processing concepts, organized under the scheme of the GAPS, I concentrated on synergistic ecphory, the idea that the outcome of a single discrete act of memory is determined jointly by storage and retrieval processes, or by the interaction between the engram and the ecphory. The concept deserves attention because of its possibly far-reaching implications and consequences for the understanding of not only human memory but learning and memory in other species as well. One such consequence is the idea that storage and retrieval, or the engram and its ecphory, cannot be studied and characterized independently of one another.

Among the classificatory concepts, I discussed current ideas about memory systems, concentrating on perceptual priming, because of its novelty, and the distinction between episodic and semantic memory, because of the changes that these two concepts have undergone since their introduction. Perceptual priming is subserved by the PRS, an early system that operates on perceptual identification of objects, a vital prerequisite for an organism's interaction with its world. With respect to the distinction between episodic and semantic memory, recent work and thought have suggested that the two systems are interdependent in the sense that acquisition of episodic information depends on an intact semantic system, but that semantic information can be acquired even by people without functioning episodic systems. A recent study of new semantic learning in a densely amnesic subject, K.C., has reinforced other similar recent findings, and suggests that in some amnesic patients semantic memory is at least partially, or perhaps even wholly, preserved. The concept of codetermination of tasks by systems, when consistently applied to the findings from neuropsychological analyses of memory disorders, helps to clarify issues in classification of memory as well as issues in memory disorders.

It has been fashionable to declare that the ultimate objective of research on memory is the construction of a general theory of memory, or the working out of the chemical basis, or cellular basis, or neuroanatomical basis of memory. The theme of the discussion presented in this chapter has been that there is no such single *thing* as memory. Instead, there exist a number of different brain/behavior/cognition systems and processes that, through cooperation and interaction with one another, make it possible for their possessor to benefit from past experience and thereby promote survival. The known and as yet unknown memory systems deal with and operate on different aspects of the organism's environment, they function according to different principles, and they follow their own specialized laws of processing. To understand memory means to comprehend the structures and the underlying processes of this totality.

Acknowledgement: The preparation of this paper has been supported by the Natural Sciences and Engineering Research Council of Canada, Grant No. A8632.

Notes

1. The concepts of engram and ecphory were originally proposed by Richard Semon, a German biologist, whose then unappreciated work anticipated many modern developments in memory research. For the story of Semon's life and contributions to the science of memory, see Schacter (1982) and Schacter, Eich, and Tulving (1978).

2. In experiments in which the target events can be reproduced with a high degree of fidelity, latencies (reaction times) of reproductive responses can also provide useful information.

3. In a popular task used to study perceptual priming, the lexical decision task, a string of letters is presented to the subject, and the objective is to determine, as rapidly as possible, whether the string represents a word or not. In this categorization task the determination of the string's identity constitutes just an intermediate stage. Perceptual priming was demonstrated early with this task (e.g., Scarborough, Cortese, & Scarborough, 1977).

REFERENCES

Atkinson, R. C., & Shiffrin, R. M. (1968). Human memory: A proposed system and its control processes. In K. W. Spence (Ed.), *The psychology of learning and motivation: Advances in research and theory* (vol. 2) (pp. 89–195). New York: Academic Press.

Baddeley, A. D. (1984). Neuropsychological evidence and the semantic/episodic distinction. *Behavioral and Brain Sciences, 7*, 238–239.

Baddeley, A. D. (1986). *Working memory*. Oxford: Clarendon Press.

Baddeley, A. D., Hitch, G. J. (1974). Working memory. In G. H. Bower (Ed.), *Recent advances in learning and motivation*, (vol. VIII) (pp. 47–90). New York: Academic Press.

Barclay, J.R., Bransford, J. D., Franks, J. J., McCarrell, N. S., & Nitsch, K. (1974). Comprehension and semantic flexibility. *Journal of Verbal Learning and Verbal Behavior, 13*, 471–481.

Bowers, J. S., & Schacter, D. L. (1990). Implicit memory and test awareness. *Journal of Experimental Psychology: Learning, Memory, and Cognition, 16*, 404–416.

Buschke, H. (1987). Criteria for the identification of memory deficits: implications for the design of memory tests. In D. S. Gorfein & R. R. Hoffman (Eds.), *Memory and cognitive processes: The Ebbinghaus Centennial Conference* (pp. 331–344). Hillsdale, New Jersey: Erlbaum.

Cermak, L. S. (1984). The episodic-semantic distinction in amnesia. In L. R. Squire & N. Butters (Eds.), *Neuropsychology of memory* (pp. 55–62). New York: Guilford Press.

Cermak, L. S. (1986). Amnesia as a processing deficit. In G. Goldstein & R. E. Tarter (Eds.), *Advances in clinical neuropsychology*, (Vol. 3) (pp. 265–290). New York: Plenum.

Claparède, E. (1911). Recognition et moïté. *Archives de Psychologie, Genève, 11*, 79–90.

Cohen, N. J. (1984). Preserved learning capacity in amnesia: Evidence for multiple memory systems. In L. R. Squire & N. Butters (Eds.), *The neuropsychology of memory* (pp. 83–103). New York: Guilford Press.

Cohen, N. J. & Squire, L. R. (1980). Preserved learning and retention of pattern analyzing skill in amnesia: Dissociation of knowing how and knowing that. *Science, 210,* 207–209.

Coltheart, M. (1983). Iconic memory. *Philosophical Transactions of the Royal Society, London, B302,* 183–294.

Craik, F. I. M., & Tulving, E. (1975). Depth of processing and the retention of words in episodic memory. *Journal of Experimental Psychology: General, 104,* 268–294.

Dagenbach, D., Horst, S., & Carr, T. H. (1990). Adding new information to semantic memory: How much learning is enough to produce automatic priming? *Journal of Experimental Psychology: Learning, Memory, and Cognition, 16,* 581–591.

DeRenzi, E., Liotti, M., & Nichelli, P. (1987). Semantic amnesia with preservation of autobiographic memory. A case report. *Cortex, 23,* 575–597.

Dudai, Y. (1989). *The neurobiology of memory.* New York: Oxford University Press.

Fisher, R. P., & Craik, F. I. M. (1977). The interaction between encoding and retrieval operations in cued recall. *Journal of Experimental Psychology: Human Learning and Memory, 3,* 701–711.

Gabrieli, J. D. E., Cohen, N. J. & Corkin, S. (1988). The impaired learning of semantic knowledge following bilateral medial temporal-lobe resection. *Brain and Cognition, 7,* 157–177.

Gardiner, J. M. (1988). Functional aspects of recollective experience. *Memory & Cognition, 16,* 309–313.

Gardiner, J. M., & Java, R. I. (1990). Recollective experience in word and nonword recognition. *Memory & Cognition, 18,* 23–30.

Gardiner, J. M., & Parkin, A. J. (1990). Attention and recollective experience in recognition memory. *Memory & Cognition, 18,* 579–583.

Glisky, E. L. , & Schacter, D. L. (1988). Long-term retention of computer learning by patients with memory disorders. *Neuropsychologia, 26,* 173–178.

Glisky, E. L., Schacter, D. L., & Tulving, E. (1986a). Computer learning by memory-impaired patients: Acquisition and retention of complex knowledge. *Neuropsychologia, 24,* 313–328.

Glisky, E. L., Schacter, D. L. & Tulving, E. (1986b). Learning and retention of computer-related vocabulary in memory-impaired patients: Method of vanishing cues. *Journal of Clinical and Experimental Neuropsychology, 8,* 292–312.

Graf, P., & Mandler, G. (1984). Activation makes words more accessible, but not necessarily more retrievable. *Journal of Verbal Learning and Verbal Behavior, 25,* 553–568.

Graf, P., & Schacter, D. L. (1985). Implicit and explicit memory for new associations in normal and amnesic subjects. *Journal of Experimental Psychology: Learning, Memory, and Cognition, 11,* 501–518.

Graf, P., Squire, L. R., & Mandler, G. (1984). The information that amnesic patients do not forget. *Journal of Experimental Psychology: Learning, Memory and Cognition, 10,* 164–178.

Hamann, S. B. (1990). Level of processing effects in conceptually driven implicit tasks. *Journal of Experimental Psychology: Learning, Memory, and Cognition, 16,* 970–977.

Hashtroudi, S., Parker, E. S., DeLisi, L. E., Wyatt, R. J., & Mutter, S. A. (1984). Intact retention in acute alcohol amnesia. *Journal of Experimental Psychology: Learning, Memory, and Cognition, 10,* 156–163.

Hayman, C. A. G., & Macdonald, C. A. (1990, May). *Benefits of error-free learning in amnesia.* Paper presented at the Annual Meeting of the Canadian Psychological Association, Ottawa.

Hayman, C. A. G., & Tulving, E. (1989). Is priming in fragment completion based on a "traceless" memory system? *Journal of Experimental Psychology: Learning, Memory, and Cognition, 15*, 941–956.

Hirsh, R. (1974). The hippocampus and contextual retrieval of information from memory: A Theory. *Behavioral Biology, 12*, 421–444.

Hirst, W., & Volpe, B. (1982). Temporal order judgments with amnesia. *Brain and Cognition, 1*, 294–306.

Hyde, T. S., & Jenkins, J. J. (1969). Differential effects of incidental tasks on recall and organization of highly associated words. *Journal of Experimental Psychology, 82*, 275–292.

Jacoby, L. L., & Dallas, M. (1981). On the relationship between autobiographical memory and perceptual learning. *Journal of Experimental Psychology: General, 110*, 306–340.

Jacoby, L. L., & Witherspoon, D. (1982). Remembering without awareness. *Canadian Journal of Psychology, 32*, 300–324.

Johnson, M. K. (1990). Functional forms of human memory. In J. L. McGaugh, N. M. Weinberger, & G. Lynch (Eds.), *Brain organization and memory: Cells, systems, and circuits* (pp. 106–134). New York: Oxford University Press.

Kesner, R. P., & DeMattia, B. V. (1984). Posterior parietal association cortex and hippocampus: Equivalency of mnemonic function in animals and humans. In L. R. Squire & N. Butters, *The neuropsychology of memory* (pp. 385–398). New York: Guilford Press.

Kinsbourne, M., & Wood, F. (1975). Short-term memory processes and the amnesic syndrome. In D. Deutsch & J. A. Deutsch (Eds.), *Short-term memory* (pp. 258–291). New York: Academic Press.

Kinsbourne, M., & Wood, F. (1982). Theoretical considerations regarding the episodic-semantic memory distinction. In L. S. Cermak (Ed.), *Human memory and amnesia* (pp. 194–217). Hillsdale, New Jersey: Erlbaum.

Kirsner, K., & Dunn, J. C. (1985). The perceptual record: A common factor in repetition priming and attribute retention. In M. I. Posner & O. S. Marin (Eds.), *Mechanisms of attention: Attention and performance, XI*, (pp. 547–566). Hillsdale, New Jersey: Erlbaum.

Kovner, R., Mattis, S., & Goldmeier, E. (1983). A technique for promoting robust free recall in chronic organic amnesia. *Journal of Clinical Neuropsychology, 5*, 65–71.

Light, L. L., Singh, A., & Capps, J. L. (1986). Dissociation of memory and awareness in older adults. *Journal of Clinical and Experimental Neuropsychology, 8*, 62–74.

Locke, D. (1972). *Memory*. New York: Macmillan.

Markowitsch, H. J., & Pritzel, M. (1985). The neuropathology of amnesia. *Progress in Neurobiology, 25*, 189–287.

Mathews, R. C. (1977). Semantic judgements as encoding operations: The effects of attention to particular semantic categories on the usefulness of interitem relations in recall. *Journal of Experimental Psychology: Human Learning and Memory, 3*, 160–173.

Mattis, S., & Kovner, R. (1984). Amnesia is as amnesia does: Toward another definition of the anterograde amnesias. In L. R. Squire & N. Butters (Eds.), *Neuropsychology of memory* (pp. 115–121). New York: Guilford Press.

Mayes, A. R., Meudell, P. R., & Pickering, A. (1985). Is organic amnesia caused by a selective deficit in remembering contextual information? *Cortex, 21*, 167–202.

Mayr, E. (1982). *The growth of biological thought*. Cambridge, Massachusetts: Harvard University Press.

McAndrews, M. P., Glisky, E. L., & Schacter, D. L. (1987). When priming persists: Long-lasting implicit memory for a single episode in amnesic patients. *Neuropsychologia, 25*, 497–506.

McKoon, G., Ratcliff, R., & Dell, G. S. (1986). A critical evaluation of the semantic-episodic distinction. *Journal of Experimental Psychology: Learning, Memory and Cognition, 12*, 295–306.

Melton, A. W. (1963). Implications of short-term memory for a general theory of memory. *Journal of Verbal Learning and Verbal Behavior, 2*, 1–21.

Meyer, D. E., & Schvaneveldt, R. W. (1971). Facilitation in recognizing pairs of words: Evidence of a dependence between retrieval operations. *Journal of Experimental Psychology, 90*, 227–234.

Milner, B., Corkin, S., & Teuber, H. L. (1968). Further analysis of the hippocampal amnesic syndrome: 14 year follow-up study of H.M. *Neuropsychologia, 6*, 215–234.

Milner, B., Petrides, M., & Smith, M. L. (1985). Frontal lobes and the temporal organization of memory. *Human Neurobiology, 4*, 137–142.

Mitchell, D. B. (1989). How many memory systems? Evidence from aging. *Journal of Experimental Psychology: Learning, Memory and Cognition, 15*, 31–49.

Morris, C. D., Bransford, J. D., & Franks, J. J. (1977). Levels of processing versus transfer appropriate processing. *Journal of Verbal Learning and Verbal Behavior, 16*, 519–533.

Morton, J. (1979). Facilitation in word recognition: Experiments causing changes in the logogen models. In P. A. Kolers, M. E. Wrolstead, & H. Bouma (Eds.), *Processing of visible language*. New York: Plenum.

Musen, G., & Treisman, A. (1990). Implicit and explicit memory for visual patterns. *Journal of Experimental Psychology: Learning, Memory and Cognition, 16*, 127–137.

Naito, M. (1990). Repetition priming in children and adults: Age-related dissociation between implicit and explicit memory. *Journal of Experimental Child Psychology, 50*, 462–484.

Neely, J. H. (1977). Semantic priming and retrieval from lexical memory: Roles of inhibitionless spreading activation and limited-capacity attention. *Journal of Experimental Psychology: General, 106*, 226–254.

Neville, H. J., Kutas, M., Chesney, G., & Schmidt, A. L. (1986). Event-related brain potentials during initial encoding and recognition memory of congruous and incongruous words. *Journal of Memory and Language, 25*, 75–92.

Nielsen, J. M. (1958). *Memory and amnesia*. Los Angeles: San Lucas Press.

Nissen, M. J., Knopman, D. S., & Schacter, D. L. (1987). Neurochemical dissociation of memory systems. *Neurology, 37*, 789–794.

Olton, D. A. (1984). Comparative analysis of episodic memory. *Behavioral and Brain Sciences, 7*, 250–251.

Parkin, A. J., & Streete, S. (1988). Implicit and explicit memory in young children and adults. *British Journal of Psychology, 79*, 361–369.

Petersen, S. E., Fox, P. T., Posner, M. I., Mintum, M., & Raichle, M. E. (1988). Positron emission tomographic studies of the cortical anatomy of single-word processing. *Nature, 331*, 585–589.

Ratcliff, R., & McKoon, G. (1986). More on the distinction between episodic and semantic memories. *Journal of Experimental Psychology: Learning, Memory and Cognition, 12*, 312–313.

Reiff, R., & Scheerer, M. (1959). *Memory and hypnotic age regression*. New York: International Universities Press.

Richardson-Klavehn, A., & Bjork, R. A. (1988). Measures of memory. *Annual Review of Psychology, 39*, 475–543.

Roediger, H. L., III. (1984). Does current evidence favor the episodic/semantic distinction? *Behavioral and Brain Sciences, 7*, 252–254.

Roediger, H. L., III. (1990a). Implicit memory: A commentary. *Bulletin of the Psychonomic Society, 28*, 373–380.

Roediger, H. L., III. (1990b). Implicit memory: Retention without remembering. *American Psychologist, 45*, 1043–1056.

Roediger, H. L., III, & Blaxton, T. A. (1987). Retrieval modes produce dissociations in memory for surface information. In D. S. Gorfein & R. R. Hoffman (Eds.), *Memory and cognitive processes: The Ebbinghaus Centennial Conference* (pp. 349–379). Hillsdale, New Jersey: Erlbaum.

Roediger, H. L., III, Weldon, M. S., & Challis, B. H. (1989). Explaining dissociations between implicit and explicit measures of retention: A processing account. In H. L. Roediger, III & F. I. M. Craik (Eds.), *Varieties of memory and consciousness: Essays in honour of Endel Tulving* (pp. 3–42). Hillsdale, New Jersey: Erlbaum.

Rozin, P. (1976). The psychobiological approach to human memory. In M. R. Rosenzweig & E. L. Bennett (Eds.), *Neural mechanisms of learning and memory* (pp. 3–46). Cambridge, Massachussetts: MIT Press.

Ruggiero, F. T., & Flatt, S. F. (1976). Do animals have memory? In D. L. Medin, W. Roberts, & R. T. Davis (Eds.), *Processes of animal memory* (pp. 1–19). New York: Wiley.

Scarborough, D. L., Cortese, C., & Scarborough. (1977). Frequency and repetition effects in lexical memory. *Journal of Experimental Psychology: Human Perception and Performance, 3*, 1–17.

Schacter, D. L. (1982). *Stranger behind the engram: Theories of memory and the psychology of science.* Hillsdale, New Jersey: Erlbaum.

Schacter, D. L. (1985). Multiple forms of memory in humans and animals. In N. M. Weinberger, J. L. McGaugh, & G. Lynch (Eds.), *Memory systems of the brain* (pp. 351–379). New York: Guilford Press.

Schacter, D. L. (1987a). Implicit expressions of memory in organic amnesia: Learning of new facts and associations. *Human Neurobiology, 6*, 107–118.

Schacter, D. L. (1987b). Implicit memory: History and current status. *Journal of Experimental Psychology: Learning, Memory, and Cognition, 13*, 501–518.

Schacter, D. L. (1990). Perceptual representation systems and implicit memory: Toward a resolution of the multiple memory systems debate. In A. Diamond (Ed.), Development and neural bases of higher cognitive functions. *Annals of the New York Academy of Sciences, 608*, 543–571.

Schacter, D. L., Cooper, L. A., & Delaney, S. M. (1990). Implicit memory for unfamiliar objects depends on access to structural descriptions. *Journal of Experimental Psychology: General, 119*, 5–24.

Schacter, D. L., Delaney, S. M., & Merikle, E. P. (1990). Priming of nonverbal information and the nature of implicit memory. In G. H. Bower (Ed.), *The psychology of learning and motivation* (Vol. 26) (pp. 83–123). New York: Academic Press.

Schacter, D. L., Eich, J. E., & Tulving, E. (1978). Richard Semon's theory of memory. *Journal of Verbal Learning and Verbal Behavior, 17*, 721–743.

Schacter, D. L., Harbluk, J., & McLachlan, D. (1984). Retrieval without recollection: An experimental analysis of source amnesia. *Journal of Verbal Learning and Verbal Behavior, 23*, 593–611.

Shallice, T. (1988). *From neuropsychology to mental structure.* Cambridge: Cambridge University Press.

Shallice, T., & Warrington, E. K. (1970). Independent functioning of the verbal memory stores: A neuropsychological study. *Quarterly Journal of Experimental Psychology, 22*, 261–273.

Sherry, D. F., & Schacter, D. L. (1987). The evolution of multiple memory systems. *Psychological Review, 94*, 439–454.

Shimamura, A. P. (1986). Priming effects in amnesia: Evidence for a dissociable memory function. *Quarterly Journal of Experimental Psychology, 38A*, 619–644.

Shimamura, A. P., Janowsky, J. S., & Squire, L. R. (1990). Memory for the temporal order of events in patients with frontal lobe lesions and amnesic patients. *Neuropsychologia, 28,* 803–813.

Shimamura, A. P., & Squire, L. R. (1987). A neuropsychological study of fact memory and source amnesia. *Journal of Experimental Psychology: Learning, Memory, and Cognition, 13,* 464–473.

Shimamura, A. P., & Squire, L. R. (1988). Long-term memory in amnesia: Cued recall, recognition memory, and confidence ratings. *Journal of Experimental Psychology: Learning, Memory, and Cognition, 14,* 763–770.

Sloman, S. A., Hayman, C. A. G., Ohta, N., Law, J., & Tulving, E. (1987). Forgetting in primed fragment completion. *Journal of Experimental Psychology: Learning, Memory, and Cognition, 14,* 223–239.

Smith, M. E., & Halgren, E. (1989). Dissociation of recognition memory components following temporal lobe lesions. *Journal of Experimental Psychology: Learning, Memory, and Cognition, 15,* 50–60.

Snodgrass, J. G., & Feenan, K. (1990). Priming effects in picture fragment completion: Support for the perceptual closure hypothesis. *Journal of Experimental Psychology: General, 119,* 276–296.

Squire, L. R. (1986). Mechanisms of memory. *Science, 232,* 1612–1619.

Squire, L. R. (1987). *Memory and brain.* New York: Oxford University Press.

Squire, L. R., & Cohen, N. J. (1984). Human memory and amnesia. In J. L. McGaugh, G. Lynch, & N. M. Weinberger (Eds.), *The neurobiology of learning and memory* (pp. 3–64). New York: Guilford Press.

Squire, L., Shimamura, A. P., & Amaral, D. G. (1989). Memory and the hippocampus. In J. Byrne & W. Berrys (Eds.), *Neural models of plasticity* (pp. 208–239). New York: Academic Press.

Srinivas, K., & Roediger, H. L., III (1990). Classifying implicit memory tests: Category association and anagram solution. *Journal of Memory and Language, 29,* 389–412.

Thomas, G. J. (1984). Memory: Time binding in organisms. In L. R. Squire & N. Butters (Eds.), *The neuropsychology of memory* (pp. 374–384). New York: Guilford Press.

Thomson, D. M., & Tulving, E. (1970). Associative encoding and retrieval: Weak and strong cues. *Journal of Experimental Psychology, 86,* 255–262.

Tulving, E. (1972). Episodic and semantic memory. In E. Tulving & W. Donaldson (Eds.), *Organization of memory* (pp. 381–403). New York: Academic Press.

Tulving, E. (1982). Synergistic ecphory in recall and recognition. *Canadian Journal of Psychology, 36,* 130–147.

Tulving, E. (1983). *Elements of episodic memory.* Oxford: Clarendon Press.

Tulving, E. (1984a). Multiple learning and memory systems. In K. M. J. Lagerspetz & P. Niemi (Eds.), *Psychology in the 1990's* (pp. 163–184). North Holland: Elsevier Science Publishers B.V.

Tulving, E. (1984b). Relations among components and processes of memory. *Behavioral and Brain Sciences, 7,* 257–268.

Tulving, E. (1985a). How many memory systems are there? *American Psychologist, 40,* 385–398.

Tulving, E. (1985b). Memory and consciousness. *Canadian Psychology, 26,* 1–26.

Tulving, E. (1985c). On the classification problem in learning and memory. In L.-G. Nilsson & T. Archer (Eds.), *Perspectives on learning and memory* (pp. 67–95). Hillsdale: New Jersey: Erlbaum.

Tulving, E. (1986). What kind of a hypothesis is the distinction between episodic and semantic memory? *Journal of Experimental Psychology: Learning, Memory, and Cognition, 12,* 307–311.

Tulving, E. (1987). Multiple memory systems and consciousness. *Human Neurobiology, 6,* 67–80.

Tulving, E. (1989). Memory: Performance, knowledge, and experience. *European Journal of Cognitive Psychology, 1,* 3–26.

Tulving, E., Hayman, C. A. G., & Macdonald, C. A. (1991). Long-lasting perceptual priming and semantic learning in amnesia: A case experiment. *Journal of Experimental Psychology: Learning, Memory and Cognition, 17,* 595–617.

Tulving, E., & Osler, S. (1968). Effectiveness of retrieval cues in memory for words. *Journal of Experimental Psychology, 77,* 593–601.

Tulving, E., & Pearlstone, Z. (1966). Availability versus accessibility of information in memory for words. *Journal of Verbal Learning and Verbal Behavior, 5,* 381–391.

Tulving, E., Risberg, J., & Ingvar, D. H. (1988, November). *Regional cerebral blood flow and episodic memory retrieval.* Paper presented at the Annual Meeting of the Psychonomic Society, Chicago.

Tulving, E., & Schacter, D. L. (1990). Priming and human memory systems. *Science, 247,* 301–306.

Tulving, E., Schacter, D. L., McLachlan, D. R., & Moscovitch, M. (1988). Priming of semantic autobiographical knowledge: A case study of retrograde amnesia. *Brain and Cognition, 8,* 3–20.

Tulving, E., Schacter, D. L. & Stark, H. A. (1982). Priming effects in word-fragment completion are independent of recognition memory. *Journal of Experimental Psychology: Learning, Memory and Cognition, 8,* 352–373.

Tulving, E., & Thomson, D. M. (1973). Encoding specificity and retrieval processes in episodic memory. *Psychological Review, 80,* 352–373.

Warrington, E. K. (1975). The selective impairment of semantic memory. *Quarterly Journal of Experimental Psychology, 27,* 635–657.

Warrington, E. K. (1979). Neuropsychological evidence for multiple memory systems. *Brain and Mind: Ciba Foundation Symposium* (Vol. 69, new series) (pp. 153–166). Amsterdam: Excerpta Medica.

Warrington, E. K., & Shallice, T. (1969). The selective impairment of auditory verbal short-term memory. *Brain, 92,* 885–896.

Warrington, E. K., & Taylor, A. M. (1978). Two categorical stages of object recognition. *Perception, 7,* 695–705.

Warrington, E. K., & Weiskrantz, L. (1968). New method of testing long-term retention with special reference to amnesic patients. *Nature, 217,* 972–974.

Warrington, E. K., & Weiskrantz, L. (1970). Amnesic syndrome: Consolidation or retrieval? *Nature, 228,* 628–630.

Warrington, E. K., & Weiskrantz, L. (1974). The effect of prior learning on subsequent retention in amnesic patients. *Neuropsychologia, 12,* 419–428.

Watkins, M. J., & Tulving, E. (1975). Episodic memory: When recognition fails. *Journal of Experimental Psychology: General, 104,* 5–29.

Waugh, N. C., & Norman, D. A. (1965). Primary memory. *Psychological Review, 72,* 89–104.

Weinberger, N. M. (1990). Neuromnemonics: Forms and contents. In J. L. McGaugh, N. M. Weinberger, & G. Lynch (Eds.), *Brain organization and memory: Cells, systems, and circuits* (pp. 137–144). New York: Oxford University Press.

Weiskrantz, L. (1985). On issues and theories of the human amnesic syndrome. In N. M. Weinberger, J. L. McGaugh, & G. Lynch (Eds.), *Memory systems of the brain* (pp. 380–415). New York: Guilford Press.

Weiskrantz, L. (1987). Neuroanatomy of memory and amnesia: A case for multiple memory systems. *Human Neurobiology, 6,* 93–105.

Weizkrantz, L. (1990). Problem of learning and memory: One or multiple memory systems? *Philosophical Transactions of the Royal Society, London, B329,* 99–108.

Zacks, R. (1984). Review of *Elements of Episodic Memory. Psychology Today, 29,* 615–616.

I

Distribution of Learning-Induced Brain Activity

2

Insights into Processes of Visual Perception from Studies in the Olfactory System

WALTER J. FREEMAN

> The certainty of ideas is not the foundation of the certainty of perception but is, rather, based on it—in that it is perceptual experience which gives us the passage from one moment to the next and thus realizes the unity of time. In this sense all consciousness is perceptual, even the consciousness of ourselves.
> MAURICE MERLEAU-PONTY, *The Primacy of Perception* (1946)

> If the doors of perception were cleansed everything would appear to man as it is, infinite.
> WILLIAM BLAKE, *The Marriage of Heaven and Hell* (1793)

Memory begins and ends with perception. That which is stored is not the raw stimulus but the congeries of appurtenant stimulus-induced activities that are assembled in the cerebral cortex. That which is recalled serves to guide and shape the cortical activities that are induced by a stimulus that is to be perceived. In order to learn the neural basis of associative memory, we must discern the neurophysiological space–time attributes of the information that is to be memorized, which is a percept, not a stimulus. In order to learn the neural basis for what we experience as retrieval or ecphoria, we must observe how the activity that is induced by a stimulus interacts with stored information to form a percept. The experimental studies that are summarized in this chapter indicate that these neural events of storage and recall take place in primary sensory cortexes where stimulus-induced activity first reaches the cortical mantle, and they depend on the effects of prior learning. My particular aims are to infer from studies of olfactory perception what may be guiding principles of visual perception as the basis for understanding visual learning and memory, and to describe some critical experiments that serve to validate those principles.

Vision and olfaction are commonly perceived as the farthest apart on a spectrum of the senses encompassing hearing, proprioception, touch, and taste. Vision is characterized by a dichotomy of receptor types; three primary color components; wide dynamic range of intensity coding in spike frequencies; intricate local processes of feature extraction that concentrate discrete forms of information into pulse trains of single neurons in successive layers; topographic order within each layer; and well defined mappings and spatial transforms from each layer to the next. Olfaction is characterized by absence of verified primary odorants; lack of tuning of individual receptors or central neurons to one or a few odorants; narrow ranges of concentration sensitivity, so that multiple cells are required to convey information about each odorant over its dynamic range of detectability; lack of well defined criteria for measuring similarity among stimuli or for making generalization gradients and hierarchical classification trees; poor to absent topographic order within layers or mappings from each layer to the next; and exquisite sensitivity to familiar but chemically undefined mixtures.

Substantial effort has been expended over the past four decades to apply lessons from visual physiology to the study of olfaction. These include the search for primaries, for local mechanisms of contrast enhancement and feature extraction by interneuronal inhibitory feedback, and for representation of odorants by topographically organized spatial patterns of neural activity. Evidence has been sought of increased selectivity of central neurons over receptors to single odorants, as the basis for olfactory feature extraction. Modest success has been achieved in finding spatial pattern specificity among receptors in the mucosa and among interneurons in the outer layer of the olfactory bulb (e.g., Lancet, Greer, Kauer, & Shepherd, 1982), but not in the deeper layers or in other structures to which the bulb projects (Haberly, 1985). In the main the olfactory system has been refractory to attempts (Shepherd, 1972) to model its architectural and dynamic properties on those of the visual system.

In contrast, there have been major advances in understanding the analytical mechanisms by which visual images are decomposed into points, lines, local and global movements, and color patches, and how these features are mapped into arrays of single neurons in multiple cortical receiving areas (e.g., Ts'o, Frostig, Lieke, & Grinvald, 1990). However, there is little comprehension of how these many kinds of information are rapidly and reliably synthesized into global percepts that provide the bases for behavioral pattern recognition and decisive action.

One approach to this so called "binding problem" in both visual and olfactory psychophysiology has been to construct models of the neural bases of perception and to test these models on problems of artificial pattern classification and recognition. Examples are Daugman's (1990) convolution of visual images with Gabor filters in order to compress the data into manageable strings, and Marr's (1982) development of schemata for assembling information from feature detectors into structures that are guided by top-down expectations of the nature of objects in the visual world. These and many other models (e.g., Anderson, Silverstein, Ritz, & Jones, 1977;

Grossberg, 1990) are derived from and driven by insights gained from anatomical and electrophysiological studies of the visual system. A comparable attempt in olfaction has been to model the functional olfactory architecture and the nonlinear dynamics of olfactory neural activity, and then to test the model for its capabilities in classifying spatial patterns of various kinds (Freeman, Yao, & Burke, 1988; Yao & Freeman, 1990).

Given the relatively advanced state of the applications of nonlinear dynamics in studies of olfactory perception, it is reasonable to ask: what can be predicted and learned about visual perception from studies of the olfactory system? In this chapter I will: (a) give a brief overview of the neurodynamics of olfactory perception; (b) present a model that embodies this view; (c) describe what further steps are required to incorporate the dynamics in an effective device for pattern classification; (d) list some predictions that have already been fulfilled regarding the nature of categorizing operations that are revealed in recordings of visual cortical neuroelectrical activity; and (e) sketch a possible mode of visual system function that it built on, but also somewhat removed from, models currently shared among most workers in neural and artificial vision.

PHYSIOLOGICAL BASES OF OLFACTORY PERCEPTION

A key premise for the study of central olfactory processing is the concept that neural information coexists in microscopic and macroscopic forms. Sensory input to the bulb takes the form of trains of action potentials on single afferent axons. These are point processes that have precise locations in time and space, and they serve to define information univocally in terms of the firing rates of specified neurons. This form holds also for the output of the bulb to its several target structures, and therefore for the bulbar mitral cells that generate that output.

Simultaneously there is a macroscopic form of information, which is carried in the instantaneous spatial ensemble averages of local neighborhoods of neurons, and which is coordinated by cooperative dynamics over the entire olfactory system. This macroscopic form of information is the self-organized perceptual activity of the bulb as distinct from its evoked sensory activity. It is continuously distributed over the entire surface of the bulb, and it is uniform in spatial density. It is temporally segmented into brief epochs by the actions of other parts of the brain onto the bulb. This perceptual activity is shaped by past and present input through learning, and it determines the spatiotemporal firing patterns of mitral cells. Microscopic and macroscopic activities similarly coexist in the anterior olfactory nucleus and prepyriform cortex. The interactions between these parts by forward and feedback pathways serve to generate and regulate the ongoing activity of the entire olfactory system, which is revealed in the so-called "spontaneous" activities observed both in spike trains of central axons and the dendritic currents that give rise to the local field potentials (LFPs) also known as electroencephalograms (EEGs).

Sensory information is encoded in the spatial patterns of neural activity of both axons and dendrites. Odorants activate subsets of receptors that are inhomogenously distributed in the mucosa and therefore provide for transduction of chemical stimuli into spatially patterned neural firings. Similarly, discrete patches of odorant induced activity are seen in the outer (glomerular) layer of the olfactory bulb by means of metabolic labeling (Lancet et al., 1982). The perceptual information takes the form of amplitude modulation of an oscillation in neural activity that is common to the entire bulb. The carrier wave is characteristically aperiodic, and from several converging lines of evidence it can be described as the output of a deterministic chaotic system (Freeman & Skarda, 1985; Skarda & Freeman, 1987). Under the influence of centrally controlled variables such as the respiratory cycle and the state of motivation, the bulbar mechanism undergoes repeated state changes that we believe constitute bifurcations. These state changes demarcate the bulbar output into time segments or frames. Each frame contains a burst of oscillation, which has a unique pattern of phase of the oscillation unrelated to odorants (Freeman & Baird, 1987), and it usually has a reproducible pattern of amplitude that constitutes perceptual information (Freeman & Grajski, 1987; Freeman & Viana Di Prisco, 1986).

The forms of these spatial patterns are peculiar to each animal. They are formed under reinforcement by synaptic modification in accordance with use dependency as predicted by Hebb (1949). The nerve cell assemblies that emerge during training are not in themselves sufficient for pattern classification by bulbar output. Instead, they sensitize the bulbar mechanism to particular learned classes of input, so that each nerve cell assembly can guide bulbar activity into a standard spatial pattern of activity. Each pattern serves to signal an odorant on which the nerve cell assembly was formed during training. The nerve cell assembly serves as a kind of manager to direct the flow of bulbar traffic when it is activated by its stimulus.

A MODEL THAT SIMULATES OLFACTORY DYNAMICS

The simulation of the spatiotemporal activity patterns of the bulb, anterior olfactory nucleus, and prepyriform cortex has been based on physiological measurements of the properties of local populations of neurons within these structures (Freeman, 1975, 1987a). Under very deep anesthesia an "open loop" state appears, in which there are no spontaneous or induced oscillations, and in which the evoked potential on stimulation of axonal tracts is an extracellularly recorded compound excitatory postsynaptic potential (EPSP). Its finite rise and decay times can be modeled with the solution to a linear second order ordinary differential equation. In the normal "closed loop" state the linear operation of integration is followed by a nonlinear operation at the trigger zones of the neurons. In the populations within each structure this takes the form of a static sigmoid curve (Eeckman & Freeman, 1990; Freeman, 1975, 1979). Both the delays and the nonlinearities endow the populations with inherent tendencies to instability in feedback interactions. Partly this instability is due to the delay that is introduced by synapses and by the cable properties of dendrites. More importantly it is promoted by the sigmoid function (Freeman, 1975; Eeckman & Freeman, 1991), because its maximal slope (gain) is displaced to the excitatory side, so that the sensitivities of the populations are enhanced by any excitatory input. More gain brings more activity and yet more gain, so that the population is always on the positive slope of an explosive increase in self-regenerative activity. This asymmetry of the sigmoid function is the basis for bifurcation on input in the olfactory system and also in the model that simulates it.

The architecture of the model conforms to that of the several main parts of the olfactory system. Populations of excitatory neurons and inhibitory neurons are massively interconnected in parallel within and between serial layers and have massively parallel input and output lines. Negative feedback between excitatory and inhibitory neural populations gives rise to the oscillations of the system in the gamma range of the EEG (20–100 Hz, including the well known "40 Hz" band). The long-range mutually excitatory connections enable the formation of large-scale stable patterns. It is these connections that are modified to form nerve cell assemblies over training trials. In conjunction with the sigmoid function, these connections enhance the regenerative feedback, which induces oscillation by bifurcation upon presentation of a learned odorant in a test trial. The model indicates further that mutual inhibition must also be present in order to account for the observed frequencies of oscillation and for the stabilization of the system in the absence of learned odorant input.

Feedback is also global from the anterior olfactory nucleus and from prepyriform cortex back to the bulb. There are both dispersion and long delays in the feedback pathways, and the feedback is directed to both excitatory and inhibitory neurons in the bulb. Each of the three structures has its characteristic frequency, which is incommensurate with the others. The couplings with delays constitute the conditions that lead to the appearance of chaotic activity in the intact system (Freeman, 1987b). The excitatory feedback drives the system away from rest, whereas the inhibitory feedback tends to suppress it, but normally the incommensurate frequences and the delays prevent it from ever settling to equilibrium.

One of the most dramatic physiological findings is the disappearance of background activity in all three structures (bulb, nucleus, and prepyriform) when the lateral olfactory tract is inactivated pharmacologically or surgically (Freeman, 1975). This finding demonstrates that the basal unit and EEG activities of these structures are indeed global properties, and they are not the sums of locally generated activity as has long been believed.

The visual cortex is similar to the olfactory cortex in important ways, including the dense interconnections of large numbers of excitatory and inhibitory neurons, the laminar architecture of these populations, and the massively parallel input and output axonal pathways. The activities of both structures show sustained oscillations, particularly under conditions of sensory stimulation. The question is: what do these properties have to do with self-organization and perception in olfaction and vision? To approach an answer, we model odor perception as an operation in pattern classification.

APPLICATION OF THE MODEL TO PATTERN CLASSIFICATION

The model based on these experimental findings from the olfactory system has been tested extensively in both hardware (Eisenberg, Freeman, & Burke, 1989) and software versions (Freeman et al., 1988) with artificially generated data sets. More interesting has been our experience with data sets supplied by the manufacturer (Buckley, 1978) of a device for the rapid and reliable classification of large numbers of small objects that are screened for quality prior to use in automated assembly lines (Yao, Freeman, Burke, & Yang, 1991).

The process for inspection might well be called machine vision, were it not for the fact that the method relies not on light but on ultrasound. Each object is shot through a field of 40 kHz ultrasound that contains an array of 12 photocells in the path of travel. Each photocell triggers an array of eight microphones to read the sound intensity and phase. We reduce the phase data to an 8×8 array of 0's and 1's by discarding a third of the triggered traces, centering the phase distributions at 0, and binarizing above and below the mean for each of the 64 readings. A 64×1 binary column vector is formed for each of 20 objects already known to lie within desired specifications and 20 others known to lie outside.

A subset of two to five objects in each class is used to train a software version of the system on a Cray MXP by strengthening the mutually excitatory connections among 64 coupled oscillators to form a template that is equivalent to a nerve cell assembly for each class. The overlap of the two templates is removed by setting the input connection strengths of the overlapping oscillators to zero. The system is tested by measuring the spatial pattern of output when a step input is given to the 64 coupled oscillators. The step input is amplitude-modulated by the column vector of each member of the training and test sets. The output is calculated as a 64×1 column vector of response amplitudes. Each component in the vector from a burst is an amplitude along one of 64 coordinate axes, so that the vector specifies a point in a 64-dimensional "graph." A collection of bursts from one odorant gives as a "cloud" of points. The centroid is calculated for the set of points from each training set, and a distance measure is calculated for its radius expressed in units of standard deviation. The classification is made by determining the minimal of two Euclidean distances for each point in the test set.

Each input is given to the system when it is in a stationary chaotic state with low amplitude. The input amplitude is nonzero across the entire array, with a fixed additional increment for each nonzero input channel. The system undergoies bifurcation to a high-amplitude narrow-band chaotic oscillation that converges to a stationary pattern within about 50 simulated milliseconds with common components of d.c. shift and oscillation. On termination of the input step the system returns to the same chaotic basal state, as determined by visual inspection of the phase portrait of the activity taken from two or more selected elements among the oscillators (Yao et al., 1991).

The system has been tested on four sets of objects that are graded in difficulty of classification from easy to very difficult. The same sets of objects have also been classified by other techniques, including a Bayesian approach, a Hopfield (1982) model, a PDP system with back propagation (Rumelhart & McClelland, 1986), and a simpler version of our model that employs a Hopf bifuraction on input from a prestimulus equilibrium state to a limit cycle that is induced by the step input (Freeman et al., 1988). The systems do equally well on the easier objects, but only the system with chaotic dynamics solves the problem with the most difficult objects, which have the largest variability of input image.

We do not know the mechanism by which the chaotic dynamics provide this superior classificatory capability. The task of solving the 584 first order differential equations at 0.5 ms steps by numerical techniques on a digital computer is sufficiently time consuming to preclude vigorous and detailed exploration of the performance characteristics of the system in its present form. Our intent was merely to find the circumstances in which a biologically derived dynamic model might function at least as well as theoretically derived systems for pattern classification, and we are not prepared fully to explain or defend the outcome, merely to present what we have found as an incentive for further study of chaotic dynamical systems in this application.

VERIFIED PREDICTIONS AND EXTENSIONS FOR VISUAL PROCESSES

The prediction was made (Freeman & van Dijk, 1987) that visual information would be found in the spatial patterns of the visual cortical EEG activity, and that it would be found in the gamma range of frequencies. The prediction was tested by recording from a 5×7 array of 35 electrodes placed subdurally over the primary visual cortex of a rhesus monkey that had already been trained in a visual discrimination task (Dagnelie, 1986). The cortical EEG was recorded from 16 channels across the 750 ms required for the performance of the task, filtered to remove activity below 20 Hz and above 50 Hz, and displayed as an unaveraged time series for each trial. Four EEG segments were selected from each trial: first, prior to the arrival of a conditioned stimulus (CS); second, between the CS and the onset of a conditioned response (CR); third, during the CR when the gaze of the monkey shifted from the target on a screen to the juice spout for its reward (UCS); and fourth, after the performance of the unconditioned response (UCR).

The durations of the segments averaged 120 ± 22 ms. Each segment was subjected to principal components analysis and reduced to a 16×1 column vector of the factor loadings of the dominant component. The vector was used successfully to classify the EEG segments retrospectively into CS and CR groupings, showing that behavioral information was present in oscillations at a common instantaneous frequency over the entire array. In conformance with our experience in olfaction the activity was intrinsically aperiodic but band-limited to the gamma range. As in the olfactory bulb the percentage of the variance that was incorporated by the dominant component averaged 65% but ranged from 20% to over 80% in different segments and trials. The commonality of oscillation in phase was found to hold over the full array dimensions of 28 mm × 36 mm, an area roughly an order of magnitude greater than the extent of spatial coherence over the entire olfactory bulb.

The olfactory model gave predictions (Freeman, 1975, 1987a) that unit activity of neocortical neurons would be found to show the same sigmoid saturation function as that found throughout the olfactory system (Eeckman & Freeman, 1990), and strong oscillations in firing probability at frequencies of the cortical gamma EEG. Several investigators have now confirmed and significantly extended these predictions for visual cortical neurons (Eckhorn et al., 1988; Gray, Koenig, Engel, & Singer, 1989). In both anesthetized and waking cats the pulse trains of selected neurons, which are activated by moving line segments projected onto the retina, show oscillations in firing probability in the gamma range. These pulse probability waves are approximately in phase with the concomitant fluctuation in cortical EEG at the same frequency. When a line segment is passed across two receptor fields having approximately the same orientation and direction specificity, the pulse trains of the two cortical neurons are strongly correlated even at distances up to 7 mm apart between the two recording sites. The frequency of oscillation, while not uncommonly near the nominal "40 Hz" (Sheer, 1976), is variable both within and between periods of induced oscillation, though the usual methods of autocorrelation and spike-triggered averaging tend to obscure the variation within trials. Thus at present there is strong evidence for fundamental likeness in significant aspects of the dynamics of the olfactory and visual systems.

ASPECTS OF A PROPOSED MODEL FOR VISUAL PERCEPTION

The greatest difference between the olfactory and visual systems lies in the respective amounts of sensory preprocessing, for it is meager in olfaction apart from dynamic range compression and some degree of spatial coarse graining in the glomerular layer. Yet olfaction does have minimal homologies with the operations in the retina and lateral geniculate nucleus that serve to extract local spatial and temporal derivatives and color gradients, to compress the data in proportion to the ratio of numbers of receptors to ganglion cells, and to establish detailed relations between the two inputs bilaterally. Moreover, in both systems there are strong tendencies for vigorous firing in the presence of a pertinent stimulus and not otherwise. We suggest that this property may constitute a step of binarization (as in our model) of the sensory input to the bulb and to the visual cortex. This preprocessing step makes sense when it is seen as a transformation, in which microscopic input carried by the activity of a small number among many millions of afferent axons serves to guide the emergence of an appropriate macroscopic pattern of cortical activity. When a small fraction of the immense number of afferents is activated, it would seem desirable that they be strongly active, because the cortical neurons integrating over many thousands of input neurons might be insensitive to fine gradations of activity on single lines. This insight comes from viewing the cortex as a massively interconnected neuropil rather than as a discrete network abstracted in the manner of Golgi preparations, in which small gradations of activity might be significant on single axons.

Although the taking of local temporal and spatial derivatives leads to the appearance of point, line, edge, and motion sensitivities among retinal and cortical neurons having well defined receptor fields, the philosophical step of labeling these cells as "feature detectors" can have misleading consequences. There is no question that the gradients of images projected onto arrays of receptors constitute information that is enhanced by the central neural machinery, but it need not follow that these geometric constructs are the "primitives" from which triangles, cubes, eyes, faces, etc. are elaborated and identified. These features exist in the minds of observers and may or may not exist in the brains of experimental subjects.

An important lesson we have learned from our experience with industrial data is that we do not and cannot know what the features of the training objects are that our system has extracted and codified, nor is this necessary. A self-organizing system creates its own frames of reference through Hebbian or possibly other mechanisms of learning and by generalization over examples. The features used by a monkey that inspects a juice spout or by a machine that receives numbers from the sound waves reflected by a screw driver bit are not reducible to analytic geometries or hierarchical trees, because the frames of reference are internally devised and applied by the categorizing system. An act of perception involves an enormous data compression over the receptor space and over past experience that has been incorporated into cortical synaptic modifications. The essence of this compression can be described as the replacement of an infinitely dimensioned flow of microscopic information from receptors with a finitely dimensioned chaotic macroscopic activity pattern. Furthermore, in our experience with the olfactory bulb the spatial patterns of gamma EEG activity reflect the meanings of the odorants and not the stimuli per se. We have shown this in several ways, most effectively by changing the reinforcement contingencies of CSs. The same odorants then induce new spatial patterns of bulbar EEG activity (Freeman & Grajski, 1987; Freeman & Viana Di Prisco, 1986). Such findings reinforce the conclusion, long established in visual physiology, that neuronal responses to stimuli depend as much on past experience as on the stimuli. If the determinants of neuronal responses are meanings rather than stimuli, then the utility of the concept of "features" is called into question.

Moreover, an understanding of the nature of features, that is, whether the meanings are endogenous (subject oriented) or exogenous (observer oriented), is critical for an approach to the "linkage" problem, whereby an array of feature detectors that is stimulated by a visual image is coupled into an organized pattern of cortical activity (Eckhorn et al., 1988; Gray et al., 1989; Hubel & Wiesel, 1962). Are the features made of points and directed line segments that are coupled into more complex geometric entities, or do they consist of visual gestalts without analytical forms, which are the raw materials for object recognition? Does the requisite learning occur mainly in developmental critical periods in which local networks are organized for extracting local spatial and temporal gradients, or does it take place mainly in adults during the induction of widespread synaptic changes in associational learning from empirical examples accompanied by reinforcement?

Physiologists who conceive the linkage problem at the micro level (e.g., Eckhorn et al., 1988; Gray et al., 1989) emphasize the formation of discrete networks of small numbers from the myriads of cortical neurons. In the macro view the linkage problem is solved by a bifurcation, in which a global pattern of cortical activity involving *all* visual cortical neurons is selected by an exemplary input that directs the system into a preformed basin of attraction. All of the information from receptors is disseminated among pyramidal cells by corticocortical excitatory synaptic connections that have been weighted during past experience. The cortex is conceived to be operating as a global entity in a highly active but stabilized state, such that numerous learned basins of attraction are available to it almost instantly. All that is needed is a stimulus from a learned class to push the whole system across a separatrix into the basin of an attractor corresponding to that class. This view subsumes but is not limited to the concept of the linkage of pairs of neurons, which are the basis for Hebbian learning, and which are accessible to observers with microelectrodes. The synaptic pair is an essential component for the concept of a macroscopic cortical spatial pattern that is accessed with macroelectrodes, but the number of pairs is unmeasurably large.

In the macro view the distributed oscillation or "wave packet" (Freeman, 1975) is not a sensory response that is evoked by a stimulus. It is a perceptual state that is induced or selected by a stimulus from a previously experienced class. It is characterized by a homogeneous information density across the cortex. That is, the value of the information expressed by each neuron is not proportional to its firing rate (black is no less important in a pattern than white, for both are necessary), and no one neuron conveys any more or less information than any other, whether it fires rapidly or not at all.

There is a common carrier wave that typically is not periodic, and it need not be so because the state transitions are not based on resonance or entrainment. The instantaneous frequency is the same everywhere, even though the spectrum is broad over short time segments. The phase at the common frequency may be distributed over a range bounded by a quarter cycle (Freeman, 1990). Otherwise neither of these variables is heavily restricted, and it appears that they can and do vary substantially in the visual cortex, as they do in the olfactory system. The dissemination of information can be likened to the property of a hologram, which can be broken into parts, each having the whole scene though at reduced resolution. Furthermore, inspection of a holographic pattern in its stored form is meaningless to human observers until the information is retrieved by the inverse transform, and the appearance of the spatial patterns of cortical activity that convey percepts are just as shapeless and meaningless for the human eye (Freeman & van Dijk, 1987), but in the cortex there is no inverse transform, nor need there be one.

The macro view is entirely compatible with the experimental data that support the micro view, because the two kinds of information coexist in recordings of cortical activity. Each kind is accessed by a different method. Microscopic activity that manifests sensory stimuli is extracted by time ensemble averaging, in which the time base is locked to the time of stimulus onset. Macroscopic activity is accessed with spatial ensemble averaging, in which the common carrier is extracted from an array of time series that is simultaneously recorded from multiple electrodes spaced to capture the highest spatial frequency of the patterns sought. Time ensemble averaging across trials tends to degrade the macroscopic information, because the frequencies and times of onset of wave packets tend to vary unpredictably in the manner of self-organized events.

The macro view can also solve the problem of allocation of the output of visual cortex to multiple structures (e.g., the pulvinar, lateral geniculate nucleus, colliculus, inferotemporal cortex, frontal areas, etc). We conceive that the same information is transmitted to every structure to which the visual cortex projects at a resolution that is proportional to the fraction of the whole output that each target receives. Each target structure can extract whatever cortical output is appropriate for its task. This problem is intractably complex for the micro view because of the combinatorial problem of the number of feature-linking networks and the diversity of targets. It is simple and self-evident in the macro view.

The process of extraction of perceptual information by target areas receiving visual cortical output can be seen to reside in the spatial integration that characterizes most corticocortical projections, owing to divergence in transmission and convergence in reception. Each target neuron is conceived to integrate in real time the outputs of neurons widely dispersed over the visual cortex and thereby to extract the cortical activity at the common instantaneous frequency and phase, within the above prescribed tolerances. Other activity is smoothed out to the extent that it is dispersed in phase and frequency. In essence the cooperative activity of the visual cortex becomes the signal, and other persisting local activity is treated as noise and is removed. Hence spatial divergence in central axonal transmission tends to act as a laundry to enhance the reception of the cooperative activity that is generated for cortical transmission.

CONCLUSION

This description is less a model than a set of guidelines for future studies in visual perception. The recently widespread interest in oscillations opens new opportunities for experimental work and modeling, and may help to break the rigid mold in which most visual physiological studies have been constrained for the past two decades. Emphasis should be placed on the nonlinear dynamics of large populations of cortical neurons, which differ substantially from the dynamics of single neurons and parts of neurons (Freeman, 1975, 1987a,b). More information is needed about the generic types of feedback within and between neural populations, including mutual excitation, mutual inhibition, and negative feedback. Methods are needed for identifying the actions of individual neurons as excitatory or inhibitory, not merely whether they are excited or inhibited by particular stimuli.

Most pressing is the need for simultaneous multichannel recording of neural activity from widely separated electrodes, both at the micro and macro levels. Serious efforts are needed to analyze, comprehend, and verify the results from recordings of summed dendritic potentials in the extracellular spaces and at the surface of the visual cortex. These manifestations of the flow of synaptic currents through the tissue provide the best access to the local mean fields of cortical populations, because in the proper circumstances they constitute a local spatial ensemble average of the activity of a neighborhood of neurons. These observable phenomena known also as LFPs give us our best direct access to the macro states of cortical populations. Ongoing developments in nonlinear dynamics and the theory of chaos have provided us with the tools needed to make this sign of cortical activity less the "roar of a crowd at a football game" and more the macroscopic brain language of perception to supplant the "grandmother cell." As such, this sign provides an essential key to comprehending and modeling cortical function in perception and to applying this knowledge in clinical neurology and in artificial intelligence.

REFERENCES

Anderson, J. A., Silverstein, J. W., Ritz, S. R., & Jones, R. S. (1977). Distinctive features, categorical perception, and probability learning: Some applications of a neural model. *Psychological Review, 84*, 413–451.

Blake, W. (1793). *The marriage of heaven and hell. Modern Library Edition (1947)* (p. 657). New York: Random House.

Buckley, S. (1978). Phase monitoring for automated inspection, positioning and assembly. *Transactions of the Society of Manufacturing Engineering, 6*, 56–63.

Dagnelie, G. (1986). *Pattern and motion processing in primate visual cortex. A study in visually evoked potentials.* Unpublished thesis, University of Amsterdam.

Daugman, J. G. (1990). An information-theoretic view of analog representation in striate cortex. In E. L. Schwartz (Ed.), *Computational neuroscience* (Ch. 13, pp. 403–423). Cambridge, Massachussetts: MIT Press.

Eckhorn, R., Bauer, B., Jordan, W., Brosch, M., Kruse, W., Munk, M., & Reitboeck, H. J. (1988). Coherent oscillations: A mechanism of feature linking in visual cortex? *Biological Cybernetics, 60*, 121–130.

Eeckman, F. H., & Freeman, W. J. (1990). Correlations between unit firing and EEG in the rat olfactory system. *Brain Research, 528*, 238–244.

Eeckman, F. H. & Freeman, W. J. (1991). Asymmetric sigmoid non-linearity in the rat olfactory system. *Brain Research, 557*, 13–21.

Eisenberg, J., Freeman, W. J. & Burke, B. (1989). Hardware architecture of a neural network model simulating pattern recognition by the olfactory bulb. *Neural Networks, 2*, 315–325.

Freeman, W. J. (1975). *Mass action in the nervous system.* New York: Academic Press.

Freeman, W. J. (1979). Nonlinear gain mediating cortical stimulus-response relations. *Biological Cybernetics, 33*, 237–247.

Freeman, W. J. (1987a). Techniques used in the search for the physiological basis of the EEG. In A. Gevins & A. Remond (Eds.), *Handbook of electroencephalography and clinical neurophysiology* (Vol. 3A, Part 2, Ch. 18). Amsterdam: Elsevier.

Freeman, W. J. (1987b). Simulation of chaotic EEG patterns with a dynamic model of the olfactory system. *Biological Cybernetics, 56*, 139–150.

Freeman, W. J. (1990). On the problem of anomalous dispersion in chaoto-chaotic phase transitions of neural masses, and its significance for the management of information in brains. In H. Haken & M. Stadler (Eds.), *Synergetics of cognition* (pp. 126–143). Berlin: Springer-Verlag.

Freeman, W. J. (1991). The physiology of perception. *Scientific American, 264*, 78–85.

Freeman, W. J. & Baird, B. (1987). Relation of olfactory EEG to behavior: Spatial analysis. *Behavioral Neuroscience, 101*, 393–408.

Freeman, W. J., & Grajski, K. A. (1987). Relation of olfactory EEG to behavior: Factor analysis. *Behavioral Neuroscience, 101*, 766–777.

Freeman, W. J., & Skarda, C. A. (1985). Spatial EEG patterns, non-linear dynamics and perception: The neo-Sherringtonian view. *Brain Research Reviews, 10*, 147–175.

Freeman, W. J., & Van Dijk, B. (1987). Spatial patterns of visual cortical fast EEG during conditioned reflex in a rhesus monkey. *Brain Research, 422*, 267–276.

Freeman, W. J., & Viana Di Prisco, G. (1986). Relation of olfactory EEG to behavior: Time series analysis. *Behavioral Neuroscience, 100*, 753–763.

Freeman, W. J., Yao, Y., & Burke, B. (1988). Central pattern generating and recognizing in olfactory bulb: A correlation learning rule. *Neural Networks, 1*, 277–288.

Gray, C. M., Koenig, P., Engel, A. K., & Singer, W. (1989). Oscillatory responses in cat visual cortex exhibit intercolumnar synchronization which reflects global stimulus properties. *Nature, 338*, 334–337.

Grossberg, S. (1990). Content-addressable memory storage by neural networks: A general model and global Liapunov method. In E. L. Schwartz (Ed.), *Computational neuroscience* (Ch. 6, pp. 56–65). Cambridge, Massachusetts: MIT Press.

Haberly, L. B. (1985). Neuronal circuitry in the olfactory cortex: anatomy and functional implications. *Chemical Senses, 10*, 219–238.

Hebb, D. O. (1949). *The organization of behavior: A neuropsychological theory.* New York: Wiley.

Hopfield, J. J. (1982). Neuronal networks and physical systems with emergent collective computational abilities. *Proceedings of the National Academy of Sciences, U.S.A., 81*, 3058–3092.

Hubel, D., & Weisel, T. (1962). Receptive fields, binocular interactions, and functional architecture in the cat's visual cortex. *Journal of Neurophysiology, 160*, 106–154.

Lancet, D., Greer, C. A., Kauer, J. S. & Shepherd, G. M. (1982). Mapping of odor-related neuronal activity in the olfactory bulb by high-resolution 2-deoxyglucose autoradiography. *Proceedings of the National Academy of Sciences, U.S.A., 79*, 670–674.

Marr, D. (1982). *Vision: A computational investigation into the human representation and processing of visual information.* New York: Freeman.

Merleau-Ponty, M. (1946). *The primacy of perception and other essays* (p. 13). Trans. by J. M. Edie (1964). Chicago, Illinois: Northwestern University Press.

Rumelhart, D. E., & McClelland, J. L. (1986). *Parallel distributed processing* (Vol. 1). Cambridge, Massachusetts: MIT Press.

Sheer, D. (1976). Focussed arousal and 40-Hz EEG. In R. M. Knights & D. J. Baker (Eds.), *The neuropsychology of learning disorders: Theoretical approaches* (pp. 71–87). Baltimore, Maryland: University Park Press.

Shepherd, G. (1972). Synaptic organization of the mammalian olfactory bulb. *Physiological Review, 52*, 864–917.

Skarda, C. A., & Freeman, W. J. (1987). How brains make chaos in order to make sense of the world. *Behavioral and Brain Sciences, 10*, 161–195.

Ts'o, D. Y., Frostig, R. D., Lieke, E. E., & Grinvald, A. (1990). Functional organization of primate visual cortex revealed by high resolution optical imaging. *Science, 249*, 417–420.

Yao, Y., & Freeman, W. J. (1990). Model of biological pattern recognition with spatially chaotic dynamics. *Neural Networks, 3*, 153–170.

Yao, Y., Freeman, W. J., Burke, B., & Yang, Q. (1991). Pattern recognition by a distributed neural network: An industrial application. *Neural Networks, 4*, 103–121.

3

Optical Imaging of Architecture and Function in the Living Brain

AMIRAM GRINVALD
TOBIAS BONHOEFFER
DOV MALONEK
DORON SHOHAM
EYAL BARTFELD
A. ARIELI
RINA HILDESHEIM
EUGENE RATZLAFF

Two optical imaging techniques offer unique advantages that may be particularly suitable to explore higher cognitive brain functions in experimental animals and in the human, including the neuronal basis of learning and memory. In this chapter we briefly review our recent work regarding the development and applications of these novel techniques to explore simpler information processing systems, mostly the visual system.

It appears that these two optical imaging techniques begin to shed more light on the organization and function of the cortex, because activity of millions of neurons is imaged simultaneously, rather than activity of a single neuron at a time. The first method uses voltage sensitive dyes to image the flow of neuronal activity from one cortical site to the next in real time. In cortical tissue, optical imaging based on voltage-sensitive dyes reflects mostly the inputs impinging on the fine dendrites of cortical cells, rather than the spike activity in the cell somata. It therefore often yields pictures very different from those obtained with conventional techniques. Indeed, our optical experiments begin to reveal extensive long-range interactions between cortical modules, much larger than those predicted from retinotopic or somatotopic maps, and consistent with the strong effect of long-range horizontal connections and inter- and intracortical connections. The results suggest a much larger degree of distributed processing relative to previous estimates.

We define a neuronal assembly as a large group of cells that are coherently active while performing a given neuronal computation. To test the hypothesis that coherent activity in large cell assemblies plays an important role in encoding and decoding sensory input, we combined real-time optical imaging with single-unit electrical recordings. This combination facilitated, for the first time, the visualization of neuronal assemblies rather than mixed populations of active neurons.

We investigated both ongoing activity (without a stimulus) and activity in response to a visual stimulus. In each case we found oscillatory spatiotemporal patterns at multiple frequencies of 3–25 Hz. Our studies indicated that oscillations exist also without a stimulus. Furthermore, the amplitude of ongoing oscillations was often nearly as large as that of evoked activity. We therefore concluded that oscillations are an intrinsic property of functioning cortex probably also related to thalamic inputs. Furthermore, ongoing electroencephalograph (EEG)-like activity must strongly interact with sensory evoked activity. While the oscillations were detected at several frequencies (mostly around 3, 11, and 25 Hz), surprisingly, the spatial patterns at different temporal frequencies revealed striking frequency-dependent spatial structures of the neuronal activity. Interestingly, we also found that several recurring spatiotemporal patterns were very similar during both ongoing and evoked activity. These results suggest that intrinsic ongoing oscillations in neuronal assemblies play an important role in shaping spatiotemporal patterns evoked by sensory stimuli.

The second method is based on monitoring intrinsic changes in optical properties of active brain tissue. This relatively noninvasive method permitted the high-resolution imaging of elements of the functional architecture of the visual cortex in the living brain of cats and monkeys. In addition, functional mapping was obtained through the intact dura and thinned bone. Furthermore this technique was also successfully applied to the imaging of functional architecture in the awake monkey. Recently attempts are being made to apply it for the mapping of the human brain in patients undergoing neurosurgical procedures.

With high-resolution intrinsic imaging we confirmed the functional architecture of orientation and ocular dominance columns in the visual cortex of cat and monkeys, thus establishing the validity of the technique. Since this imaging technique provides a more complete picture of the functional architecture than all alternative methodologies, we were able to find that in both cat and monkey visual cortex, the orientation domains are arranged in a pinwheel fashion around orientation centers, rather than in elongated parallel bands. We also investigated the interaction between cortical activity evoked by adjacent stimuli. While we found that even in primary visual cortex, processing is rather distributed, we also noted that the long-range interactions are not uniformly or randomly distributed, but they are probably mediated by precise highly specific long-range connections.

ADVANTAGES OF OPTICAL IMAGING

The processing of sensory information, coordination of movement, or other cognitive brain functions are carried out by millions of neurons forming elaborate networks. Individual neurons are synaptically connected to hundreds or thousands of other neurons that shape their response properties. These connections may be local, spanning a short distance, or long range, either within the same cortical area or between different cortical areas. How these neurons and their intricate connections endow the brain with its remarkable performance is one of the central questions in neurobiology.

In the mammalian brain, cells that perform a given function or share common functional properties are often grouped together (Hubel & Wiesel, 1965; Mountcastle, 1957, e.g., the orientation and ocular dominance columns of the visual cortex). Attaining an understanding of the three-dimensional functional organization of such groups of cells is a key step towards revealing the mechanisms of information processing in a given cortical region. Thus, of special importance are experimental methods that allow the visualization of the functional organization of a cortical region, particularly methods that provide high spatial and temporal resolution. Several imaging techniques have been developed that yield information about the spatial distribution of active neurons in the brain, where each technique has advantages as well as significant limitations. For example, while the 2-deoxyglucose method (2-DG) (Sokoloff, 1977) permits postmortem visualization of active brain areas, or even single cells, its time resolution is minutes or hours rather than milliseconds. Furthermore, 2-DG is a one-shot approach: only a single stimulus condition in a single animal can be assayed (although the two-isotope 2-DG method permits the mapping of activity resulting from the two-stimulus condition). Positron-emission tomography (PET) offers three-dimensional localization of active regions in the living, functioning brain, but has low temporal and spatial resolution. Other imaging techniques have also been applied in vivo with success, but they still suffer from either a limited spatial resolution, temporal resolution, or both. These methods include radioactive imaging of changes in blood flow, electroencephalography, magnetoencephalography, nuclear magnetic resonance imaging (MRI), and thermal imaging.

The visualization of cortical functional organization does not require high temporal resolution. In contrast, a complete understanding of the mechanisms of cortical information processing, at the level of neuronal assemblies, demands methods that can monitor the flow of neuronal signals from one group of neurons to the next on a millisecond time basis. To date, single-unit techniques have provided the best tools to study the functional response properties of single cortical neurons. These methods, however, are not optimal for a detailed study of neuronal networks and of neuronal assemblies that are responsible for these response properties. It is apparent, considering the tremendous effort required for the careful analysis of neuronal networks of simple invertebrate ganglia and the slow progress attained with multiple microelectrode recordings, that new approaches must be used. Although multielectrode techniques offer promise, the size and placement of these electrode arrays pose severe problems. In addition, multiple recordings are only practical extracellularly, thus obscuring essential information contained in subthreshold synaptic potentials.

Optical imaging of cortical activity is a particularly attractive technique for providing new insights into the development, organization, and function of the mammalian brain. Among its advantages over other methodologies are: (a) the direct recording of the summed intracellular activity of neuronal populations, including the fine dendritic and axonal processes; (b) the imaging of spatiotemporal patterns of activity of neuronal populations with submillisecond time resolution both in vitro and in the living brain, including the selective visualization of neuronal assemblies; and (c) the possibility of repeated measurements from the same cortical region with different experimental or stimulus conditions over an extended time.

OPTICAL IMAGING OF NEURONAL ACTIVITY WITH DYES

The development of suitable voltage-sensitive dyes has been the key to the successful application of optical recording, because different preparations often require dyes with different properties (Cohen & Lesher, 1986; Grinvald, Frostig, Lieke, & Hildesheim, 1988; Ross & Reichardt, 1979). The preparation under study is first stained by bath application of the dye. The dye molecules bind to the external surface of excitable membranes and act as molecular transducers that transform changes in membrane potential into optical signals (Cohen & Lesher, 1986; Grinvald et al., 1988). The resulting changes in the absorption or the emitted fluorescence occur in microseconds and are linearly correlated with the electrical activity of the stained neurons. These changes are then monitored with light measuring instrumentation. By using an array of photodetectors positioned in the microscope image plane, the activity of many individual targets can be detected simultaneously.

Figure 3.1 depicts the diode array apparatus for optical monitoring of neuronal activity from 100 to 128 sites (Cohen & Lesher, 1986; Grinvald, Cohen, Lesher, & Boyle, 1981; Grinvald et al., 1988). The optical chamber mounted above the exposed cortex is shown in Figure 3.2. Optical imaging with voltage sensitive dyes permits the visualization of cortical activity with a submillisecond time resolution and a spatial resolution of 50–100 μm. The instrumentation to record these fast optical signals with a higher spatial resolution over a large area requires fast detectors with many more pixels

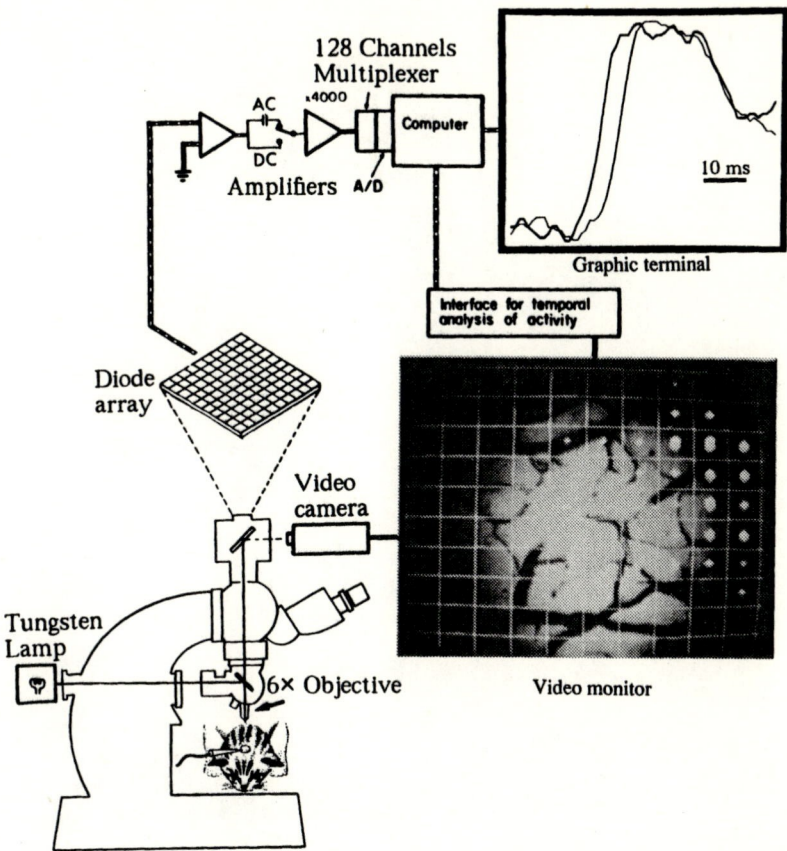

FIGURE 3.1. Optical apparatus for real-time imaging of electrical activity with a photodiode array. The monitor screen shows an image of the exposed cortical area. Time sections (frames) of the optically detected neuronal activity are superimposed on that image and can be visualized in slow motion. The frame shown illustrates the development of seizure activity in cat visual cortex after topical application of bicuculline. Inset: comparison between the time course of interictal event in the anterior (bold trace) and posterior (thin trace) portion of the imaged cortical area (3 × 3 mm). (Modified from Grinvald, Manker, & Segal, 1982)

and is currently expensive. It is important to note that optical signals recorded from the cortex are different from those recorded from single cells or their individual processes and thus should be interpreted with care. In simpler preparations, where single cells are distinctly visible, the optical signal looks just like an intracellular electrical recording. In optical recordings from cortical tissue, however, single cell activity is not resolved and the optical signal represents the sum of intracellular membrane potential changes, in both pre- and postsynaptic neuronal elements, as well as a possible contribution from the depolarization of neighboring glial cells. Since the

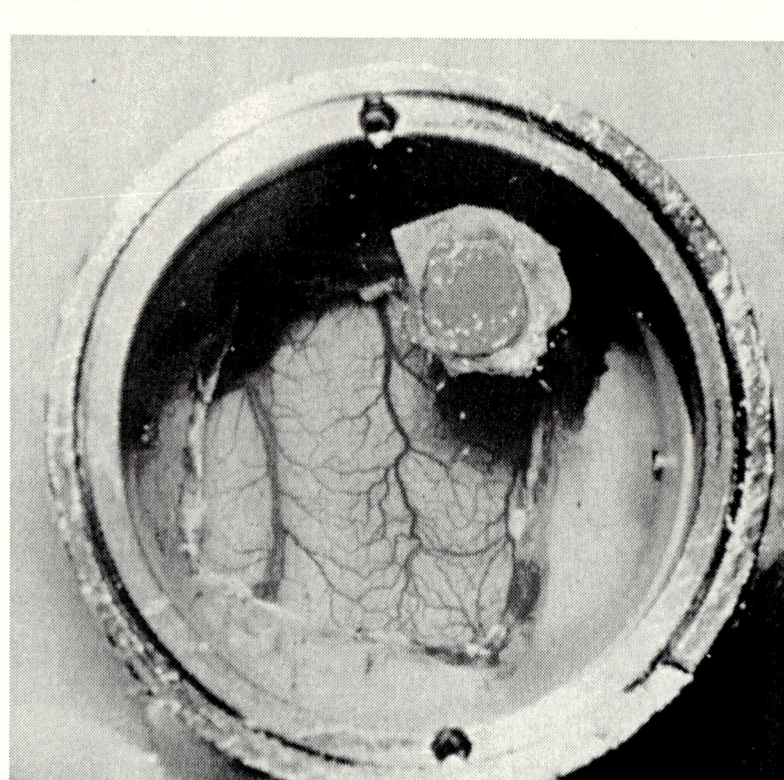

FIGURE 3.2. The mounted sealed optical chamber. A 13mm × 13mm exposed patch of monkey striate cortex as seen through the transparent glass window on top of the sealed chamber mounted on the monkey skull with the aid of dental cement. This oil-filled chamber dramatically reduces pulsation due to respiratory and heartbeat movements. The lunate sulcus is underneath the large vertical blood vessel to the left. The pancake-like structure at the top right is a rubber septum, permitting electrical recordings to be made simultaneously with optical imaging. (Modified from Lieke, Frostig, Ratzlaff, & Grinvald, 1988)

optical signals measure the integral of the membrane potential changes (integrating membrane area as well as time), slow subthreshold synaptic potentials in the extensive dendritic arborization are easily detected by optical recording. Thus optical signals, when properly dissected (Grinvald et al., 1988), can provide information about aspects of neuronal processing that is usually not available from single-unit recordings. Limitations of the use of dyes are briefly discussed in the section on pages 78–79.

OPTICAL IMAGING BASED ON INTRINSIC SIGNALS

A second imaging strategy is based on the slower intrinsic changes in the optical properties of active brain tissue and permits visualization of active cortical regions at high spatial resolution and without some of the problems associated with voltage sensitive dyes. Possible sources for these activity-dependent intrinsic signals include either changes in physical properties of the tissue itself or changes in the absorption, fluorescence or other optical properties of intrinisic molecules having significant absorption or fluorescence. The existence of small intrinsic optical changes associated with metabolic activity in many tissues has been known since the pioneering experiments of Kelin and Millikan on the absorption of cytochromes (Kelin, 1925) and hemoglobin (Millikan, 1937). The first optical recording of neuronal activity was made more than 40 years ago by Hill and Keynes (1949) who detected light scattering changes in active nerves. Changes in absorption and fluorescence of intrinsic chromophores where extensively investigated by Chance and his colleagues (Chance, Cohen, Jobsis, & Schoener, 1962), and Jobsis and his colleagues (Jobsis, Keizer, LaManna, & Rosental, 1977). However, the intrinsic optical signals are usually very small and therefore until recently, the optical measurement of intrinsic signals was not applied to the imaging of spatial patterns of neuronal activity (for reviews see Chance et al., 1962; Cohen, 1973; Jobsis et al., 1977; Mayevsky & Chance, 1982).

The remainder of this chapter will first provide examples of work that illustrate the types of experimental strategies and results that have been obtained from optical imaging with voltage-sensitive dyes in vivo. The next series of examples demonstrates the imaging of the functional organization of the cortex using the intrinsic signals. Finally, the relative merits of each imaging method will be discussed. The technical details of optical imaging techniques cannot be presented here but are nevertheless crucial for optimizing these techniques and evaluating the feasibility of new types of experiments. Additional information is available in earlier reviews (Cohen & Lesher, 1986; De Weer & Salzberg, 1986; Grinvald et al., 1988; Grinvald, 1985; Loew, 1987; Orbach, 1987; Salzberg, 1983; Tasaki & Warashina, 1976; Waggoner, 1979; Waggoner & Grinvald, 1977).

STUDIES OF THE ORGANIZATION AND FUNCTION OF NEURONAL POPULATIONS USING VOLTAGE-SENSITIVE DYES

The detection of spatiotemporal patterns of activity in mammalian brain slices (Grinvald, Manker, & Segal, 1982) suggested that optical imaging techniques could prove to be a useful tool for the study of the mammalian brain in vivo. However, preliminary experiments in rat visual cortex in 1982 revealed several complications for in vivo optical imaging, which included large noise due to respiratory and heartbeat motion. In addition, the relative opacity and the packing density of the cortex limited the penetration of the excitation light and the ability of available dyes to stain deep layers of the cortex. Better dyes (e.g., RH-414) were developed at the Weizmann Institute and proved useful in extensive dye screening experiments on rat cortex. In addition, an effective remedy for the large heartbeat noise was found by synchronozing the data acquisition with the electrocardiogram (ECG) and substracting a no-stimulus trial. These improvements facilitated the in vivo real-time imaging of the whisker barrels in rat somatosensory cortex (Orbach, Cohen & Grinvald, 1985), the retinotopic responses in the frog optic tectum (Grinvald, Anglister, Freeman, Hildesheim, & Manker, 1984), and the experiments on the salamander olfactory bulb (Kauer, 1988; Orbach & Cohen, 1983). More hydrophilic dyes have also been developed that provide better performance in cat and monkey visual cortex (e.g., RH-704 and RH-795; Grinvald, Gilbert, Hildesheim, Lieke, & Wiesel, 1985; Grinvald, Lieke, Frostig, Gilbert, & Wiesel, 1986).

Topographical Mapping of Sensory-Evoked Responses

Among the first applications of in vivo real-time optical imaging using the voltage-sensitive dyes were experiments that visualized the topographic distribution of sensory responses. The frog retinotectal connections are one such system that is topographically organized. The optical signals obtained from the tectum in response to discrete visual stimuli corresponded well to the known retinotopic map of the tectum. However, in addition to a focus of excitation, the spatial distribution of the signals showed smaller, delayed activity (3–20 ms) covering a much larger area than expected from classical single unit mapping (Grinvald et al., 1984). Similar mapping experiments were performed in the rat somatosensory cortex, where the simple organization of the whisker barrels offered a convenient preparation for testing new strategies. When the tip of a whisker was gently moved, optical signals were observed in the corresponding cortical barrel field. However, a discrepancy was noted between the size of an individual barrel recorded optically (1300 μm) and the histologically defined barrel (300–600 μm in layer IV of the cortex). This difference is reasonable considering that most of the optical signal originates from the superficial cortical layers (I–III) and that barrel neurons extend long processes to neighboring barrels (Orbach et al., 1985).

Retinotopic imaging experiments in monkey striate cortex (Lieke, Frostig, Ratzlaff, & Grinvald, 1988; Lieke, Frostig, Hildesheim, & Grinvald, manuscript in preparation) also showed activity over a cortical area much larger than predicted from standard receptive field analysis (Figures 3.3 and 3.4) but consistent with the anatomical finding of long-range horizontal connections in visual cortex (Gilbers & Wiesel, 1983).

These optical imaging experiments on the topographic distribution of sensory processing all demonstrated a central focus of excitation corresponding

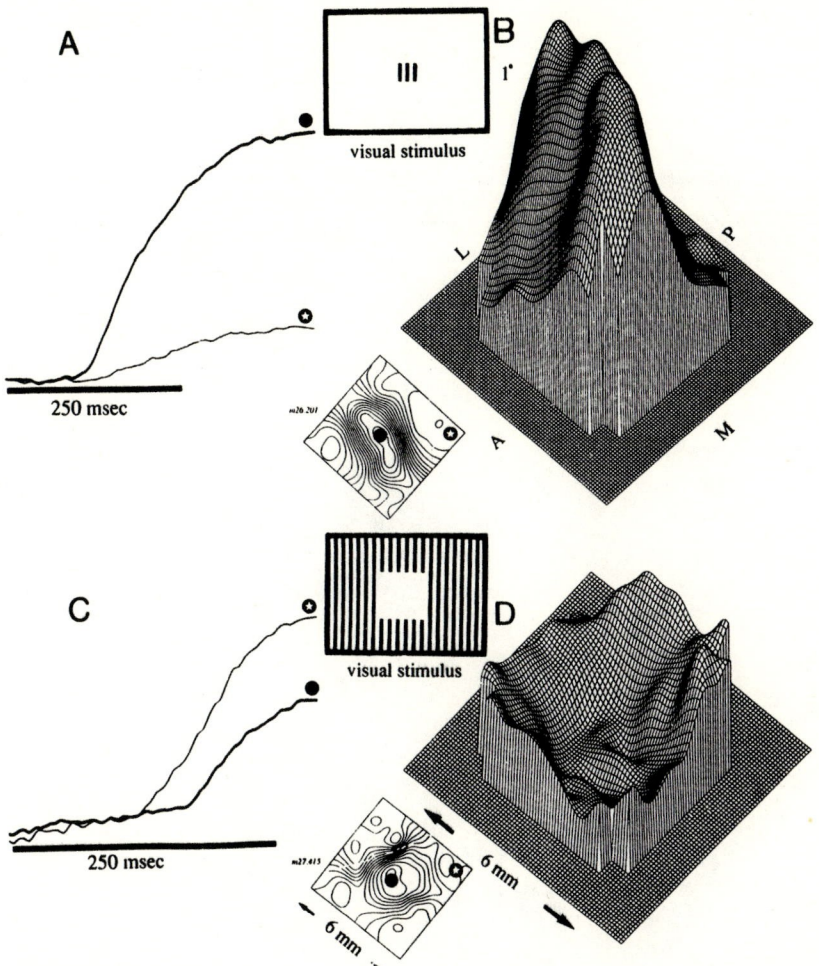

FIGURE 3.3.   The spatiotemporal spread of the optical signal beyond its retinotopic origin. (A) Optical signals from the center (bold) of the photodiode-array and the periphery (star) elicited by a small (0.5°) moving grating ("center-only" stimulus). (C) Optical signals elicited by a large moving grating with a "hole" in the center ("surround" stimulus). The hole was 3° in diameter, so that the cells activated by the stimulus were at least 6 mm away from the center of activity elicited by the "center-only" stimulus. The center of the monitored cortical area was activated 48 ms after the edge, consistent with a conduction velocity of 0.07–0.15 m/s (nearly identical in each direction). (B, D) three-dimensional (3-D) picture of the spatial patterns of the two signals from one frame, corresponding to 350 ms after the stimulus onset. The insets display the stimuli (top) and contour maps of the signals (bottom) at that time. The star and the bold circle on the contour map show the optical recording sites for the traces shown in the left part of this figure. (Modified from Lieke, Frostig, Ratzlaff, & Grinvald, 1988)

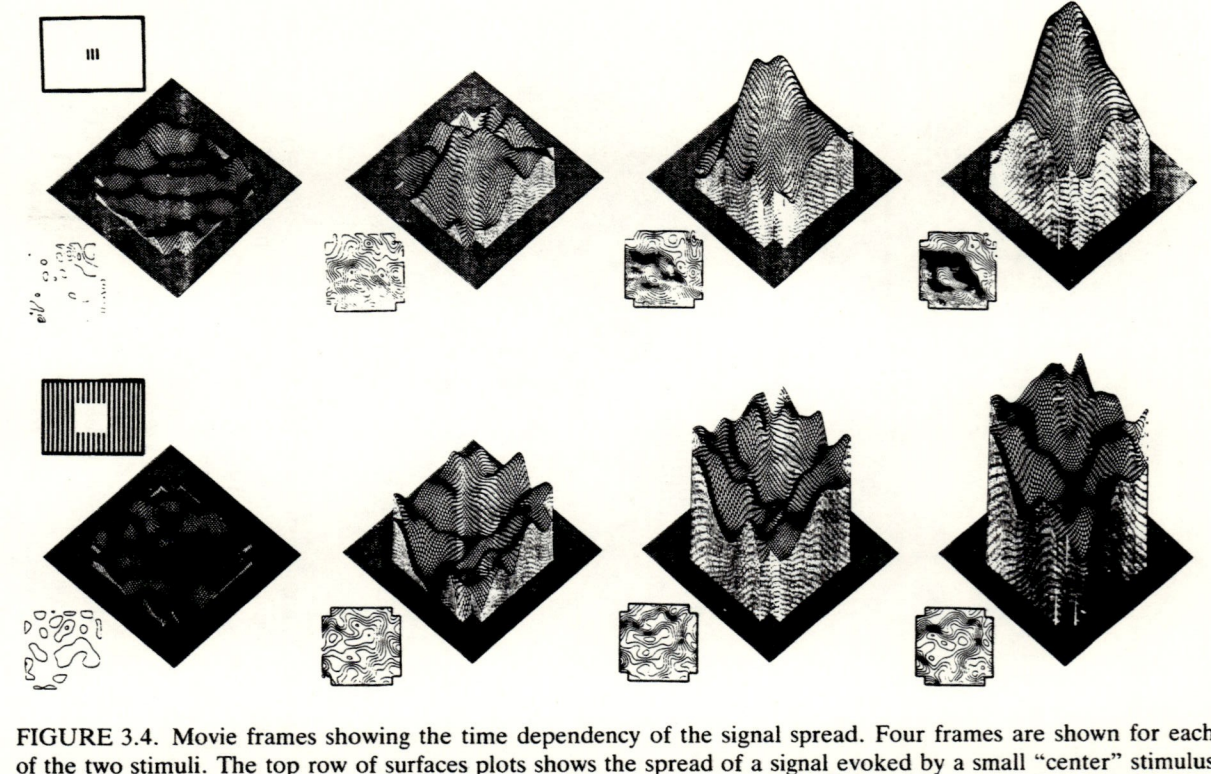

FIGURE 3.4. Movie frames showing the time dependency of the signal spread. Four frames are shown for each of the two stimuli. The top row of surfaces plots shows the spread of a signal evoked by a small "center" stimulus that retinotopically activated only the center portion of the 6 mm x 6 mm imaged area. The bottom row of frames shows the activity resulting from the "surround" stimulus, which spreads from the surround of the imaged cortical area to its center. (Modified from Lieke, Frostig, Ratzlaff, & Grinvald, 1988)

to the applied stimulus, and a surrounding area of cortical activity larger than predicted by single unit recording (Figure 3.3). Possible explanations for the expanded area of optically detected activity include: (a) the optical pick-up of axonal activity in long-range horizontal connections that spread far beyond the directly activated area, (b) a large contribution from subthreshold excitation of postsynaptic dendrites at the regions where most neurons are not actually firing in response to the given stimulus, (c) a smearing of neuronal signals by slower glial signals (Lev-Ram & Grinvald, 1986; Konnerth & Orkand, 1986) that spread across the electrically coupled glial synsitium, and (d) a large contribution from layer I whose functional organization is not well characterized. While additional experiments are required to clarify the origin of the signal spread, we suspect that the predominant dye-signal source is the cortical neuropil.

Surround Inhibition Revealed by Optical Imaging

Although the amplitude of optical signals is linearly related to the membrane potential change, the detection of positive optical signals in a given cortical region does not necessarily imply that inhibition is not present. For example, a strong inhibition may not be accompanied by marked hyperpolarization and furthermore it may be masked by a larger depolarization at other neuronal sites. In addition, action potentials in inhibitory axons may also mask the small hyperpolarization in the postsynaptic cells. Thus, it was important to determine whether the surround activity in the topographic mapping experiments discussed above had any inhibitory component. The surround signals were tested with more revealing stimulus paradigms and with the use of pharmacological agents that block inhibitory synapses.

On presenting a second spot of light that was delayed and displaced (26°) from a preceding spot of light, optical imaging of the frog tectum showed that the activity evoked by a second flash was inhibited by the first flash (by 60%). When a single light spot was used, application of the amino butiric acid (GABA) blocker bicuculline led to a 10-fold increase in the region of excitation, consistent with the notion that inhibitory interactions shape the excitation area. It was also noted that the conduction velocity of the bicuculline-induced excitation spread from the excitation focus was faster along the rostral–caudal axis than the medial–lateral axis, implying a possible asymmetry in the lateral surround connections (Grinvald et al., 1984).

In the studies of the rat somatosensory cortex, stimulation of two whiskers that were relatively far apart (e.g., A1 and D4) evoked responses in two circumscribed areas. A large overlap in the response area was obtained when neighbouring whiskers were stimulated, but the responses could be resolved if they were activated with some delay (< 20 ms). Activity evoked by one whisker often inhibited the activity evoked by another whisker when the interstimulus interval was 20–120 ms, indicating a surround inhibition extending 2–4 mm in the rat somatosensory cortex (Orbach et al., 1985).

Inhibitory center-surround interactions were also revealed by optical

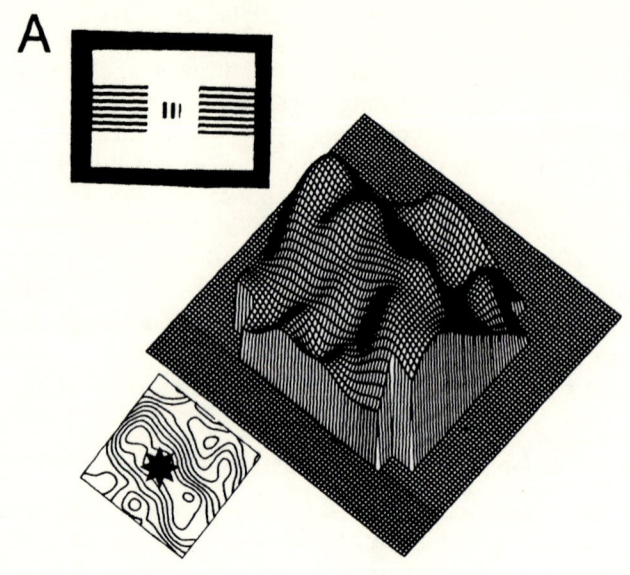

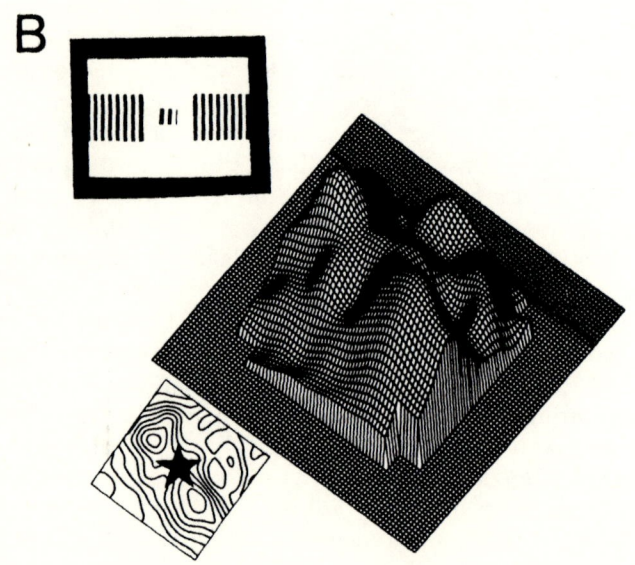

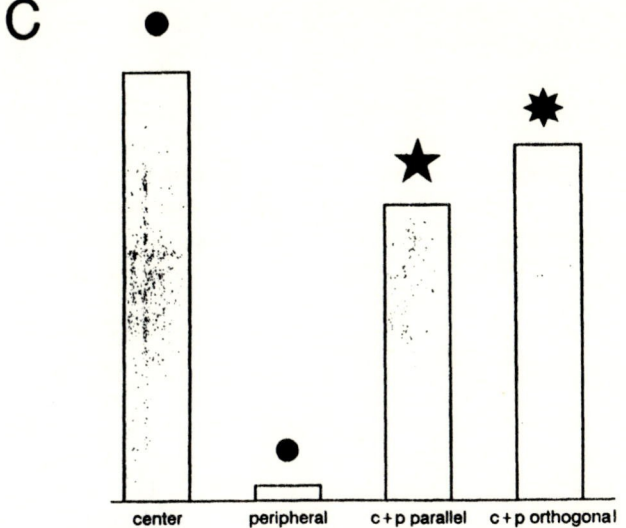

FIGURE 3.5. Center surround inhibitory interactions. 3-D pictures of the optical signals 350 ms after stimulus onset for each of the two different stimuli, both containing center and surround stimuli, but the surround orientation varying in the two experiments. When the surround orientation matches that of the center, there is greater inhibition of activity evoked by the center stimulus (B) than when the surround orientation is orthogonal to that of the center (A). The histogram (C) compares the amplitude of the responses at a position in the center of the exposed cortex. The responses to the center + surround stimuli are smaller than that to the "center only" condition. Note that inhibition was larger when the two stimuli had the same orientation. This histogram summarizes the results for the center detector of the array only. From each experiment, which lasts about 30 min, 30,000 histograms were obtained; such results are best shown in a movie. (Modified from Lieke, Frostig, Ratzlaff, & Grinvald, 1988)

imaging of a 6 mm × 6 mm region of monkey striate cortex. Four interlaced visual patterns of moving gratings were presented, stimulating either a small center field or the surround alone, or both together, with center and surround gratings having either matching or orthogonal orientation. The small (0.5–2°) center gratings alone yielded activity in the surrounding cortical area that was delayed relative to the center and had a smaller amplitude. An annular surround grating, instead, produced activity in the center that was smaller and delayed relative to the directly evoked activity in the periphery. Presenting the center and surround gratings together yielded center and surround cortical signals that were both smaller (~50%) and slower relative to signals from either grating alone, and were smallest when the center and surround gratings had the same orientation. These results (Figure 3.5) indicate that the interactions between center and surround have a strong inhibitory component (Lieke et al., 1988; Lieke et al., in preparation). However these experiments do not rule out the existence of lateral excitation between specific cortical sites as has been shown by other physiological and anatomical studies (e.g., Nelson & Frost, 1985; Ts'o, Gilbert & Wiesel, 1986). This apparent discrepancy illustrates that different techniques may reveal different aspects of cortical interactions. The use of different stimulus conditions may help to clarify this issue. Local injections of drugs that block either excitation or inhibition may also improve such studies as well as nail down the contribution of intracortical connections to the observed interactions (additional information will be described by Lieke et al., manuscript in preparation).

Selective Visualization of Neuronal Assemblies in Cat Visual Cortex

A neuronal assembly may be defined as a group of neurons that cooperate to perform a specific computation required for a specific task. The activity of cells in an assembly is timelocked (coherent). However, the cells that comprise an assembly may be spatially intermixed with cells in other neuronal assemblies that are performing different computational tasks. Therefore, techniques that can visualize only the average population activity in a given cortical region may not be adequate to study neuronal assemblies. What is needed, therefore, is a method to discriminate between the operations of several colocalized assemblies. We found a promising approach to solve this problem by using the timelocked activity of the assembly neurons, to visualize selectively only that assembly. The firing of a single neuron that is a member of the assembly served as the source of synchronization for this selective visualization.

Thus we combined single-unit recordings and subsequent spike-triggered averaging of the optical recordings to study the spatiotemporal organization of neuronal assemblies. With sufficient averaging, the activity of neuronal assemblies not containing the reference neuron was averaged out, enabling the selective visualization of the reference neuron's assembly. The visual cortex (area 18) of an anesthetized cat was stained with the dye RH-795, and either ongoing (spontaneous) or evoked activity were recorded continuously for 70 s. We recorded simultaneously optical signals from 124 sites, together with electrical recordings of local field potentials (LFP) and single-unit recordings (1–3 isolated units recorded with the same electrode). The spike-triggered averaging analysis confirmed that single units had a tendency to fire at the positive peak of the local EEG (e.g., Frost, 1986). In addition, the averaged optical signal at the electrode site had a peak that also coincided with the occurrence of a peak in the local field potential (LFP). This result indicates that many neurons next to the electrode site had coherent firing patterns (Arieli, Frostig, Lieke, Hildesheim, & Grinvald, 1987; Arieli & Grinvald, 1988; Arieli, Shoham, Hildesheim, & Grinvald, 1990). However, surprisingly the optically observed signals were very heterogeneous in the field of view of 2 mm × 2 mm of cortex (Figure 3.6), indicating that optical recording provides a better spatial resolution relative

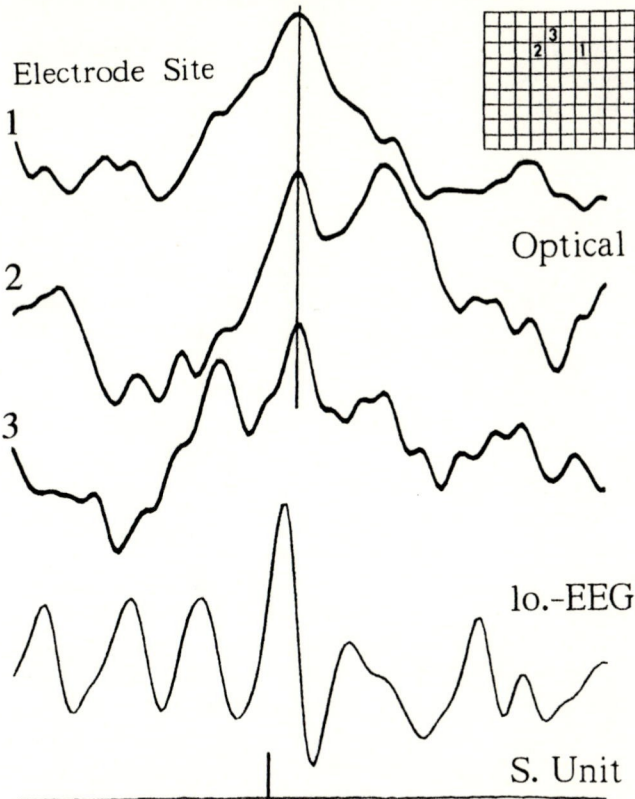

FIGURE 3.6.   Optical imaging of coherent activity in cat cortex. Single-unit activity and local field potentials were recorded via an electrode placed at site 1 (see inset). Spike-triggered averaging of spontaneous activity was performed using 78 spikes. The bottom trace shows the time of the trigger event. The averaged local field potential (lo.-EEG) indicated that this unit had a large probability of firing 7 ms prior to a large peak in the local field potential. Three optical traces from different cortical loci are shown at the top of the figure. The uppermost trace shows the large coincident activity that was optically recorded from the same site as the single-unit and lo.-EEG recordings. The two remaining optical traces show activity with peaks of preceding, coincident, and delayed firing relative to the firing of this reference cell, recorded from a neighboring cortical loci, 200–400 μm apart. (Modified from Arieli & Grinvald, 1988)

to field potential recordings. (At present, we recorded from 128 cortical sites simultaneously. We are currently testing a new design of a fast imaging system with which the number of sites will increase to 4096, allowing better spatial resolution and/or investigation of larger cortical area.)

Oscillations of Ongoing and Evoked Activity in Neuronal Assemblies

We investigated spatiotemporal patterns of neuronal assemblies either during ongoing activity (without a stimulus) or in response to a visual stimulus. In each case we found oscillatory spatiotemporal patterns at multiple frequencies of 3–25 Hz. Our studies indicated that oscillations also exist without a stimulus. Furthermore, often the amplitude of ongoing oscillations was nearly as large as that of evoked activity. Thus we concluded that at least some oscillations are an intrinsic property of functioning cortex rather than related to the stimulus (probably also mediated by thalamic inputs). Because of the large amplitude of the ongoing oscillations in dendritic membrane potential we conclude that ongoing EEG-like activity must strongly interact with sensory evoked activity. While the oscillations were detected at several frequencies (mostly around 3, 11, and 25 Hz), surprisingly the spatial patterns at different temporal frequencies revealed striking frequency-dependent spatial structures of the neuronal activity. Interestingly, we also found that several recurring spatiotemporal patterns were very similar during both ongoing and evoked activity (e.g., frame 1, 4, or 7 in Figure 3.7; here activity was evoked with a drifting grating of a given orientation). The spatial patterns of both ongoing and evoked oscillations did not always show a clear correspondence to the orientation columns. These results suggest that intrinsic ongoing oscillations in neuronal assemblies play an important role in shaping spatiotemporal patterns evoked by sensory stimuli. We are currently testing a working hypothesis that an important strategy used by the brain to perceive sensory input is to detect how ongoing spatiotemporal patterns (perhaps a representation of a given percept) are modulated by the evoked activity (rather than detecting the evoked activity itself, which is somehow coded and perceived.

OPTICAL IMAGING OF ACTIVITY USING INTRINSIC SIGNALS

Although considerable progress has been made in the study of various neuronal systems with extrinsic signals originating from voltage-sensitive dyes, the use of intrinsic signals has several distinct advantages. Since no dye is required, the measurement of intrinsic signals is less invasive, can be made for an indefinite period of time and is free of several technical complications associated with the use of dyes (e.g., photodynamic damage, bleaching, and pharmacological side-effects; see Grinvald et al., 1988). The existence of changes in optical properties associated with metabolic or electrical activity in many tissues, including brain, has been known for many years. The primary disadvantage of the use of slow intrinsic signals is the lack of the millisecond time resolution achievable with the use of voltage-sensitive dyes. However, the solution of many neurophysiological questions does not demand high temporal resolution and these questions can be pursued with the imaging of intrinsic signals. Blasdel and Salama (1986) stated that intrinsic signals were not useful for mapping the functional

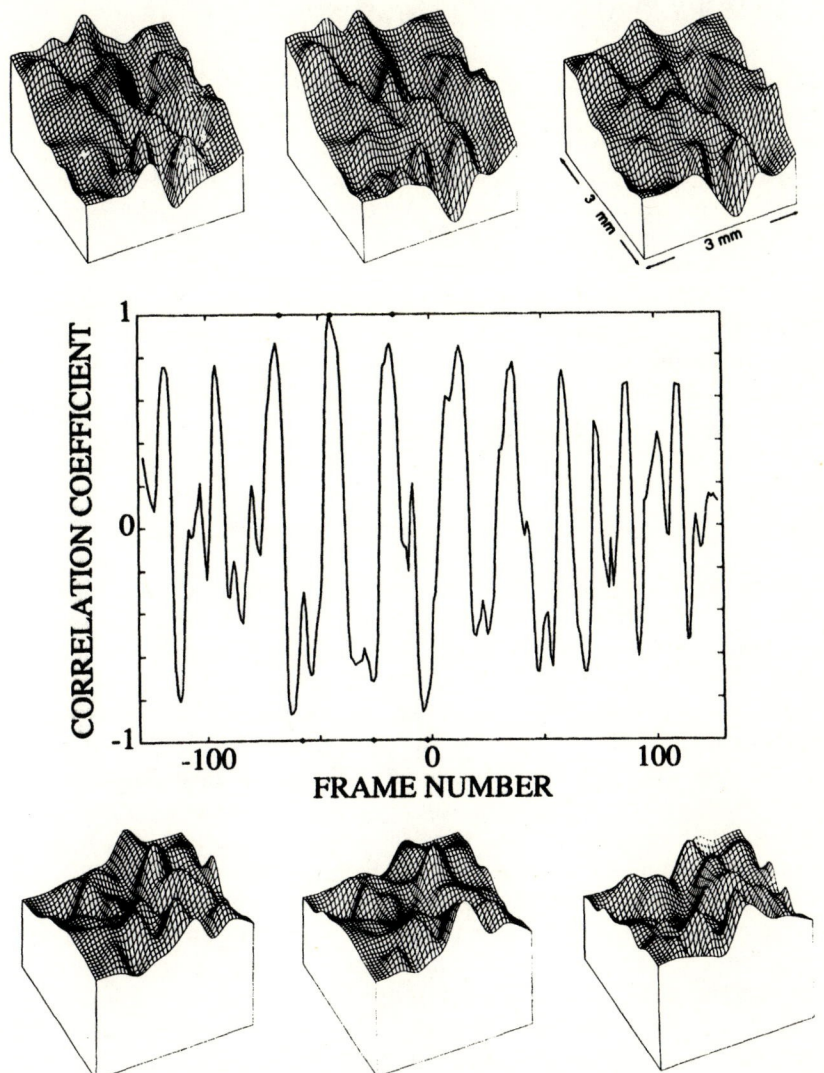

FIGURE 3.7. Real-time optical imaging of brain wave oscillations. The 3-D figures show the amplitudes of the dendritic depolarization in a 3 mm × 3 mm region of cat visual cortex. To visualize the dynamic behavior of a given neuronal assembly, from the vangage point of a single neuron, 250 action potentials of a single reference cell were used for spike-triggered averaging of the corresponding optical data. The result is a movie, in which each frame depicts the patern of cortical activity at a certain distance in time (in 3 ms intervals) from the occurrence of the spike. A dominant feature of the movie is an oscillation between two recurring patterns, having nearly opposite polarity (top and bottom images), at a frequency of 11 Hz (which is characteristic for the alpha rhythm). The top three 3-D figures show three separate occurrences of one of these patterns, and the bottom three figures show three separate occurrences of the other. The graph shows the similarity (as measured by the correlation coefficient) between each frame of the movie and a representative frame of the first pattern. The oscillation between the two patterns is clearly seen in the graph. (From Shoham, Arieli, & Grinvald, unpublished results)

organization of monkey striate cortex. In contrast we have found that the intrinsic signals have proved to be well suited for mapping in the monkey striate cortex, as well as in other preparations. For example, in rat somatosensory cortex, the map of a whisker barrel was observed using a photodetector array to monitor the decreases in reflected light intensity that correspond to cortical activation from a single whisker stimulation. An identical map was later obtained with the voltage-sensitive dye signals, confirming the map obtained with the slow intrinsic signal. Thus, although the intrinsic signal was at least two orders of magnitude slower than dye signals, neverthelesss it was useful for mapping known functional components of the cortex (Frostig, Lieke, T'so, & Grinvald, 1990; Grinvald et al., 1986; Ts'o, Frostig, Lieke, & Grinvald, 1990).

Determining the Source and Nature of the Intrinsic Signals

Experiments on the nature of the intrinsic signals useful for functional imaging have revealed at least three major components. One component of the intrinsic signal originates from changes in blood volume that are probably due to local capillary recruitment or dilatation of venules or increased concentration of blood cells in the capillaries in an activated area. These changes appear as an increase in hemoglobin absorption. A detailed characterization of the time course and saturation of this component of the optical signal may help to improve the performance of PET imaging, presumably based on a similar mechanism (Fox et al., 1986), or MRI functional imaging based on similar mechanisms (Moonen, Van-Ziji, Frank, Le-Biham, & Beckjer, 1990). The second component of the intrinsic signal originates from activity-dependent changes in the oxygen saturation level of hemoglobin resulting either from metabolic demands or changes in blood flow affecting the relative amounts of hemoglobin and oxyhemoglobin. This component probably dominates the signal at 600–650 nm. The third component to the intrinsic signal originates from the light-scattering changes that accompany cortical activation (originating from ion and water movement, expansion and contraction of extracellular spaces, capillary expansion, and neurotransmitter release; see review by Cohen, 1973). The microcirculation-related components of the intrinsic signal dominate at the short wavelength range, while the light-scattering component probably becomes more significant in the near infrared region above 800 nm. These three components have different time courses. Nevertheless, maps of functional organization obtained in both regions of the spectrum were identical either in area 17 of the macaque monkey or area 18 of the cat. Thus each component can be used for functional mapping.

These experiments have also shown that the proper control of depth of field is an important factor in optical imaging of cortical activity. Since near infrared light penetrates the cortex deeper than visible light, it should facilitate the imaging of deeper cortical structures. In addition, the confocal microscope or other optical sectioning techniques may improve the depth resolution. Thus infrared imaging may prove more useful for three-dimensional confocal imaging than visible light (additional information is described in Frostig et al., 1990).

Mapping of Functional Organization in Cat Cortex using a Diode Array

A prominent feature of the visual cortex is the arrangement of cells with similar orientation forming preference into columns or bands (Hubel & Wiesel, 1962). The optical imaging of the orientation columns with the aid of intrinsic signals required the separate collection of signals for each of two presented moving gratings of orthogonal orientation, and subsequent analytical comparison. A moving grating stimulus evoked intrinsic signals over a large region of cortex. However, at each cortical site the signals evoked by the optimal stimulus orientation were somewhat larger than the signals evoked by the orthogonal orientation (Figure 3.8A). The spatial distribution of the regions preferring the horizontal stimulus is shown as a two-state coded map in Figure 3.8B, and the raw data in Figure 3.8C. To obtain a more precise map of the orientation columns the results from vertical and horizontal stimulus presentations were combined with results from presentations at orientations of 45° and 135°. The resulting map is shown in Figure 3.8D. The orientation map was confirmed, using a double-blind procedure, by making a series of 42 electrode penetrations (Grinvald et al., 1986). Also in cat visual cortex, when a similar strategy to visualize the orientation columns was used with the fast voltage-sensitive-dye signals, the resulting orientation maps were identical to those obtained with the aid of the slow intrinsic signals (Lieke et al., manuscript in preparation).

Increasing the Spatial Resolution: Imaging with a CCD Camera

Blasdel and Salama (1986), Gross, Loew, & Webb (1985), Gross & Webb (1984), and Kauer (1988) have demonstrated, in imaging experiments with dyes, that standard video techniques may be used economically to permit higher spatial resolution optical imaging at the expense of time resolution. However, in addition to the poorer time resolution relative to photodiode arrays, a standard video camera also has a poor signal-to-noise ratio, usually no better than 100:1. A slowscan CCD camera (Figure 3.9) offered improved signal-to-noise ratios (e.g., 1400:1), while retaining the advantages of higher spatial resolution and moderate cost and complexity. We have employed such a CCD camera for the optical imaging at high spatial resolution of the intrinsic signals, where the millisecond time resolution of photodiode arrays is not required (additional information is described in Ts'o, Frostig, Lieke, & Grinvald, 1988; Ts'o et al., 1990).

Imaging Functional Architecture of Primate Visual Areas 17 and 18

CCD imaging of the intrinsic signals has enabled us to image directly several of the features of the functional organization of monkey visual areas 17 and

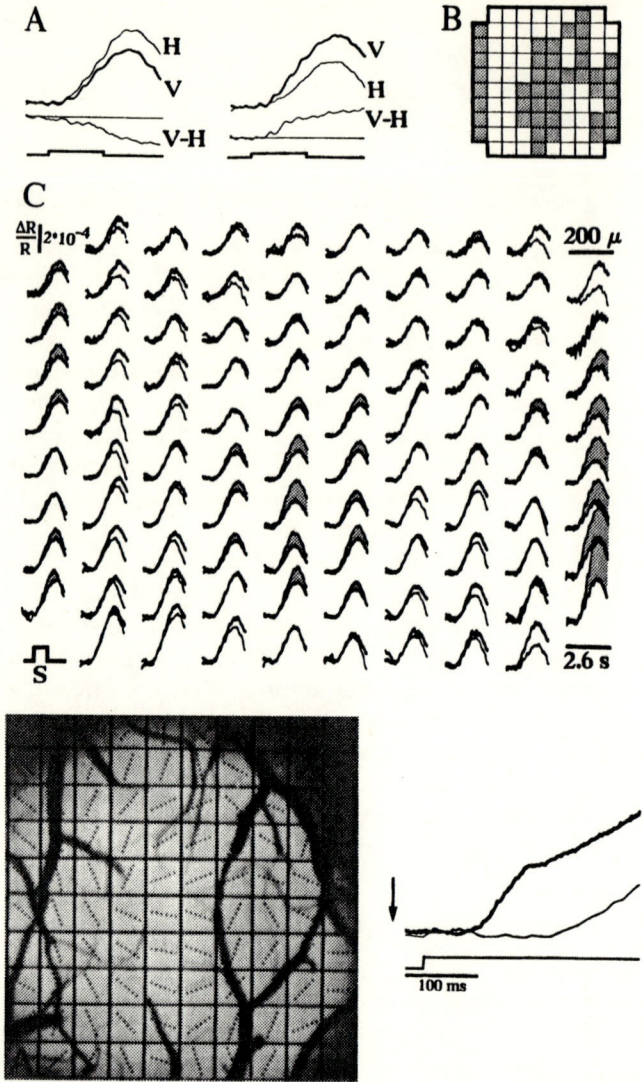

FIGURE 3.8. "Intrinsic imaging" of the orientation columns in cat visual cortex using a diode array. (A) In one cortical site (left traces), single units preferentially responded to gratings with horizontal orientation. The corresponding intrinsic signal (thin trace) was larger than that obtained in response to the vertical stimulus (thick trace). In a second cortical site (right), single units had preferential responses to the gratings with vertical orientation and the opposite result was obtained. Stimulus duration: 1 s(B) The spatial distribution of cortical regions preferring the horizontal stimulus (shaded area). (C) The raw data showing the distribution of the signals in 96 cortical sites for horizontal (thin traces) and vertical stimuli (thick traces). Bottom left: Superimposed on the picture of the exposed cortex are dashed bars showing the optimal stimulus orientation for each cortical site as determined by the angle resulting from vectorial addition of each the responses using four different stimulus orientations. Bottom right: A comparison between the time course of the voltage-sensitive-dye signal (thick trace) and an intrinsic signal (thin trace). (Modified from Grinvald, Lieke, Frostig, Gilbert, & Wiesel, 1986)

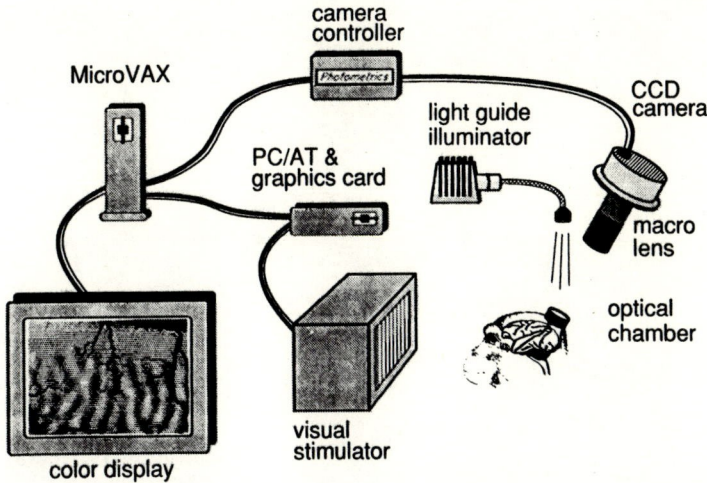

FIGURE 3.9.   Setup for high-resolution imaging based on intrinsic signals. A sealed chamber having a transparent glass window is implanted over an exposed cortical region. The monkey is visually stimulated with gratings moving on a CRT screen (visual stimulator). The brain is illuminated with light of 630 nm wavelength. A CCD camera is used to take high-resolution images from the exposed brain region. These pictures carrying information about neural activity are digitized and sent to a computer where they are analytically compared. The resulting activity maps are then displayed on an RGB video display monitor. (From Ts'o, Frostig, Lieke, & Grinvald, 1988)

18 in vivo (Ts'o et al., 1990). In each type of experiment, a separate set of frames from the CCD camera is collected for each of several opponent visual stimulus conditions (e.g., vertical vs. horizontal orientation, left eye vs. right eye) and the resulting sets of frames are compared analytically. This procedure has revealed the orientation columns in areas 17 and 18. Similar success has been obtained in imaging the ocular dominance columns (Figure 3.10) and the blobs (color selective, mostly monocular neurons) in area 17. In area 18 we were able to image the thick and thin stripes usually only visualized with postmortem cytochrome oxidase histology (for more details see Ts'o et al., 1990).

One problem in earlier optical imaging experiments has been the large blood vessels artifacts apparent in the functional maps (e.g., Figure 3.10) and thus often hampering subtle interpretations of the observed results. Recently, we found that by using a shallow depth of field lens (Ratzlaff & Grinvald, 1991) and by focusing 300 μm below the cortical surface (Malonek, Shoham, Ratzlaff, & Grinvald, 1990), the vasculature artifacts virtually disappear. An example for the improvement we achieved is illustrated in Figure 3.11.

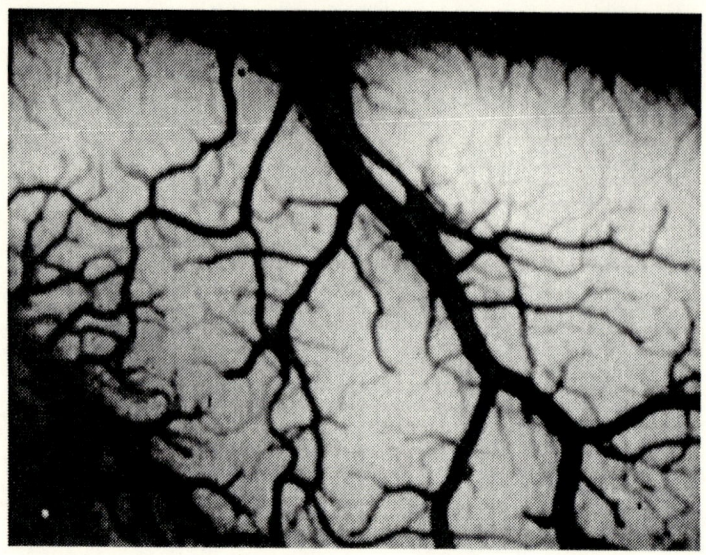

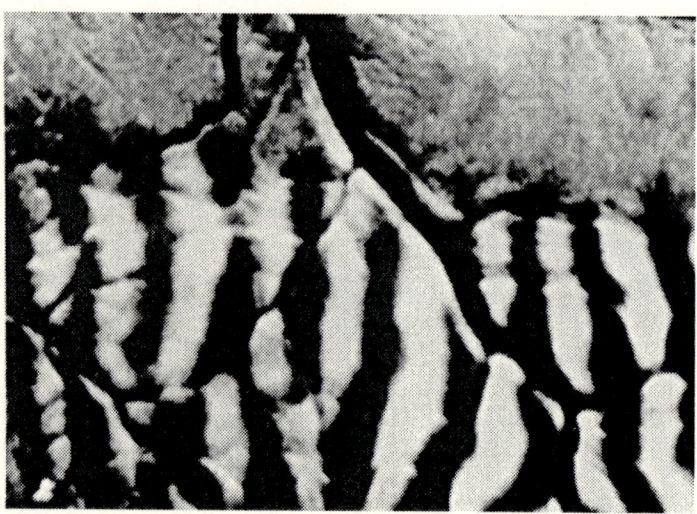

FIGURE 3.10. Ocular dominance columns in monkey striate cortex. The frames show an area of 9 mm × 6 mm. Top: CCD picture of the exposed cortex showing the vasculature of the imaged brain area. The 17/18 border was about 2 mm from the top. Bottom: The ocular dominance columns, obtained by presenting moving gratings of various orientations to the right and left eye individually, averaging the optically recorded frames for each eye, and subtracting the two sets of frames. Note the lack of columnar organization in area 18. This map was confirmed by comparison with cytochrome oxidase histology. (From Ts'o, Frostig, Lieke, & Grinvald, unpublished)

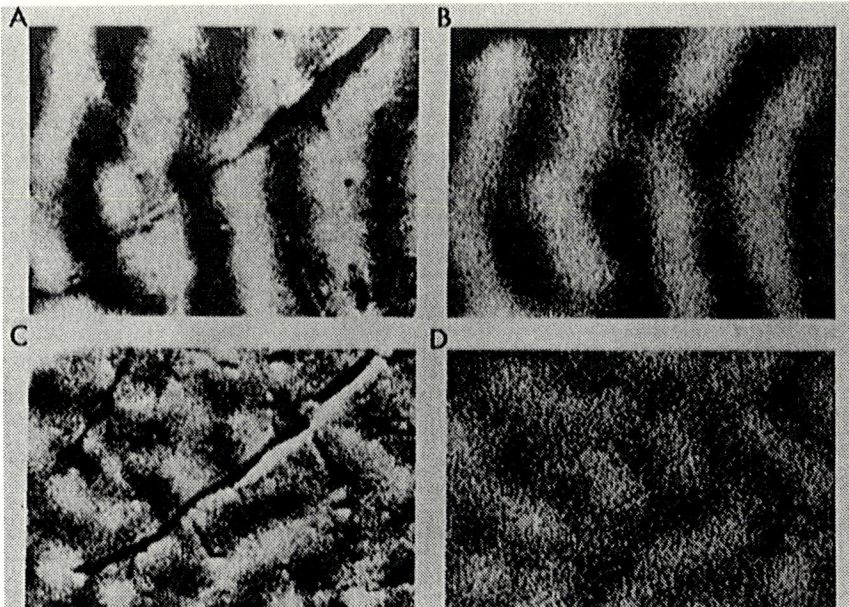

FIGURE 3.11. Elimination of the vascular artifact with the tandem macroscope. Images of ocular dominance and orientation columns from monkey striate cortex. The left images containing vascular artifact were recorded from the surface of cortex. The right images shows ocular dominance (top) and orientation maps recorded from 300 μm below the surface where the vascular artifact virtually disappeared. (Modified from Malonek, Shoham, Ratzlaff, & Grinvald, 1990, and Ratzlaff & Grinvald, 1991)

Studies of Cortical Interactions Between Adjacent Visual Stimuli

We also continued the exploration of interaction between cortical responses evoked by two adjacent stimuli (along the line pursued with voltage sensitive dyes; Lieke et al., 1988). We again used center and surround bars or gratings of either matched or orthogonal orientations. In all cases studied, an addition of a surround stimulus had an inhibitory effect on responses evoked by the center stimulus alone. Interestingly, we observed with intrinsic imaging that a small stimulus evoked clear responses also outside the retinotopically activated cortical region. Unlike the results observed with voltage-sensitive dyes, the high resolution of the intrinsic imaging technique facilitated the visualization of patchy activation of the cortex rather than a uniform activation observed with the low-resolution diode array measurements. We could then test if the patches of laterally activated cortical regions are best tuned for a matched orientation of the adjacent stimulus or not. By comparing the orientation maps obtained with a large stimulus to the patches, we concluded that the laterally activated area mostly contained neurons that are best tuned for the same orientation rather than the orthogonal one. This result supports the notion (Gilbert & Weisel, 1983; Ts'o et al., 1986) that long-range horizontal connections have a strong excitatory effect at least at some of their first monosynaptic connections (Grinvald & Gilbert, unpublished results).

Imaging of the Functional Architecture of Cat Areas 17 and 18

In another set of experiments we took advantage of the fact that one can obtain multiple maps from one cortical region to examine whether "directionality columns" exist in cat visual cortex. Such columns have been reported in cat area 17 (Payne, Berman, & Murphy, 1980; Tolhurst, Dean, & Thompson, 1981) and area 18 (Swindale, Matsubara, & Cynader, 1987), but these results remain controversial. By directly comparing high-resolution activity maps obtained with a grating moving in one direction with those obtained with the same grating moving in the opposite direction, we could determine whether cells are sorted into columns according to preferred direction of motion. In experiments on 13 hemispheres such comparisons invariably revealed that the same cortical area is activated by the two stimuli (implying that there are no directionality columns).

Besides our interest in directionality columns, we also wanted to clarify the detailed organization of orientation preference. There has been a great deal of debate about how orientation columns are spatially organized in cat visual cortex. While they were originally described as "parallel" bands (Hubel, Wiesel, & Stryker, 1977, 1978; Löwel, Freeman, & Singer, 1987), some authors later claimed that the data of Hubel and Weisel could just as well be explained by a radial organization (Braitenberg & Braitenberg, 1980; Seelen, 1970; Swindale, 1982). Since all the previously performed experiments lacked either sufficient resolution (electrode recordings) or the benefit of having data from many different orientations (2-DG experiments; Sokoloff, 1977) we used our new method to take a closer look at the organization of orientation preference in cat area 18.

The unique advantage of optical imaging of intrinsic signals is that one can obtain many maps from one patch of cortex, repeatedly. Two 2-DG-like orientation columns maps obtained by optical imaging are shown in Figure 3.12. To derive a much more complete picture of the overall organization of orientation preference, we made use of this advantage of optical imaging and combined the data from eight different orientations. Data of this kind are presented in Figure 3.13, which then provide the complete orientation map, which appears patchy as opposed to banded as one might have expected from 2-DG studies and from Figure 3.2 of the present work.

A prominent feature of these maps is that orientation preferences seem to be organized around points that we termed "orientation centers." Areas with different preferred orientation are ordered in a pinwheel-like fashion around the orientation centers. We found, on average, 1.2 of these pinwheels per mm². In Figure 3.14 four typical pinwheels are shown at a higher

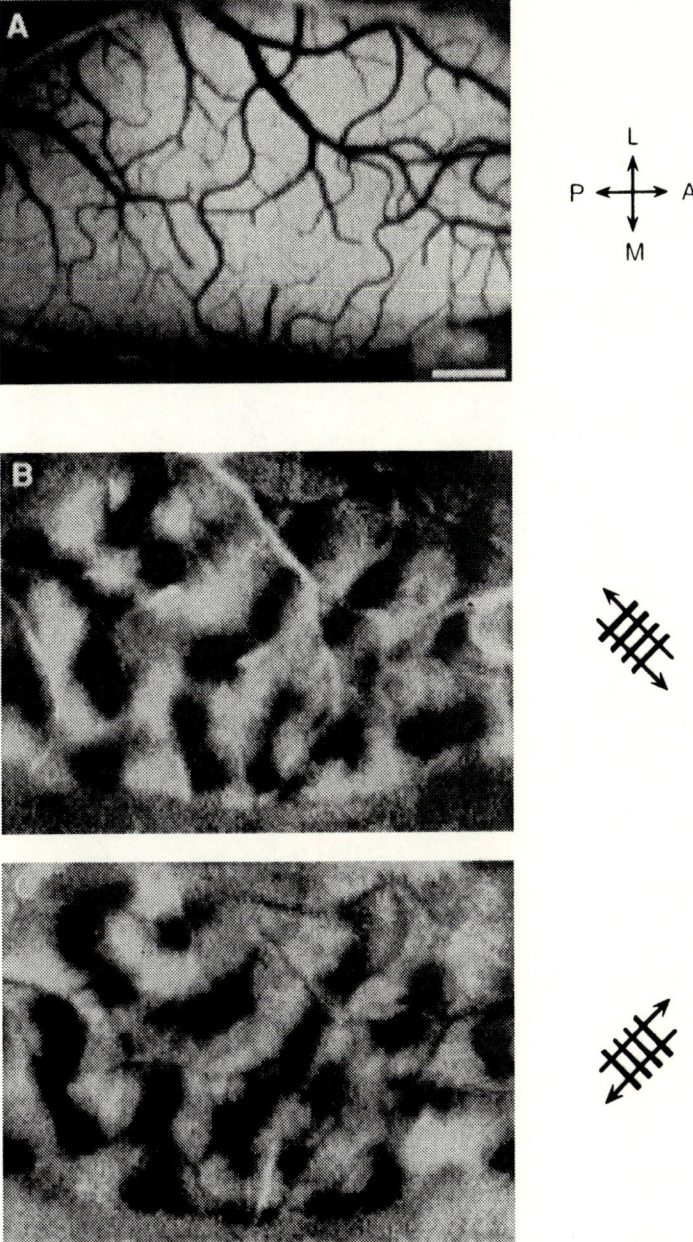

FIGURE 3.12. Imaging of orientation columns from a 6 mm × 9 mm piece of cat visual cortex (area 18). (A) Image of the cortical surface showing the blood vessels pattern of the recorded region. (B) Activity map recorded with an oblique moving grating as stimulus. Dark areas in the map denote areas of stronger absorption and hence higher activity. (C) Activity map obtained with the orthogonal stimulus. By comparing part B to part C of this figure one can see how regions strongly activated by one stimulus are only weakly activated by the orthogonal one. Scale bar is 1 mm. (Modified from Bonhoeffer & Grinvald, 1991)

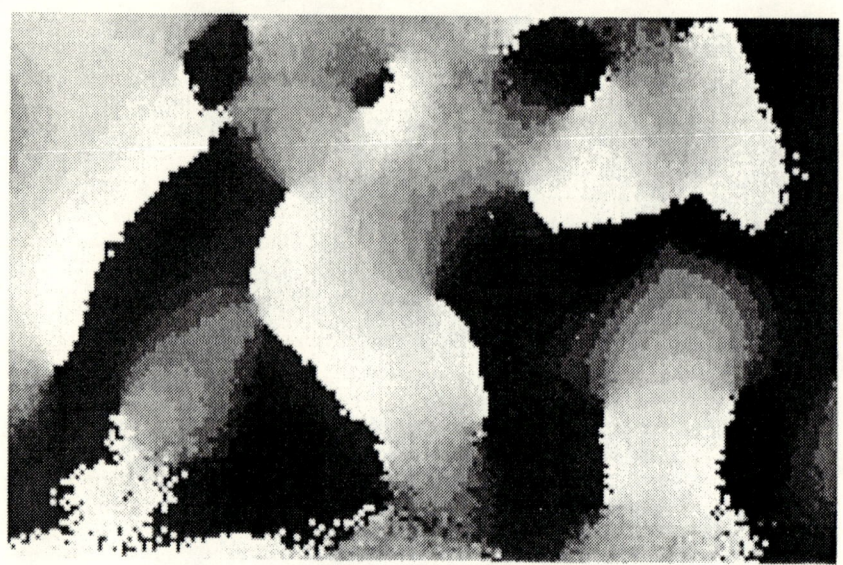

FIGURE 3.13.   High-resolution CCD imaging of orientation columns in cat areas 17 and 18. Map of orientation columns obtained by vectorial addition, performed in a similar manner to that discussed in Figure 3.8. The optimal orientation tuning is coded as different gray levels where white corresponds to the vertical orientation. (Modified from Bonhoeffer & Grinvald, 1991)

magnification. Different orientation domains encircle the orientation centers. Every orientation appears once around an orientation center (additional information is described in Bonhoeffer & Grinvald, 1991).

The Functional Organization of Orientation Tuning in Monkey Striate Cortex

The above result obtained for the organization of orientation domains in cat cortex, together with the technical improvements in our mapping approach, prompted us to re-examine the organization of orientation tuning in the monkey. This topic was first investigated with optical imaging by Blasdel and Salama (1986) and Ts'o et al. (1988, 1990). In recent experiments we found that: (a) in the monkey also, pinwheels and orientation centers are the predominant features of the organization of orientation tuning (Figure 3.15); (b) the pinwheels' centers lie along the center of ocular dominance columns; and (c) the iso-orientation domains cross the boundary of ocular dominance columns at right angles. More details will be described by Bartfeld et al. (manuscript in preparation).

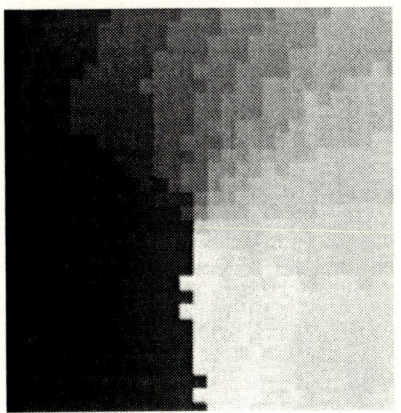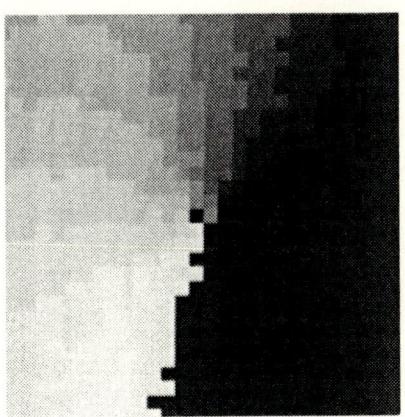
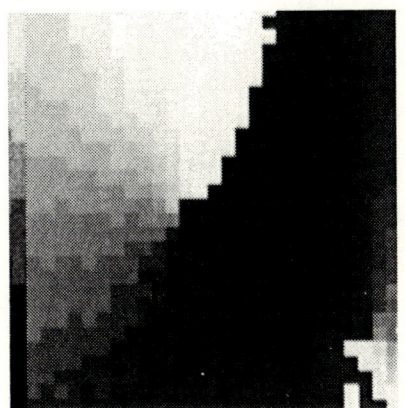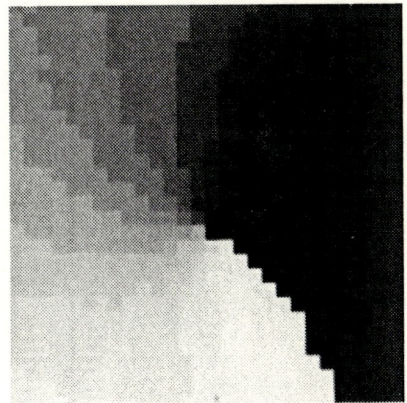

FIGURE 3.14.   Close-up pictures of four "pinwheels" in cat cortex. Two "clockwise" and two "counterclockwise" pinwheels are shown. The optimal orientation tuning is coded as different gray levels where white corresponds to the vertical orientation. Scale bar is 300 mm. (Modified from Bonhoeffer & Grinvald, 1991)

Infrared Imaging of Functional Organization Through the Intact Dura

A particularly promising result of studies of the nature and wavelength-dependence of the intrinsic signals, as discussed above, is the ability optically to image cortical activity through the normally opaque dura covering the brain. Because of its penetrating power and lack of absorption by hemoglobin, near infrared light has allowed us to image, using the CCD camera, the orientation columns of the cat through the intact dura (Frostig et al., 1990). The maps obtained proved to be identical to maps obtained after the dura

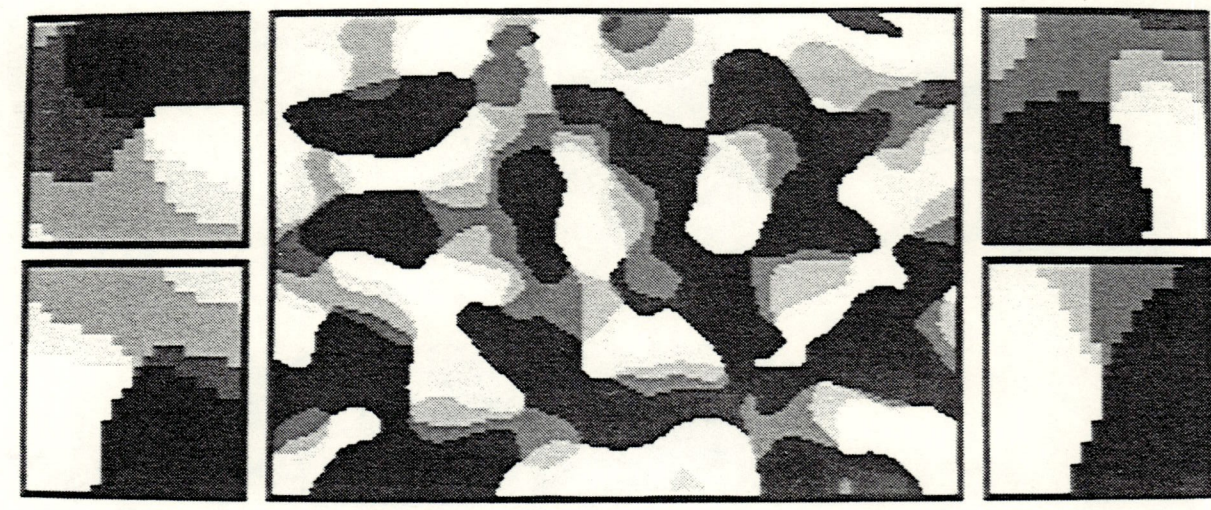

FIGURE 3.15. "Pinwheels" around orientation centers in monkey striate cortex. The organization of orientation tuning, "clockwise," and "counterclockwise" pinwheels is shown. The optimal orientation tuning is coded as different gray levels where white corresponds to the vertical orientation. Scale bar is 300 mm. (From Bartfeld, Malonek, Ts'o, & Grinvald, unpublished)

was removed (Figure 3.16). This ability to image the functional organization of cortex through the dura will be advantageous for long-term studies in various animal preparations.

High-Resolution Optical Imaging of Cortical Activity in the Awake Monkey

Experiments in awake monkeys offer many advantages for the study of higher cognitive functions. We established that imaging based on intrinsic signals is suitable for exploring the brain of behaving primates. We designed a chronic sealed chamber, which was mounted on the monkey skull over the primary visual cortex and facilitated imaging experiments through a glass window, 3 months after implantation. We found that restriction of head position by a solid head holder was sufficient to eliminate movement noise in the awake animal. Furthermore, functional maps could be obtained without the noise reduction procedure previously obtained by synchronizing the animal respiration to the ECG and triggering the data acquisition on the ECG. We found that the wavelength dependency and time course of the intrinsic signals were similar in anesthetized and awake monkeys, indicating that the signal sources were similar. High-resolution imaging of the ocular dominance and the blobs was achieved simply by taking pictures of the exposed cortex while the awake monkey was viewing video movies (Figure 3.17). We speculate, therefore, that future studies using this technique should be quite productive in exploring functional organization related to higher brain functions of the primate. It should also provide a diagnostic tool for delineating the functional cortical borders and for assessing proper cognitive functions of human patients in certain neurosurgical situations. (Additional information is described in Grinvald, Siegel, Bartfeld, & Frostig, in press).

COMPARISON OF OPTICAL IMAGING WITH AND WITHOUT VOLTAGE-SENSITIVE DYES

The principal advantage of cortical mapping using voltage-sensitive dyes is its millisecond time resolution, in contrast to the time resolution of the intrinsic signals, which is of the order of seconds. This time resolution is important for a detailed understanding of flow of information and its processing at different cortical sites. For example, in rat somatosensory cortex the area of the observed barrel 15 ms after stimulation of a single whisker is about half the size of that seen after 20 ms (Orbach et al., 1985). The trade-off for this good time resolution is a loss in spatial resolution. It is much easier to obtain a good signal-to-noise ratio if signals are slow (a measurement of small slow signals with a risetime of a second rather than a millisecond may yield a 33-fold improvement in the signal-to-noise ratio, owing to the square-root relationship between the number of samples and signal-to-noise ratio). The spatial resolution of optical imaging of the cortex

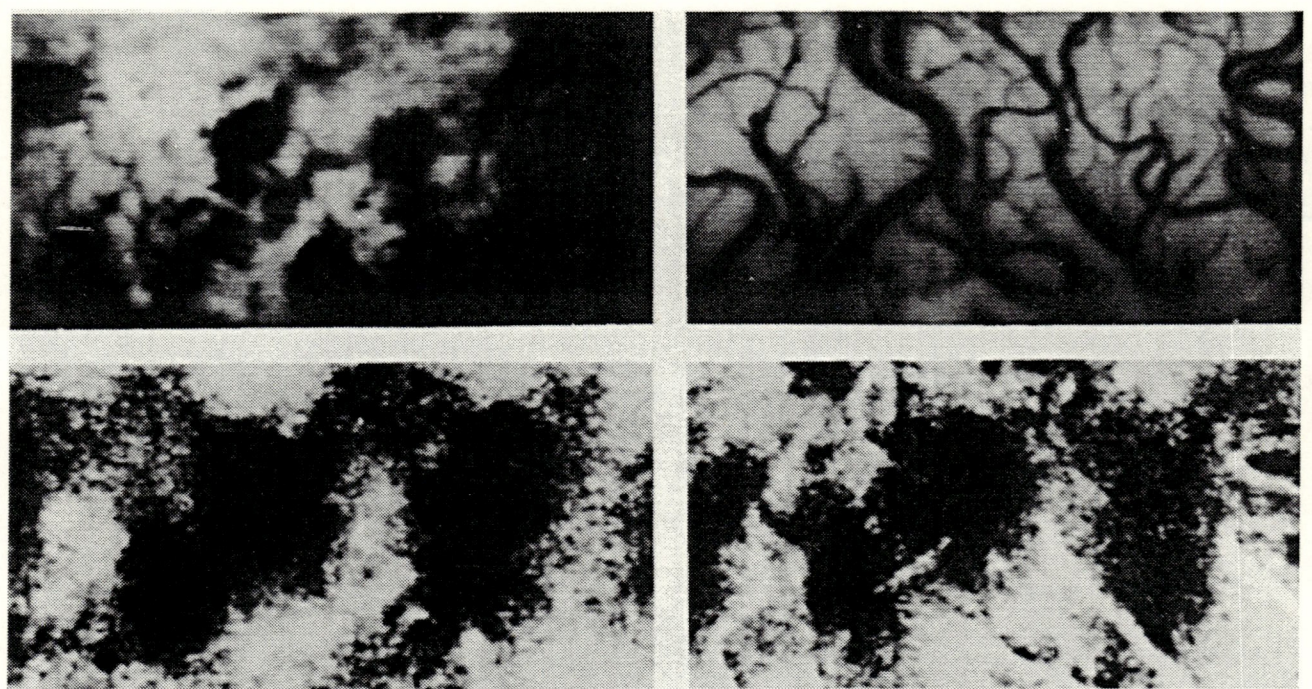

FIGURE 3.16. Infrared imaging of the orientation columns through the intact dura in cat cortex. Left top: CCD picture of the intact dura illuminated with green light. Left bottom: Imaging of the orientation columns through the intact dura using infrared light illumination (810 nm). Right top: Underlying visual cortex under green light after the dura was removed. Right bottom: The same orientation map was obtained after the dura was removed. (Modified from Frostig, Lieke, T'so, & Grinvald, 1990)

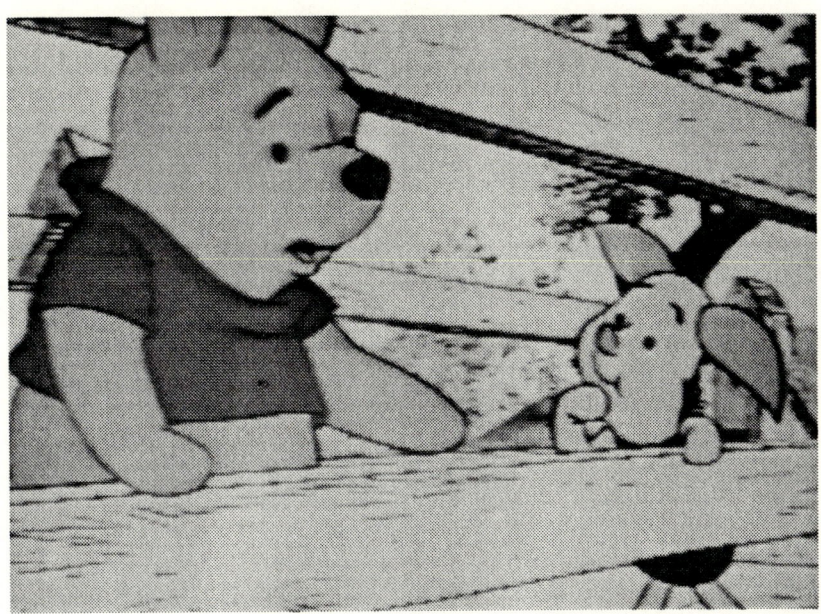

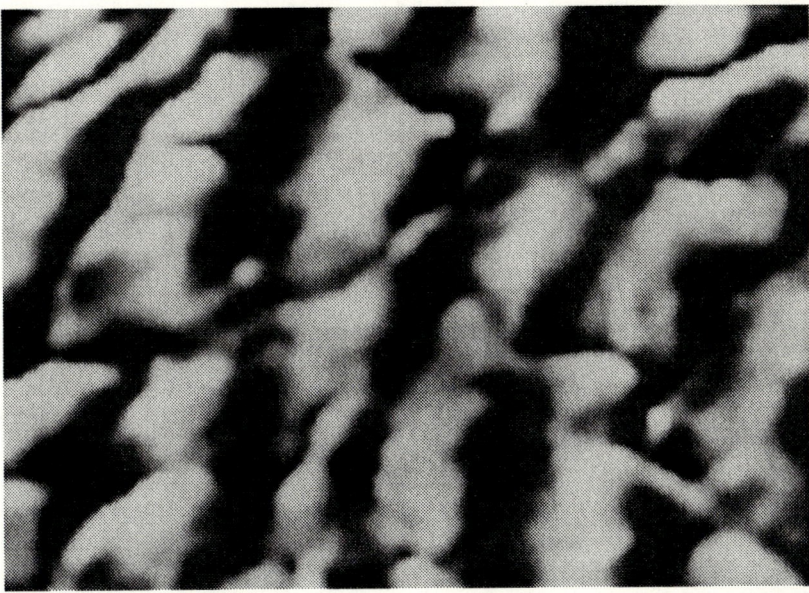

FIGURE 3.17. Optical imaging in an awake primate cortex. A map of the ocular dominance columns was obtained when the awake primate was watching a VCR movie with the right and left eye alternating. The top shows a frame from the movie used for visual stimulation. (From Grinvald, Bartfeld, Siegel, & Frostig, in press)

with the current voltage-sensitive dyes is not ultimately limited by the number of pixels of the photodetector or the available computer and instrumentation capabilities, but instead is limited by obtainable signal size and concomitant photodynamic damage. Without a significant improvement in the quality of the present dyes, we estimated that a resolution of 50–100 µm is close to the usable limit. In addition to the photodynamic damage associated with the dyes on prolonged or intense illumination, the use of dyes has other difficulties such as bleaching, limited depth of penetration into the cortex, and possible pharmacological side-effects. While the extent of pharmacological side-effects on cortical function has not been carefully evaluated, it was evident that stained cortical cells still maintained their intricate response properties.

Since imaging of intrinsic optical signals makes no use of dyes, the technique does not suffer from the possibility of photodynamic damage and can currently achieve higher spatial resolution. The slow time course of the intrinsic signals further facilitates the use of more economical cameras (e.g., video, CCDs) to achieve the higher spatial resolution. Optical imaging with intrinsic signals is less invasive and can therefore be repeated over a long period of time. As we have shown, the imaging of the intrinsic signals may also be performed through the intact dura in the cat, a very promising prospect that would probably be quite difficult to implement with dyes. These advantages suggest that optical imaging with intrinsic signals may also have clinical applications.

Although the spatial resolution of optical imaging techniques clearly depends on the number of pixels as well as the resolution of the optics used, these elements may not always present the limiting factors in real experiments. There are sources of biological noise and artifacts that can be averaged out through multiple trials (e.g., heartbeat and respiratory movements). A more subtle source of artifacts may be the accumulation of systematic errors that are not effectively reduced by averaging (e.g., activity-related signals originating from the microvasculature that spread far beyond the activated cortical region; slow changes in oxygenation level of the microvasculature). Therefore, signal-to-noise ratio and reproducibility of the optical images of activity are necessary, but not sufficient, criteria. Controls for a lack of systematic distortions as well as a satisfactory signal-to-noise ratio may obviate such pitfalls.

Recently we found that by imaging below the cortical surface with a shallow depth of field, blood vessel artifacts can be nearly eliminated (Malonek et al., 1990). Imaging with a shallow depth of field was achieved with the aid of a home-made tandem lens macroscope having a relatively large numerical aperture at low magnification (Ratzlaff & Grinvald, 1991). Using this macroscope we also evaluated the prospects of three-dimensional optical imaging from different cortical layers. We found that imaging from layers at a depth of at least 700 µm was feasible with an illumination wavelength of 750 mm. However, we estimate that a three- to five-fold improvement of the signal-to-noise ratio in the imaging experiments is still required to achieve three-dimensional optical sectioning capability in the intact brain (Malonek et al., 1990).

CONCLUSIONS

There is a growing perception (or perhaps a naive hope) in brain research that understanding of the complex function of the brain will require simultaneous recordings from many sites. This idea has led to a considerable effort in the design of arrays of extracellular electrodes. We feel that optical imaging and multielectrode techniques are very complementary and that a combination of the two techniques will form the basis of particularly promising studies in the investigation of cortical function. Several technical difficulties still complicate the use of optical imaging for the study of neuronal activity. Possible solutions to many of the technical problems have been outlined in previous reviews. Further technical improvements are likely to shorten the duration of the measurements dramatically (for example, in one case we were able to image the monkey ocular dominance columns in 13 seconds). Once achieved, this should facilitate the use of this technique, in certain neurosurgical situations, and is also likely to improve our understanding of higher brain functions in the human.

Novel findings and concepts have already begun to emerge from studies using optical imaging. Our studies indirectly suggest that it would also be worthwhile to use optical imaging for the study of cortical development, plasticity or recovery of function after injury or lesions, or as a result of transplantation. Similarly, the use of awake primates and optical imaging can contribute both to the study of the function of primary sensory area, as well as greatly assisting in in vivo studies of higher brain functions such as attention, motivation, memory and learning, etc. The spatial resolution of functional maps achieved in our experiment using the awake primate indicate that this approach will be particularly useful as a clinical mapping tool in certain neurosurgical situations on human patients. It should provide precise maps of invisible functional borders on the cortical surface of human patients of regions that need to be spared during microsurgical removal of tumors, or during neurosurgical treatment of vascular and neoplasmic lesions. Optical imaging may also be useful in the intraoperative evaluation of epileptic foci.

Looking beyond these technical issues, however, it is clear that new methods to handle and analyze the large amount of data need to be developed, as well as new conceptual frameworks that will aid in the design of experimental paradigms and the interpretation of the resulting data. These needs call for additional multidisciplinary efforts to advance our understanding of the development and organization of the central nervous system and the fascinating strategies it uses for performing higher cognitive functions.

Acknowledgements: We thank Dr L. Katz for his useful comments on an earlier version of the manuscript, and Drs Frostig, Lieke, Ts'o, Gilbert and Wiesel for the performance of several joint experiments. Our work was supported by IBM and grants from the Riklis Foundation, the NIH (NS 14716), the U.S.-Israel Binational Science Foundation, the U.S. Air Force, Klingenstein Foundation, and Dupont.

REFERENCES

Arieli, A., Frostig, R. D., Hildesheim, R., & Grinvald, A. (1987). Cortical correlates of the EEG revealed by real-time optical imaging of neuronal activity in cat cortex. *Society of Neuroscience Abstracts, 13*, 52.

Arieli, A., & Grinvald, A. (1988). Dynamic patterns of on-going coherent activity in neuronal assemblies revealed by real-time optical imaging in cat cortex. *Society of Neuroscience Abstracts, 14*, 1122 (manuscript in preparation).

Arieli, A., Shoham, D., Hildesheim, R., & Grinvald, A. (1990). Oscillations of on-going and evoked activity in neuronal assemblies revealed by real time optical imaging in cat visual cortex. *Society of Neuroscience Abstracts, 16*, 1220.

Blasdel, G. G., & Salama, G. (1986). Voltage-sensitive dyes reveal a modular organization in monkey striate cortex. *Nature, 321*, 579–585.

Bonhoeffer, T., & Grinvald, A. (1990). Orientation preference are arranged in pinwheel-like structure in area 18 in cat visual cortex. *Society of Neuroscience Abstracts, 16*, 292.

Bonhoeffer, T., & Grinvald, A. (1991). Functional architecture of orientation tuning in areas 17 and 18 in cat visual cortex. *Nature, 353*, 429–431.

Braitenberg, V., & Braitenberg, C. (1980). Geometry of orientation columns in the visual cortex. *Biological Cybernetics, 33*, 179–186.

Chance, B., Cohen, P., Jobsis, F., & Schoener, B. (1962). Intracellular oxidation-reduction states in vivo. *Science, 137*, 499–508.

Cohen, L. B. (1973). Changes in neuron structure during action potential propagation and synaptic transmission. *Physiological Review, 53*, 373–418.

Cohen, L. B., & Lesher, S. (1986). Optical monitoring of membrane potential: methods of multisite optical measurement. *Society of General Physiologists Series, Vol. 40*, 71–99. New York: Wiley.

De Weer, P., & Salzberg, B. M. (Eds.) 1986. Optical methods in cell physiology. *Society of General Physiologists Series, Vol. 40*. New York: Wiley.

Egger, M. D., & Petran, M. (1967). New reflected light microscope for viewing unstained brain and ganglion cells. *Science, 157*, 305–307.

Fox, P. T., Mintun, M. A., Raichle, M. E., Miezin, F. M., Allman, J. M., & van Essen, D. C. (1986). Mapping human visual cortex with positron emission tomography. *Nature, 323*, 806–809.

Frost, J. D. (1986). EEG-intracellular potential relationships in isolated cerebral cortex. *Electroencephalography and Clinical Neurophysiology, 24*, 434–443.

Frostig, R. D., Lieke, E. E., Ts'o, D. Y., & Grinvald, A. (1988). Infra-red imaging of functional organization of visual cortex through the intact dura using a CCD camera. *Society of Neuroscience Abstracts, 14*, 897.

Frostig, R. D., Lieke, E. E., Ts'o, D. Y., & Grinvald, A. (1990). Cortical functional architecture and local coupling between neuronal activity and the microcirculation revealed by in vivo high-resolution optical imaging of intrinsic signals. *Proceedings of the National Academy of Sciences, U.S.A., 87*, 6082–6086.

Gilbert, C. D. & Wiesel, T. N. (1983). Clustered intrinsic connections in cat visual cortex. *Journal of Neuroscience, 3*, 1116–1133.

Grinvald, A. (1984). Real time optical imaging of neuronal activity: from single growth cones to the intact brain. *Trends in Neuroscience, 7*, 143–150.

Grinvald, A. (1985). Real-time optical mapping of neuronal activity: from single growth cones to the intact mammalian brain. *Annual Review of Neuroscience, 8*, 263–305.

Grinvald, A., Anglister, L., Freeman, J. A., Hildesheim, R., & Manker, A. (1984). Real time optical imaging of naturally evoked electrical activity in the intact frog brain. *Nature, 308*, 848–850.

Grinvald, A., Cohen, L. B., Lesher, S., & Boyle, M. B. (1981). Simultaneous optical monitoring of activity of many neurons in invertebrate ganglia, using a 124 element 'Photodiode' array. *Journal of Neurophysiology, 45*, 829–840.

Grinvald, A., Frostig, R. D., Lieke, E., & Hildesheim, R. (1988). Optical imaging of neuronal activity. *Physiological Review, 68*, 1285–1366.

Grinvald, A., Frostig, R. D., Siegal, R. M., & Barfeld, E. (1991). High resolution optical imaging of functional architecture in the awake monkey. *Proceedings of the National Academy of Sciences*, U.S.A.

Grinvald, A., Gilbert, C. D., Hildesheim, R., Lieke, E., & Wiesel, T. N. (1985). Real time optical mapping of neuronal activity in the mammalian visual cortex in vitro and in vivo. *Society of Neuroscience Abstracts, 11*, 8.

Grinvald, A., Hildesheim, R., Farber, I. C., & Anglister, L. (1982). Improved fluorescent probes for the measurement of rapid changes in membrane potential. *Biophysical Journal, 39*, 301–308.

Grinvald, A., Lieke, E., Frostig, R. D., Gilbert, C. D. & Wiesel, T. N. (1986). Functional architecture of cortex revealed by optical imaging of intrinsic signals. *Nature, 324*, 361–364.

Grinvald, A., Manker, A., & Segal, M. (1982). Visualization of the spread of electrical activity in rat hippocampal slices by voltage sensitive optical probes. *Journal of Physiology, 333*, 269–291.

Grinvald, A., & Segal, M. (1983). Optical monitoring of electrical activity; detection of spatiotemporal patterns of activity in hippocampal slices by voltage-sensitive probes. In R. Dingledine (Ed.), *Brain Slices* (pp. 227–261). New York: Plenum Press.

Gross, D., Loew, L. M., & Webb, W. W. (1985). Spatially resolved optical measurement of membrane potential distribution in single cells. *Biophysical Journal, 47*, 270a.

Gross, D., & Webb, W. W. (1984). Molecular counting in small clusters of LDL on cell surfaces by fluorescence intensity quantization. *Biophysical Journal, 45*, 269a.

Hill, D. K., & Keynes, R. D. (1949). Opacity changes in stimulated nerve. *Journal of Physiology, 108*, 278–281.

Hubel, D. H., & Wiesel, T. N. (1962). Receptive fields, binocular interactions and functional architecture in the cat's visual cortex. *Journal of Physiology, 160*, 106–154.

Hubel, D. H., & Wiesel, T. N. (1965). Receptive fields and functional architecture in two non-striate visual areas (18 and 19) of the cat. *Journal of Neurophysiology, 28*, 229–289.

Hubel, D. H., Wiesel, T. N., & Stryker, M. P. (1977). Orientation columns in macaque monkey visual cortex demonstrated by the 2-deoxyglucose autoradiographic technique. *Nature, 269*, 328–330.

Hubel, D. H., Wiesel, T. N., & Stryker, M. P. (1978). Anatomical demonstration of orientation columns in macaque monkey. *Journal of Comparative Neurology, 177*, 361–380.

Jobsis, F. F., Keizer, J. H., LaManna, J. C., & Rosental, M. J. (1977). Reflectance spectrophotometry of cytochrome aa_3 in vivo. *Journal of Applied Physiology, 43*, 858–872.

Kauer, J. S. (1988). Real-time imaging of evoked activity in local circuits of the salamander olfactory bulb. *Nature, 331*, 166–168.

Kelin, D. (1925). On cytochrome, a respiratory pigment, common to animals, yeast, and higher plants. *Proceedings of the Royal Society of London, 98*, 312–339.

Konnerth, A., & Orkand, R. K. (1986). Voltage sensitive dyes measure potential changes in axons and glia of frog optic nerve. *Neuroscience Letters, 66*, 49–54.

Lev-Ram, V., & Grinvald, A. (1986). Ca^{2+} and K^+ dependent communication between central nervous system myelinated axons and oligodendrocytes revealed by voltage-sensitive dyes. *Proceedings of the National Academy of Sciences, U.S.A., 83*, 6651–6655.

Lieke, E. E., Frostig, R. D., Hildesheim, R., & Grinvald, A. (1992). Center/surround inhibitory interaction in macaque V1 revealed by real time optical imaging (manuscript in preparation).

Lieke, E. E., Frostig, R. D., Ratzlaff, E. H., & Grinvald, A. (1988). Center/surround inhibitory interaction in macaque V1 revealed by real time optical imaging. *Society of Neuroscience Abstracts, 14*, 1122.

Loew, L. M. (1987). *Optical measurement of electrical activity.* Boca Raton: CRC Press.

Löwel, S., Freeman, B., & Singer, W. (1987). Topographic organization of the orientation column system in large flat-mounts of the cat visual cortex: a 2-deoxyglucose study. *Journal of Comparative Neurology, 255*, 401–415.

Malonek, D., Shoham, D., Ratzlaff, E., & Grinvald, A. (1990). In vivo three dimensional optical imaging of functional architecture in primate visual cortex. *Society of Neuroscience Abstracts, 16*, 292.

Mayevsky, A., & Chance, B. (1982). Intracellular oxidation-reduction state measured in situ by a multichannel fiber-optic surface flurometer. *Science, 217*, 537–540.

Milikan, G. A. (1937). Experiments on muscle hemoglobin in vivo; the instantaneous measurement of muscle metabolism. *Proceedings of the Royal Society of London, 123*, 218–241.

Moonen, C. T., Van-Ziji, C. M., Frank, J. A., Le-Biham, D., & Baeckjer, E. D. (1990). Functional magnetic resonance imaging in medicine and physiology. *Science, 250*, 53–61.

Mountcastle, V. B. (1957). Modality and topographic properties of single neurons of cat's somatic sensory cortex. *Journal of Neurophysiology, 20*, 408–434.

Nelson, J. I., & Frost, B. J. (1985). Intracortical facilitation among co-oriented, co-axially aligned simple cells in cat striate cortex. *Experimental Brain Research, 61*, 54–61.

Orbach, H. S. (1987). Monitoring electrical activity in rat cerebral cortex. In L. M. Loew (Ed.), *Optical measurement of electrical activity.* Boca Raton: CRC Press.

Orbach, H. S. & Cohen, L. B. (1983). Simultaneous optical monitoring of activity from many areas of the salamander olfactory bulb. A new method for studying functional organization in the vertebrate CNS. *Journal of Neuroscience, 3*, 2251–2262.

Orbach, H. S., Cohen, L. B., & Grinvald, A. (1985). Optical mapping of electrical activity in rat somatosensory and visual cortex. *Journal of Neuroscience, 5*, 1886–1895.

Payne, B. R., Berman, N., & Murphy, E. H. (1980). Organization of direction preferences in cat visual cortex. *Brain Research, 211*, 445–450.

Ratzlaff, E. H., & Grinvald, A. (1991). A Tandem-lens epifluorescence macroscope: Hundred-fold brightness advantage for wide field imaging. *Journal of Neuroscience Methods, 36*, 127–137.

Ross, W. N., & Reichardt, L. F. (1979). Species-specific effects on the optical signals of voltage sensitive dyes. *Journal of Membrane Biology, 48*, 343–356.

Salzberg, B. M. (1983). Optical recording of electrical activity in neurons using molecular probes. In J. Barber & J. McKelvy (Eds.), *Current methods in cellular neurobiology* (pp. 139–187). New York: J. Wiley.

Salzberg, B. M., Obaid, A. L., & Gainer, H. (1985). Large and rapid changes in light scattering accompany secretion by nerve terminals in the mammalian neurohypophysis. *Journal of General Physiology, 86*, 395–411.

Seelen, W. von (1970). Zur Informationsverarbeitung im visuellen System der Wirbeltiere. *Kybernetik, 7*, 89–106.

Sokoloff, L. (1977). Relation between physiological function and energy metabolism in the central nervous system. *Journal of Neurochemistry, 19*, 13–26.

Swindale, N. V. (1982). A model for the formation of orientation columns. *Proceedings of the Royal Society of London, B215*, 211–230.

Swindale, N. V., Matsubara, J. A., & Cynader, M. S. (1987). Surface organization of orientation and direction selectivity in cat area 18. *Journal of Neuroscience, 7*, 1414–1427.

Tasaki, I., & Warashina, A. (1976). Dye membrane interaction and its changes during nerve excitation. *Photochemistry and Photobiology 24*, 191–207.

Tolhurst, D. J., Dean, A. F., & Thompson, I. D. (1981). Preferred direction of movement as an element in the organization of cat visual cortex. *Experimental Brain Research, 44*, 340–342.

Ts'o, D. Y., Frostig, R. D., Lieke, E. E., & Grinvald, A. (1988). Functional organization of visual area 18 of macaque as revealed by optical imaging of activity-dependent intrinsic signals. *Society of Neuroscience Abstracts, 14*, 898.

Ts'o, D. Y., Frostig, R. D., Lieke, E. E., & Grinvald, A. (1990). Functional organization of primate visual cortex revealed by high resolution optical imaging. *Science, 249*, 417–420.

Ts'o, D. Y., Gilbert, C. D., & Wiesel, T. N. (1986). Relationships between horizontal interactions and functional architecture in cat striate cortex as revealed by cross correlation analysis. *Journal of Neuroscience, 6*, 1160–1170.

Waggoner, A. S. (1979). Dye indicators of membrane potential. *Annual Review of Biophysics and Bioenergetics, 8*, 47–63.

Waggoner, A. S., & Grinvald, A. (1977). Mechanisms of rapid optical changes of potential sensitive dyes. *Annals of the New York Academy of Sciences, 303*, 217–242.

4

Modular Organization of Information Processing in the Normal Human Brain: Studies with Positron Emission Tomography

MARCUS E. RAICHLE

Substantial evidence supports the hypothesis that the human brain is structurally and functionally modular. One of the great challenges in neuroscience is to understand how this modularity is organized in support of mental activity. Such an understanding must at least accompany, if not precede, a knowledge of how specific components of a mental operation are implemented in individual modules (e.g., local ensembles of neurons). Modern imaging techniques substantially improve our ability to identify and study widely distributed component modules supporting specific mental operations. One approach is the measurement of local brain blood flow with positron emission tomography (PET). Changes in neuronal activity are accompanied by rapid (<1 s) changes in local blood flow and metabolism in the brain (Raichle, 1987). Positron emission tomography accurately and rapidly measures changes in local blood flow (Raichle, 1983, 1986). Assuming all mental activity is accompanied by changes in local blood flow, PET is ideally suited to accomplish the task of relating changes in local neuronal activity to mental activity. These studies reveal the distributed, modular nature of mental activity implemented in the normal human brain (Petersen, Fox, Posner, Mintun, & Raichle, 1988, 1989; Petersen, Fox, Snyder, & Raichle, 1990). This technique is especially important because it permits an examination of these distributed modular relationships in the normal human brain.

In this chapter I outline briefly a strategy employing PET measurements of *changes* in local brain blood flow. These measurements are obtained by subtracting measurements made in a control state from those made in a functionally activated state in the same subject. These measurements are then averaged across subjects (and occasionally within a subject) to improve the signal-to-noise properties of the resulting image. From such data emerges a map of the distributed modular brain organization underlying normal human cognition and emotion. Using PET measurements of local blood flow and strategies for accurately localizing these changes, the general topography of systems concerned with the analysis of words is presented.

THE TECHNIQUE

Emission tomography is a technique that produces an image of the distribution of a previously administered radionuclide in any desired section of the body. Positron emission tomography uses the unique properties of the annihilation radiation that is generated when positrons are absorbed in matter (Raichle, 1983) to provide an image that is a highly faithful representation of the spatial distribution of the radionuclide at a selected plane through the tissue. Such an image is effectively equivalent to a *quantitative tissue autoradiogram* obtained with laboratory animals, but PET has the added advantage that it is noninvasive, hence studies are possible in living animals, including humans. It has been used in humans to measure brain blood flow, blood volume, metabolism of glucose and oxygen, acid–base balance, receptor pharmacology, and transmitter metabolism (for an introduction to this literature see Raichle, 1986). In this chapter I will focus on the measurement of brain blood flow and its use in mapping the local functional activity within the normal human brain.

Our strategy for the functional mapping of neuronal activity in the human brain with PET is composed of a number of important elements. These include the deliberate selection of blood flow measured with the PET adaptation of the Kety autoradiographic technique (Herscovitch, Markham, & Raichle, 1983; Herscovitch, Raichle, Kilbourn, & Welch, 1987; Raichle, Martin, Herscovitch, Mintun, & Markham, 1983), or estimated from the radioactive counts accumulating in brain tissue during 40 s following the intravenous bolus administration of $H_2^{15}O$ (Fox, Perlmutter, & Raichle, 1985), as the most accurate and flexible signal of changes in local neural activity that can be detected with PET Fox, Raichle, Mintun, Dence, 1988). Linearly scaled images of blood flow or radioactive counts in a control state are subtracted from images obtained during functional activation in each subject (i.e., paired image subtraction). The control state and the stimulated state are carefully chosen so as to isolate, as far as possible, a single mental operation (e.g., Petersen, Fox, Posner, Mintun, & Raichle, 1988). By subtracting blood flow measurements made in the control state from each task state it is possible to identify those areas of the brain concerned with the mental operations unique to the task state. This extends to our work a strategy first introduced to psychology by Donders in 1868, in which reaction time was used to dissect out the components of mental operations (Donders, 1969). In our work we can now do so in terms of specific regions of the brain. These subtraction images form the basis of a data set that is composed of averaged responses across many individual subjects or across many runs in the same individual. Image averaging dramatically enhances the signal-to-noise properties of such data. This enables us to detect even low-level responses associated with mental activity (Fox, Mintun, Reiman, & Raichle, 1988; Mintun, Fox, & Raichle, 1989).

FUNCTIONAL MAPPING STUDIES

For several years now we have been examining the cortical anatomy of single-word processing (Petersen et al., 1988; Petersen, Fox, Posner, Mintun, & Raichle, 1989; Petersen et al., in press) as an initial step in the study of language. Because of the great complexity of language, restriction of our efforts to an understanding of the processing of individual words seemed warranted. Furthermore, the design of tasks appropriate for such studies with PET was greatly aided by extant knowledge in cognitive psychology, linguistics, and clinical neurology (e.g., Coltheart, 1985; Damasio, 1984; LaBerge & Samuels, 1974).

In this project we used four behavioral conditions in each subject to form a three-level subtractive hierarchy in which each task state was intended to add a small number of mental operations to those of its subordinate (control) state.

In the *first level* comparison the visual presentation of single words without a lexical task was compared with visual fixation on a small cross-hairs on a television monitor without word presentation. Words were presented for 150 ms at the rate of once per second on a television screen during the 40 s measurement of blood flow. No motor output or volitional lexical processing was required in this task; rather, simple sensory input and involuntary word-form processing were targeted by this subtraction.

The areas of brain identified as active during the passive viewing of words appear to support two different computational levels: one of passive sensory processing in primary visual cortex, and a second level of modality-specific word-form processing in extrastriate areas. The main regions activated (Figure 4.1, triangles labeled P) were in striate cortex bilaterally (P5,6; Figure 4.1) and three extrastriate areas, one on the left (P1, Figure 4.1) and two on the right (P2,4, Figure 4.1), extending to the temporal–occipital boundary on the right. The primary striate responses were similar to those produced by simple sensory stimuli such as the checkerboard annuli used in our earlier experiments (Fox et al., 1986; Fox, Meizen, Allman, Van Essen, & Raichle, 1987). The regions in extrastriate cortex became candidates for a network of cortical modules that code for visual word form. Subsequent experiments (Petersen, Fox, Snyder, & Raichle, 1990) demonstrated that the area located at P1 (Figure 4.1) was activated by words and non-words obeying rules of English and not by consonant letter strings or false fonts (Figure 4.2). Taken together the several regions of striate and extrastriate cortex activated by passive visual words appear to combine, functionally, to

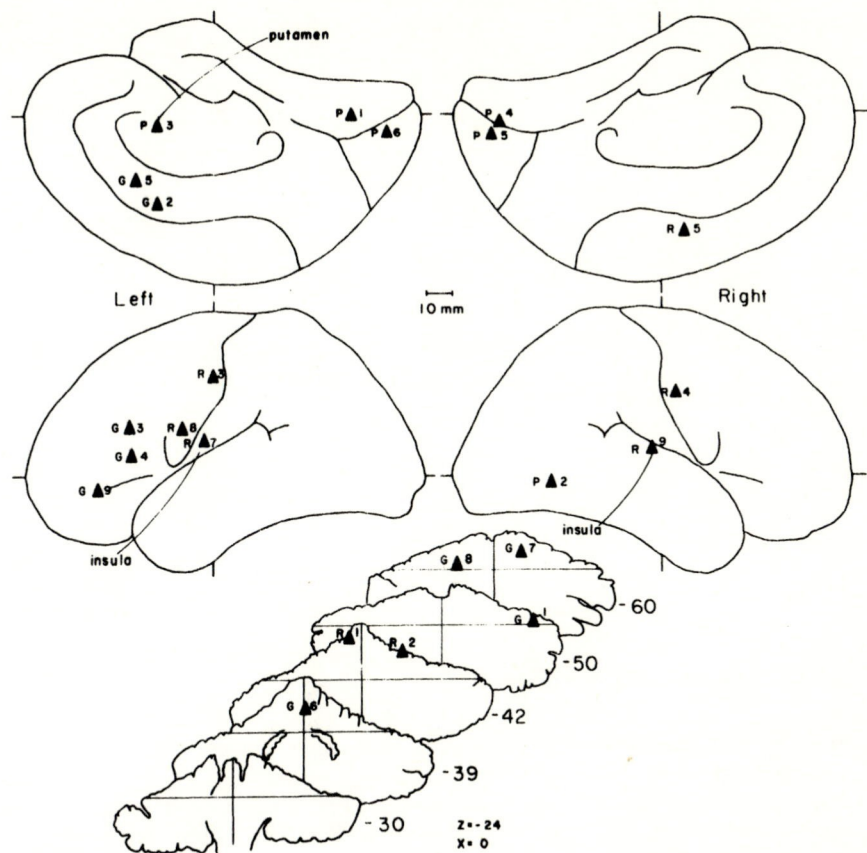

FIGURE 4.1.   Location of averaged local blood flow changes during the processing of single visual words in normal adult subjects. Three different task states were studied in each subject: passive presentation of visual words (symbols denoted P), repeating visual words (symbols denoted R), and generating a verb for a presented noun (symbols denoted G). The words, common English nouns, were presented on a television monitor at the rate of 1 Hz. The control state for the passive viewing of nouns was looking at a fixation point on the monitor. The control state for repeating nouns was the passive presentation of the same nouns. Finally, the control state for generating verbs was repeating nouns. The relative magnitude of each response within conditions is shown to the right of the symbol. The cerebral hemisphere fiducial markers represent the zero planes for the Z (horizontal) and Y (vertical) axes of the Talairach stereotaxic system (Talairach & Szikla, 1967). These data are replotted from Petersen, Fox, Posner, Mintun, & Raichle (1988).

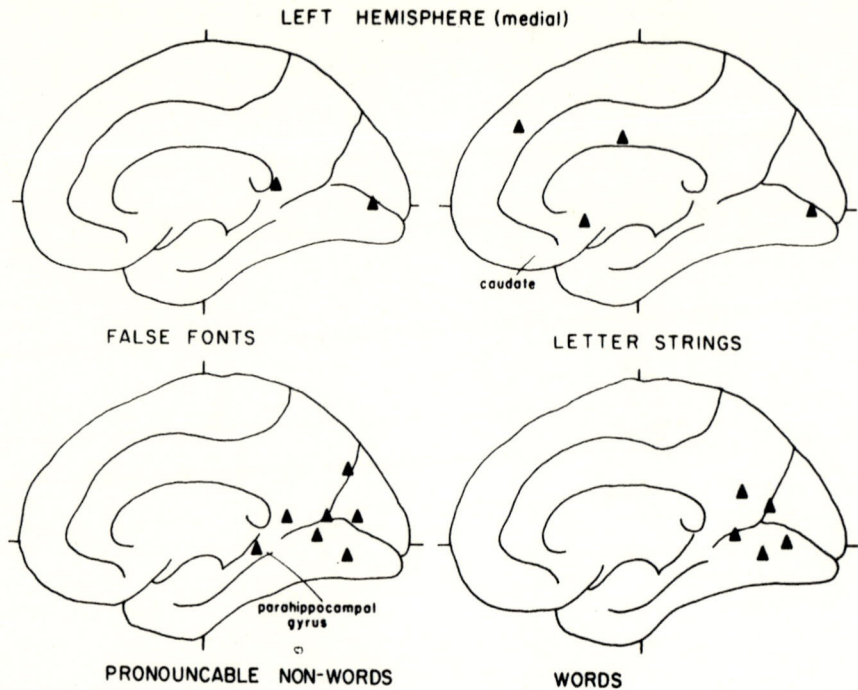

FIGURE 4.2. Location of averaged local blood flow changes during the passive viewing of false fonts (upper left), consonant letter strings (upper right), pronounceable non-words (lower left), and words (lower right). The control state for each task was passive viewing of a fixation point on a monitor. The presentation rate of the stimuli was 1 Hz on the same monitor. Note the striking increase in the number of responses in the area of calcarine cortex, lingual, and fusiform gyrii during the presentation of words and pronounceable non-words indicating that the normal human brain has learned to make a distinction between symbols that obey the English spelling rules and those that do not, even though the latter have identical visual features. (For more details about this experiment see Petersen, Fox, Snyder, & Raichle, in press.)

analyze visual symbols that behave according to rules of the English language. As such they must represent a learned response.

Words presented auditorily with subjects passively fixating on the visual cross-hairs activated an entirely separate set of areas in temporal cortex bilaterally (not shown in Figure 4.1; see Petersen et al., 1988, 1989). Areas in left posterior temporal cortex (appropriate candidates for Wernicke's area) were clearly seen with auditory presentation but were conspicuous by their absence during the presentation of words visually. Only when subjects were asked to judge whether pairs of visual words rhymed were responses seen in these areas (Petersen et al., 1988, 1989) emphasizing the functionally flexible nature of these modular relationships.

In the *second level* comparison, subjects were asked to repeat the words presented auditorily or visually. The control state for the PET blood flow subtraction was the passive presentation of auditory or visual words. Areas related to motor output and articulatory coding were activated. In general, similar regions were activated for visual (responses labeled R, Figure 4.1) and auditory presentation (not shown). Responses occurred in primary sensorimotor mouth cortex bilaterally (R3,4, Figure 4.1), the supplementary motor area of SMA (R5, Figure 4.1) and in insular cortex bilaterally (R7, 9, Figure 4.1). The left insular response is near Broca's area, a region often viewed as specifically serving language output. However, similar insular activation was also found when subjects were instructed simply to move their mouths and tongues (unpublished data), arguing against specialization of this region for speech output.

In the *third* and final *level* of comparison, subjects were asked to speak a verb for each noun presented, either auditorily or visually, again while monitoring a fixation point. Responses were identified in two areas of cerebral cortex as well as for both auditory (not shown) and visual word presentation (labeled G, Figure 4.1). A left inferior prefrontal areas (G2, 5, Figure 4.1) was identified that participates, in an undefined way, in the process of semantic association. The second area in the anterior cingulate gyrus (G2,5, Figure 4.1) is probably part of an anterior attentional system engaged in selection for action. This localization of function was suggested by the performance of converging experiments detailed elsewhere (Pardo, Pardo, Janer, & Raichle, 1990; Posner, Petersen, Fox, & Raichle, 1988). An additional area (left posterior temporal cortex in the area of the middle temporal gyrus) only became active when, on subsequent experiments (unpublished data), we increased the interstimulus interval to 1500 ms from 1000 ms. This finding would be consistent with this area serving as a verbal memory buffer. Further experiments are under way to establish more exactly its precise role.

Responses in the cerebellum (G1,6,7,8, Figure 4.1), especially in the right lateral cerebellar hemisphere (G1, Figure 4.1) were also detected in this task. Because we had subtracted the motoric aspects of simply saying words, this result strongly suggests that the cerebellum plays an important role in high-level information processing involving a novel task that engages the left prefrontal cortex. This is the first direct evidence in support of the hypothesis that the cerebellum plays an important role in high-level information processing in humans, as suggested by others (Berntson & Torello, 1984; Bracke-Tolkmitt et al., 1989; Leiner, Leiner, & Dow, 1989).

Finally, one additional preliminary (unpublished) observation may be of importance in understanding the information processing role of the responses observed in this task. Specifically, the responses in left prefrontal cortex and anterior cingulate cortex were only present when subjects were first exposed to this task (i.e., when it was novel and required active attention). Practice generating verbs to a specific list of nouns resulted in disappearance of the left inferior prefrontal and anterior cingulate responses. These results suggest a role for these areas of cortex in the *learning* of a new skill, in this case linguistic.

What do such results suggest about the modular organization of the human brain for tasks associated with single-word processing? They suggest a *flexible* modular organization consisting of multiple routes. For example, there is no activation in any of our visual tasks near Wernicke's area or the angular gyrus in posterior temporal cortex unless a specific phonological judgement must be made (i.e., rhyme judgment). Visual information from occipital cortex appears to have access to output coding without undergoing phonological recoding in these areas in the posterior temporal cortex. Furthermore, tasks calling for semantic processing of single words activate frontal cortices (i.e., left prefrontal and anterior cingulate). The role of the left posterior temporal cortex in semantic processing remains to be determined. As mentioned above, preliminary experiments indicate that it becomes active as the interstimulus interval is lengthened, suggesting a role as a verbal memory buffer. Finally, sensory-specific information appears to have independent access to semantic and output codes; simple repetition of a presented word failed to activate the left frontal semantic areas.

CONCLUSIONS

This brief review is intended to demonstrate that a combination of cognitive and neurobiological approaches to the study of normal human subjects, aided by modern imaging techniques, can give us important new information about the flexible, distributed, modular organization of cognition and emotion in the human brain. Progress in our evolving understanding of the implementation of mental activities in the human brain will be dependent on an appreciation of the distributed nature of the processing. Inferences drawn about the role of specific local neuronal ensembles in particular mental activities must be guided by the knowledge that an ensemble may be only a part of a very distributed network in which local areas of the brain contribute highly specialized component functions. Continued progress in this type of work should serve to enlighten us about the solution to the problem of mind–brain interaction, which has intrigued us for so long. Finally, one must hope that the insights gained will provide a more rational basis for the understanding and treatment of some of humankind's most devastating diseases.

Acknowledgements: This work was supported by NS 06833, HL 13851, and the MacArthur Foundation.

REFERENCES

Berntson, G. G., & Torello, M. W. (1984). The paleocerebellum and the integration of behavioral function. *Physiological Psychology, 10*, 2–12.

Bracke-Tolkmitt, R., Linden, A., Canavan, A. G. M., Rockstroh, B., Scholz, E., Wessel, K., & Diener, H-C. (1989). The cerebellum contributes to mental skills. *Behavioral Neuroscience, 103*, 442–446.

Coltheart, M. (1985). Cognitive neuropsychology and the study of reading. In M. I. Posner & O. S. M. Marlin (Eds.), *Attention and performance XI* (pp. 3–37). Hillsdale, New Jersey: Lawrence Erlbaum.

Damasio, A. R. (1984). The neural basis of language. *Annual Review of Neuroscience, 7*, 127–147.

Donders, F. C. (1969). On the speed of mental processes. Reprinted in *Acta Psychologica, 30*, 412–431.

Fox, P. T., Meizen, F. M., Allman, J. M., Van Essen, D. C., & Raichle, M. E. (1987). Retinotopic organization of human visual cortex mapped with positron emission tomography. *Journal of Neuroscience, 7*, 913–922.

Fox, P. T., Mintun, M. A., Raichle, M. E., Meizen, F. M., Allman, J. M., & Van Essen, D. C. (1986). Mapping human visual cortex with positron emission tomography. *Nature, 323*, 806–809.

Fox, P. T., Mintun, M. A., Reiman, E. M., & Raichle, M. E. (1988). Enhanced detection of focal brain responses using intersubject averaging and distribution analysis of subtracted PET images. *Journal of Cerebral Blood Flow and Metabolism, 8*, 642–653.

Fox, P. T., Perlmutter, J., & Raichle, M. E. (1985). A stereotactic method of anatomical localization for positron emission tomography. *Journal of Computer Assisted Tomography, 9*, 141–153.

Fox, P. T., Raichle, M. E., Mintun, M. A., & Dence, C. (1988). Nonoxidative glucose consumption during focal physiologic neural activity. *Science, 241*, 462–464.

Herscovitch, P., Markham, J., & Raichle, M. E. (1983). Brain blood flow measured with intravenous $H_2^{15}O$. I. Theory and error analysis. *Journal of Nuclear Medicine, 24*, 782–789.

Herscovitch, P., Raichle, M. E., Kilbourn, M. R., & Welch, M. J. (1987). Positron emission tomographic measurement of cerebral blood flow and permeability surface area product of water using ^{15}O-water and ^{11}C-butanol. *Journal of Cerebral Flow and Metabolism, 7*, 527–542.

LaBerge, D., & Samuels, S. J. (1974). Toward a theory of automatic information processing in reading. *Cognitive Psychology, 6*, 293–323.

Leiner, H. C., Leiner, A. L., & Dow, R. S. (1989). Reappraising the cerebellum: What does the hindbrain contribute to the forebrain? *Behavioral Neuroscience, 103*, 998–1008.

Mintun, M. A., Fox, P. T., & Raichle, M. E. (1989). A highly accurate method of localizing regions of neuronal activation in the human brain with positron emission tomography. *Journal of Cerebral Blood Flow and Metabolism, 9*, 96–103.

Pardo, J. V., Pardo, P. J., Janer, K. W., & Raichle, M. E. (1990). The anterior cingulate cortex mendiates processing selection in the stoop attentional conflict paradigm. *Proceedings of the National Academy of Sciences, U.S.A., 87*, 256–259.

Petersen, S. E., Fox, P. T., Posner, M. I., Mintun, M. A., & Raichle, M. E. (1988). Positron emission tomographic studies of the cortical anatomy of single-word processing. *Nature, 331*, 585–589.

Petersen, S. E., Fox, P. T., Posner, M. I., Mintun, M. A., & Raichle, M. E. (1989). Positron emission tomographic studies of the processing of single words. *Journal of Cognitive Neuroscience, 1*, 153–170.

Petersen, S. E., Fox, P. T., Snyder, A. Z., & Raichle, M. E. (1990). Activation of extrastriate and frontal cortical areas by visual words and word-like stimuli. *Science, 249*, 1041–1044.

Posner, M. I., Petersen, S. E., Fox, P. T., & Raichle, M. E. (1988). Localization of cognitive functions in the human brain. *Science, 240*, 1627–1631.

Raichle, M. E. (1983). Positron emission tomography. *Annual Review of Neuroscience,* 6, 249–268.

Raichle, M. E. (1986). Neuroimaging. *Trends in Neuroscience, 9,* 525–529.

Raichle, M. E. (1987). Circulatory and metabolic correlates of brain function in normal humans. In V. B. Mountcastle & F. Plum (Eds.), *Handbook of physiology: Vol. V. The nervous system* (pp. 643–674). Bethesda: American Physiological Society.

Raichle, M. E., Martin, W. R. W., Herscovitch, P., Mintun, M., & Markham, J. (1983). Brain blood flow measured with $H_2{}^{15}O$. II. Implementation and validation. *Journal of Nuclear Medicine, 24,* 790–798.

Talairach, J., & Szikla, G. Atlas d'anatomie stereotaxique du telencephale. Paris, Masson & Cie, 1967.

5

Structures in the Human Brain Participating in Visual Learning, Tactile Learning, and Motor Learning

PER E. ROLAND
BALÁZS GULYÁS
RÜDIGER J. SEITZ

Learning in a neurobiological context most often means the processing and storage of information. The information that is stored is stored in specific memory systems or, more specifically, in distributed memories, from which it can be retrieved by addressing the memories in a specific way. From studies of patients with cognitive memory deficits resulting from circumscribed lesions of the brain, it is known that the integrity of the hippocampal formation and adjacent parts of the medial temporal lobe, together with the midline and dorsal parts of thalamus, are important for the storage of visual and auditory events, patterns, and experiences, but these brain structures are themselves not part of the storage sites (Scoville & Milner, 1957; Squire & More, 1979). Patients with lesions of these structures have no trouble learning new motor skills (Corkin, 1968). This led to the hypothesis that storage and memory for motor skills and those for cognitive information make use of different anatomical brain structures, and a distinction was made between motor memory and cognitive (declarative) memories (Squire, 1987). Lesions of anatomical structures in the brain important for the generation of voluntary movements, such as the cerebellum, certain brain stem nuclei, and the motor cortical areas, impair the acquisition of motor skills (Brinkman & Porter, 1983; Sasaki & Gemba, 1982). But since motor skills can only be revealed through voluntary motor activity, lesions are unable to reveal if any distinction exists between anatomical structures participating in learning of a skill and those participating in the execution of the skill during learning and after learning has taken place.

Studies of patients with circumscribed lesions can only identify where damage to a particular brain area interferes with a brain function such as memory. We decided to explore which brain structures are active in the living human brain during learning, recall, and recognition of visual patterns, during tactile learning of the shapes of objects, and during learning and mastery of a motor skill. The regional cerebral blood flow (rCBF) in a normal brain is an indicator of activity and metabolism in synaptic regions (Ginsberg, Dietrich, & Busto, 1987; Greenberg, Hand, Sylvestro, & Reivich, 1979). This is fortunate, because changes in synaptic activity are supposed to be crucial for all types of learning. In mammals, the changes in synaptic efficacy that are supposed to be the mechanism of learning are not confined to single neurons. In nonlearning situations the brain works by activating larger fields and larger dispersed synaptic populations in the cortex and subcortical structures. This is the cortical field activation hypothesis (Roland, 1985). There is reason to assume that the brain, during storage of information, will also work the same way. Therefore learning and retrieval processes in the brain have a chance to be visualized by the use of in vivo tracer methods in combination with positron emission tomography (PET). Results from such experiments rely on the assumption that learning, recall, and recognition change the activity in synaptic regions to such an extent that the metabolism, and thereby the rCBF, changes significantly. In this chapter, results from PET experiments are reported, which show the anatomical structures engaged in storage and retrieval visual memories, tactile memories, and the structures modulating their activity during learning of a motor skill. The methods and the equipment are described in recent reports (Roland, Eriksson, Stone-Elander, & Widén, 1987; Roland, Eriksson, Widén, & Stone-Elander, 1989; Roland, Gulyás, Seitz, Bohm, & Stone-Elander, 1990) and therefore only a brief summary is given here.

METHODS

In all learning studies the rCBF was measured as an indicator of regional synaptic activity in normal volunteers who inhaled 50 mCi of the freely diffusible tracer, $^{11}CH_3F$ in a single breath (Holden et al., 1981; Roland et al., 1987). The arterial concentration of tracer was determined continuously (Eriksson, Bohm, Kesselberg, & Holte, 1988). From the arterial concentration of $^{11}CH_3F$ and the PET measurements of the concentrations of tracer in the brain, the rCBF was determined pixel by pixel during the first 80 s by the dynamic method described by Roland et al. (1987) using the algorithm of Koeppe, Holden, & Ip (1985). The four-ring seven-slice PC384-7B PET camera with an in-plane resolution of 7.6 mm and slice thickness of 11.5 mm and 8 mm (cross slices) (Litton, Bergström, Eriksson, Bohm, & Blomqvist, 1984) was used for all measurements. The single-scan frames were reconstructed with a filter of 4 mm. The final images of rCBFR were filtered with a spatial Gaussian filter of 4 mm (full with half maximum). The rCBF images were then corrected for differences in arterial partial pressure of CO_2 between control measurements and test rCBF measurements by 4% per mm mercury (Olesen, Paulson, & Lassen, 1971).

For determination of the brain anatomy of each subject and the final standardization of the PET images, each subject was equipped with the fixation helmet of Bergström, Boetius, Eriksson, Greitz, & Widén (1981) and had a high-resolution magnetic resonance tomographic scan taken (Seitz, Bohm, et al., 1990). This helmet is also used for stereotactic surgery. The computerized adjustable atlas of Bohm and Greitz (Bohm et al., 1986; Greitz, Bohm, Holte, & Eriksson, 1991; Seitz, Bohm, et al., 1990) was then adapted to the individual magnetic tomographic image of the brain by linear and nonlinear elastic transformations as described by Seitz, Bohm, et al., (1990) and Greitz et al. (1991). Thereafter all images were transformed into a standard brain anatomy as described by Seitz, Bohm, et al. (1990). The main feature of this atlas is that one can construct pictures of the change in rCBF between rest and other PET measurements in which the brains are all of the same shape and size irrespective of the different shapes and sizes of the individual brains. This allows construction of pictures of the mean changes in rCBF between rest and the test measurements or between different test measurements. The accuracy and precision of these procedures were evaluated (Seitz, Bohm, et al., 1990). For central structures, such as the globus pallidus and putamen, the standard deviation of localization is around 1 mm in the x-direction and 2 mm in the y-direction. The mean rCBF changes during the different learning tests were localized to anatomical structures from the database of the atlas. With this technique, active synaptic regions can be localized with a precision beyond the spatial resolution of the PET camera (Seitz, Bohm, et al., 1990).

Each subject was measured in one control state, a rest state defined by Roland and Larsen (1976). During all measurements, arterial pCO_2, EEG, eye movements recordings, electromyogram (EMG), and video monitoring were performed, which is standard in our laboratory. The galvanic skin conductance and the intra-arterial blood pressure were, however, not measured. In addition three PET measurements were taken during different stages of learning, recall, and recognition. The rCBF from the control state was subtracted from that of the test state to give individual subtraction images. These were reformatted by the adjustable computerized atlas into standard size and shape and subsequently averaged to give mean ΔrCBF images. In addition, mean rCBF images for each test were created from the individual rCBF images. The pixel ΔrCBF was tested for being distributed according to a Gaussian distribution by plots on normality paper and Q–Q plots (Johnson & Wichern, 1982; Seitz, Bohm, et al., 1990). Paired descriptive t-values were then calculated pixel by pixel corresponding to the mean ΔrCBF images (Seitz, Bohm, et al., 1990). According to preliminary investigations the spatial correlation between pixel values of ΔrCBF extends for 8 mm after which it becomes negligible (Urodal et al., unpublished observations). Pixels 8 mm apart were therefore regarded as uncorrelated in practice. An a priori arbitrarily set numerical level of 2.3 was set to dichotomize the pixels of the t-images. This value was chosen on the basis of an examination of the distribution of noise and signal in rest and test images in the study of Seitz, Bohm, et al. (1990). With 10 degrees of freedom each uncorrelated pixel would have an average probability of 0.04 of exceeding a numerical value 2.3. If all changes in rCBF between the test and control were due to random fluctuations, the probability of getting 2, 3, and 4 uncorrelated pixels exceeding a numerical value of 2.3 in a sample of 9 uncorrelated pixels can be estimated from an upper limit to the hypergeometrical distribution (Feller, 1968) to be less than 0.05, 0.005, and 0.0005, respectively. In the study of Seitz, Bohm, et al. (1990) it was shown that the background noise in the mean ΔrCBF images did not exceed a numerical value of 3.0 ml/100 g/min. For this reason all mean ΔrCBF values exceeding a numerical value of 5.0 ml/100 g/min were examined in a resampled population of the subjects participating in the test. One subject was removed according to a table of random numbers and a picutre of the mean ΔrCBF computed. In this picture all spots having ΔrCBF exceeding 5.0 ml/100 g/min were listed as potential areas of change. The procedure was then repeated until every subject had been removed once. In addition the group of subjects was randomly assigned into two groups with five subjects each. It was then analyzed whether all spots having a mean ΔrCBF exceeding 5.0 ml/100 g/min appearing in the first group were also present in the second group. Only spots having ΔrCBF values consistently exceeding 5.0 ml/100 g/min in all resampled populations were considered in the further analysis. Post hoc it was examined which of the spots being consistently activated in all resampled populations coincided with areas having $t > 2.3$ and all such spots were localized to the anatomical structures by the computerized atlas. In the study of Seitz, Bohm, et al. (1990) it was shown that the number of (correlated 1.275 mm $\times$ 1.275 mm) pixels in a cluster with noise exceeding 1.0 ml/100 g/min never exceeded 8. For these reasons we regarded activation as having taken place in an area encompassing at least two uncorrelated pixels and having a spot for which ΔrCBF was consistently larger than 5.0 ml in all resampled populations (Roland et al., 1990). These areas are listed in the tables. It is impossible with any of the present statistical methods to give exact significance limits for each of these activations, but the statistical significance increases the more uncorrelated pixels the activation comprises.

In the case of tactile learning the mean ΔrCBF values were obtained from regions of interest drawn independently on pictures of the regional cerebral oxidative metabolism (see Roland et al., 1989, for details). In the case where the mean rCBF picture of visual learning was subtracted from the mean rCBF during motor learning, the sectors of the brain subjected to analysis were delimited a priori on the basis of the results from the separate studies of visual learning and motor learning, respectively.

MOTOR LEARNING

Learning of a complicated motor sequence with the fingers of the right hand was studied by Seitz, Roland, Bohm, Greitz, & Stone-Elander (1990). The task was conducted with the right hand and consisted in letting the thumb briefly touch the ring finger once, the index finger twice, the long finger once, the little finger twice, and then again the little finger twice, the ring finger three times, the long finger once and then the index finger twice... then again the ring finger once... and so on continuously until the subject was stopped. A full sequence (from start until the ring finger was touched once again), when perfectly learned, should be carried out in less than 5 s without errors. The subjects were blindfolded and were initially instructed verbally and by moving the appropriate fingers. This is an example of motor learning in which an internal representation of the task must be effectively translated into motor commands.

At the initial learning state, when the subjects knew exactly what to do but had very little practice, their finger movements were carried out with a rather low frequency, 1.8 ± 0.4 Hz. The subjects at this stage tended to guide their performance by internal counting of how many times the thumb had to touch each of the other fingers. This was reflected in the rCBF increases in Broca's area and its right hemisphere homologue. The anatomical structures participating in this initial stage of motor learning could be grouped into (a) the structures participating in voluntary motor activity, i.e., the premotor areas, the supplementary motor areas, the primary motor hand area, the basal ganglia, possibly the ventrolateral thalamus, and the cerebellum; (b) structures participating in the analysis of somatosensory information, i.e., the (left) somatosensory hand area in the postcentral gyrus, the somatosensory association areas in the anterior part of the superior parietal lobule, the supplementary sensory area, and the cortex in the intraparietal sulcus; (c) structures participating in the production of language: the left and right inferior frontal gyrus. Quite remarkably the rCBF decreased in the midsector of the putamen and the globus pallidus and presumably in the regions of the red nucleus and pons (Table 5.1).

The subjects were further trained and, as learning proceeded, after an hour the initially strongly activated fields in the somatosensory association cortices diminished progressively in intensity and extent. This took place most drastically ipsilaterally to the finger movements in the right hemisphere. The activated fields in the inferior frontal gyrus and the superior temporal gyrus disappeared (Table 5.1). At this point the finger movements were faster (2.6 ± 0.5 Hz) and the subjects said that they did not count internally the number of times the fingers should touch the thumb any more. Finally, 2 h after the initial training when the subjects were executing perfectly the sequence in less than 5 s, the changes in brain activations concentrated on the motor structures. The individual finger movements were now executed with a frequency of 3.2 ± 0.4 Hz. When the sequence was learnt, the decreases in the basal ganglia, red nucleus zone, and pons disappeared and

TABLE 5.1 Brain Regions Changing rCBF During Motor Learning. Mean Changes in ml/100 g/min ± SD (9 Subjects)

Region	Initial Learning		Advanced Learning		Skilled Performance	
	cm³	ΔrCBF mean	cm³	ΔrCBF mean	cm³	ΔrCBF mean
Insula R	1.9	−10.1*†	1.9	−7.1†	1.9	−8.2†
Temporal pole R	1.9	−7.4	1.9	−4.4	1.9	−3.4
Temporal pole L	1.9	−5.3	1.9	−9.9†	1.9	−9.9*†
G. cinguli ant. R	2.2	−7.9†	2.2	−4.2	2.2	−3.8
Pons L	0.5	−8.3†	0.5	−8.7†	0.5	−6.4
Lob. ant. cerbell. R	1.4	9.1*†	1.6	10.8*†	2.1	9.4*†
N. ruber region L	0.3	−11.6†	0.3	−8.1	0.3	−5.9
Thalamus ventral L	1.9	5.5†	1.4	4.9†	1.4	5.1†
Putamen-pallidus R	2.4	−5.4†	2.4	−4.8	1.8	2.9
Putamen-pallidus L	2.4	−7.6*†	1.8	−4.3	1.8	1.8
Motor hand area L	3.2	19.0*†	4.3	19.1*†	4.5	23.5*†
Premotor area L	2.4	9.2*†	2.5	8.2*†	2.7	11.5*†
Supplementary mot. L	1.9	9.0*†	2.6	10.0*†	2.6	9.4*†
Somatosensory hand L	2.0	12.4*†	2.3	10.6*†	2.5	10.5*†
Supplementary sens. R	2.3	8.6*†	2.0	5.5†	2.3	5.6
Supplementary sens. L	1.0	7.1*†	1.0	7.4	1.0	6.3
Intraparietal ant. R	4.2	9.5*†	1.5	4.9	1.5	2.7
Intraparietal ant. L	2.3	8.2*†	2.3	3.9	2.3	3.2
G. front. inf. p. oper. L	2.9	5.6†	1.6	4.0	1.6	0.6

R: right; L: left; g: gyrus; ant: anterior; lob: lobulus; N: nucleus; inf: inferior; p: pars; oper: opercularis. * Areas of change for which $t > 2.3$ or $t < -2.3$. † Area of change in which a spot was found with changes consistently larger than 5 ml/100 g/min. The volume of the areas of change is also listed.

were replaced by neutral rCBF (rCBF as is in rest). Throughout all three phases, the rCBF tended to decrease in limbic and paralimbic structures: the insular cortex, the temporal pole, and the cingulate cortex (Table 5.1).

The pattern of synaptic activity, as reflected in the rCBF, thus undergoes radical changes during the course of learning. In the initial phase of learning there are activations of cortical motor areas and cerebellum, but de-activations of the basal ganglia. These motor sectors of the brain are assisted by activation of structures that provide information to the cortical areas: anterior language areas and somatosensory association areas. As learning proceeded, the activated fields in the somatosensory association areas shrank and diminished in intensity and the anterior language areas disappeared. Concurrently the subjects no longer counted the number of touches internally. The frequency of finger movements increased beyond the point where they could be guided by feedback of somatosensory information from the skin, joints, and muscles of the moving fingers (Freund, 1986). The anterior language areas and the somatosensory association areas might inject information into the motor sectors of the brain at the early phase of motor learning, but are no longer of any use when the motor programme has been established and is executed in a feed forward manner.

Perhaps the most conspicuous finding was the modulation of the synaptic activity in the midsector of the putamen and globus pallidus. In monkeys the corresponding sector contains neurons firing in relation to arm and hand movements (DeLong, 1972). The initial decrease in rCBF means an intial decrease of synaptic activity. Subsequently this effect tapered off and the synaptic activity returned to rest level when the learning was accomplished. The decrease in synaptic activity in the arm sector could be due to reduction of excitation. In accordance with this idea, Hikosaka and Wurtz (1983) found that neurons in the reticular part of substantia nigra, having high spontaneous activity, decreased the firing when a monkey had to make a saccade to a remembered target, but did not change their firing if the target was still on.

Apart from a very small transient increase in rCBF in the right posterior lobe of cerebellum confined to the learning phase, Seitz, Roland, et al. (1990) found no changes of rCBF in the cerebellum. The increases in the right anterior lobe were of the same intensity throughout the course of learning. This does not mean that there was no modulation of synaptic activity here. Initially the finger movement sequences were carried out at 1.8 Hz and during the course of learning the frequency almost doubled. This must have increased the afferent input to the cerebellar hand area in the anterior lobe, and yet the total rCBF was of the same increase throughout learning. The relative metabolic expense per single movement, therefore, was much higher during the initial phase of learning compared with the fast and perfect performance.

The most interesting problem still remains: where in the brain is the motor program stored? Logically the program should be stored within the structures active during the flawless performance of the program, that is, within the following structures: the motor cortices, the motor arm sectors of the basal ganglia, the cerebellum, and the ventrolateral thalamus. Whether the program is distributed within all these structures or only in a few is uncertain. When Roland, Larsen, Lassen, & Skinhöj (1980) let their subjects recall the motor sequence, but not execute it, only the supplementary motor areas were active among the cortical regions. However, the technique used by Roland et al. (1980) did not allow any measurements in the basal ganglia, thalamus, or cerebellum.

TACTILE LEARNING

The tactile sense organ is a moving sense organ, but learning of somatosensory information is not confounded by simultaneous learning of the exploratory movements. The exploratory movements are established once, early in life, but thereafter they do not seem to change (Roland & Mortensen, 1987).

In a recent experiment we (Roland et al., 1989) measured rCMRO$_2$ (the regional cerebral metabolic rate of oxygen) and rCBF in 20 young volunteers during rest, tactile learning, and tactile recognition of complicated geometrical objects (Figure 5.1). The subjects used their right hand. During the learning the objects were presented one by one in random order. The subjects were instructed to learn the shape of the objects and they knew that they later would go through a recognition test for evaluation of what had been learned. In the early phase of tactile learning of these objects the subjects explored the objects with a movement frequency of the fingers of about 1.1 Hz. The rCBF increased in the anatomical structures shown in Table 5.2. The active anatomical structures can be grouped into (a) structures and divisions of structures subserving motor functions: the premotor areas, the supplementary motor areas, and the ventral thalamus; (b) the cerebellum: the right anterior and both posterior lobes of the cerebellum; (c) structures and divisions of the brain devoted to the analysis of somatosensory information: the ventral-posterolateral thalamus, the hand area of gyrus postcentralis, fields in the supplementary sensory area, the superior parietal lobule and S II (the secondary somatosensory area); (d) limbic and paralimbic structures: hippocampus-amygdala, the posterior and anterior insular cortex, the orbitofrontal cortex and the anterior parts of gyrus cinguli; (e) prefrontal fields; and (f) the striatum: the head of the (left) caudate nucleus and the mid-sector of the caudate and putamen. Most of these activated structures were also engaged in somatosensory discrimination of shape (Roland & Larsen 1976; Seitz et al., 1991) in which no learning of somatosensory information occurs. In fact only the secondary somatosensory area and the anterior part of gyrus cinguli were not activated in somatosensory discrimination.

After 2 h and 10 min of learning it was evaluated how much information was retained by each subject in a recognition test in which the learnt objects were mixed with new objects (Figure 5.1). Four recognition tests were

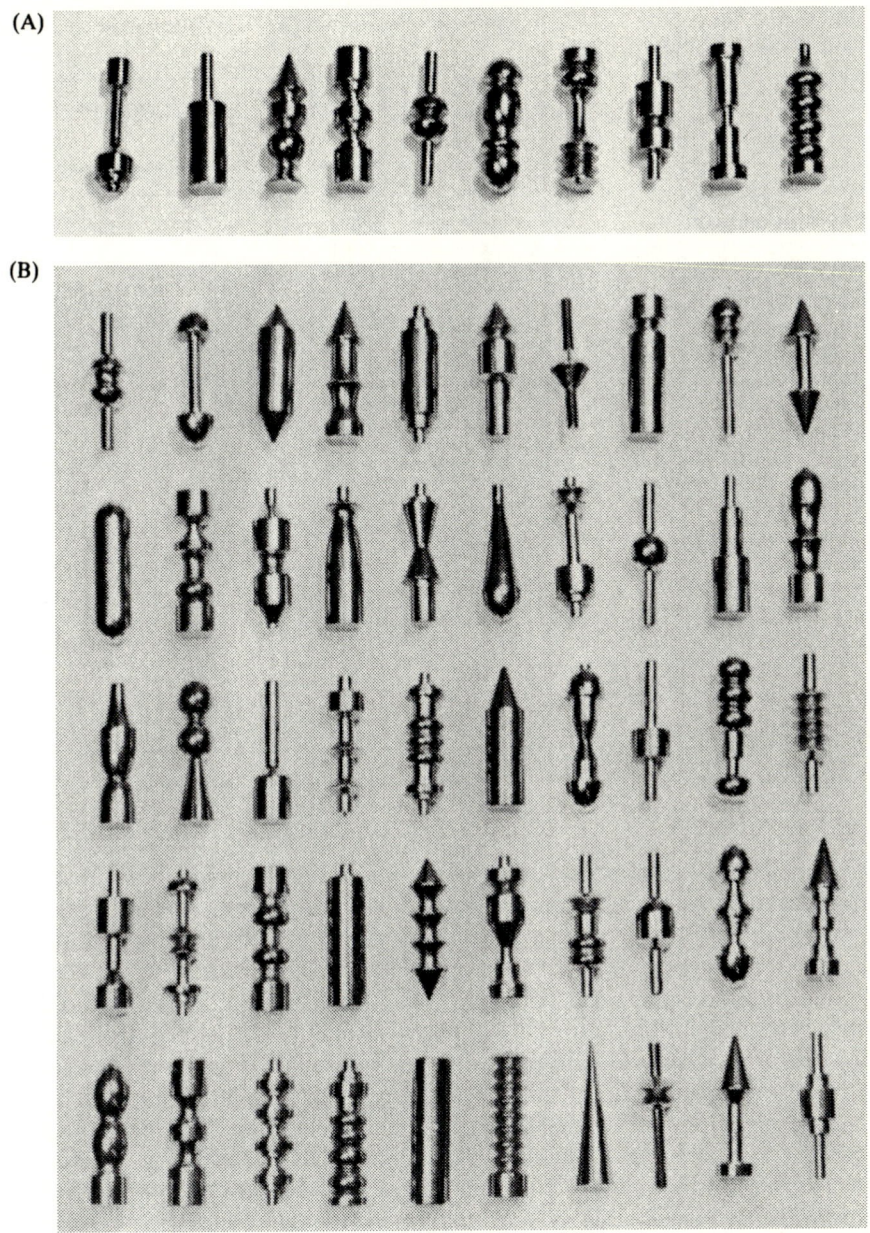

FIGURE 5.1. (A) Tactile stimuli used in the learning experiment. Each object is examined tactually by the right hand for 3.2 s. All objects are made of the same material. They have identical surface and thermal properties and approximately identical weight. Each object is characterized by a specific occurrence of geometrical "letters." (B) The objects that were mixed with the learned objects in the recognition tests. (From Roland, Eriksson, Widén, & Stone-Elander, 1989, by permission of Oxford University Press)

TABLE 5.2 Brain Regions Changing rCBF During Tactile Learning. Mean changes in ml/100 g/min ± SD (8 Subjects)

Region	Right Hemisphere		Left Hemisphere	
	Mean	SD	Mean	SD
Orbitofrontal post.	9.3	7.5	7.6	5.7
Insula ant.	11.0	4.9	10.7	6.9
Insula post.	5.5	6.9	10.5	8.7
Hippocampal compl.	10.0	3.4	6.6	3.7
G. cinguli ant.	16.6	6.5	16.6	6.5
Caudate head	5.7	3.7	13.1	10.7
Caudate-putamen	6.8	6.5	12.8	6.3
Thalamus ventral	10.6	13.2	14.3	12.7
SI hand area	3.1	5.3	16.0	12.0
Supplementary. sens. area	11.4	5.5	10.5	4.8
Lobul. parietalis sup.	6.8	4.3	11.1	4.4
MI hand area	5.7	5.7	21.6	8.8
Supplementary mot. area	8.8	7.4	15.3	8.9
Premotor	12.7	6.4	17.3	7.1
Cerebellum lob. ant.	14.6	7.8	5.6	5.5
Cerebellum lob. post.	11.05	6.8	10.4	4.4
G. frontalis med. 1	6.1	7.9	8.0	6.9
G. frontalis med. 2	7.8	6.1	10.5	10.7
G. frontalis med. 3	9.1	8.2	0.00	8.2
G. frontalis sup.	11.6	5.4	10.3	6.5

post: posterior; ant: anterior; g: gyrus; mot: motor; lob: lobulus; sens: sensory; med: medius; sup: superior.

performed which showed that the subjects retained much, but not all, information (Figure 5.2). There was no learning during the recognition sessions. One PET measurement of rCBF was performed when the volunteers were recognizing the objects. During tactile recognition the frequency of exploratory movements went up to 1.5 Hz. Accordingly $rCMRO_2$ and rCBF was now higher in the motor cortical areas (Roland et al., 1989; Table 5.3). However, the structures being active were, with minor exceptions, the same as those activated during tactile learning. Most remarkable were the quantitative differences between learning and recognition. The caudate and putamen showed statistically significant higher rCBF in learning. The same was the case for the anterior cingulate cortex, and the posterior orbitofrontal cortex (Table 5.3). In the posterior lobes of the cerebellum the $rCMRO_2$ and rCBF were significantly higher during the learning phase, despite the fact that frequency of movements was less during learning. This was interpreted as an extra metabolic demand in the neocerebellar cortex during the learning phase. The process that is most energy demanding in the cerebellar cortex is to restore the ionic equilibrium after climbing fibre activation of the Purkinje cell dendrites (Roland et al., 1989).

The rCBF and $rCMRO_2$ changes preferentially mark the active synaptic

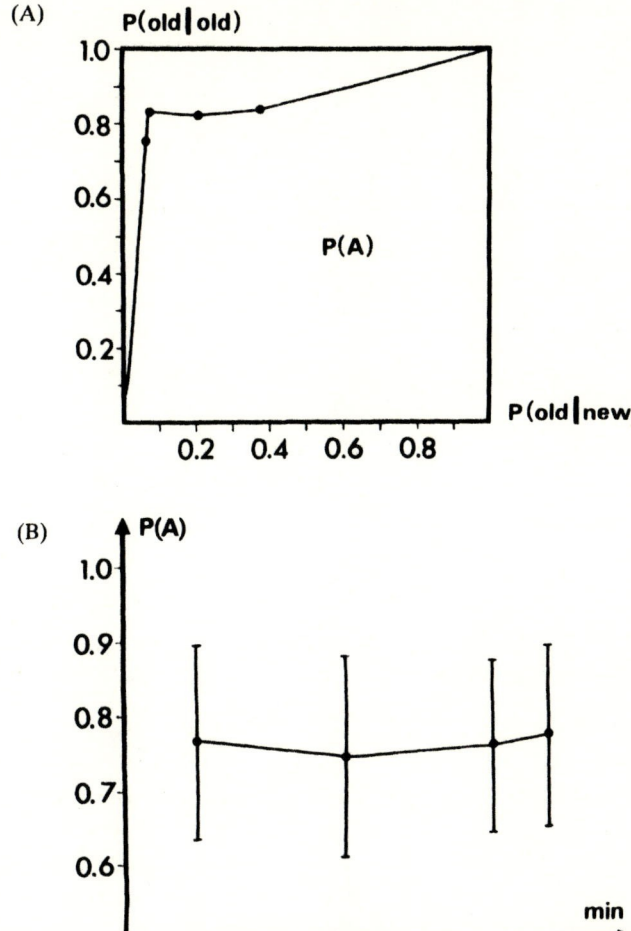

FIGURE 5.2. (A) Receivers operating characteristic from one subject in the four recognition tests. The conditional probabilities were calculated from each recognition session. The amount of retained information was calculated as the area P(A) under the receivers operating characteristic (Green & Swets, 1966). (B) Mean amount of retained information as a function of time during the four recognition tests. Time separations were 40 min, 40 min, and 15 min between tests. (From Roland, Eriksson, Widén, & Stone-Elander, 1989, by permission of Oxford University Press)

sites. The synapses can be activated by intrinsic axon terminals belonging to the anatomical structure increasing its rCBF or $rCMRO_2$, or the synapses can be activated because of increased activity in extrinsic afferents. In the latter case the activated synaptic populations in the cortex and subcortical structures are parts of circuits. Presumably most of the synaptic activation in the cortex, striatum, thalamus, and cerebellum is due to activity in

TABLE 5.3   Differences in rCBF Between Tactile Learning and Tactile Recognition (Positive Values: rCBF More During Learning). Mean Changes in ml/100 g/min ± SD (8 Subjects)

Region	Right Hemisphere		Left Hemisphere	
	Mean	SD	Mean	SD
Oribitofrontal post.	14.3	7.1	5.4	8.1
Hippocampal compl.	2.8	2.0	−2.6	4.0
G. cinguli ant.	6.3	4.8	6.3	4.8
Caudate-putamen	5.5	5.3	4.7	10.1
Thalamus ventral	−0.6	5.7	3.0	7.4
SI hand area	−0.8	6.1	−5.7	6.9
Supplementary sens.	5.9	5.2	3.4	5.5
MI hand area	−8.7	10.4	−4.6	7.9
Supplementary mot.	−5.7	7.0	−1.8	6.5
Premotor	−6.1	7.0	6.7	3.1
Cerebellum lob. post.	5.7	3.6	3.6	5.5

g: gyrus; ant: anterior; mot: motor; sens: sensory; post: posterior.

afferents. If this is the case, one can hypothesize that corticostriatal circuits, corticolimbic circuits, and corticocerebellar circuits are engaged in tactile learning.

VISUAL LEARNING

Very recently, we (Roland et al., 1990) tried to separate the anatomical structures engaged in learning of colored geometrical visual patterns, from those engaged in recall and recognition of the learnt patterns. As in the tactile learning, instruction trials were first given with other stimuli for the purpose of eliminating any learning of the task procedures during the actual experiment. In the actual experiment, during the learning sessions, the subjects looked at 10 colored geometrical patterns with the purpose of learning them. Each pattern was exposed for 10 s covering the field of view. The patterns were always presented in the same order. The PET measurement during learning was made during the second learning session, which took place 3–4 min after the start of the experiment. After 15 learning sessions extending over 50 min, the subjects with their eyes closed recalled the patterns in color in the order they were exposed. In a recognition experiment during which old patterns were mixed with new in ratios between 0.15 and 0.35, it was subsequently evaluated how much information was stored during the learning.

The structures changing rCBF during learning of colored complex geometrical patterns can be divided into (a) the primary visual area in and around the calcarine sulcus; (b) visual association areas; rCBF increases covering the rest of the cuneus, the posterior part of precuneus, the lingual gyrus, the fusiform gyrus, the occipital gyri, the angular gyrus, and the posterior part of the superior parietal lobule; (c) prefrontal cortical regions, especially the cortex lining the superior frontal sulcus and the frontal eye field; (d) limbic and paralimbic structures: the anterior hippocampal formation (but not the posterior), the mediodorsal thalamus (decrease), the anterior cingular cortex, temporal pole, and anterior sector of insula; and (e) the anterior midpart of the neostriatum. These areas are listed in Table 5.4. Learning thus activated the visual areas participating in visual perception and which are responsible for a construction of representation of properties of the stimulus pattern.

When the subjects with their eyes closed *recalled* the images this was accompanied by (a) rCBF increases restricted to the posterior parietal lobe in the precuneus, the superior parietal lobule and the angular gyrus. These areas were a small subset of those activated during learning of the patterns. Neither the primary visual area, nor the remaining visual association areas showed any changes in rCBF. The differences between this nonactivation during recall and the activation during visual learning were statistically significant; (b) prefrontal regions, which, with the exception of the frontal eye fields, were other than those activated during learning; and (c) in contrast to the changes during learning, both the anterior cingulate cortex, posterior cingulate cortex, and the posterior hippocampus were activated. The remote visual association areas in the posterior parietal lobe extending from the precuneus on the mesial side over the posterior part of the superior parietal lobule to the angular gyrus on the lateral side were activated as the only visual areas. These remote visual association areas were the only visual areas activated during both learning and recall. The increased rCBF in these remote visual association areas is a measure of increased synaptic metabolism here during recall. This increase is most likely related to the recall of the stored visual patterns, because recall of familiar surroundings also selectively activates these fields among the visual areas in man (Roland & Friberg, 1985; Roland et al., 1987). It is therefore tempting to suggest that they constitute the storage sites for the learned patterns.

From the synaptic populations activated during visual learning one can assume that corticolimbic circuits and corticostriatal circuits were active during visual learning. Furthermore, it is obvious that recall of the stored patterns must rely on different mechanisms than learning of the patterns, since the anatomical sectors engaged in the recall differed from those engaged during learning, with the exceptions of the possible storage sites, the anterior cingulate cortex, and the frontal eye fields.

DIFFERENCES BETWEEN MOTOR LEARNING AND COGNITIVE LEARNING

If one accepts motor sequence learning as a typical exponent for skill learning and visual learning of colored patterns a typical exponent for

TABLE 5.4   Mean Change in rCBF During Visual Learning, Recall, and Recognition in 11 Subjects

Region	Learning (L)			Recall (RC)			Recognition (RN)		
	cm³	ΔrCBF	SD	cm³	ΔrCBF	SD	cm³	ΔrCBF	SD
Calcarine R	6.5	20.8	2.4*†	6.5	2.6	2.7	6.5	8.7	3.4*†
Calcarine L	3.4	19.4	1.9*†	3.4	−0.2	1.6	3.4	9.9	2.9*†
Cuneus R§	10.5	12.0	2.2*†	10.5	1.3	1.9	7.4	7.4	2.7*†
Cuneus L§	13.2	12.3	2.1*†	13.2	0.9	2.4	10.4	7.6	2.5*†
Gyri occipitales R§	11.3	8.0	1.8*†	11.3	1.2	2.1	9.1	6.4	1.6*†
Gyri occipitales L§	9.4	8.3	1.6*†	9.4	1.5	1.8	8.3	6.6	1.7*†
Sulc. parieto-occ. R§	13.1	9.0	1.6*†	13.1	1.5	1.9	6.3	8.0	1.9*†
Sulc. parieto-occ. L§	10.9	8.6	1.9*†	10.9	2.6	2.0	9.4	7.8	2.0*†
Precuneus R§	3.4	7.1	1.9*†	3.4	1.8	2.8	3.4	2.7	3.0
Precuneus L§	3.4	6.5	1.3*†	3.4	1.5	2.0	3.4	6.3	0.9*†
Lobulus parietalis sup. post. part R§	7.9	8.4	1.6*†	2.9	7.2	1.2*†	5.9	8.3	2.0*†
Lobulus parietalis sup. post.part L§	8.4	7.4	1.3*†	1.2	6.3	0.9*†	5.8	6.8	1.7*†
Gy. temp. inf. post part + fusiform gyrus R§	11.7	6.8	1.1*†	11.7	1.4	1.3	11.7	7.6	1.1*†
Gy. temp. inf. post part + fusiform gyrus L§	6.6	5.7	1.8*†	6.6	3.0	2.0	6.6	6.6	1.9*†
Angular gyrus R	5.0	6.9	0.8*†	1.2	7.8	1.2*†	1.2	6.4	1.3*†
Angular gyrus L	5.3	6.8	0.3*†	2.0	7.5	0.8*†	2.0	7.6	0.6*†
Temporal pole R	2.5	6.9	1.1*†	2.5	2.3	2.7	2.5	4.5	1.2
Temporal pole L	3.7	8.6	1.3*†	3.7	3.6	1.6	3.7	−1.9	2.7

Gyrus cinguli ant. R	1.6	5.9	0.7*†	1.6	7.7	1.5*†	1.6	6.7	1.8*†
Gyrus cinguli ant. L	2.5	5.2	2.3	2.5	8.2	1.4*†	2.5	5.7	0.5*†
Gyrus cinguli post. R	1.3	4.9	1.0	1.3	7.1	0.8*†	1.3	7.3	0.4*†
Gyrus front. medius R	3.4	4.4	0.8	3.4	7.1	0.4*†	3.4	5.7	0.3*†
Gyrus front. medius L	2.8	4.0	0.4	2.8	6.7	0.3*†	2.8	5.7	0.3*†
Sup. frontal sulcus	1.8	6.9	1.5†	1.8	3.7	0.9	1.8	4.1	0.8
Sup. frontal sulcus	2.1	5.9	0.9*	2.1	4.0	0.7	2.1	2.4	0.4
Frontal eye field R	1.6	2.3	2.2	1.6	6.5	1.2†	1.6	5.4	1.6*
Frontal eye field L	3.1	5.7	0.9*†	2.4	7.5	0.9*†	2.4	7.3	1.5*†
Frontoparietal operculum R§	9.3	−3.8	2.2	9.3	−4.2	1.3†	9.3	−7.4	1.5*†
Frontoparietal operculum L§	7.8	−2.9	2.4	7.8	−2.4	1.4	7.8	−5.6	0.9*†
Thalamus dorsomed. R	1.5	−4.5	1.2*†	1.5	−0.6	2.6	1.5	1.0	1.9
Thalamus dorsomed. L	1.2	−4.1	1.3†	1.2	0.9	0.6	1.2	2.2	0.5
Thalamus post. R	1.5	0.9	1.7	1.5	3.4	1.2	1.5	6.8	1.1*†
Thalamus post. L	1.2	3.1	1.0	1.2	4.9	2.6	1.2	6.9	1.7*†
Caudate nucl. R	2.1	−4.8	0.3*†	2.1	−1.4	1.4	2.1	0.1	3.2
Caudate nucl. L	1.0	−3.6	1.3	1.0	4.6	1.3	1.0	−2.3	0.2
Putamen R	1.0	−4.1	0.4*†	1.0	−1.0	2.0	1.0	−0.3	2.2
Putamen L	1.8	−6.2	0.4*†	1.8	−1.4	0.9	1.8	−0.9	2.2
Hippocampal formation ant. R	1.8	7.8	1.0*†	1.8	1.9	1.4	1.8	3.7	1.6
Hippocampal formation ant. L	1.9	7.0	1.8*†	1.9	1.3	1.1	1.9	4.6	1.5
Hippocampal formation post. R	1.0	1.9	3.2	1.0	5.4	0.8*†	1.0	4.6	0.7*†
Hippocampal formation post. L	1.0	1.8	1.8	1.0	5.5	0.6*†	1.0	5.3	0.3*†

R: right; L: left; sup: superior; post: posterior; inf: inferior; ant: anterior; sul: sulcus; gy: gyrus; front: frontal; nucl: nucleus. * Areas of change having t > 2.3 between rest and test; † Areas of change in which a spot of activity was found with mean changes consistently > 5.0 ml/100 g/min in all resampled populations. The SD denotes the standard deviation of the mean changes across 0.5 cm^3 voxels. § Denotes a composite region consisting of several activated fields. The total volume of activated tissue is shown for each structure.

cognitive learning, the computerized atlas version of the data permit a direct subtraction between the mean rCBF picture during visual learning and the mean rCBF picture during motor learning. Both measurements were performed at the same level of learning, approximately 3 min after the start of learning. Differences between the two conditions can occur because of decreases or increases of rCBF in one of the conditions. Of course, the major differences between the two conditions were that motor cortical areas were activated in motor learning and visual cortical areas in visual learning. More interesting were the differences in limbic, paralimbic and subcortical sectors of the brain. For the present evaluation descriptive *t*-maps were made of the subtraction picture and the analysis concentrated on limbic, striatal, and cerebellar regions, which were predefined in the previous evaluation of the changes in motor learning and visual learning (Tables 5.1 and 5.4). All regions covered more than three independent pixels and changes were considered significant if the *t*-value exceeded 2.3 throughout the predefined region.

The structures which had *increases* of rCBF in *visual learning* but not in motor learning were: the hippocampus–parahippocampal gyrus, the temporal pole, the anterior cingular cortex, and the ventral striatum. Although the decreases in rCBF in these structures were not all significant during motor learning, the difference between motor learning and visual learning was significant. This deactivation in motor learning and activation in visual learning is a strong indication of the different roles of these limbic and paralimbic structures in motor learning and cognitive learning.

One structure which *selectively increases* rCBF during *motor learning* but in which rCBF was unchanged during visual learning was the right anterior lobe of cerebellum. This demonstrates the selectivity of the corticocerebellar circuit in motor learning. The right anterior lobe of the cerebellum and the left ventrolateral thalamus were selectively activated in motor learning. These structures are probably part of a circuit extending from the motor cortices in the left hemisphere to the right anterior lobe of cerebellum, to the ventrolateral thalamus and back to the primary motor cortex.

Finally, the putamen and globus pallidus showed decreases in motor learning, as well as in visual learning. However, in the subtraction picture the center of the decrease in visual learning was 5 mm anterior to the center of the decrease in motor learning. Taking the accuracy of the localization in the mean pictures into account (see methods section) one may conclude that different sectors of the striatum change activity in visual and motor learning and that the sector modulating activity in motor learning may be the arm–hand sector, which is thus posterior to the sector involved in visual learning. Thus, during motor learning the putamen–pallidum decreases its activity initially, probably as a part of the motor cortex–putamen–pallidum–ventralis lateralis loop. That cognitive learning may also make use of a prefrontal striatal loop is remarkable and not foreseen in the current theories of cognitive learning. There is, however, an observation by Buerger,

Gross, & Rocha-Miranda (1974) showing that destruction of the putamen impaired visual discrimination learning in monkeys.

Striatal changes in rCBF or rCMR (regional cerebral metabolic rate) are not specific for learning (Mazziotta, Phelps, & Wapenski, 1985; Roland et al., 1987, 1989; Seitz, Roland, Bohm, Greitz, & Stone-Elander, 1989). Since the rCBF and rCMR measurements during learning by necessity are taken before the measurements during recognition of the learnt material, one might think that changes in attention might explain the differences between learning and recognition. However, the EEG recordings showed no differences in attentive parameters between learning and recognition. The changes in rCBF and rCMR recorded in motor learning, tactile learning, and visual learning took place during the 1–1.5 h period during which the material to be learned became stored in the brain. Exposure of similar stimuli that were already learnt or execution of movements already learnt did not cause the quantitative changes in the striatum revealed during the learning phase (Roland et al., 1987, 1989, 1990; Seitz et al., 1989). Moreover, the modulations of rCBF and rCMR were limited to structures in the limbic, striatal, and cerebellar divisions of the central nervous system. The limbic structures showed no modulation during motor learning and neither did the cerebellar structures during visual learning, recall, and recognition. It is thus reasonable to assume that the structures modulating their activity in the time period of the visual learning phase had something to do with the governing of the storage of visual cognitive information. Similarly it is reasonable to propose that the structures modulating their activity during the motor learning phase promoted the storage of the final successful motor program. According to current views there are many parallel corticostriatal circuits. The spatial resolution of the computerized atlas makes it possible to identify different sectors of the striatum engaged in cognitive and motor learning. Still higher resolution is required to dissect the major divisions of the thalamus.

In summary, motor learning of the type examined here relies on two sets of anatomical structures organized in a corticostriatothalamocortical circuit and a corticocerebellorubrothalamic circuit. Visual learning relies on limbic circuits involving the (anterior) hippocampal region, the temporal pole and the cingular cortex, and probably a corticostriatal circuit as well. The parts of the striatum engaged in visual learning and motor learning are separate. Tactile learning seemed to be a transitional form between motor learning and cognitive learning, since it relied upon corticocerebellar circuits, corticostriatal circuits, as well as corticolimbic circuits.

Acknowledgments: The research reported in this chapter was supported by grants from the Soderberg Foundation, The Karolinska Institute, and Deutsche Forschungs-gemeinshaft.

REFERENCES

Bergström, M., Boetius, J., Eriksson, L., Greitz, T., & Widén, L. (1981). Head fixation device for reproducible position alignment in transmission CT and positron emission tomography. *Journal of Computer Assisted Tomography, 5,* 136–141.

Bohm, C., Greitz, T., Blomqvist, G., Fardoe, L., Forsgren, P. O., & Kingsley, D. (1986). Applications of a computerized adjustable brain atlas in positron emission tomography. *Acta Radiologica Supplementum, 369,* 449–452.

Brinkman, C., & Porter, R. (1983). Supplementary motor area and premotor area of monkey cerebral cortex: functional organization and activities of single neurons during performance of a learned movement. *Advances in Neurology, 39,* 393–420.

Buerger, A. A., Gross, C. G., & Rocha-Miranda, C. E. (1974). Effects of ventral putamen lesions on discrimination learning in monkeys. *Journal of Comparative and Physiological Psychology, 86,* 440–466.

Corkin, S. (1968). Acquisition of motor skill after bilateral medial temporal excision. *Neuropsychologia, 6,* 255–265.

DeLong, M. (1972). Activity of basal ganglia neurons during movement. *Brain Research, 40,* 127–135.

Eriksson, L., Bohm, C., Kesselberg, M., & Holte, S. (1988). An automated blood sampling system used in positron emission tomography. *Nuclear Sciences Applications, 3,* 133–143.

Feller, W. (1968). *An introduction to probability theory and its applications.* (p. 508). New York: Wiley.

Freund, H. H. (1986). Time control of hand movements. *Progress in Brain Research, 64,* 287–294.

Ginsberg, M. D., Dietrich, W. D., & Busto, R. (1987). Coupled forebrain increases of local cerebral glucoze utilization and blood flow during physiologic stimulation of a somatosensory pathway in the rat: demonstration by double-label autoradiography. *Neurology, 37,* 11–19.

Green, D. M., & Swets, J. A. (1966). *Signal detection theory and psychophysics.* (p. 465). New York: Wiley.

Greenberg, J., Hand, P., Sylvestro, A., & Reivich, M. (1979). Localized metabolic-flow couple during functional activity. *Acta Neurologica Scandinavica, 60,* (Suppl. 72), 12–13.

Greitz, T., Bohm, C., Holte, S., & Eriksson, L. (1991). A computerized brain atlas: construction, anatomical content, and some applications. *Journal of Computer Assisted Tomography, 15,* 26–38.

Hikosaka, O., & Wurtz, R. H. (1983). Visual and oculomotor functions of the monkey substantia nigra pars reticulata. III. Memory contingent visual and saccade responses. *Journal of Neurophysiology, 49,* 1268–1285.

Holden, J. E., Gatley, S. J.., Hichwa, R. D., Ip, W. R., Shaughnessy, W. J., Nickles, R. J., & Polcyn, R. E. (1981). Cerebral blood flow using PET measurements of fluoromethane kinetics. *Journal of Nuclear Medicine, 22,* 1084–1088.

Johnson, R. A., & Wichern, D. W. (1982). *Applied multivariate statistical analysis.* (p. 420). New Jersey: Englewood Cliffs.

Koeppe, R. A., Holden, J. E., & Ip, W. R. (1985). Performance of parameter estimation techniques for the quantification of local cerebral blood flow by dynamic positron computed tomography. *Journal of Cerebral Blood Flow and Metabolism, 5,* 224–234.

Litton, J-E., Bergström, M., Eriksson, L., Bohm, C., & Blomqvist, B. (1984). Performance study of the PC384 positron camera system for emission tomography of the brain. *Journal of Computer Assisted Tomography, 8,* 74–87.

Mazziotta, J., Phelphs, M. E., & Wapenski, J. A. (1985). Human cerebral motor system in health and disease. *Journal of Cerebral Blood Flow and Metabolism, 5,* (Suppl. 1), S213–214.

Olesen, J., Paulson, O., & Lassen, N. A. (1971). Regional cerebral blood flow in man determined by the initial slope of the clearance of interarterially injected ^{133}Xe. *Stroke, 2,* 519–540.

Roland, P. E. (1985). Application of imaging of brain blood flow to behavorial neurophysiology: the cortical field activation hypothesis. In L. Sokoloff (Ed.), *Brain imaging and brain function.* (pp. 87–106). New York: Raven Press.

Roland, P. E., Eriksson, L., Stone-Elander, S., & Widén, L. (1987). Does mental activity change the oxidative metabolism of the brain? *Journal of Neuroscience, 7,* 2373–2389.

Roland, P. E., Eriksson, L., Widén, L., & Stone-Elander, S. (1989). Changes in regional cerebral oxidative metabolism induced by tactile learning and recognition in man. *European Journal of Neuroscience, 1,* 3–18.

Roland, P. E., & Friberg, L. (1985). Localization of cortical areas activated by thinking. *Journal of Neurophysiology, 53,* 1219–1243.

Roland, P. E., Gulyás, B., Seitz, R. J., Bohm, C., & Stone-Elander, S. (1990). Functional anatomy of storage, recall, and recognition of a visual pattern in man. *NeuroReport, 1,* 53–56.

Roland, P. E., & Larsen, B. (1976). Focal increase of cerebral blood flow during stereognostic testing in man. *Archives of Neurology, 33,* 551–558.

Roland, P. E., Larsen, B., Lassen, N. A., & Skinhöj, E. (1980). Supplementary motor area and other cortical areas in the organization of voluntary movements in man. *Journal of Neurophysiology, 43,* 118–136.

Roland, P. E., & Mortensen, E. (1987). Somatosensory detection of icrogeometry, macrogeometry and kinesthesia in man. *Brain Research Reviews, 12,* 1–42.

Sasaki, K., & Gemba, H. (1982). Development and change of cortical field potentials during learning processes of visually initiated hand movements. *Experimental Brain Research, 48,* 429.

Scoville, W. B., & Milner, B. (1957). Loss of recent memory after bilateral hippocampal lesions. *Journal of Neurology, Neurosurgery and Psychiatry, 20,* 11–21.

Seitz, R. J., Bohm, C., Greitz, T., Roland, P. E., Eriksson, L., Blomqvist, G., Rosenqvist, G., & Nordell, B. (1990). Accuracy and precision of the computerized brain atlas programme for localization and quantification in positron emission tomography. *Journal of Cerebral Blood Flow and Metabolism, 10,* 443–457.

Seitz, R. J., Roland, P. E., Bohm, C., Greitz, T., & Stone-Elander, S. (1991). Somato-sensory discrimination of shape: Tactile exploration and cerebral activation. *European Journal of Neuroscience, 3,* 481–492.

Seitz, R. J., Roland, P. E., Bohm, C., Greitz, T., & Stone-Elander, S. (1990). Motor learning in man: a positron emission tomographic study. *NeuroReport, 1,* 57–60.

Squire, L. R. (1987). *Memory and brain.* (p. 315). New York: Oxford University Press.

Squire, L. R., & More, R. Y. (1979). Dorsal thalamic lesion in a noted case of human memory dysfunction. *Annals of Neurology, 6,* 503–506.

6

Does Synaptic Selection Explain Auditory Imprinting?

HENNING SCHEICH
E. WALLHÄUSSER-FRANKE
K. BRAUN

Ever since it was recognized that synaptic plasticity could be a basic correlate of learning and memory, "growth theories" have dominated this field of research (see McGeer, Eccles, & McGeer, 1978, chapter 15; Rosenzweig, Møllgaard, Diamond & Bennet, 1972). It appears to be common intuition that storage of new information in the brain should correspond to some "additive process" at the substrate level, anything from synaptic strengthening to formation of new synapses. Seminal theories like Hebb's (1949) favored this view. Findings, such as long-term potentiation (LTP) (Bliss & Lømo, 1973; Gustafsson and Wigström, 1988), synaptic learning in *Aplysia* (Abrams & Kandel, 1988), and cortical synapse formation after environmental enrichment (Greenough & Bailey, 1988) have strengthened the point. Consequently, computer models of associative networks have adopted differential strengthening of connections as a basic mechanism (Hopfield, 1982; Linsker, 1988; Palm, 1981; Sejnowski & Rosenberg, 1987).

Nevertheless, it has been pointed out that information could also be specified and stored by subtractive processes at synaptic sites, from weakening of transmission to loss of connectivities (Changeux & Danchin, 1976; Changeux, Heidmann, & Patte, 1984; Rosenzweig et al., 1972). Recent results in cortex slices suggest that long-term depression (LTD) is a phenomenon as common after tetanization of inputs as long-term potentiation (LTP) (Artola, Bröcher, & Singer, 1990). This chapter focuses on the working hypothesis that, at least for imprinting, regression of synapses is an integral if not the most significant aspect of the synaptic changes that accompany this type of learning as it could explain the largely irreversible nature of imprinting.

Since the classical description by Lorenz (1935), imprinting is considered *a juvenile learning process by which an individual acquires a lasting behavioral preference for a stimulus pattern through experience during a sensitive phase.*

Imprinting as a special type of learning has received broad attention from ethologists (for reviews see Bateson, 1981; Hess, 1973; Immelmann & Suomi, 1981; Marler, 1987). In visual and auditory filial imprinting in birds (for reviews see Bradley & Horn, 1987; Horn, 1985; Scheich, 1987; Scheich & Braun, 1988) and in vocal learning in song-birds (for reviews see Arnold, Bottjer, Nordeen, Nordeen, & Sengelaub, 1987; Konishi, 1985, Margoliash, 1987; Nottebohm, 1984; Scheich & Braun, 1988), progress has been made in defining relevant brain circuits and neural correlates of this learning type.

Several of Lorenz's numerous criteria for distinguishing filial imprinting from other types of learning are not generally applicable to the different imprinting phenomena that are hitherto known. Following in part revisions made by Lorenz (Bateson, 1979, 1981, 1987; Immelmann & Suomi, 1981; Rauschecker & Marler, 1987; Scheich, 1987), we emphasize here four behavioral criteria, for reasons which will become apparent in the sections on brain mechanisms:

1. *Stimulus selection occurs on the basis of temporal priority during a sensitive phase.* As it matters chiefly to which pattern an individual is exposed first, there seems to be lack of behavioral feedback confirming or disproving species-specific usefulness of the pattern. In some forms of imprinting (sexual imprinting, song learning, olfactory imprinting in salmon), this is emphasized by a long interval between stimulus learning and its first control of the specific behavior.
2. *For each species and each imprinting phenomenon a more or less species-specific disposition exists*, which guides the choice of an imprinting stimulus beside priority. In that way each individual develops a preference for relatively narrow stimulus specifications within a broader species-relevant frame of options.
3. *Once a stimulus is selected by an individual a strong preference is established after the sensitive phase.* Later experiences may replace the imprinted stimulus to some extent but if the individual has the choice the earlier preference reappears (irreversibility). Revision of earlier preference due to new stimuli is optional, however, under some circumstances during the sensitive phase.
4. *Schedule and duration of the sensitive phase depend on the type of imprinting*—for example, filial, olfactory, sexual imprinting, auditory phase of song learning, and so forth—and are species specific. While the beginning of the sensitive phase is governed by internal, presumably genetic, mechanisms, the duration of the time window also depends on external influences.

While these four criteria together make imprinting a separate category of learning, it appears that phenomena under this heading are quite heterogeneous and some are far more complex than an establishment of a stimulus–response relationship. It awaits clarification in each behavioral complex that is modified by imprinting whether criteria of the numerous other forms of memory that have been proposed are also applicable, for example, associative versus nonassociative, procedural versus declarative memory (Squire, 1982), habit versus memory (Hirsh, 1974), and so forth (see Sherry & Schacter, 1987). For instance, learning by simple exposure as seen in imprinting is reminiscent of episodic memory (Tulving, 1985). Operational criteria such as *sensitive phase, learning by first exposure*, and *resistance against revision* are stringent and may be as useful for a search of underlying mechanisms of imprinting as *critical stimulus pairing* and *extinction* are for Pavlovian conditioning, or *delayed discrimination* is for cognitive learning (Mishkin & Petri, 1983). Especially the largely irreversible nature of the result of imprinting after the sensitive phase suggests radical events at the synaptic level.

AUDITORY FILIAL IMPRINTING IN 2-DEOXYGLUCOSE EXPERIMENTS

Auditory imprinting of Guinea fowl and domestic chicks can be achieved simply by playing a rhythmic pure tone for extended periods to social groups of hatchlings kept together in a nest. Individual chicks subsequently run in a Y-shaped maze towards a loudspeaker emitting the imprinted sound (approach test) and prefer the imprinted sound over a discrimination stimulus presented simultaneously from the other loudspeaker (discrimination test: stimulus with different frequency and rhythm) (Braun, 1980; Maier & Scheich, 1983, 1987; Wallhäusser & Scheich, 1987). The sensitive phase for auditory imprinting of this type is 4 days after hatching. Rhythmic pure tones are adequate stimuli provided they are below 1 kHz in domestic and below 3 kHz in Guinea fowl chicks.

Imprinting with such simple tone patterns opened up the possibility to search the auditory system for neuronal correlates of learning as the tonotopic organization of central nuclei of the auditory pathway is well known in gallinaceous birds (Bonke, Scheich, & Langner, 1979; Heil & Scheich, 1985; Scheich, 1991; Scheich, Bonke, Bonke, & Langner, 1979). At present the most comprehensive way to analyze representation of tones in tonotopic maps is the 2-deoxyglucose (2-DG) autoradiographic method introduced by Sokoloff (1975). Glucose consumption of neurons chiefly depends on the activity of the sodium pump, thus on their electrical activity (Mata et al., 1980). The glucose analogue 2-DG is not distinguished by the membrane transport mechanisms of neurons and is therefore incorporated into cells dependent on its relative concentration in the blood. Upon phosphorylation, further 2-DG metabolism is blocked. 2-DG accumulates intracellularly with time as a function of neural activity and can be measured autoradiographically with sufficient resolution in brain sections when 2-DG is tagged with ^{14}C. The method has been used in a number of mammals and birds to study tonotopic maps (Heil & Scheich, 1985; Ryan, Woolf, & Sharp, 1982; Scheich et al., 1979; Webster, Servière, Crewther, & Crewther,

1984). After an exposure of 45–90 min, repetitive tones at one frequency are represented as a labeled frequency band lamina of increased 2-DG activity in those structures of a brain where best frequencies of neurons are laid out in an orderly fashion (tonotopy).

The application of the method in our studies covered various age groups of securely imprinted Guinea fowl and domestic chicks to which their imprinting stimulus was played back in 2-DG experiments after extensive behavioral tests (Maier & Scheich, 1983, 1987; Scheich, 1987; Wallhäusser & Scheich, 1987). Chicks were stimulated separately for 45 min under ambient lighting in small pens placed in sound-proof boxes. Naive controls of the same age listened to the imprinting stimulus of the corresponding experimental groups. In none of these groups was a clear difference of tonotopic labeling found between experimental and control animals. The chief target of this analysis was field L, which is the auditory cortex analogue of birds in the caudal telencephalon (Bonke, Bonke, & Scheich, 1979; Heil & Scheich, 1986; Karten, 1968). Field L showed a similarly prominent tone-induced frequency band lamina of 2-DG activity in experimental and control animals. We concluded from this result that the primary auditory system does not contain a "memory trace" detectable with the 2-DG method after auditory imprinting. This is remarkable, as the whole auditory pathway, including auditory cortex, showed a frequency-specific increase of 2-DG uptake in the rat after classical aversive tone conditioning (Gonzalez-Lima & Scheich, 1984, 1986).

In contrast to the auditory system, several rostral areas of the telencephalon with hitherto undetermined functional properties showed patterns of increased 2-DG uptake in imprinted chicks but not in naive controls (Figure 6.1). The strongly labeled rostral forebrain areas are: (a) the rostral Wulst, covering the layers hyperstriatum accessorium dorsally through hyperstriatum dorsale in the depth (together termed HAD); (b) a medial part of rostral neostriatum including a small strip of dorsally adjacent hyperstriatum ventrale (MNH); and (c) an area in neostriatum and hyperstriatum ventrale located dorsally and laterally adjacent to the visual ectostriatum (LNH). A few other brain structures, connected to MNH, showed moderate increase of 2-DG uptake at Day 7 in related experiments (see below).

After imprinting on the day of hatching, playback of tones to the chicks induced strong labeling patterns in MNH, LNH, and HAD reliably by Day 7 (after the sensitive phase) but rarely by Day 4 or earlier. Interestingly, playback of the tones to "unimprintable" chicks, which failed in tests (usually 30%) but had all the stimulus experience, did not produce the strong labeling patterns on Day 7. In this sense they were similar to naive controls on Day 7 (Maier & Scheich, 1983). Also, the labeling in the three areas was weaker when in controls a tone pattern was used for playback with a rhythm and a frequency somewhat different from the imprinted pattern. The labeling patterns in the rostral forebrain in mediolateral and rostrocaudal directions

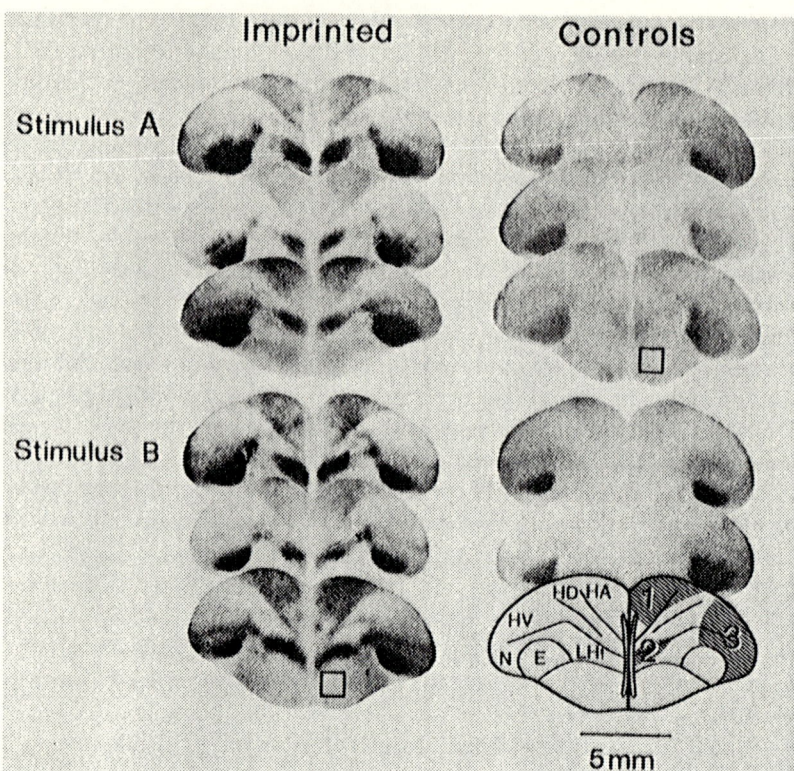

FIGURE 6.1. 2-Deoxyglucose labeling of rostral brain areas of 7-day-old socially raised domestic chicks after listening 45 min to rhythmic tones of 400 Hz (row A) and 900 Hz (row B). Transverse sections are shown from six imprinted chicks and five naive controls. Imprinted animals listened to their imprinting stimulus while controls listened to the same stimulus for the first time. Areas with significant labeling differences are hatched in the scheme at the bottom right: 1, HAD; 2, MNH; 3, LNH. Other symbols are: E, visual ectostriatum; N, lateral neostriatum; HV, hyperstriatum ventrale; LH, lamina hyperstriatica separating neostriatum and HV; HD, hyperstriatum dorsale; HA, hyperstriatum accessorium, both in the Wulst. (From Wallhäusser & Scheich, 1987)

had sharp boundaries (Figures 6.1 and 6.2), even though they cut dorsoventrally across some cytoarchitectural divisions that are traditionally used to parcellate the noncorticate bird telencephalon (see below).

FUNCTIONAL PROPERTIES AND CONNECTIONS OF MNH

Of the three areas, MNH showed the strongest labeling on playback of the imprinted tone pattern. Several lines of evidence from our laboratory suggest that it is the structure most relevant for the auditory aspects of the imprinting

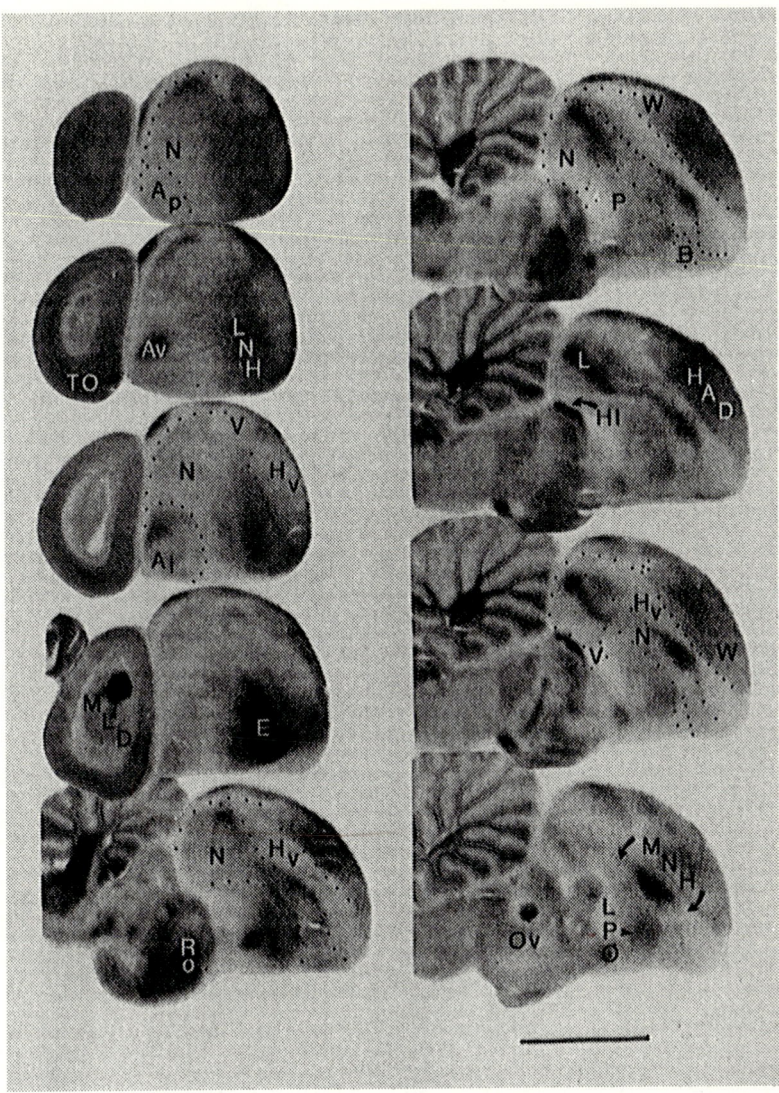

FIGURE 6.2.   2-DG autoradiographs of serial sagittal sections through one hemisphere of a 7-day-old chick exposed from a distance to the sight and vocalizations of a group of known cage mates. Order from top left to bottom right corresponds to lateromedial sequence. The emphasis is on the rostrocaudal location of the strongly labeled MNH (between arrows) in the last two sections on the right. Laminae separating subdivisions of the forebrain are indicated by pointed lines. Other symbols are: LPO, lobus parolfactorius; Ov, auditory nucleus ovoidalis in thalamus; W, wulst; Hv, hyperstriatum ventrale; N, neostriatum; V, ventricle; Hl, lateral habenula; HAD, specifically labeled Wulst-layers; L, auditory field L; P, palaeostriatum; B, nucleus basalis; Ro, visual thalamic nucleus rotundus; E, visual ectostriatum; MLD, mesencephalic auditory nucleus; Ai, archistriatum intermedium; TO, tectum opticum; Av, archistriatum ventrale; Ap, archistriatum posterius; LNH, specifically labeled lateral neostriatum. Scale bar 1 cm. (From Müller, 1987)

paradigm. Microelectrode recordings in awake domestic chicks (M. Sperl, in Scheich, 1987) revealed auditory units in MNH that were preferentially tuned to frequencies below 1kHz, the range relevant for auditory imprinting (Figure 6.3). Other units showed high spontaneous and often bursting activity. They responded with initial suppression and delayed excitation to a wide range of frequencies. Still other units fired concomitant with the chick's own distress vocalizations, which naturally serve in acoustic communication with a mother or siblings out of sight.

2-DG experiments in unilaterally blindfolded chicks with cage mates serving as natural visual and acoustic stimuli produced asymmetric labeling of HAD and LNH but symmetric labeling of MNH in the two hemispheres (Figure 6.4). Visual activity in HAD and LNH is not surprising as parts of these areas include, and are rostrally adjacent to, ectostriatal belt and visual Wulst, targets of the two telencephalic visual pathways in birds (Shimizu & Karten, 1991). In contrast, playback of cage mate vocalizations to chicks in the dark produced strong bilateral labeling of MNH and reduced labeling of HAD and LNH. This suggests that HAD and LNH receive a visual input, while MNH is the chief target of auditory information (Müller, 1987; Müller & Scheich, 1986; Scheich, 1987).

It follows from these results on differential sensory input to the three areas, that playback of the auditory stimulus pattern to chicks imprinted on an acoustic stimulus alone should have activated MNH but not necessarily the two other more visually driven areas. That coactivation takes place in the absence of a visually imprinted stimulus may be an indication of interesting system properties which gear these areas together by direct or indirect connections. In a biological sense this is meaningful as both visual and auditory cues together usually secure the contact of a chick to a parent (Dyer & Gottlieb, 1990).

The functional role of MNH within a system of brain structures that learn the relevant stimulus pattern and control the behavior (following) has been further elucidated with pathway tracing and lesion techniques. Four main connections of MNH (Figure 6.5) were found (Wallhäusser-Franke, 1989; Wallhäusser-Franke & Scheich, in preparation). There is a strong input from dorsomedial thalamic nuclei (DMP/DMA). Inputs from DMP/DMA to the area of MNH have also been reported from other bird species (Kitt & Brauth, 1982; Wild, 1987a). The input from dorsomedial thalamus is also most relevant in the sense that it defines the spatial extent of the neostriatal part of MNH (Figure 6.6). Thus, the 2-DG labeling pattern and the thalamic input converge and allow an exact localization of MNH (compare Figures 6.2 and 6.6). Other inputs are from scattered cells in the midbrain reticular formation including locus coeruleus. The chief output structures of MNH are the intermediate archistriatum (Ai), presumably a motor area (Zeier & Karten, 1971), and a dorsocaudal area in the neostriatum (Ndc), which receives input from the auditory field L (Bonke, Bonke, & Scheich, 1979). Ndc also projects back to MNH and therefore may be the source of its auditory input. Ndc is probably an association/premotor area (Wallhäusser-

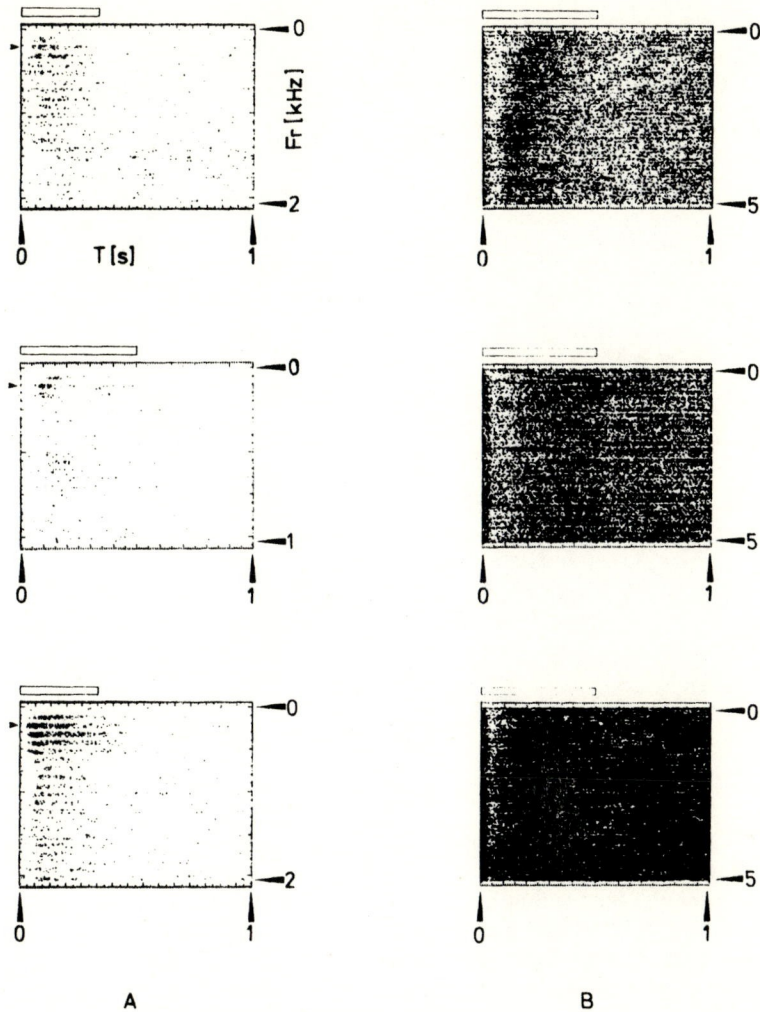

FIGURE 6.3. Frequency responses of auditory units found in MNH of awake young chicks. Point plots represent spike events during a period of 1 s, which starts with a 300 or 500 ms presentation of different tone frequencies. Upper frequency limits of tests were 1, 2, or 5 kHz in the different insets. Presentation of tones was in pseudorandom order with four repetitions each. First row of points (0 kHz) represents spontaneous activity. To the left (A), three units with on-responses and narrow tuning to frequencies below 500 Hz are shown. Bars above insets represent tone duration. To the right (B), three units are shown with high spontaneous activity, short on-suppression of activity followed by delayed on-activation. Such units were often "burster" and the lever of response was not frequency specific but the duration of the on-suppression (first and third unit) (M. Sperl, unpublished data).

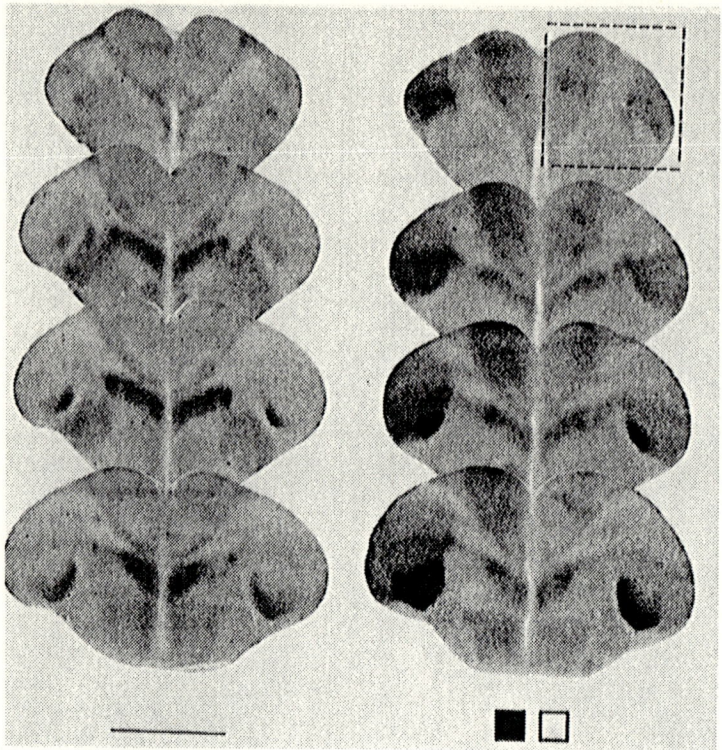

FIGURE 6.4. 2-DG autoradiographs of serial transverse sections through the rostral forebrain of two 7-day-old socially raised chicks. Rostral to caudal from top to bottom. (Left) Stimulation in the dark with vocalizations of cage mates. Note strong labeling of MNH and background labeling in LNH and HAD. Some activity in ventral parts of the visual ectostriatum is still present. (Right) Chick exposed from a distance to the sight and vocalizations of cage mates while having the left eye covered. Note asymmetric labeling of HAD and LNH and symmetric labeling of MNH. Scale bar 5 mm. (From Müller, 1987)

Franke, 1989). Concerning the functional nature of the DMP/DMA input to MNH, it is interesting that these thalamic nuclei receive afferents from medial hyperthalamic areas (Berk & Butler, 1981). Therefore, the DMP/DMA pathway to MNH may carry, at least in part, information from the limbic system.

On the basis of these connectivities there is some analogy of MNH to the magnocellular nucleus of the neostriatum (MAN), a vocal-motor nucleus which is prominent in song birds and controls vocal learning (Bottjer, Miesner, & Arnold, 1984; Nottebohm, Stokes, & Leonard, 1976). The MNH projection areas Ai and Ndc as well as the lobus parolfactorius (LPO) were found to be distinctly 2-DG labeled in addition to MNH, LNH, and

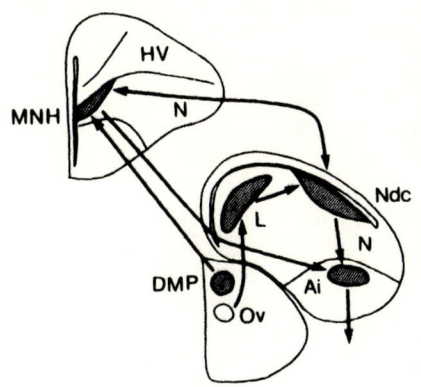

FIGURE 6.5. Scheme of inputs and outputs of MNH in transverse sections as obtained from several tracing studies (see text). Symbols: HV, hyperstriatum ventrale; N, neostriatum; Ndc, neostriatum dorsocaudale; L, field L; Ai, archistriatum intermedium; Ov, nucleus ovoidalis thalami; DMP, nucleus dorsomedialis posterior thalami. (After Wallhäusser-Franke, 1989)

HAD in a social separation paradigm (Müller, 1987; Müller & Scheich, 1986). There, single chicks were separated from cage mates during the 2-DG session but could maintain auditory and visual contact. These chicks relentlessly tried to approach the mates with all signs of distress, similar to a situation when they are separated from a mother hen, thus supporting the notion that chicks also imprint on each other (Dyer & Gottlieb, 1990).

Furthermore, studies in male zebra finches have shown that arousing exposure to females and courting during a 2-DG session produces strong labeling in regions comparable to those previously described in chicks, including the area in and around MAN (Bischof & Herrmann, 1986, 1988). In general, topology and connections of the circuit in chicks are strongly reminiscent of the forebrain system of distinct vocal-motor nuclei in songbirds (Nottebohm et al., 1976) with the following correspondences of structures: MNH/MAN, Ndc/HVc, Ai/RA. Thus, these forebrain nuclei and their circuit in songbirds may be a specialization for auditory–vocal imprinting (song learning) and song-dependent social interactions on the basis of a phylogenetically older system of areas, as present in gallinaceous birds, which control auditory filial imprinting and other acoustic social interactions. It should also be mentioned, yet in a more speculative sense, that MNH, receiving its main input from dorsomedial thalamus, and from (presumably dopaminergic) midbrain reticular neurons (Figure 6.7), bears some analogy to prefrontal cortex in mammals.

Lesion studies with small injections of kainic acid bilaterally in MNH aimed to determine which aspect of imprinting behavior could be blocked in the Y-maze tests (unpublished data). Chicks securely imprinted the first day were lesioned after the sensitive phase between Days 4 and 7. After the effects of anesthesia had worn off, they were observed the same day in the Y-maze during approach and discrimination tests. Most chicks showed strong deterioration of the following behavior, either running aimlessly in the start area of the arena or choosing the goal boxes at random. However, the next morning this effect had disappeared and most chicks passed the tests again.

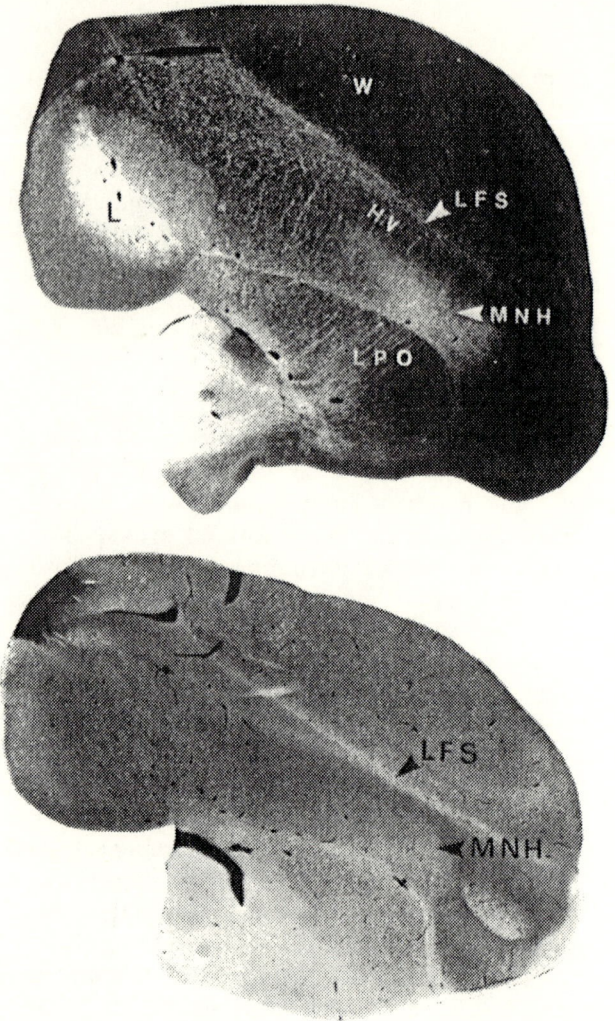

FIGURE 6.6.   Afferent connections of the neostriatal part of MNH and its definition by calretinin immuno-reactivity. (A) Dark field autoradiograph of a medial sagittal section of guinea chick forebrain showing fiber tracts and terminal labeling after a 3H-proline injection into the dorsomedial thalamus. Rostral is to the right. This large injection beyond the limits of DMP/DMA into the underlying auditory nucleus ovoidalis was made to identify the full spatial extent of neostriatal MNH as defined by its thalamic input. Therefore, the auditory projection to field L in caudal neostriatum (L) and various other fiber systems connecting the lamina frontalis superior (LFS) below the Wulst (W) are also shown. Note labeled fiber bundles cursing through LPO into MNH and terminal network in its neostriatal part. The hyperstriatal part of MNH contains mostly fibers of passage to LFS. (B) Dark field view of a medial sagittal section of domestic chick forebrain stained with a calretinin antibody. Note zone of dense staining (terminal fibers) in neostriatal MNH, the extent of which corresponds to afferent fiber terminals in (A).

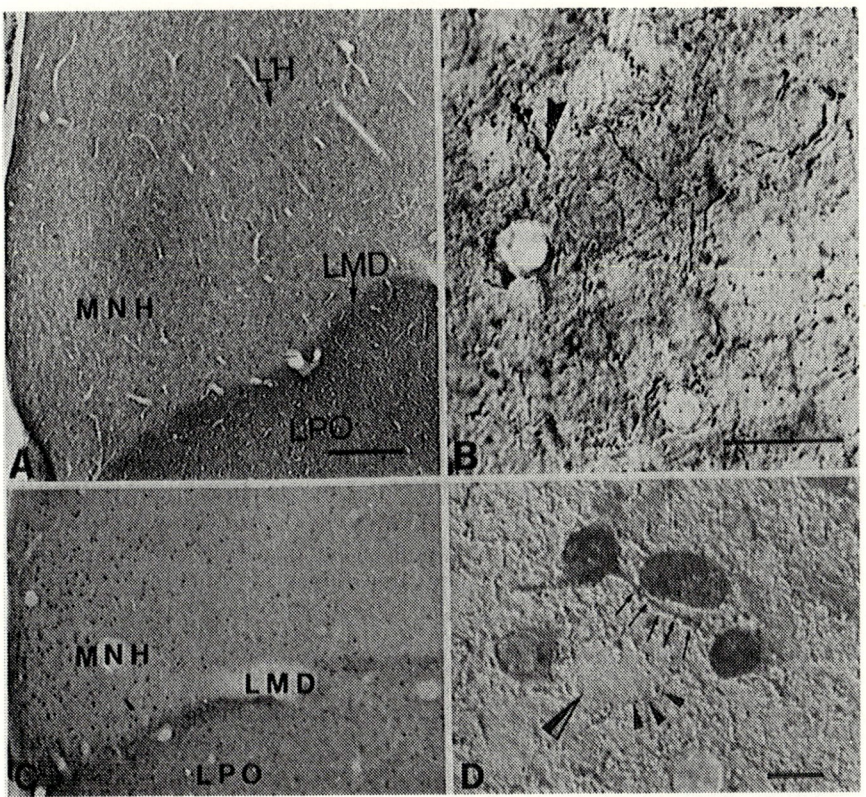

FIGURE 6.7. Dopamine and GABA immunoreactivity in right MNH of 7-day-old domestic chicks. The midline is to the left. (A) The dopamine antibody stains fibers in both the neostriatal and hyperstriatal part of MNH. (B) High magnification of dopaminergic neuropil surrounding unstained somata (from Kalogirou, 1988). (C) The GABA antibody stains neuronal somata and processes in MNH. The density of cells is less than the density of parvalbumin-positive neurons (compare Figure 6.12). (D) High magnification showing several GABA-immunostained small neurons with processes (small arrows). Note terminal boutons (black arrowheads) on the soma of an unstained neuron (mixed arrowhead. (From S. Braun, 1987)

In contrast, chicks lesioned right after hatching could rarely be imprinted (only about 10% of the animals passed the test later on). These preliminary results indicate that MNH is important for memory acquisition. Once the memory is securely formed, MNH functions are no longer necessary for the following behavior in the arena. Thus, storage of the imprinted sound may be widespread in the system. Here again an analogy is found to the vocal-motor nucleus MAN of songbirds, the lesion of which does not disrupt maintenance of song but prevents song learning (Bottjer et al., 1984).

GOLGI STUDIES OF NEURONS IN THE NEOSTRIATIAL PART OF MNH

On the basis of the large changes of activity in MNH after imprinting as seen with the 2-DG method, it appeared promising to pursue the analysis of plasticity at the morphological level in domestic chicks (Wallhäusser & Scheich, 1987). A Golgi method was used as it would also provide a basic classification of neuron types. A previous Golgi analysis in the forebrain vocal control system of mynah birds had revealed changes of spine density and dendritic morphology concomitant with vocal imprinting (Rausch, 1985; Rausch & Scheich, 1982; Scheich & Braun, 1988; see last section).

As a functional method similar to electrophysiology, the 2-DG method has the power to reveal whether a brain structure is more or less responsive to a given stimulus independent of its responsiveness to other stimuli. This made it possible, for instance, to raise chicks socially, to imprint them on tones, and to test responsiveness of MNH to the tones later in a playback experiment. However, in a morphological study the cause of an observed change, such as alteration of synaptic morphology, cannot be directly inferred. This is because possible effects of other stimuli, to which the animal might have been exposed, cannot be separated afterwards. Therefore, chicks designated for Golgi analysis were primarily excluded from any social and other experiences that could interfere with imprinting stimuli.

Hatchlings assigned for Golgi analysis were kept separately up to 20 days in the neutral environment of lighted sound-proof boxes with some noise level. Thus, chicks were socially but not sensorily deprived. The only interruption of these conditions in one subgroup of the chicks was intermittent stimulation with rhythmic tones and the test in the Y-maze, during which precautions were taken to exclude other visual and auditory cues suitable for imprinting. Another subgroup remained in the isolation boxes.

As a further control of the state of MNH after isolation, a third subgroup of isolates was exposed for the first time on Day 7 in a 2-DG experiment with the standard rhythm of 400 Hz tones. While field L was tonotopically labeled, MNH did not show any increased uptake to the very first stimulus presentation. This lack of 2-DG uptake in MNH is similar to socially raised 7-day-old control chicks of previous experiments (Maier & Scheich, 1983, 1987; Wallhäusser & Scheich, 1987) which had not experienced the imprinting stimulus earlier. Thus, social isolation per se does not introduce alterations of metabolic responsiveness to a new auditory stimulus in MNH (Wallhäusser-Franke & Scheich, unpublished observations).

Golgi-Cox analysis of imprinted chicks and controls was carried out on neurons in the neostriatal part of MNH of 7-day-old chicks (i.e., after the normal sensitive phase; Wallhäusser & Scheich, 1987). Essentially three Golgi types of neurons were found: (a) a large type with polymorphic soma and up to four dendritic branchings and high spine frequency (Type I), (b) a medium-size isomorphic neuron with fewer branchings and high spine frequency (Type II), and (c) a small neuron with many basal dendrites and few dendritic spines (Type III).

The study revealed a remarkable 47% difference of dendritic spine frequency on Type I neurons between tone imprinted and nonimprinted cases (Figures 6.8 and 6.9). Unexpectedly, it was the imprinted animals that had fewer dendritic spines. Spine frequency counts were quite homogeneous in Type I neurons within each group and the magnitude of the difference was similar in all dendritic segments except basal ones (Figure 6.9). Because this finding suggested a loss rather than a proliferation of spine synapses with imprinting, some form of synaptic selection was suspected to be an underlying mechanism.

This hypothesis was specifically addressed by extending the Golgi analysis

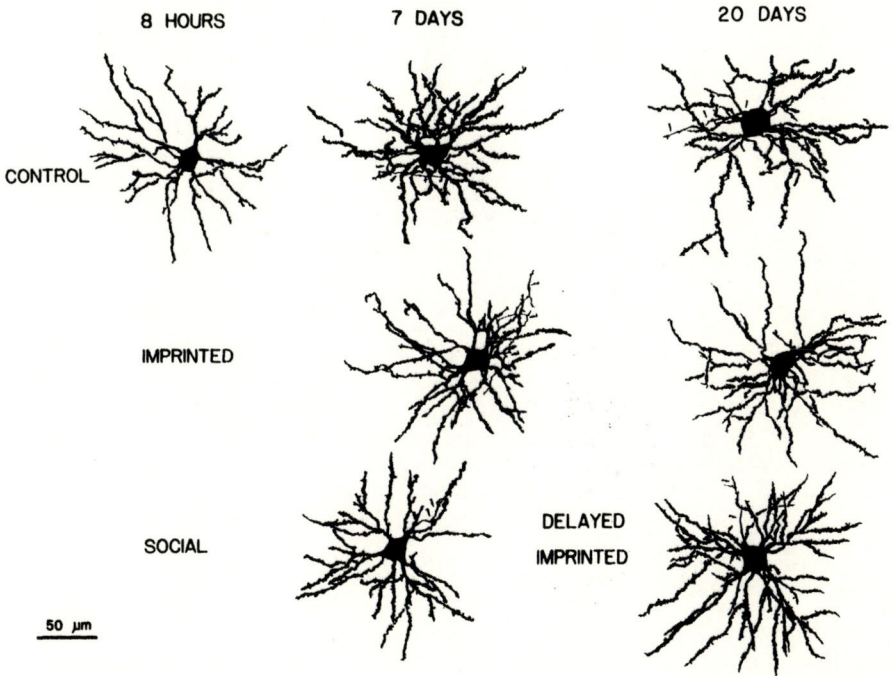

FIGURE 6.8. Representative Golgi impregnated Type I neurons in the neostriatal part of chick MNH from different ages and experimental situations as described in the text. Camera lucida drawings. In the first row, neurons from socially deprived controls sacrificed at various ages are shown. In the second row chicks were imprinted on 400 Hz tones on the first day and sacrificed at 7 days or 20 days of age. In the third row the neuron from the social chick was naturally incubated by and imprinted on a hen and sacrificed on Day 7. The delayed imprinted chicks were imprinted on tones at Day 8 (after the normal sensitive phase) and sacrificed at Day 20. Low spine density of the neuron from the 8 h control and of neurons in the second row from chicks imprinted on the (improverished) tone pattern are obvious even at this small magnification. (After Wallhäusser-Franke, 1989)

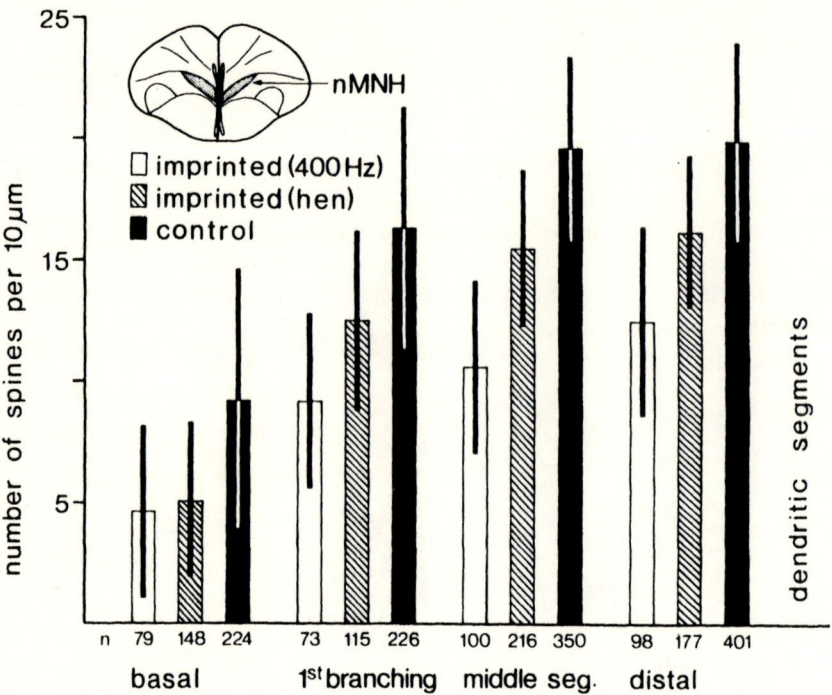

FIGURE 6.9. Histogram showing the average spine density of 10 large MNH neurons per chick. Data are from two animals imprinted on 400 Hz, five animals imprinted on a living hen, and seven controls. Numbers (n) at the bottom refer to 10 μm dendritic segments included in each column. Thick bars represent ±SD. Since there were no pronounced differences within each group, values from individuals in a group were pooled. Dendrites were divided into four segments: basal, behind first branching, middle, and distal. Except for the basal segments in two imprinted groups, all differences were highly significant (Mann-Whitney U-test, $p < .0001$). (From Wallhäusser & Scheich, 1987)

of MNH neurons (a) to stages earlier and later than 7 days of age, (b) to a different imprinting stimulus, and (c) by a manipulation of the sensitive phase. Type I MNH neurons showed lower spine densities on the day of hatching than in 7-day-old isolated controls (Figure 6.10). Densities in hatchlings were similar, however, to 7-day-old chicks that had been imprinted on rhythmic 400 Hz tones. Thus, at first glance there is the paradox that imprinting seems to leave spine density unaltered during the first week while isolation increases the density. This interpretation must be rejected, however, considering results in 7-day-old chicks that were imprinted on and followed a broody hen in a farm (Figure 6.10). In these chicks, which probably had experienced an optimum of imprintable species-specific calls, spine density was intermediate (e.g., 22% higher than in 1-day-old chicks and 33% higher than in 7-day-old chicks imprinted on rhythmic tones). Consequently, an

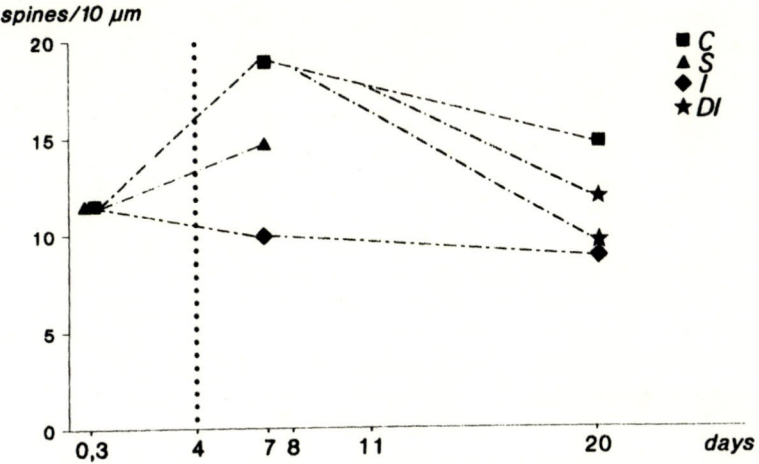

FIGURE 6.10. Age-dependent profiles of average spine frequency (across all dendritic segments) in control chicks and different experimental groups. Type I neurons in neostriatal MNH. Values from the same experiment carry the same symbol and are connected by lines. C, socially deprived controls; S, social chicks incubated by a hen and imprinted on this hen; I, socially deprived and imprinted on the (impoverished) stimulus of 400 Hz tones; DI, socially deprived and delayed imprinted at Days 8 and 11 (after the normal sensitive phase) on 400 Hz tones. All differences at Day 7 and differences between controls and imprinted chicks are significant at Day 20 ($p < .01$). (From Wallhäusser-Franke, 1990)

increase of spine density with imprinting above the level of 1-day-old chicks is a normal alternative with naturally complex stimulation. Therefore, the lack of a net increase with tone imprinting appears to be a consequence of extremely impoverished input.

Taking these results together, their most plausible interpretation is the presence of two counteracting processes:

1. A developmental proliferation of spine synapses independent of imprinting stimuli, as illustrated by the large increase between Days 1 and 7 in isolated controls.
2. A specific reduction of spine synapses dependent on the occurrence of imprinting stimuli. The degree of reduction of irrelevant synapses may be larger the simpler the imprinted sound pattern. In the extreme case of tone imprinting the nonspecific proliferation after Day 1 may be numerically abolished by reduction.

In order to determine more of the time course of the two assumed dynamic processes spine frequencies of naive and 400 Hz imprinted chicks were analyzed at Day 20. Even after this long time the tone-imprinted chicks showed but a small 17% reduction of spine frequency compared with Day 7 and there was only a 28% drop in spine frequency in isolated controls

(Figures 6.10 and 6.11). This means that the result of imprinting, that is, the difference between imprinted and nonimprinted chicks, remains large between Days 7 and 20. Spine frequency differences are not related to changing size of the dendritic tree, as measurements of the diameter have shown no difference between Days 1 and 7 in any group and a 13% increase between Days 7 and 20 but no difference between imprinted animals and controls (Figures 6.8 and 6.11).

As an important consequence, the control results suggest that most of the abundant, presumably nonspecific, spine synapses of isolated chicks remain in some "waiting" state at least until Day 20. This possibility encouraged us to test imprintability in such animals. Indeed, 20–40% of isolated chicks could still be imprinted on 400 Hz tones at Days 8 and 11 (i.e., long after the normal sensitive phase) and passed tests in the Y-arena. Some of these animals were subjected to a Golgi analysis. Their spine frequencies conformed to the hypothesis of specific spine reduction. By Day 20, counts in chicks imprinted at Day 8 were similar to the low values of 20-day-old chicks that were imprinted on tones the first day posthatch (Figure 6.10). Counts in chicks imprinted even later, e.g., at Day 11, showed intermediate values by Day 20.

This latter result seems to be significant in several respects. It demonstrates that under conditions of isolation, when suitable stimuli are withheld, the sensitive phase can be extended (Bateson, 1979, 1987). The end of the

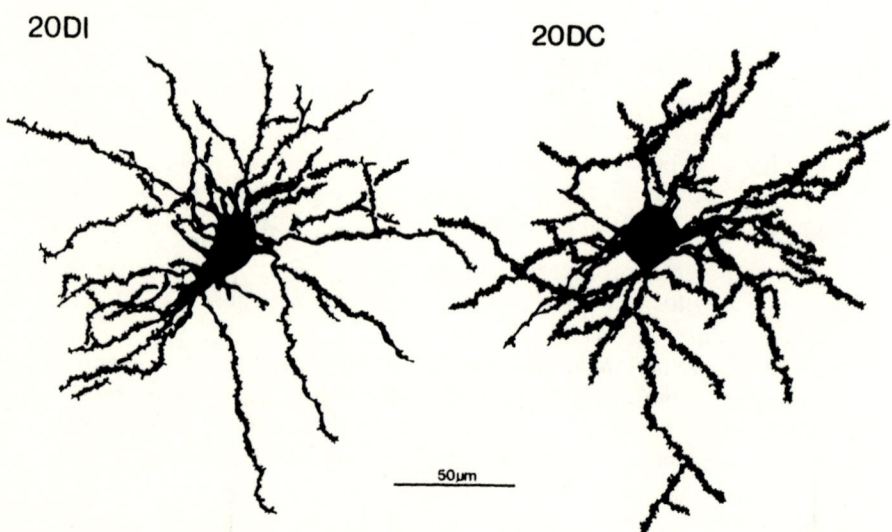

20DI **20DC**

50μm

FIGURE 6.11. Representative Golgi impregnated Type I neurons from 20-day-old chicks. 20DI, socially deprived chick imprinted on the 400 Hz stimulus; 20DC, socially deprived control chick without imprinting experience. Note high spine frequency in the control chick even at this late stage.

phase does not obey internal rules but appears to depend directly or indirectly on some undetermined sensory input. Furthermore, a causal relationship between imprinting and spine loss is established by this experiment. Early imprinting allows only indirect conclusions on the specific mechanism due to apparent interference of proliferative and regressive changes during the first days. Imprinting after the normal sensitive phase isolates the regressive mechanism since spine loss starts from a more stable level of high spine density.

The results described, in our opinion, support the hypothesis that during auditory filial imprinting, Type I MNH neurons are subject to some type of synaptic selection. In a general form this could be envisaged as a four-stage process:

1. Proliferating spines of Type I neurons are occupied in a preliminary and more or less random fashion by terminals that constitute labeled lines for different information. Such inputs, extrinsic or relayed by other MNH neurons, are thought to cover the possible range of species-relevant information as options for imprinting.
2. Any specific stimulus presented at the time of imprinting will activate only a subset of these inputs. The more complex a stimulus the more inputs it needs to be specified. After their use spine synapses will be stabilized.
3. Owing to stabilization of some synapses, mechanisms will be activated that eliminate nonstabilized spine synapses. The simpler the imprinted stimulus the more synapses may be eliminated.
4. The influence of the remaining specific connections on the whole MNH network may initially be relatively weak but may become stronger through some functional strengthening of remaining network connectivities. This is suggested by the delayed increase of 2-DG uptake in MNH at Day 7 after imprinting the first day (Maier & Scheich, 1987) and by the findings of an LTP-like potentiation mechanisms (see below).

Our favored idea of consolidation of relevant spine synapses and subsequent elimination of irrelevant synapses as a mechanism of information storage is based on the assumption that the selection process takes place on spines that carry presynapses. We have no systematic electron microscopic data as yet to show this. However, using arguments that newly formed spines are occupied at an early stage (Greenough & Bailey, 1988; Westrum, Hugh Jones, Gray, & Barron, 1980), it would appear that chicks should have reached that stage at least between Days 7 and 20, where we could isolate the regressive changes most clearly.

However, theoretical alternatives could still be (a) that spines which are reduced after imprinting were not initially occupied by presynapses, or (b) that the loss of spines reflects a transformation of occupied spine synapses to dendritic shaft synapses. While resolution of these alternatives need electron microscopic investigations, they both appear less compatible with some of our results on spine dynamics. For example, if nonoccupied spines were reduced in general there should be no difference in the net result whether chicks were imprinted on simple (tones) or enriched stimuli (hen). If transformation into shaft synapses were the mechanism, one would expect that imprinting on simple stimuli would lead to a smaller spine loss than imprinting on enriched stimuli, which was the converse in our results. Therefore, the above-described selection hypothesis appears to be the most plausible one.

Consolidation and elimination of spines require a molecular machinery that controls differentially the changes in the corresponding synaptic compartments. Relevant synapses by definition are those by which activity is passed to the postsynaptic neuron when an imprinting stimulus is presented. Irrelevant synapses are those that at the same time do not pass activity. Irrelevant synapses are thus defined by the fact that relevant synapses on the same postsynaptic neurons were active and probably retain some molecular traces of this activation. In order to identify the nonactivated spine synapses, one possible way may be the generation of a message starting with the activation of some spines and spreading intracellularly in the postsynaptic neuron. Where the messenger encounters a nonactivated spine (without an activity-dependent molecular trace) it may be eliminated. It should be noted that this assumed differential mechanism is not following Hebbian rules in a strict sense (Hebb, 1949), as its crucial point, elimination of irrelevant synapses, does not directly depend on local pre- and postsynaptic interactions. However, other mechanisms of identifying and eliminating nonactivated synapses are also conceivable.

CORRELATES OF INTRACELLULAR CALCIUM CONTROL AND LTP IN MNH

The search for local postsynaptic messengers has led us to the discovery of molecular specializations of MNH (and of the vocal motor system in birds) with respect to calcium control (Braun, Scheich, Braun, Rogers, & Heizmann, 1991; Braun, Scheich, Heizmann, & Hunziker, 1991; Braun, Scheich, Schachner, & Heizmann, 1985a, b; Scheich & Braun, 1988). In several systems with pronounced functional plasticity of synapses, like hippocampus, cortex, and the Aplysia gill reflex pathway, it has been shown that calcium plays an important role as messenger in the intracellular chain of events finally leading to changes of synaptic transmission (Abrams & Kandel, 1988; Gustafsson & Wigström, 1988). Especially tetanic stimulation, as in LTP, leads to calcium influx into neurons (Dunwiddie & Lynch, 1979). The calcium current seems to pass through voltage-controlled and NMDA-receptor dependent calcium channels (Gustafsson & Wigström, 1988). A high density of such channels has been demonstrated in LTP-producing structures such as hippocampus and cortex.

From these considerations it appears that neurons during learning-related activity are likely to be loaded with calcium. Therefore, membrane calcium channels and special intracellular calcium control could be indicators, among other possibilities, of synaptic plasticity. In MNH of chicks a correlation between a very high density of neurons immunoreactive to antibodies against the calcium-binding protein parvalbumin (PV) and of enhanced ligand binding for voltage-dependent calcium channels has been found (Figure 6.12) (Braun, Scheich, Heizmann, & Hunziker, 1991; Scheich & Braun, 1988). The high density of PV-positive neurons in MNH is remarkable and concentrated in the neostriatal part of MNH, largely sparing the hyperstriatal part which is labelled in addition by 2-DG in imprinting experiments (Figure 6.1). However, unlike 2-DG labeling and terminal distribution of thalamic inputs from dorsomedial thalamus, which define MNH in three dimensions, the PV staining pattern is most intense there but extends beyond the rostrocaudal limits of MNH.

The neostriatal part of MNH exhibits strong labeling with both [125]J-Jodipine, the 1,2'-dihydropyridine receptor ligand, and ^{3}H-desmethoxyvera-pamil, the phenylalkylamine receptor ligand of voltage-controlled calcium channels (Figure 6.12). Such ligands also have a high affinity for dendritic fields of granule cells in the dentate gyrus and of pyramidal cells in the hippocampus proper (Mourre, Cervera, & Lazdunki, 1987; Murphy, Gould & Snyder, 1982; Quirion, 1983). Thus, similar to the hippocampal formation, where evidence for learning-related electrophysiological plasticity is over-whelming, calcium influx into MNH neurons appears to be pronounced.

The neuron-specific calcium-binding protein parvalbumin (PV) is related to calmodulin, the ubiquitous calcium-binding protein in eucaryotic cells. In contrast to calmodulin, PV exchanges calcium ions for magnesium ions. Different from calmodulin, PV is localized only in distinct neuron populations in structures including hippocampus, cortex, cerebellum, parts of auditory and visual pathways, and in all nuclei of the vocal motor system of songbirds (Braun, Scheich, Schachner, & Heizmann, 1985a,b; Celio & Heizmann, 1981; Stichel, Kägi, & Heizmann, 1986; for reviews see Braun, 1990; Heizmann & Braun, 1990).

A differential role of PV for intracellular calcium control is implicated by its nonhomogeneous distribution in different parts of the neuron. The song control nucleus HVc exhibits multiple signs of physiological and morphological plasticity (Konishi, 1985; Margoliash, 1987; Nottebohm, 1984) including learning-related spine loss (Rausch & Scheich, 1982). The nucleus shows strong binding of [125]J-Jodipine beside numerous PV-positive cells (Scheich & Braun, 1988). In HVc, PV is present primarily in the soma and in dendrites of HVc neurons, and less frequently in myelinated axons and terminals as seen at the electron microscopic level (Zuschratter, Scheich, & Heizmann, 1985). In fact, the dense staining pattern of HVc is chiefly determined by dendrites containing PV. In MNH of the chick the PV staining pattern is determined by high density of positive somata and neuropil (Figure 6.13) (Braun, Scheich, Braun, Rogers, & Heizmann, 1991). In some nuclei of the visual system, PV was found only in somata and terminal boutons (Braun, 1990); in other areas of the mammalian brain it can be

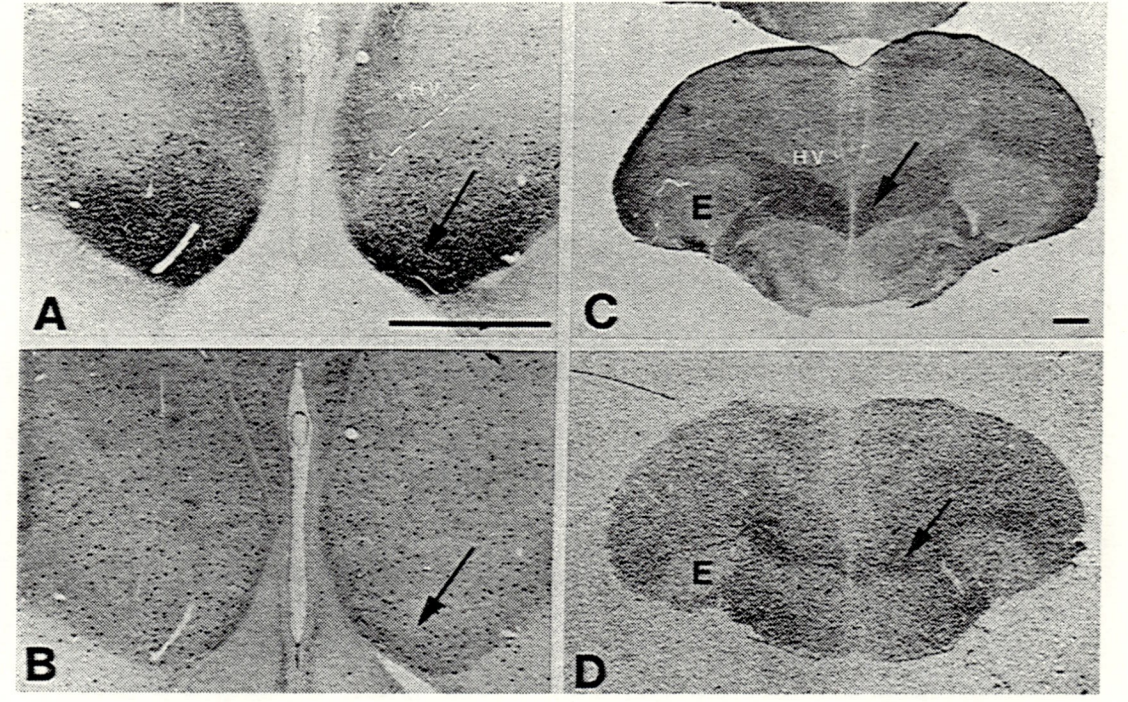

FIGURE 6.12. Comparison of parvalbumin and calbindin-D-28K immunostaining, and density of voltage-dependent calcium channels (C and D) in the neostriatal part of MNH. The staining patterns of parvalbumin (A) and calbindin-D-28K (B) in adjacent frontal sections are illustrated. The neostriatal part of MNH (arrows) displays a high density of binding sites for ^{125}J-labeled jodipine (C) and for ^{3}H-labeled desmethoxyverapamil (D), two ligand types for voltage-dependent calcium channels. HV, hyperstriatum ventrale. Bars are 500 μm. (From Scheich & Braun, 1988)

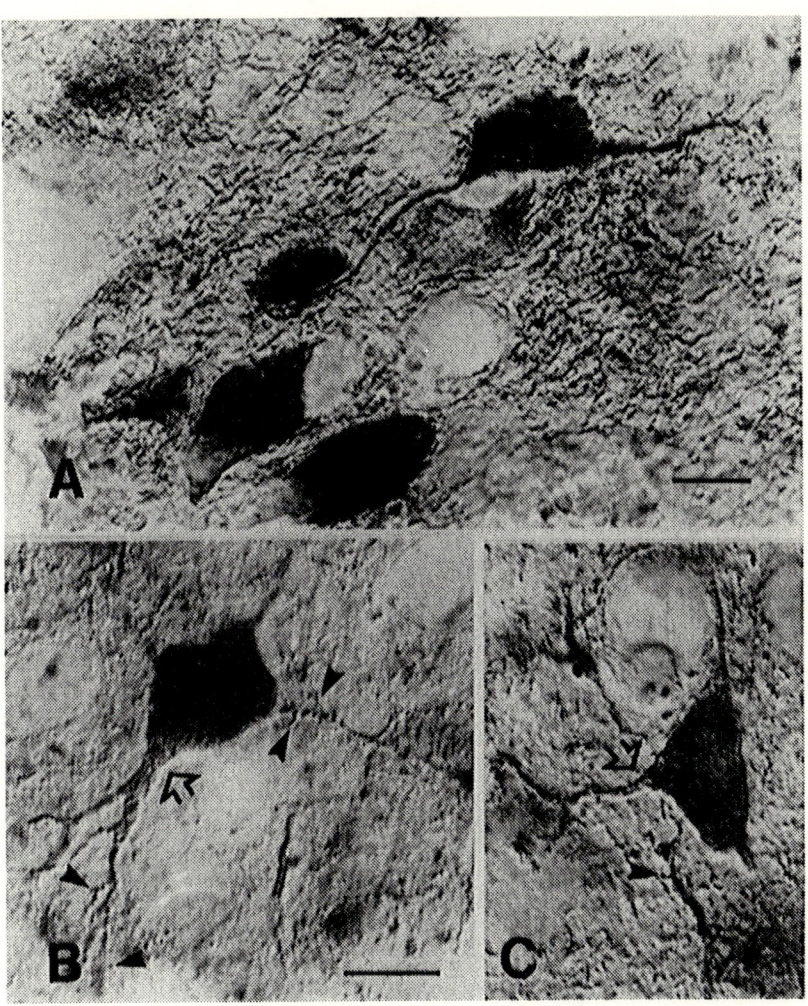

FIGURE 6.13. Morphology of parvalbumin-immunoreactive neurons in the neostriatal part of MNH. The large, heavily stained neurons are characterized by a multipolar shape of the soma leading to the basal dendrites (open arrows in B and C). Dendrites taper and show reduced and patchy immunostaining towards the more distal dendritic segments. It is not clear whether the small immunoreactive structures that occasionally emerge from the dendrites (small arrowheads in B and C) are spines or terminal boutons. Note the characteristic dense PV-immunoreactive neuropil in (A). Calibration bars are 10 μm.

restricted to axons and terminals of otherwise unlabeled neurons (Celio, 1990).

In MNH, another population of neurons, which contain the calcium-binding protein calbindin-D28K (CaBP) is found (Figures 6.12 and 6.14), as well as a dense fiber network and a few somata, which contain the calcium-binding protein calretinin (CaR) (Figures 6.6 and 6.15) (Braun, Scheich, Braun, Rogers, & Heizmann, 1991).

It appears that CaR immunoreactivity mainly labels afferent fibers ascending into the neostriatal part of MNH (Figure 6.6B). In fact, the outline of the CaR-labeled terminal network in this area corresponds to the terminal field of afferents, which is obtained by anterograde transport of

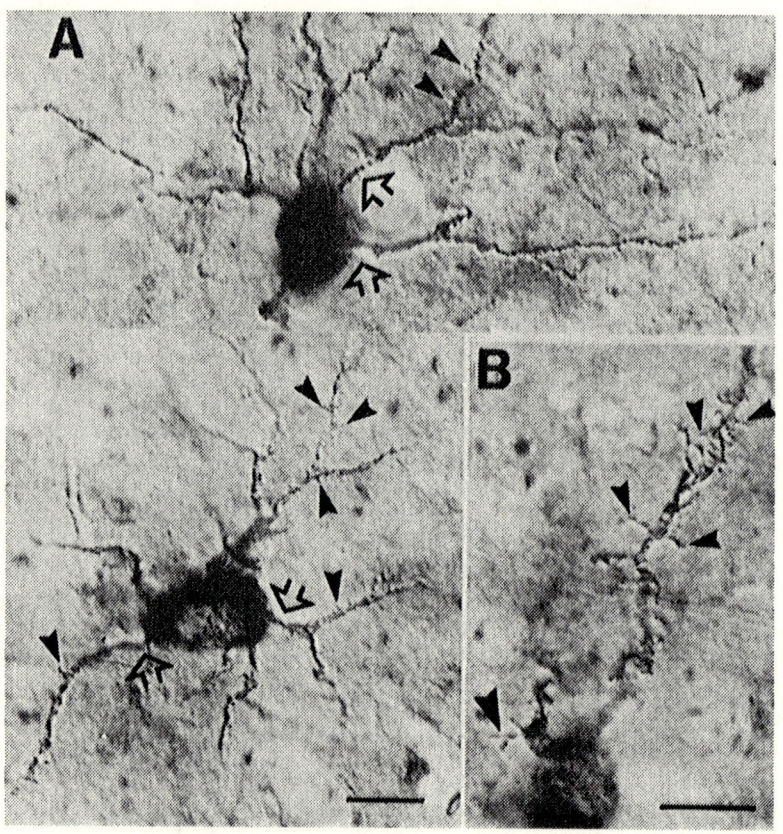

FIGURE 6.14. Morphology of calbindin-D-28K (CaBP) immunoreactive neurons in the neostriatal part of MNH. The slender dendritic trees of the CaBP-positive neurons emerge from an isopolar and often ovoid soma (open arrowheads in A). Dendrites are immunoreactive throughout most of their length. They are studded with spines (arrowheads), which occasionally may reach considerable length and may be branched (B). Calibration bars are 10 μm.

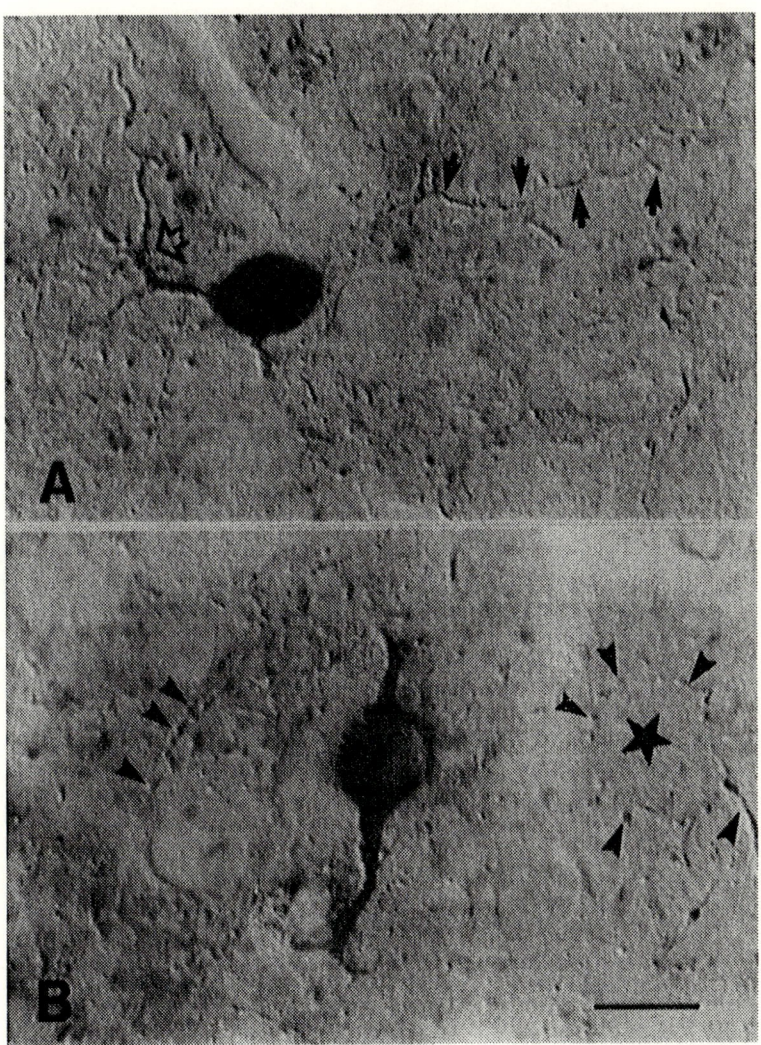

FIGURE 6.15.   Morphology of calretinin-immunoreactive neurons in the neostriatal part of MNH. The scarce calretinin-positive neurons occasionally show immunostained araborized dendrites (open arrow in A). In some cases a long, thin, and branched process can be observed (small arrowheads in A), which presumably represents the axon. The remainder of the dense neuropil lying between the few immunoreactive cells consists of varicose fibers (arrowheads in B), which often surround large unstained somata (asterisk). Bar is 10 μm.

^{3}H-proline from dorso-medial thalamic nuclei (Figure 6.6A). Therefore, CaR fiber staining can be used as a molecular marker of the neostriatal part of MNH.

Soma sizes of neurons with either one of the three calcium-binding proteins overlap (Figure 6.16), and according to their soma size and dendritic morphology they cover both Golgi Type I and Type II neurons. A proportion of PV-positive neurons, however, are extremely large and their multipolar morphology corresponds to Golgi Type I neurons. PV-positive neurons show patchy immunostaining in their dendrites and it is not clear whether they express PV immunoreactivity in the spines (Figure 6.13).

In contrast, CaBP-immunoreactive neurons show a relatively even labeling of dendritic trees, which also includes spines (Figure 6.15). According to the size and isopolar shape of soma and their dendritic morphology, CaBP-neurons most likely belong to the spine-conserving Golgi Type II neurons, with the exception of a few large ones which may contribute to the population of the spine-loosing Type I neurons. Scarce CaR-immunoreactive neurons in MNH (Figures 6.6 and 6.15) may also contribute to the Type I population.

In view of the wide overlap of soma sizes of the PV-, CaBP-, and CaR-neurons (Figure 6.16) it is not likely that anyone of these immunocytochemical types completely matches one of the three described Golgi types. Therefore, it appears that immunocytochemistry of calcium-binding proteins goes beyond morphological criteria and labels neurons with similar, yet to be defined, functional characteristics. Although the role of either of the three calcium-binding proteins is still unknown, some hypothesees in the context of other functional findings may be developed.

One feature of PV-positive neurons in MNH could be the ability to express fast-spiking activity. In fact, it has been demonstrated that the PV-immunoreactive interneurons in the hippocampal formation display fast-spiking patterns (Kawaguchi, Katsumara, Kosaka, Heizmann, & Hama, 1987). The striking correlation of PV-rich brain areas with high enzymatic activities and high 2-DG uptake (Braun et al., 1985a,b) may reflect the high energy demand of these cells. The high density of voltage-dependent calcium channels in MNH may be indirect evidence for an involvement of calcium currents in these specialized activities.

Furthermore, the expression or concentration of PV-immunoreactivity is upregulated by neuronal activity, as has been shown in the hippocampal formation, where kindling stimulation leads to an increase of PV immunoreactivity in neurons and especially in neuropil (Kamphuis, Huisman, Wadman, Heizmann, & Lopez da Silva, 1989).

In the hippocampal formation the vast majority of the PV-positive fast-spiking interneurons are GABAergic, but in MNH, as well as in some visual nuclei (Braun et al., 1988; Braun, Rogers, & Rubel, 1990), PV-positive neurons greatly outnumber GABA-positive neurons (compare Figures 6.7 and 6.12). Also, GABAergic neurons in MNH have, on the average, smaller

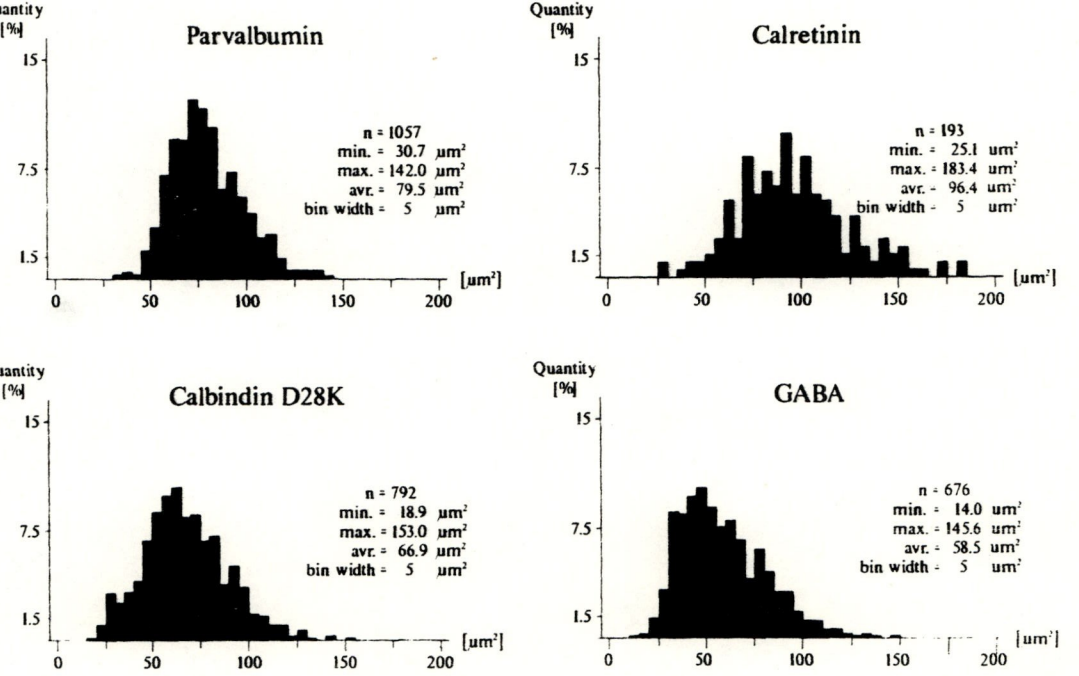

FIGURE 6.16. Soma area histograms of parvalbumin-, calbindin-D-28K-, calretinin-, and GABA-positive neurons in the neostriatal part of MNH. None of the four histograms corresponds to a normal distribution (Kolmogorow-Smirnov), which suggests heterogeneous populations. Note strongest overlap in the distribution of GABA- and calbindin-positive neurons. (From Braun, Scheich, Braun, Rogers, & Heizmann, 1991)

soma sizes than PV cells (Figure 6.16). Therefore, PV-related functional properties, in principle, must be transmitter-independent.

In contrast to PV, CaBP immunoreactivity seems to be correlated with relatively low electrical and metabolic activities (Celio, Schärer, Morrison, Norman, & Bloom, 1986) and its expression or concentration seems to be downregulated by high electrical stimulation. CaBP immunoreactivity in dentate granule cells decreased significantly after kindling stimulation (Baimbridge & Miller, 1984).

CaR immunoreactivity is also regulated by neuronal activity: after blockade of eighth nerve activity, the neurons and axons in the second and third order auditory brain stem nuclei reduce CaR immunoreactivity (Braun, Rogers & Rubel, 1990).

In summary, owing to their differential activity-dependent intracellular regulation, PV, CaBP, and CaR immunoreactivities represent useful markers of the calcium-controlled activity levels and/or activity patterns of neuronal structures in the MNH network.

Probably a major step forward in understanding the initiation of changes during the learning process in MNH is the recent finding of a long-term potentiation-like phenomenon (LTP). This result may also represent the connecting link to some of the signs of elaborate calcium control reported above. LTP is easily produced in the neostriatal part of MNH in brain slices in which the afferent fiber bundles to MNH (see Figure 6.6) are tetanized by stimulation electrodes in lobus parolfactorius (LPO) (Babinsky, 1990). During extracellular recordings, evoked compound action potentials were potentiated with a time course (Figure 6.17) similar to LTP studies in mammalian hippocampus and cortex (Gustafsson & Wigström, 1988). At the same sites in the slices, the converse (i.e., long-term depression (LTD)) was produced. Intracellular recordings showed lowering of threshold for spike initiation as a relevant mechanism for LTP (Wang, unpublished observations).

The hypothesis, that LTP-like changes are mediated by calcium signals and that they represent a first step in the chain of events leading to regressive changes, is under present investigation. The abundance of PV-positive neurons in MNH, and of voltage-dependent calcium channels, together with CaBP-positive neurons, and a dense CaR-positive fiber network suggest that this area is indeed specialized with respect to calcium-dependent processes. The intracellular role of these calcium-binding proteins is not known at present. Therefore, it remains to be shown, how various calcium-binding protein containing structures are linked with each other and how they interact during the imprinting process in the MNH network.

VISUAL IMPRINTING AND PECKING AVOIDANCE RELATED TO PLASTICITY IN THE HYPERSTRIATUM VENTRALE

There are two other lines of memory research in young chicks, visual imprinting (for a review see Horn, 1985) and visually guided pecking

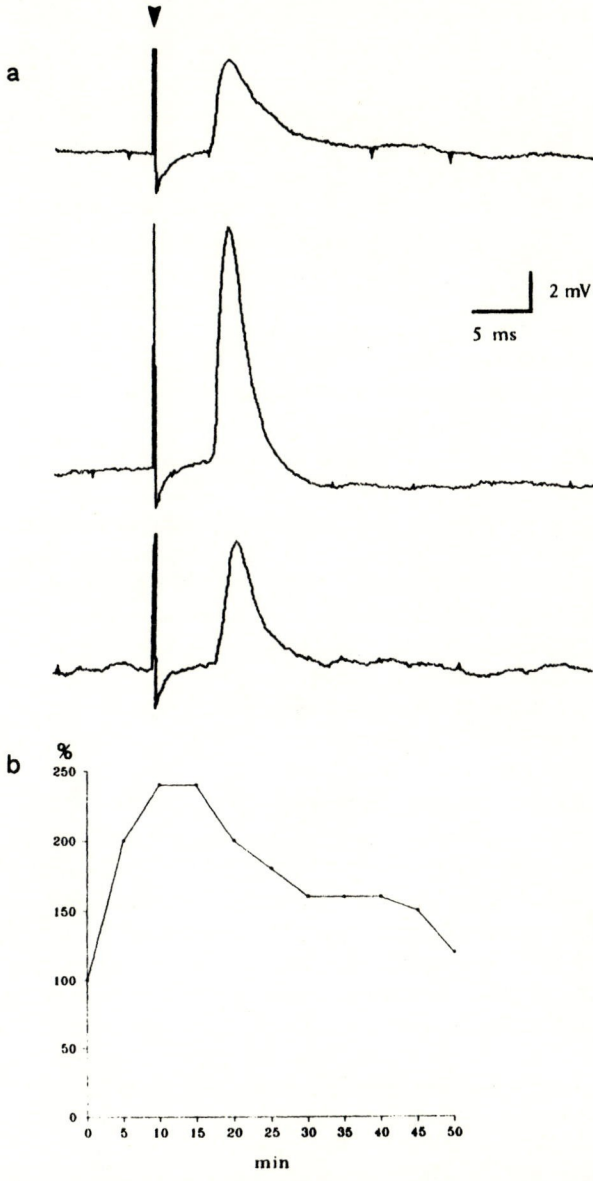

FIGURE 6.17. Long-term potentiation (LTP-like) in the neostriatal part of MNH. (a) Extracellular compound action potentials after one 100 μs stimulation pulse (arrowhead) to fiber bundles in LPO, which are afferent to MNH (see Figure 6.6). First trace is the initial response, second trace is 15 min after tetanus (50 Hz, 5 × 1 s), and third trace is 50 min after tetanus. (b) Time course of potential amplitude during the experiment in percentage of initial value (Wang & Babinsky, unpublished data).

avoidance (for reviews see Rose, 1989; Stewart, 1990), which have focused on the intermediate and medial hyperstriatum ventrale (IMHV) as an apparently common region of relevant plasticity. As this region belongs to brain systems different from the chiefly neostriatal MNH, in our studies it is not mandatory that the numerous learning-related changes reported from IMHV follow the same systems logic as reported for MNH. The common feature of all three paradigms is early posthatch learning, that is, a period of extensive structural remodeling (Wolff, Leutgeb, Holzgraefe, & Teuchert, 1989). Sensitive phase learning as a common denominator is less certain in the case of pecking avoidance. The essential difference is auditory learning in our case compared with visual learning in the other two paradigms. Therefore, it is of general interest to delineate, where feasible, similarities and differences between the findings in neostriatum and hyperstriatum ventrale. As forebrain organization of birds is still largely a matter for specialists, we have also attempted to tie into the discussion some general considerations on this organization.

One common result of all three learning paradigms seems to be that some brain areas show increased 2-DG uptake after learning. In IMHV and in the lateral-rostral neostriatum, enhanced metabolic activity was seen autoradiographically after exposure of imprinted chicks to their visual imprinting stimulus (Kohsaka, Takamatsu, Aoki, & Tsukada, 1979). During a period of 2-DG exposure, which included first experience of a bitter tasting object and later tests of pecking avoidance the posterior hyperstriatum ventrale, palaeostriatum augmentatum and LPO showed increased autoradiographic labeling (Kossut & Rose, 1984). In a subsequent experiment with homogenized brain samples, a predominance of 2-DG uptake was found in medial hyperstriatum ventrale and LPO of the left hemisphere, which could be further differentiated with the time of 2-DG exposure after learning (Rose & Csillag, 1985). After playback of an imprinted sound or by exposing chicks from a distance to their cage mates, increased 2-DG uptake was seen in MNH, LNH (both chiefly neostriatum but including a small strip of hyperstriatum ventrale), and furthermore in HAD, Ndc, Ai, and LPO (our studies, Figures 6.1, 6.2, and 6.4). These 2-DG results lend support to the belief that all three learning paradigms sooner or later after acquisition lead to some increased neuronal activity in several brain areas. There appears to be an overlap in areas that are not yet the main focus of research (LNH and LPO).

However, spatial identification of what has been referred to as IMHV in these and subsequent reports seems to be difficult. IMHV was defined autoradiographically by Horn, McCabe & Bateson (1979) on the basis of incorporation of radioactive uracil into the hyperstriatum ventrale (HV) of visually overtrained chicks. Dividing the forebrain (and HV) in the rostrocaudal direction into quartiles of equal thickness it would appear from Horn's Figure 1 (1983) that IMHV is located in the third quartile counting from the rostral pole of the forebrain. According to Figure 1 in Kohsaka et al. (1979) their visual-imprinting-related labeling is in the second quartile, not only in hyperstriatum ventrale but evidently also in the neostriatum below. In Figure 1 of Kossut and Rose (1984) increased labeling is located in the posterior hyperstriatum ventrale above the auditory field L (i.e., in the fourth quartile). From Figure 1 and the description of dissecting methods in Rose and Csillag (1985) it follows that the medial hyperstriatum ventrale was in the third quartile presumably extending into the fourth. Consequently, there is a large discrepancy in the location of what is called IMHV in the current literature.

MNH as shown here in transverse and sagittal sections is located chiefly in the neostriatum and precisely in the second quartile of the brain (Figures 6.1, 6.2, 6.4, and 6.6). The location of its neostriatal part is defined by congruent patterns of 2-DG activity and thalamic inputs (Figure 6.6). As a further landmark it may be said that MNH is centered to the level of the rostral half of the ectostriatum in transverse sections (Figures 6.1 and 6.4). Immunocytochemical markers such as PV and CaBP antibodies or calcium channel ligands are confined to the neostriatum but do not provide a sharp boundary of MNH rostrocaudally. However, the dense CaR immunoreactive fiber network clearly distinguishes the neostriatal part of MNH from the surrounding neostriatum and hyperstriatum ventrale (Figure 6.6). It is interesting that topological similarities appear to exist between two labeled areas in the visual imprinting study of Kohsaka et al. (1979) and our results on auditory imprinting. In both studies the lateral rostral neostriatum is 2-DG labeled, and the area called IMHV overlaps with MNH, all in the second quartile.

The question of exact IMHV location and, in connection with this, the need for a more detailed topography of its connectivities with the visual system (Bradley, Davies, & Horn, 1985; Horn, 1983) results from the very nature of the organization of the hyperstriatum ventrale of which IMHV must be one part. The reason is that the bird forebrain above the level of basal ganglia cytoarchitecturally shows only few subdivisions in rostrocaudal and mediolateral directions but, in a simplified view, corresponds to a stack of multiple horizontal divisions traditionally named striata (Figures 6.1 and 6.2). The more dorsal striata, starting with the neostriatum and overlying hyperstriatum ventrale followed by multiple layers of the Wulst, appear to be neocortical equivalents. This is not in the sense of modality-specific cortical fields like AI or Area 17 but more like neocortical layers and (or) in the sense of broader definitions like striate cortex, extrastriate cortex, association cortex, and so forth (Karten, 1969; Shimizu & Karten, 1991; Scheich, 1991). Consequently, each striatum is not one functional unit but contains numerous areas functionally specified by individual connectivities.

The neostriatum is one of the subdivisions that receives multiple direct thalamic and other ascending inputs to separate areas. Along the rostrocaudal course of the neostriatum known subdivisions (Figure 6.2) are the beak representation area nucleus basalis (Veenmann & Gottschaldt, 1986), the visual ectostriatum (Karten & Hodos, 1970), the neostriatal part of MNH with its assumed involvement in acoustic social interaction and auditory learning (Wallhäusser-Franke, 1989), a somatosensory area (Faber, Braun, Zuschratter, & Scheich, 1989; Wild, 1987), and the auditory field L (Bonke, Bonke, & Scheich, 1979; Karten, 1968). Nucleus basalis, ectostriatum, and field L also represent landmarks in the neostriatum as they are cytoarchitecturally distinct nuclei in Nissl stain. Similar to the definition of these other neostriatal areas by long ascending inputs, the neostriatal part of MNH is specified by its strong thalamic input from DMP/DMA as well as by a dense CaR-positive network (Figure 6.6).

The HV, dorsally adjacent to the neostriatum through the length of the forebrain, does not contain obvious cytoarchitectural landmarks, in contrast to the neostriatum. This is in line with several transmitter immunocytochemical, receptor autoradiographic, and histochemical studies, which may highlight HV as a whole, or show gradients of intensity within HV, but so far do not demarcate a sector in the rostrocaudal direction that could help to identify IMHV as a subarea in HV (Braun, Scheich, & Braun, 1988; Dietl, Cortés, & Palacios, 1988a,b; Dietl & Palacios, 1988; Faber et al., 1989; Reiner, Brauth, Kitt, & Quirion, 1989; Csillag et al., 1989; Stewart et al., 1988; Wächtler, 1985).

Unfortunately, the natural lack of structural definition in HV is aggravated by a general neglect of this lamina in bird pathway tracing studies (for reviews see Pearson, 1972; Benowitz, 1980; Showers, 1982; Shimizu & Karten, 1991). The impression from the few observations available is that HV has chiefly intratelencephalic connections, for instance with neighboring neostriatum and Wulst layers (Bonke, Bonke, & Scheich, 1979; Bradley, Davies, & Horn, 1985; Bradley & Horn, 1987). Reports on direct inputs to IMHV from optic tectum (Horn, 1983) are at variance with detailed analyses of visual pathways in birds (Shimizu & Karten, 1991).

Hyperstriatal areas may be 2-DG labeled when the underlying areas of neostriatum are strongly active. This is the case with MNH and also with LNH, where the corresponding neostriatal area is ectostriatum, including its belt (Figures 6.1 and 6.4). But even in the sense of straightforward sensory processing it has been shown by electrophysiology, pathway tracing, and 2-DG technique that the auditory neostriatal field L interacts with the overlying HV through mechanisms of a common tonotopic gradient (Bonke, Bonke, & Scheich, 1979; Bonke, Scheich, & Langner, 1979; Scheich, 1991; Theurich, Müller & Scheich, 1984). These aspects suggest a function of HV as an association layer, an idea mentioned by Horn (1983). But more specifically, local associations in different parts of HV may be related to functions in the underlying neostriatum. Therefore, a future clue to a more precise definition of IMHV as part of a functional brain system could be the analysis of the connectivities with its underlying neostriatal area. Once localization and functional connectivity issues are settled a more meaningful comparison of neostriatal and hyperstriatal mechanisms of early learning would be possible.

In spite of these structural–functional insecurities about IMHV, morphological plasticity in areas of the hyperstriatum ventrale is obvious consequent on pecking avoidance learning (for a review see Stewart, 1990). Hyperstriatal neurons impregnated by Golgi showed increased spine frequency of up to 113% in the left and 69% in the right hemisphere (Patel & Stewart, 1988). In chicks with taste aversion the significant hemispheric asymmetry in spine frequency of nonavoiding water-trained controls (frequency is higher in the right than in the left) was abolished, so that both hemispheres finally had a similar (increased) spine frequency. Furthermore, spine head diameter increased and spine stem length decreased in the left hemisphere of avoiding chicks. Interestingly, recall of the aversive taste experience can be abolished by electroshocks after training and the corresponding chicks did not show the increase of spine frequency reported above (Patel, Rose, & Stewart, 1988).

Electron-microscopic analysis of synapses on hyperstriatal neurons was also performed with the avoidance paradigm. The length of postsynaptic thickening, volume of presynaptic boutons, and the number of synaptic vesicles per synapse increased after avoidance training, all in the left hemisphere (Stewart, King, & Rose, 1983; Stewart, Rose, King, Gabbott, & Bourne, 1984). However, no change of synaptic numbers was found in either hemisphere, which is in discrepancy with the spine frequency measurements, but may be explained by global counting of synapses in contrast to spine frequency measurements on an identified cell type.

Posttraining electrophysiological changes of activity of neurons (Mason & Rose, 1988) also point to the involvement of the hyperstriatum ventrale in the learning process. Finally, posttraining lesions of the hyperstriatum ventrale did not abolish the memory but were only effective if made pretraining (Patterson et al., cited in Stewart, 1990).

In the visual imprinting paradigm an increase in the mean length of the postsynaptic density (PSD) profiles of axospinous synapses in the left hyperstriatum ventrale was found after learning (Bradley, Horn, & Bateson, 1981; Horn, Bradley, & McCabe, 1985). This suggests an improved synaptic transmission as glutamic acid binding to N-methyl-D-aspartate (NMDA) receptors is increased on the left side after training (McCabe & Horn, 1988).

These results, and other less important ones in this context (Horn, 1985; Rose, 1989; Stewart, 1990), demonstrate the involvement of hyperstriatum ventrale in this type of learning, but there are two that need specific attention with reference to our data: hemispheric asymmetries and increase of spine frequency after learning. Hemispheric asymmetries were not seen in any of our numerous 2-DG studies. On the basis of this we did not actively pursue a search for asymmetries in the Golgi results. As asymmetries were not present in the 2-DG labeling it might be that asymmetries found in the other two paradigms are related to lateralization in the visual system in contrast to auditory processing. Alternatively, hyperstriatal versus neostriatal mechanisms may be responsible for the difference.

Contrary to a superficial view, increase of spine frequency as reported in avoidance learning is compatible with our data and theory of imprinting. Indeed, we could demonstrate an increase of spine frequency with imprinting on an enriched stimulus (natural hen) between Days 1 and 7 (Figure 6.10). However, with respect to deprived controls, to imprinting with impoverished stimuli (tones), and to the late imprinting after extension of the sensitive phase, it was concluded that spine frequency increases during the sensitive phase are the result of proliferative and stimulus-specific regressive changes. The results of Patel and Stewart (1988) during the first days could therefore be a reflection of a behaviorally relevant (enriched) and to-be-avoided stimulus, where proliferative changes are expected to dominate, versus a less interesting (impoverished stimulus) in controls, where regressive changes are expected to dominate, all within our frame of reasoning on selection. Therefore, it would have been interesting to include in the study chicks deprived of any relevant pecking experience as a baseline control. On the other hand it is entirely possible that hyperstriatal learning mechanisms are different from those in neostriatal MNH, especially since pecking avoidance is not considered a type of imprinting and may be expected in adult birds.

COMPARATIVE EVIDENCE FOR EPIGENETIC SPECIFICATION OF NETWORKS BY REGRESSIVE PHENOMENA

The central issue of this article is whether regressive synaptic changes explain imprinting and, namely, the largely irreversible nature of this type of learning. We believe that regression of spine synapses in chick MNH occurs after initial nonspecific proliferation of these synapses followed by activity-dependent selection and maturation of a proportion of them. The data, especially on the extension of the sensitive phase, in our opinion, provide evidence that structural regression is caused by imprinting.

An open question still appears to be the significance of this phenomenon for storage (structural specification) of new information in MNH. It could be argued that regressive changes represent secondary reorganizational phenomena concomitant with changing behavior or with storage in other brain systems, for instance in the projection areas Ndc or Ai. This is suggested by the finding that MNH lesions do not interfere permanently with the already imprinted behavior. On the other hand, lesions prevent imprinting (see also lesions in hyperstriatum ventrale [Stewart, 1990], and in MAN [Bottjer et al., 1984]). Therefore, regressive changes in MNH may initiate and may be the prerequisite for specifications to occur in addition in Ndc, Ai, or other brain areas.

At this point comparative arguments are useful form nervous systems where regressive changes are known to specify networks in an experience-dependent fashion. It has previously been pointed out that epigenetic developmental changes have several traits in common with imprinting (Bischof, 1985; Rauschecker & Marler, 1987). Epigenetic influences are seen or suspected in postnatal periods in nervous system development when extensive remodeling of the structure and redistribution of synapses occur as a general phenomenon. Remodeling of neural connections is apparently based on proliferative processes and markedly on regressive processes (Purves & Lichtman, 1980; Patterson & Purves, 1982, chapter 11; Wolff et al., 1989).

Structural regression is not a peculiar property of some bird systems but is also found in mammalian systems when postnatal remodeling occurs. After initial proliferation some spine or synaptic loss in visual cortex starts postnatally and reaches into adulthood (Cragg, 1975; Feldman & Dowd, 1975; Lund, Boothe, & Lund, 1977; Ruiz-Marcos & Valverde, 1969; Schüz, 1981; Wolff et al., 1989). Even though a correlation of the onset of loss with the end of the sensitive phase for postnatal reorganization of the visual system has been noted (Lund et al., 1977), to our knowledge no systematic attempts have been made to relate these changes directly to stimulus-specific plasticity or visual memory. There are partial exceptions in social keeping versus deprivation experiments with adult rats in which nubbin (N-type) spines showed specific differences in number (Connor & Diamond, 1982). Interestingly, it was the social and not the deprived rats in which frequency of this spine type was lower, suggesting some parallel to our experiments in MNH. In contrast, increases of spine and synaptic numbers have also been reported in the cortex of adult rats kept in enriched environments and were related to learning following a "growth concept" of memory (Greenough & Bailey, 1988).

Obviously, during learning as well as during development are the relative weights of proliferative and regressive synaptic changes difficult to separate. Therefore, our argument on the specific role of regression for structural specification and learning must be based on more lucid cases. These are formation (a) of ocular dominance columns in visual cortex, (b) of adult callosal connections of the hemispheres, (c) of motor units of skeletal muscle, and (d) of acquisition of a vocal repertoire in the vocal motor system of songbirds.

Ocular Dominance Columns in Visual Cortex

Development of binocular mechanisms in area 17 of cat visual cortex became known through the classical observations of Wiesel and Hubel (1965) and was subsequently identified in cat and monkey as a sequence of proliferation and regression of connectivities during a sensitive phase (Hubel & Wiesel, 1970; LeVay, Stryker, & Shatz, 1978; LeVay, Wiesel, & Hubel, 1980; Shatz & Stryker, 1978). At birth thalamic axons with corresponding retinotopy of the two eyes have established random overlapping connections at cortical target cells. By 8 weeks after birth inputs are redistributed in an orderly fashion. Eighty per cent of units are dominated to different degrees by one or the other eye. Left and right eye dominated units are found spatially segregated in alternating ocular dominance columns. The underlying regression of thalamic terminals is demonstrated by anterograde tracing of connections from either eye, which produces terminal labeling in periodic bands of visual cortex layer IV. The segregation into ocular dominance columns still occurs, yet is more fuzzy, when kittens are reared in complete darkness (i.e., when spontaneous but no structured visual input reaches the cortex from the two eyes). Column formation does not occur if any impulse traffic is blocked from both eyes by temporary injections of tetrodotoxin (Stryker & Harris, 1986). Spontaneous activity, however, is not enough to overcome competition from the other, normally experiencing eye. This is shown by various monocular deprivation experiments, which result in regression of inputs throughout layer IV from the deprived eye (Blakemore, 1978). Such deprivation experiments have identified the duration of a sensitive phase, during which normal interaction of the two eyes leads to normal ocular dominance columns, or abnormal interaction leads to distortions of organization, both permanently. Within the sensitive phase, reversal of monocular deprivation is compatible with a normal development of ocular dominance columns (Swindale, Vital-Durand, & Blakemore, 1981).

The conclusion from these physiological and anatomical experiments is that some proportion of initially random synaptic connections are given up under the influence of balanced activity from both eyes to specify the final binocular tuning of cortical units in orderly columns. These regressive changes are restricted to a sensitive phase after which the normal or abnormal result becomes largely irreversible. The formal similarity of this type of cortical plasticity to basic aspects of our results on filial imprinting in MNH is obvious. In both cases, regression of synaptic sites, which is dependent on input activity during a sensitive phase, leads to a final and stable pattern of activation.

Adult Callosal Connections of the Hemispheres

One of the most impressive examples of regression of connectivities concerns interhemispheric (callosal) projections, largely known through the work of Innocenti and coworkers (Innocenti, 1991). Transient callosal projections are exuberantly generated during development in the cat and other species and are subsequently eliminated following a specific time course. The elimination coincides with the phase of fast synaptogenesis in cortex and precedes myelination of the corpus callosum. The stabilization or elimination of visual callosal connections, for example, appears to depend on several factors. Among them are normal binocular vision during the second postnatal month, and integrity of the eyes and geniculocortical projections. Even though the local rules that determine acceptance or rejection of callosal axon terminals are not fully known, it would appear that experience-dependent functional network properties play a role.

Motor Units of Skeletal Muscle

The following examples from neuromuscular systems and song systems in birds are the most radical ones as regressive phenomena are not restricted to loss of connectivities but subsequently result in the loss of neurons. They are also most illustrative as they suggest several mechanisms leading to or preventing regression of connectivities. One case is the formation of motor units of muscle where initially convergent motor axons compete for innervation of "private" muscle fibers (Changeux et al., 1984; Oppenheim, 1981; Pittman & Oppenheim, 1979). Motor neurons are overproduced as a rule during development. Motor neuron loss results when the corresponding axon terminals have not succeeded in making enough functional synapses on muscle fibers during a sensitive phase. As a mechanism, competition of terminals for allosteric acetylcholine receptors has been proposed and modelled (Changeux & Danchin, 1976). The feed back after sufficient innervation may be provided by nerve growth factor secretion of activated muscle fibers. The retrograde transport of sufficient amounts presumably influences the fate of motoneurons (for a review see Patterson & Purves, 1982).

The other neuromuscular case covers motor neurons of the bulbocavernosus muscle controlling penile functions, a system that is sexually dimorphic. It was found that neonatal steroid secretion during a sensitive phase produces permanent sex differences in behavior by creating sex differences in the spinal cord (Arnold et al., 1987). Most of the somewhat overproduced motor neurons in males make permanent contact with the muscle fibers and survive. By contrast a massive loss of neurons results in females. This can be prevented by injecting androgens in females during the sensitive phase, which masculinizes the muscle inventory and prevents neuron loss in a male-like fashion.

Acquisition of a Vocal Repertoire in Songbirds

In the following examples, epigenetic specifications of circuits appear to merge into true learning phenomena. The so-called song system is a network of interconnected distinct nuclei in the forebrain of songbirds, which controls acquisition and maintenance of song (Nottebohm et al., 1976). Of the numerous developmental findings in this system, only those that are pertinent to our question are reported (for reviews see Arnold et al., 1987; Konishi, 1985). The sex difference in song behavior in many species reflects the much larger size of male vocal control nuclei with more and larger neurons (Gurney, 1981; Nottebohm & Arnold, 1976). These pervasive sex differences in brain and behavior are produced by neonatal estradiol secretion in males and can be artificially induced in females (Gurney & Konishi, 1980).

It is not certain, however, whether these hormone-dependent proliferative changes also reflects progress in the essential task of the system (i.e. song learning) or whether they are a prerequisite (Arnold et al., 1987). Besides the fact that increase of variables like volume of nuclei, cell number, and size of dendritic tree are not direct correlates of synaptic changes, they are not precisely post hoc events after learning during the relatively long sensitive and vocal maturation phases. Proliferative changes start before the sensitive phase for song learning and continue through the stages of song perfection.

A similar monophasic temporal profile was found for the expression of the calcium-binding protein PV, which is a characteristic marker protein of the vocal motor system (Braun, Scheich, Heizmann, & Hunziker, 1991, see above).

There are, however, two lines of research in the vocal motor system that report biphasic profiles of measured variables. They have the interesting aspect in common that structural proliferation turns to regression and that this reversal phase appears to coincide with the phase of sensory learning. It is after this phase that the initially variable vocal imitations (subsong) are autonomously reduced to the stable adult repertoire (crystallization).

One result in zebra finches is the reduction of neurons in the lateral MAN nucleus. The resemblance of MAN to MNH in chicks has already been pointed out (see section on functional inputs and outputs of MNH). In male MAN half of the neurons are lost between Day 25 when subsong is beginning and Day 53 when crystallization ensues (Bottjer et al., 1984; Bottjer, Glaessner, & Arnold, 1985). The involvement of MAN in the learning mechanism is strongly suggested by the fact that lesions of the adult nucleus do not interfere with the maintenance of song but lesions between Days 35 and 50 profoundly disrupt song development. Thus, MAN seems to have a similar "permissive" role in the process of learning as MNH (see above). It could be speculated that axon terminals of some MAN neurons in the nuclei HVc and RA may have initially transmitted important information during learning, which favors survival of their synapses. Nonactivation of synaptic sites may lead to retraction of axons and degeneration of MAN neurons. In principle, vacant postsynaptic synaptic sites in HVc or RA could then be abolished or occupied by other connections.

With respect to these two latter alternatives, the second line of research in mynah birds suggests an answer. Hatchling mynahs were trained in our laboratory to imitate sentences of human speech. The process starts with a babbling phase around the end of the 2nd month and proceeds through rhythmic and vowel imitation of a sentence to perfect reproduction, including consonants at the end of the first year (Rausch, 1985; Rausch & Scheich, 1982; Scheich & Braun, 1988). Mynahs do not learn much after the 1st year, which points to the presence of a sensitive phase. At 2 months, 5 months, 1 year, and 2 years, brains of some of these birds were Golgi-impregnated and neurons of the vocal motor nucleus HVc analyzed. The most impressive morphological changes were seen in the largest spiny neuron (Type I). Dendritic trees increased only slightly during the 1st year but became polarized and grew considerably during the 2nd year. In contrast, spine frequency (number of spines/10μm) decreased and the shape of spines changed during the 1st year, concomitant with gradual phonetic perfection. In some animals the average spine loss in intermediate segments of dendritic trees reached 66% in the 1st year. In other spiny neuron types no such change was found. This example documents again a regressive change of synaptic structures concomitant with sensitive-phase learning (similar to MNH). It cannot be decided yet whether the spine loss on Type I neurons is directly related to the degeneration of MAN neurons, reported for zebra finches (Bottjer et al., 1984), as the recipient neurons in HVc of MAN projections are not known. However, a reduction of some synaptic sites in HVc linked to MAN neuron degeneration is at least a plausible hypothesis.

SUMMARY

Some of these examples from epigenetic specifications of neural circuits during development may still appear far-fetched in their assumed similarity to imprinting. In other words, sensitive phase, selection, regression, and irreversibility in both types of events may be coincidental and independent. Nevertheless, it seems possible to show, at least theoretically, in what way imprinting is embedded in a general concept of brain ontogeny.

All developmental processes in the brain follow a tight schedule of sequential events. Both the schedule and the sequence are under genetic control. As genetic developmental steps are hierarchically building on each other, the process is unidirectional (irreversibility). Any epigenetic factor that provides additional instructive information during development must meet the schedule (sensitive phases). Any epigenetic change that occurs will subsequently be built on by adequate genetic mechanisms to continue the developmental process. In this sense epigenetic information, at large, should be foreseeable by the system. Mechanistically speaking, the system offers limited options in terms of connections that are selected by the information that is actually available from outside (selection). Irrelevant connections are subsequently reduced (regression). In this sense imprinting may bridge the gap between epigenetic instructions during development and adult learning (the latter with a different type of memory) independent of development that remains modifiable lifelong.

Acknowledgments: This work was supported by DFG, SFB 45, and SPP Dynamik und Stabilisierung neuronaler Systeme.

REFERENCES

Abrams, T. W., & Kandel, E. R. (1988). Is contiguity detection in classical conditioning a system or a cellular property? Learning in Aplysia suggests a possible molecular site. *TINS*, **11** (4), 128–135.

Arnold, A. P., Bottjer, S. W., Nordeen, E. J., Nordeen, K. W., & Sengelaub, D. R. (1987). Hormones and critical periods in behavioral and neural development. In J. P. Rauschecker & P. Marler (Eds.), *Imprinting and cortical plasticity. Comparative aspects of sensitive periods* (pp. 55–98). New York: John Wiley.

Artola, A., Bröcher, S., & Singer, W. (1990). An in vitro model of plasticity in neocortical slices. In L. R. Squire & E. Lindenlaub (Eds.), *The biology of memory* (pp. 319–328). New York: F. K. Schattauer.

Babinsky, R. (1990). *Das neuronale Substrat kognitiver Funktionen — Elektrophysiologische und pharmakologische in-vitro-Untersuchungen an einem gedächtnisrelevanten Vorderhirngebiet von Gallus domesticus.* Unpublished master's thesis, Technical University Darmstadt.

Baimbridge, K.G., & Miller, J. J. (1984). Hippocampal calcium-binding protein during commissural kindling-induced epileptogenesis: Progressive decline and effects of anticonvulsants. *Brain Research, 324*, 85–90.

Bateson, P. P. G. (1979). How do sensitive periods arise and what are they for? *Animal Behavior, 27*, 470–486.

Bateson, P. P. G. (1981). Control of sensitivity to the environment during development. In K. Immelmann, G. W. Barlow, L. Petrinovich, & M. Main (Eds.), *Behavioral development* (pp. 432–453). Cambridge: Cambridge University Press.

Bateson, P. P. G. (1987). Imprinting as a process of competitive exclusion. In J. P. Rauschecker & P. Marler (Eds.), *Imprinting and cortical plasticity. Comparative aspects of sensitive periods* (pp. 151–168). New York: John Wiley.

Benowitz, L. (1980). Functional organization of the avian telencephalon. In S. O. E. Ebbesson (Ed.), *Comparative neurology of the telencephalon* (pp. 389–421). New York: Plenum Press.

Berk, M. L., & Butler, A. B. (1981). Efferent projections of the medial preoptic nucleus and medial hypothalamus in the pigeon. *Journal of Comparative Neurology, 203*, 379–399.

Bischof, H. -J. (1985). Environmental influences on early development: A comparison of imprinting and cortical plasticity. In P. P. G. Bateson & H. P. Klopfer (Eds.), *Perspectives in ethology: Vol. 6. Mechanisms* (pp. 169–217). New York: Plenum Press.

Bischof, H. -J., & Herrmann, K. (1986). Arousal enhances ^{14}C-2-deoxyglucose uptake in four forebrain areas of the zebra finch. *Behavioral Brain Research, 21*, 215–221.

Bischof, H.-J., & Herrmann, K. (1988). Isolation-dependent enhancement of 2-[^{14}C] deoxyglucose uptake in the forebrain of zebra finch males. *Behavioral and Neural Biology, 49*, 386–397.

Bliss, T. V. P., & Lømo, T. (1973). Long-lasting potentiation of synaptic transmission in the dentate area of the anesthetized rabbit following stimulation of the perforant path. *Journal of Physiology (London), 232*, 331–356.

Blakemore, C. (1978). Maturation and modification in the developing visual system. In R. Held, H. Leibowitz, & H. L. Teuber (Eds.), *Handbook of sensory physiology: Perception* (pp. 377–436). Berlin: Springer.

Bonke, B. A., Bonke, D., & Scheich, H. (1979). Connectivity of the auditory forebrain nuclei in the guinea fowl (*Numida meleagris*). *Cell Tissue Research, 200*, 101–121.

Bonke, D., Scheich, H., & Langner, G. (1979). Responsiveness of units in the auditory neostriatum of the guinea fowl (*Numida meleagris*) to species-specific calls and synthetic stimuli. I. Tonotopy and functional zones of field L. *Journal of Comparative Physiology, 132*, 242–255.

Bottjer, S. W., Glaessner, S. L., & Arnold, A. P. (1985). Ontogeny of brain nuclei controlling song learning and behavior in zebra finches. *Journal of Neuroscience, 5*, 1556–1562.

Bottjer, S.W., Miesner, E. A., & Arnold, A. P. (1984). Forebrain lesions disrupt development but not maintenance of song in passerine birds. *Science, 224*, 901–903.

Bradley, P., Davies, D. C., & Horn, G. (1985). Connections of hyperstriatum ventrale of the domestic chick (Gallus domesticus). *Journal of Anatomy, 140*, 577–590.

Bradley, P., & Horn, G. (1987). Neural consequences of imprinting. In J. P. Rauschecker & P. Marler (Eds.), *Imprinting and cortical plasticity.*

Comparative aspects of sensitive periods (pp. 137–149). New York: John Wiley.

Bradley, P., Horn, G., & Bateson, P. (1981). Imprinting: An electronmicroscope study of chick hyperstriatum ventrale. *Experimental Brain Research, 41*, 115–120.

Braun, K. (1980). *Akustische Prägung bei Perlhuhnküken (Numida meleagris).* Unpublished master's thesis, Technical University Darmstadt.

Braun, K. (1990). *Calcium-binding proteins in avian and mammalian central nervous system: Localization, development and possible functions.* (Progress in Histochemistry and Cytochemistry Monograph No. 21/1). Stuttgart, New York: Gustav Fischer Verlag.

Braun, K., Rogers, J. H., & Rubel, E. W. (1990). Activity-dependent changes of calretinin-immunoreactivity in the auditory brainstem of the chick. *European Journal of Neuroscience, 3* (Suppl.), 153.

Braun, K., Scheich, H., Braun, S., Rogers, J. H., & Heizmann, C. W. (1991). Parvalbumin-, calretinin- and calbindin-D28K-immunoreactivity and GABA in a forebrain region involved in auditory filial imprinting. *Brain Research, 539*, 31–44.

Braun, K., Scheich, H., Heizmann, C. W., & Hunziker, W. (1991). Parvalbumin- and calbindin-(28K)-immunoreactivity as developmental markers of auditory and vocal motor nuclei of the zebra finch. *Neuroscience, 40*, 835–869.

Braun, K., Scheich, H., Schachner, M., & Heizmann, C. W. (1985a). Distribution of parvalbumin, cytochrome oxidase activity and ^{14}C-2-deoxyglucose uptake in the brain of the zebra finch. I. Auditory and vocal motor system. *Cell Tissue Research, 240*, 101–115.

Braun, K., Scheich, H., Schachner, M. & Heizmann, C. W. (1985b). Distribution of parvalbumin, cytochrome oxidase activity and ^{14}C-2-deoxyglucose uptake in the brain of the zebra finch. II. Visual system. *Cell Tissue Research, 240*, 117–127.

Braun, K., Scheich, H., Zuschratter, W., Heizmann, C. W., Matute, C., & Streit, P. (1988). Postnatal development of parvalbumin-, calbindin- and adult GABA-immunoreactivity in two visual nuclei of zebra finches. *Brain Research, 475*, 205–217.

Braun, S. (1987). *Immunohistochemische Untersuchungen von Gamma-aminobuttersäure (GABA) im prägungsrelevanten rostromedialen Neostriatum beim Haushuhnküken (Gallus gallus domesticus).* Unpublished master's thesis, Technical University Darmstadt.

Celio, M. R. (1990). Calbindin D28K and parvalbumin in the rat nervous system. *Neuroscience, 35*(2), 375–475.

Celio, M.R., & Heizmann, C. W. (1981). Calcium-binding protein parvalbumin as a neuronal marker. *Nature, 293*, 300–302.

Celio, M. R., Schärer, L., Morrison, J. H., Norman, A. W., & Bloom, F. E. (1986). Calbindin immunoreactivity alternates with cytochrome c-oxidase-rich zones in some layers of the primate visual cortex. *Nature, 323*, 717–717.

Changeux, J.-P., & Danchin, A. (1976). Selective stabilization of developing synapses as a mechanism for the specification of neuronal networks. *Nature, 264*, 705–712.

Changeux, J.-P., Heidmann, T., & Patte, P. (1984). Learning by selection. In P. Marler & H.S. Terrace (Eds.), *The biology of learning* (pp. 115–133). Heidelberg, New York: Springer-Verlag.

Connor, J. R., & Diamond, M. C. (1982). A comparison of dendritic spine number and type on pyramidal neurons of the visual cortex of old adult rats from social or isolated environments. *Journal of Comparative Neurology, 210*, 99–106.

Cragg, B. G. (1975). The development of synapses in the visual system of the cat. *Journal of Comparative Neurology, 160*, 147–166.

Csillag, A., Bourne, R. C., Kalman, M., Boxer, M. I., & Stewart, M. G. (1989). (^{3}H) Naloxone binding in the brain of the domestic chick (Gallus domesticus) determined by in vitro quantitative autoradiography. *Brain Research, 479*, 391–396.

Dietl, M. M., Cortés, R., & Palacios, J. M. (1988a). Neurotransmitter receptors in the avian brain. II. Muscarinic cholinergic receptors. *Brain Research, 439*, 360–365.

Dietl, M. M., Cortés, R., & Palacios, J. M. (1988b). Neurotransmitter receptors in the avian brain. III. GABA-benzodiazepine receptors. *Brain Research, 439*, 366–371.

Dietl, M. M., & Palacios, J. M. (1988). Neurotransmitter receptors in the avian brain. I. Dopamine receptors. *Brain Research, 439*, 354–359.

Dunwiddie, T. V., & Lynch, G. (1979). The relationship between extracellular calcium concentration and the induction of hippocampal long-term potentiation. *Brain Research, 169*, 103–110.

Dyer, A. B., & Gottlieb, G. (1990). Auditory basis of maternal attachment in ducklings (*Anas platyrhynchos*) under simulated naturalistic imprinting conditions. *Journal of Comparative Psychology, 104*, 190–194.

Faber, H., Braun, K., Zuschratter, W., & Scheich, H. (1989). System-specific distribution of zinc in the chick brain. *Cell Tissue Research, 258*, 247–257.

Feldman, M. L., & Dowd, C. (1975). Loss of dendritic spines in aging cerebral cortex. *Anatomy and Embryology, 148*, 279–301.

Gonzalez-Lima, F., & Scheich, H. (1984). Neural substrates for tone-conditioned bradycardia demonstrated with 2-deoxyglucose. I. Activation of auditory nuclei. *Behavioral Brain Research, 14*, 213–233.

Gonzalez-Lima, F., & Scheich, H. (1986). Neural substrates for tone-conditioned bradycardia demonstrated with 2-deoxyglucose. II. Auditory cortex plasticity. *Behavioral Brain Research, 20*, 281–293.

Greenough, W. T., & Bailey, C. H. (1988). The anatomy of memory: Convergence of results across a diversity of tests. *TINS, 11* (4), 142–147.

Gurney, M. (1981). Hormonal control of cell form and number in the zebra finch song system. *Journal of Neuroscience, 1*, 658–673.

Gurney, M., & Konishi, M. (1980). Hormone induced sexual differentiation of brain and behavior in zebra finches. *Science, 208*, 1380–1382.

Gustafsson, B., & Wigström, H. (1988). Physiological mechanisms underlying long-term potentiation. *TINS, 11*(4), 156–162.

Hebb, D. O. (1949). *The organization of behavior*. New York: Wiley.

Heil, P., & Scheich, H. (1985). Quantitative analysis and two-dimensional reconstruction of the tonotopic organization of the auditory field L in the chick from 2-deoxyglucose data. *Experimental Brain Research, 58*, 532–543.

Heil, P., & Scheich, H. (1986). Effects of unilateral and bilateral cochlea removal on 2-deoxyglucose patterns in the chick auditory system. *Journal of Comparative Neurology, 252*, 281–292.

Heizmann, C. W., & Braun, K. (1990). Calcium binding proteins. Molecular and functional aspects. In L. J. Anghileri (Ed.), *The role of calcium in biological systems* (Vol. V) (pp. 21–66). Boca Raton, Florida: CRC Press.

Hess, E. H. (1973). *Imprinting*. New York: Van Nostrand.

Hirsch, R. (1974). The hippocampus and contextual retrieval of information from memory. *Behavioral Biology, 12*, 421–444.

Hopfield, J. J. (1982). Neural networks and physical systems with emergent collective computational abilities. *Proceedings of the National Academy of Sciences, U.S.A., 79*, 2554–2558.

Horn, G. (1983). Information storage in the brain: A study of imprinting in the domestic chick. In J.-P. Ewert, R. R. Capranica, & D. J. Ingle (Eds.),

Advances in vertebrate neuroethology (pp. 511–541). New York: Plenum Press.

Horn, G. (1985). *Memory, imprinting and the brain. An inquiry into mechanisms.* Oxford: Clarendon Press.

Horn, G., Bradley, P. M., & McCabe, B. J. (1985). Changes in the structure of synapses associated with learning. *Journal of Neuroscience, 5,* 3161–3168.

Horn, G., McCabe, B. J., & Bateson, P. P. G. (1979). An autoradiographic study of the chick brain after imprinting. *Brain Research, 168,* 361–373.

Hubel, D. H., & Wiesel, T. N. (1970). The period of susceptibility to the physiological effects of unilateral eye closure in kittens. *Journal of Physiology, 206,* 419–436.

Immelmann, H., & Suomi, S. J. (1981). Sensitive phases in development. In K. Immelmann, G. W. Barlow, L. Petrinovich, & M. Main (Eds.), *Behavioral development* (pp. 395–431). Cambridge: Cambridge University Press.

Innocenti, G. M. (1991). Pathways between development and evolution. In B. L. Finlay, G. Innocenti, & H. Scheich (Eds.), *The neocortex: Ontogeny and phylogeny* (pp. 43–54). New York: Plenum Press.

Kalogirou, E. (1988). *Immunohistochemische Untersuchungen zur Lokalisation von Dopamin und Tyrosin-Hydroxylase im Gehirn von Haushuhnküken, unter besonderer Beachtung prägungsrelevanter Vorderhirngebiete.* Unpublished master's thesis, Technical University Darmstadt.

Kamphuius, W., Huisman, E., Wadman, W. J., Heizmann, C. W., & Lopez da Silva, F. H. (1989). Kindling induced changes in parvalbumin immunoreactivity in rat hippocampus and its relation to long-term decrease in GABA-immunoreactivity. *Brain Research, 479,* 23–34.

Karten, H. J. (1968). The ascending auditory pathway in the pigeon (*Columbia livia*). II. Telencephalic projections of the nucleus ovoidalis thalami. *Brain Research, 11,* 134–153.

Karten, H. J. (1969). The organization of the avian telencephalon and some speculations on the phylogeny of the amniote telencephalon. *Annals of the New York Academy of Sciences, 167,* 164–179.

Karten, H. J., & Hodos, W. (1970). Telencephalic projections of the nucleus rotundus in the pigeon (*Columba livia*). *Journal of Comparative Neurology, 140,* 35–52.

Kawaguchi, Y., Katsumaru, H., Kosaka, T., Heizmann, C. W., & K. Hama (1987). Fast spiking cells in rat hippocampus (CA 1-region) contain the calcium-binding protein parvalbumin. *Brain Research, 416,* 369–374.

Kitt, C. A., & Brauth, S. E. (1982). A palaeostriatal-thalamic-telencephalic path in pigeons. *Neuroscience, 7,* 2735–2751.

Kohsaka, S.-I., Takamatsu, K., Aoki, E., & Tsukada, Y. (1979). Metabolic mapping of chick brain after imprinting using [^{14}C]-2-deoxyglucose technique. *Brain Research, 172,* 539–544.

Konishi, M. (1985). Birdsong: From behavior to neuron. *Annual Review of Neuroscience, 8,* 125–175.

Kossut, M., & Rose, S. P. R. (1984). Differential 2-deoxyglucose uptake into chick brain structures during passive avoidance training. *Neuroscience, 12,* 971–977.

LeVay, S., Stryker, M. P., & Shatz, C. J. (1978). Ocular dominance columns and their development in layer IV of the cat's visual cortex: A quantitative study. *Journal of Comparative Neurology, 179,* 223–244.

LeVay, S., Wiesel, T. N., & Hubel, D. H. (1980). The development of ocular dominance columns in normal and visually deprived monkeys. *Journal of Comparative Neurology, 191,* 1–51.

Linsker, R. (1988). Development of feature analyzing cells and their columnar organization in a layered self-adaptive network. In R. Cotterill (Ed.), *Computer simulation in brain nuclei* (pp. 416–431). Cambridge: Cambridge University Press.

Lorenz, K. (1935). Der Kumpan in der Umwelt des Vogels. *Journal of Ornithology, 83*, 137–213.

Lund, J. S., Boothe, R.G., & Lund, R. D. (1977). Development of neurons in the visual cortexs (area 17) of the monkey (*Macaca nemestrina*): A Golgi study from fetal day 127 to postnatal maturity. *Journal of Comparative Neurology, 176*, 149–188.

Maier, V., & Scheich, H. (1983). Acoustic imprinting leads to differential 2-deoxy-D-glucose uptake in the chick forebrain. *Proceedings of the National Academy of Sciences, U.S.A., 80*, 3860–3864.

Maier, V., & Scheich, H. (1987). Acoustic imprinting in guinea fowl chicks. Age dependence of 2-deoxyglucose uptake in relevant forebrain areas. *Developmental Brain Research, 31*, 15–27.

Margoliash, D. (1987). Neural plasticity in birdsong learning. In J. P. Rauschecker & P. Marler (Eds.), *Imprinting and cortical plasticity. Comparative aspects of sensitive periods* (pp. 23–54). New York: John Wiley.

Marler, P. (1987). Sensitive periods and the roles of specific and general sensory stimulation in birdsong learning. In J. P. Rauschecker & P. Marler (Eds.), *Imprinting and cortical plasticity. Comparative aspects of sensitive periods* (pp. 99–135). New York: John Wiley.

Mason, R. J., & Rose, S. P. R. (1988). Passive avoidance learning produces focal elevation of bursting activity in the chick brain: Amnesia abolishes the increase. *Behavioral and Neural Biology, 49*, 280–292.

Mata, M., Fink, D. J., Gainer, H., Smith, C. B., Davidson, L., Savaki, H., Schwartz, W. J, & Sokoloff, L. (1980). Activity-dependent energy metabolism in rat posterior pituitary primarily reflects sodium pump activity. *Journal of Neurochemistry, 34*, 213–215.

McCabe, B. J., & Horn, G. (1988). Learning and memory: Regional changes in N-methyl-D-aspartate receptors in the chick brain after imprinting. *Proceedings of the National Academy of Sciences, U.S.A., 85*, 2849–2853.

McGeer, P. L., Eccles, J. C., & McGeer, E. G. (1978). *Molecular neurobiology of the mammalian brain.* New York: Plenum Press.

Mishkin, M., & Petri, H. L. (1983). Memories and habits: Some implications for the analysis of learning and retention. In N. Butters & L. R. Squire (Eds.), *The neuropsychology of memory.* New York: Guilford Press.

Mourre, C., Cervera, P., & Lazdunki, M. (1987). Autoradiographic analysis in the rat brain of the postnatal ontogeny of voltage-dependent Na^+ channels, Ca^{2+}-dependent K^+ channels and slow Ca^{2+} channels identified as receptors for tetrodotoxin, apamin, and (–)-desmethoxyverapamil. *Brain Research, 417*, 21–32.

Müller, S. C. (1987). *Neuronale Aktivitätsmuster im Gehirn von Hühnerküken während prägungsrelevanter Verhaltenssituationen.* Unpublished doctoral dissertation, Technical University Darmstadt.

Müller, S. C., & Scheich, H. (1986). Social stress increases (^{14}C)2-deoxyglucose incorporation in the rostral forebrain areas of the young chick. *Behavioral Brain Research, 19*, 93–98.

Murphy, K. M. M., Gould, R. J., & Snyder, S. H. (1982). Autoradiographic visualization of (^{3}H) nitrendipine binding sites in rat brain: Localization to synaptic zones. *European Journal of Pharmacology, 81*, 517–519.

Nottebohm, F. (1984). Birdsong as a model in which to study brain processes related to learning. *Condor, 86*, 227–236.

Nottebohm, F., & Arnold, A. P. (1976). Sexual dimorphism in vocal control areas of the song bird brain. *Science, 194*, 211–213.

Nottebohm, F., Stokes, T. M., & Leonard, C. M. (1976). Central control of song in the canary, *Serinus canarius. Journal of Comparative Neurology, 165*, 457–486.

Oppenheim, R. W. (1981). Neuronal cell death and some related regressive phenomena during neurogenesis: A selected historical review and progress report. In W. M. Cowan (Ed.), *Studies in developmental neurobiology: Essays in honor of Victor Hamburger* (pp. 74–133). Oxford, New York: Oxford University Press.

Palm, G. (1981). On the storage capacity of an associative memory with randomly distributed storage elements. *Biological Cybernetics, 39*, 125–127.

Patel, S. N., Rose, S. P. R., & Stewart, M.G. (1988). Training induced spine density changes are specifically related to memory formation processes in the chick, *Gallus domesticus. Brain Research, 463*, 168–173.

Patel, S. N., & Stewart, M. G. (1988). Changes in the number and structure of dendritic spines, 25 h after passive avoidance training in the domestic chick, *Gallus domesticus. Brain Research, 449*, 34–46.

Patterson, P. H., & Purves, D. (1982). *Readings in developmental neurobiology*, Section 6 (pp. 278–327). Cold Spring Harbor Reports in Neurosciences.

Pearson, R. (1972). *The avian brain*. London, New York: Academic Press.

Pittman, R., & Oppenheim, R. W. (1979). Cell death of motoneurons in the chick embryo spinal cord. IV. Evidence that a functional neuromuscular interaction is involved in the regulation of naturally occurring cell death and the stabilization of synapses. *Journal of Comparative Neurology, 187*, 425–446.

Purves, D., & Lichtman, J. W. (1980). Elimination of synapses in the developing nervous system. *Science, 210*, 153–157.

Quirion, R. (1983). Autoradiographic localization of a calcium channel antagonist, (^{3}H) nitrendipine, binding sites in rat brain. *Neuroscience Letters, 36*, 267–271.

Rausch, G. (1985). *Ontogenese der Vokalisation und des vokalmotorischen Kernes Hyperstriatum ventrale, pars caudalis (HVc) im Telencephalon des Beos (Gracula religiosa intermedia)*. Unpublished doctoral dissertation, Technical University Darmstadt.

Rausch, G., & Scheich, H. (1982). Dendritic spine loss and enlargement during maturation of the speech control system in the mynah bird (*Gracula religiosa*). *Neuroscience Letters, 29*, 129–133.

Rauschecker, J. P., & Marler, P. (1987). Cortical plasticity and imprinting: Behavioral and physiological contrasts and parallels. In J. P. Rauschecker & P. Marler (Eds.), *Imprinting and cortical plasticity. Comparative aspects of sensitive periods* (pp. 349–366). New York: John Wiley.

Reiner, A., Brauth, S. E., Kitt, Ch. A., & Quirion, R. (1989). Distribution of mu, delta, and kappa opiate receptor types in the forebrain and midbrain of pigeons. *Journal of Comparative Neurology, 280*, 359–382.

Rose, S. P. R. (1989). Glycoprotein synthesis and postsynaptic remodeling in long-term memory. *Neurochemistry International, 14*, 299–307.

Rose, S. P.R., & Csillag, A. (1985). Passive avoidance training results in lasting changes in deoxyglucose metabolism in left hemisphere regions of chick brain. *Behavioral and Neural Biology, 44*, 315–324.

Rosenzweig, M. R., Møllgaard, K., Diamond, M.C., & Bennet, E. L. (1972). Negative as well as positive synaptic changes may store memory. *Psychological Review, 79*, 93–96.

Ruiz-Marcos, A., & Valverde, F. (1969). The temporal evolution of the distribution of dendritic spines in visual cortex of normal and dark-reared mice. *Experimental Brain Research, 8*, 284–294.

Ryan, A. F., Woolf, N. K., & Sharp, F. R. (1982). Tonotopic organization in the central auditory pathway of the mongolian gerbil. A 2-deoxyglucose study. *Journal of Comparative Neurology, 207*, 369–380.

Scheich, H. (1987). Neural correlates of auditory filial imprinting. *Journal of Comparative Physiology, A161*, 605–619.

Scheich, H. (1991). Representational geometries of telencephalic auditory maps in birds and mammals. In B. L. Finlay, G. Innocenti, & H. Scheich (Eds.), *The neocortex. Ontogeny and phylogeny* (pp. 119–136). New York, London: Plenum Press.

Scheich, H., Bonke, B. A., Bonke, D., & Langner, G. (1979). Functional organization of some auditory nuclei in the guinea fowl demonstrated by the 2-deoxyglucose technique. *Cell Tissue Research, 204*, 17–27.

Scheich, H., & Braun, K. (1988). Synaptic selection and calcium regulation: Common mechanisms of auditory filial imprinting and vocal learning in birds. In F. G. Barth (Ed.), *Verhandlungen der Deutschen Zoologischen Gesellschaft. No. 81*, (pp. 77–95). New York, Stuttgart: Gustav Fischer Verlag.

Schüz, A. (1981). Pränatale Reifung und postnatale Veränderungen im Cortex des Meerschweinchens. Mikroskopische Auswertung eines natürlichen Deprivationsexperimentes. II. Postnatale Veränderungen. *Journal für Hirnforschung., 22*, 113–127.

Sejnowski, T., & Rosenberg, C. R. (1987). Parallel networks that learn to pronounce English text. *Complex Systems, 1*, 145–168.

Shatz, C. J., & Stryker, M. P. (1978). Ocular dominance in layer IV of the cat's visual cortex and the effects of monocular deprivation. *Journal of Physiology, 281*, 267–283.

Sherry, D. F., & Schacter, D. L. (1987). The evolution of multiple memory systems. *Psychological Review, 94*, 439–454.

Shimizu, T., & Karten, H. J. (1991). Multiple origins of neocortex: Contributions of the dorsal ventricular ridge. In B. L. Finlay, G. Innocenti, & H. Scheich (Eds.), *The neocortex. Ontogeny and phylogeny* (pp. 75–86). New York, London: Plenum Press.

Showers, M. J. C. (1982). Telencephalon of birds. In E. L. Crosby & H. N. Schnitzlein (Eds.), *Comparative correlative neuroanatomy of the vertebrate* (pp. 218–246). New York: Macmillan.

Sokoloff, L. (1975). The coupling of function, metabolism and blood flow in the brain. In D. H. Ingvar & N. A . Lassen (Eds.), *Brain work* (pp. 385–388). Copenhagen: Munksgaard.

Squire, L. R. (1982). The neuropsychology of human memory. *Annual Review of Neuroscience, 5*, 241–273.

Stewart, M. G. (1990). Morphological correlates of long-term memory in the chick forebrain consequent on passive avoidance learning. In L.R. Squire & E. Lindenlaub (Eds.), *The biology of memory* (pp. 193–215). Stuttgart, New York: F. K.-Schattner-Verlag.

Stewart, M.G., Bourne, R. C., Chmielowska, J., Kalman, M., Csillag, A., & Stanford, D. (1988). Quantitative autoradiographic analysis of the distribution of [³H] muscimol binding to GABA receptors in chick brain. *Brain Research, 456*, 387–391.

Stewart, M.G., King, T. S., & Rose, S. P. R. (1983). Stereological analysis of synapses in the brain of the domestic chick following avoidance learning. *Acta Stereologica, 2*, 227–230.

Stewart, M.G., Rose, S. P. R., King, T. S., Gabbott, P. L. A., & Bourne, R. (1984). Hemispheric asymmetry of synapses in chick medial hyperstriatum ventrale following passive avoidance training: A stereological investigation. *Developmental Brain Research, 12*, 261–269.

Stichel, C. C., Kägi, U., & Heizmann, C. W. (1986). Parvalbumin in cat brain: isolation, characterization and localization. *Journal of Neurochemistry, 47*, 46–53.

Stryker, P., & Harris, W. H. (1986). Binocular impulse blockade prevents the formation of ocular dominance columns in cat visual cortex. *Journal of Neuroscience, 6*, 2117–2133.

Swindale, N. V., Vital-Durand, F., & Blakemore, C. (1981). Recovery from monocular deprivation in the monkey. III. Reversal of anatomical effects in the visual cortex. *Proceedings of the Royal Society of London, B213*, 223–244.

Theurich, M., Müller, C. M., & Scheich, H. (1984). 2-Deoxyglucose accumulation parallels extracellularly recorded spike activity in the avian auditory neostriatum. *Brain Research, 322*, 157–161.

Tulving, E. (1985). How many memory systems are there? *American Psychologist, 40*, 385–398.

Veenmann, C. L., & Gottschaldt, K.-M. (1986). *The nucleus basalis–neostriatum complex in the goose (Anser anser L.). Advances in Anatomy, Embryology and Cell Biology* 96. New York: Springer-Verlag.

Wächtler, K. (1985). Regional distribution of muscarinic acetylcholine receptors in the telencephalon of the pigeon (*Columba livia f. domestica*). *Journal für Hirnforschung., 1*, 85–89.

Wallhäusser, E., & Scheich, H. (1987). Auditory imprinting leads to differential 2-deoxyglucose uptake and dendritic spine loss in the chick rostral forebrain. *Developmental Brain Research, 31*, 29–44.

Wallhäusser-Franke, E. (1989). *Anatomische Korrelate der akustischen Filialprägung im ZNS von Haushuhnküken (Gallus domesticus) und die Verbindungen der beteiligten Gebiete.* Unpublished doctoral dissertation, Technical University Darmstadt.

Webster, W. R., Servière, J., Crewther, D., & Crewther, S. (1984). Isofrequency 2DG contours in the inferior colliculus of the awake monkey. *Experimental Brain Research, 56*, 425–437.

Westrum, L. E., Hugh Jones, D., Gray, E.G., & Barron, J. (1980). Microtubules, dendritic spines and spine apparatuses. *Cell Tissue Research, 208*, 171–181.

Wiesel, T. N., & Hubel, D. H. (1965). Comparison of the effects of unilateral and bilateral eye closure on cortical unit responses in kittens. *Journal of Neurophysiology, 28*, 1029–1040.

Wild, J. M. (1987a). Thalamic projections to the palaeostriatum and neostriatum in the pigeon (*Columba livia*). *Neuroscience, 20*, 305–327.

Wild, J. M. (1987b). The avian somatosensory system: Connections of regions of body representation in the forebrain of the pigeon. *Brain Research, 412*, 205–223.

Wolff, J. R., Leutgeb, U., Holzgraefe, M., & Teuchert, G. (1989). Synaptic remodelling during primary and reactive synaptogenesis. In H. Rahmann (Ed.), *Fundamentals of memory formation. Neuronal plasticity and brain function* (pp. 68–82). Stuttgart, New York: Gustav Fischer Verlag.

Zeier, H., & Karten, H. J. (1971). The archistriatum of the pigeon, organization of afferent and efferent connections. *Brain Research, 31*, 313–326.

Zuschratter, W., Scheich, H., & Heizmann, C. W. (1985). Ultrastructural localization of the calcium-binding protein parvalbumin in neurons of the song system of the zebra finch, *Poephila guttata. Cell Tissue Research, 241*, 77–83.

II

Functional Roles of Brain Systems

7

Memory Representation in the Hippocampus: Functional Domain and Functional Organization

HOWARD EICHENBAUM
NEAL J. COHEN
TIM OTTO
CYNTHIA WIBLE

The first studies on the amnesic patient H.M. made it immediately clear that the hippocampus and associated medial temporal lobe structures are critical components of a functional system for long-term memory formation (Scoville & Milner, 1957). Subsequently, the focus of much research logically turned to characterizing the precise functional role played by the hippocampal system. Work on this issue has been conducted both with amnesic patients and with animals having experimental lesions in brain structures shown to be damaged in human amnesia. Progress toward a consensus either within or between species has been disappointingly slow, however, due in large measure to difficulties (and controversies) in identifying the relevant distinctions in memory processes that are "honored by the nervous system" (cf. Squire, 1987). Some of these issues were considered in detail in the first two meetings of this symposium (Lynch, McGaugh, & Weinberger, 1984; Weinberger, McGaugh, & Lynch, 1985) and to a lesser extent in the third (McGaugh, Weinberger, & Lynch, 1990), but a brief and pointed review will be offered here to frame the view of hippocampal system function that has emerged from our own work.

The results of thorough studies on H.M., confirmed by data from other patients with damage to the hippocampus and anatomically related brain structures (the hippocampal system), were striking in so clearly documenting the memory impairment as distinct from intact perceptual, cognitive, and motor capacities. Furthermore, the amnesic deficit resulting from this brain damage was found to be global, although certain "exceptions" of relatively preserved motor (Corkin, 1968) and perceptual (Warrington & Weiskrantz, 1968) learning were noted. Unfortunately, initial efforts to replicate the isolated memory impairment in nonhumans were disappointing in that animals with hippocampal system lesions succeeded quite impressively in learning most of the conventional discrimination and maze learning tasks employed (e.g., Douglas, 1967; Kimble, 1968), resulting in a sharp division between the results on humans and animals; subsequent work on human and animal amnesia proceeded in largely separate directions. However, about a decade ago, these efforts began to converge when studies on human amnesia revealed that the exceptions to the global deficit were only examples of a broad domain of spared learning capacity. Around the same time, experiments on animals with experimental lesions began to uncover a significant domain of impaired learning that contrasted with the otherwise intact learning abilities. Thus the two literatures began to converge along the theme of distinct impaired versus preserved domains of memory, with the dissociation between domains being attributed to the existence of multiple memory systems.

In the period spanning the early Irvine symposia, intense debate focused on delineating the domains of impaired and preserved capacities in both human and animal amnesics. Several laboratories generated different interpretations of the multiple memory system view, each attempting to capture the essential distinction between hippocampal-dependent and hippocampal-independent memory. Full consensus among the various investigators has not yet been reached, a state of affairs we attribute to the limited domain of the data considered by most accounts, speaking almost exclusively to either the human or the animal literature and largely restricted to one set of behavioral paradigms to the exclusion of others. Some have had remarkable success linking aspects of amnesia in human and nonhuman primates (Zola-Morgan & Squire, 1984, 1985), but no effort to date has made a clear bridge across primate and nonprimate species. Our goal is to develop a view of hippocampal function and memory that combines common threads in the accounts of human and animal amnesia, in the search for a comprehensive account. This has led us to develop assessments of hippocampal function that may be universally applicable across species and across behavioral paradigms, and to articulate a theoretical framework with a correspondingly broad scope. This chapter should be considered a progress report on this endeavor. We begin by outlining our analysis of the relevant literatures; we then summarize our own efforts to characterize the functional role of the hippocampal system in memory.

COMMON THREADS IN THE LITERATURE ON HUMAN AND ANIMAL AMNESIA

Review of the human amnesia literature of the past decade reveals a variety of multiple memory system accounts of human amnesia. These proposals explore distinctions between learning that is impaired versus that which is spared, respectively, such as "knowing that" versus "knowing how" (Ryle, 1949), "memory with record" versus "memory without record" (Bruner,

1969), "explicit memory" versus "implicit memory" (Graf & Schacter, 1985), and "declarative memory" versus "procedural memory" (Cohen & Squire, ` 1980). The list goes on (see Johnson, 1990; Squire, 1987; Squire & Butters, 1984; Weiskrantz, 1985) but, as several investigators have noted, there is a common focus on forms of awareness and cognitive mediation that qualify the domain of impaired memory; in each formulation the memory system supporting spared learning in amnesia operates without requiring such mediation. This focus seems to be most fully captured by the declarative/procedural distinction (e.g., Squire, 1987). On this view, amnesic patients are profoundly impaired in the conscious recollection of, and in the ability to verbally reflect on, prior experiences; these deficits may be observed even as amnesics express acquired performance based on the experience (Cohen, 1984; for a recent discussion see Squire 1987, pp. 151–169). Conversely, what characterizes all of the distinctions cited above is the preserved capacity of human amnesics to reinstantiate "procedures" or routines that led to successful performance. We have adopted this particular characterization of human amnesia for two major reasons. First, as discussed briefly below, this distinction incorporates a mechanism for how impaired and spared domains of memory are expressed, making them accessible to experimental observation. Second, this distinction includes an active operational role for both the impaired and spared memory systems, rather than a special process impaired in amnesia versus its absence in spared learning. Combined, the properties of the declarative/procedural dichotomy best capture the critical distinctions between impaired and spared memory in human amnesia and offer the greatest opportunity for finding connections with the literature on animals.

With regard to accounts of the pattern of performance in animals with hippocampal system damage, the following characterizations are prominent among proposals distinguishing impaired versus spared learning, respectively: "place learning" versus "taxon learning" (O'Keefe & Nadel, 1978), "contextual encoding" versus "learning along the performance line" (Hirsh, 1974), learning of "external context attributes" versus acquiring "rules" (Kesner, 1984), "configural association" versus "simple association" (Sutherland & Rudy, 1989), "memory" versus "habit" (Mishkin, Malamut, & Bachevalier, 1984), "recognition" versus "association" (Gaffan, 1974), "working memory" versus "reference memory" (Olton, Becker, & Handlemann, 1979), and "representational memory" versus "dispositional memory" (Thomas & Gash, 1986). These proposals have less of a common theme than was the case for human amnesia; on a casual inspection there does not seem to be the same level of consensus as apparent among proposals on human memory. For example, it is difficult to see what common thread might be found among such different characterizations as contextual encoding and working memory. But our analysis of these proposals, and the experiments generating them, suggested that they can be grouped into two sets and that a common thread might indeed join them all.

One set of theories focuses on the importance of hippocampal function in the representation of *configurations* among perceptually-independent cues, as explicit in representation of the spatial configurations that guide place learning and implicit in the creation of configural, conditional, or contextual cues (Hirsh, 1974, 1980; Kesner, 1984; Mishkin et al., 1984; Sutherland, Macdonald, Hill, & Rudy, 1989; Sutherland & Rudy, 1989; Winocur & Olds, 1978). The other proposals focus on views about hippocampal involvement in *temporal tagging*, a process that requires comparisons of current perceptions to prior representations. This notion is explicit in views of the hippocampus as a "comparator" (Gabriel, Foster, Orona, Saltwick, & Stanton, 1980; Gray, 1979; Gray & Rawlins, 1986; Rawlins, 1985) and implicit in its involvement in recognition (Gaffan, 1974), "representation" (Thomas & Gash, 1986), and working memory (Olton et al., 1979). What ties all these characterizations together is the requirement for comparison and manipulation of representations according to significant *relationships* among perceptually independent stimuli present at the same time (configurations), or among stimuli presented sequentially (temporal tagging). Conversely, what characterizes each view of the learning capacities spared in animals with hippocampal system damage is the intact ability to process stimuli individually, as opposed to relationally, and to acquire the association of an *individual* stimulus with a particular reward or response, without reference to other items in memory. In our view, the relational/individual distinction between forms of representation offers a comprehensive characterization of the impaired and preserved domains of memory after hippocampal system damage in animals, and provides the greatest opportunity for contact with the phenomenology of the human literature as captured by the declarative/procedural account.

How exactly do we connect the declarative-memory/procedural-memory account of human amnesia and the relational-representation/individual-representation account with regard to studies on animals, in order to achieve a comprehensive proposal about multiple memory systems? A full articulation of our rationale is beyond the scope of this chapter, so a summary must suffice here. We should start by noting that connecting these two literatures is complicated by two formidable hurdles. The first hurdle concerns the emphasis on conscious recollection and cognitive mediation in the characterization of human amnesia; these constructs must be defined or operationalized in such a manner as to be equally applicable to both human and animal work. The second hurdle involves articulating the linkage between "relational representation" and "declarative memory" and, conversely, "individual representation" and "procedural memory."

With regard to the first hurdle, some believe that the capacity for conscious recollection and cognitive mediation may not exist in animals, thereby representing a major schism between human and animal capacities. The issue of animal cognition (also discussed at length in a previous meeting of this symposium by Holland [1990], Mackintosh [1985], Macphail [1985], Rosenzweig & Glickman [1985] and Schacter [1985]), is far from resolved and, for several reasons, may not be tractable. But accepting the view that animal consciousness is nonexistent or inaccessible would seem to put a consensus on hippocampal function out of reach. More optimistically, we adopt the position that animal consciousness is possible and indeed straightforwardly, if indirectly, observable in nonverbal measures of its behavioral consequences. Such a position conforms with views articulated at earlier meetings of this symposium by Mackintosh (1985), Morris (1984b, 1985), and Nadel and Wexler (1984), and is consistent with accounts that propose the evolution of a relational memory system without reference to consciousness (Holland, 1990; Sherry & Schacter, 1987). For example, Mackintosh (1985; see also Holland, 1990) cited specific examples of reward devaluation experiments as evidence for the kind of cognitive mediation expressed in Tolman's notion of "expectancy" (see also Mishkin & Petri, 1984). More generally, Nadel and Wexler (1984) referred to the "generative" quality of "knowledge", a requirement of cognitive mediation for generating appropriate responses for situations never experienced, based on previous learning. The notion of a generative property is similar to what Cohen (1984) described as the "promiscuous" nature of declarative memories in humans, referring to the accessibility of declarative memory representations by many processing systems including those supporting verbal reflection and conscious recollection. These prototypically human capacities, then, can be seen as being among the manifestations of the generative quality and flexible nature of declarative memory, many of which can be observed in animals as well.

With respect to the second hurdle, let us now discuss the connection between relational representation and declarative memory. Our view is that these are not different descriptions of the same kind of memory or process in memory, but rather that one of them, relational representation, permits the other, declarative expression of memory. We suggest that the embodiment of relational representation, supported by the hippocampal system, can be envisioned as a multidimensional network of memories, a memory "space" with information nodes corresponding to particular items in memory and connections between nodes corresponding to significant relations among those items (for a general treatment of network memories see Andersen, 1990). The existence of different relational dimensions might be the functional consequences of a more simple associative architecture in the hippocampus (Kohonen, 1990; Marr, 1971; McNaughton & Morris, 1987; Morris, 1990), or might be anatomically constituted within the organization of hippocampal circuitry (cf. Amaral & Witter, 1989; Eichenbaum & Buckingham, 1991). Regardless of the structural basis of this relational representation, we suggest that a central property of such a network is that activation of one node leads to activation of items that are only indirectly connected and not previously active together. This property offers a mechanism for access to memories in new contexts, just as the operational requirement for declarative memory suggested above. The connection between the emphasis on comparison, the central process in constructing and maintaining relational representation, and the capacity for flexible expression was stated quite explicitly in Cohen's (1984) characterization of declarative memory: ". . . a declarative code permits the ability to compare and contrast information from different processes or processing systems; and it enables the ability to make inferences from and generalizations across facts derived from multiple processing sources. Such a common declarative code thereby provides the basis for access to facts acquired during the course of experiences and for conscious recollection of the learning experiences themselves" (p. 97). We have extended this view within this more comprehensive proposal, suggesting that comparison is a process central to creation and updating of relational representations that support declarative expression (Eichenbaum, Mathews & Cohen, 1989).

Finally, let us make the connection between the characterization of the spared procedural learning domain in human amnesics and our description of hippocampal-independent memory in animals as supported by individual representations. The defining quality of an individual representation is the isolation of each particular stimulus–response–reinforcement association from other stimuli and associations. A key consequence of this kind of representation is its *inflexibility*. To the extent that a representation is isolated from the record of other comparable (or contrastable) experiences, we might expect that learning could be revealed only in the restrictive range of stimuli and the context in which it was originally acquired. Indeed, this is just what is described in accounts of amnesia in both humans and animals. Schacter (1985) qualified preserved learning by human amnesics as the acquisition of *hyperspecific associations*. Mishkin and colleagues (1984) characterized the preserved learning capacity of monkeys with hippocampal system damage as the formation of *habits*; the inflexible "reflexive" nature of responses available within the habit system was recently contrasted with the flexible "reflective" capacities of the hippocampal-dependent memory system (Saunders & Weiskrantz, 1989). In nonprimates, inflexibility is implicit in characterizations of preserved learning as "along the performance line" (Hirsh, 1974), or the acquisition of "rules" (Kesner, 1980). More generally, the conditions for revealing this kind of representation are perhaps described most completely in Cohen's (1984) characterization of procedural learning as "expressible only through activation of the particular processing structures or procedures engaged by the learning tasks" (p. 96). Although some highly structured situations can be used to uncover the influence of procedural representations (e.g., verbal "priming"; Moscovitch, 1984), in general, individual representations are revealed only in repetition of the learning event.

AN EMPIRICAL APPROACH TO CHARACTERIZING HIPPOCAMPAL REPRESENTATION

The proposal summarized above offers a view of the hippocampus and memory that spans differences in the behavioral expression of memory across species and across experimental paradigms. Accordingly, empirical research on any number of different animal species can validate or falsify this proposal. In our own research program, we seek to confirm the characterization of hippocampal-dependent, declarative memory in terms of *relational representation*, the encoding of cues in terms of comparisons and significant relationships among multiple independent percepts, and *mnemonic flexibility*, the capacity for flexible use of memories in novel situations. While aimed at this particular characterization, our experiments are also designed to address two general and related questions about the nature of hippocampal processing. We refer to these as the *functional domain* question, which asks about the role of the hippocampal system in memory, and the *functional organization* question, which asks about the nature of hippocampal representation and its organization within hippocampal structure. We will argue below that the pursuit of these questions, asked in parallel, offer converging evidence for a view of hippocampal memory representation that spans differences in the behavioral expression of memory across species and across memory paradigms.

THE FUNCTIONAL DOMAIN OF THE HIPPOCAMPAL SYSTEM

Our insights about the functional domain of the hippocampal system have come primarily from behavioral evaluations of humans and animals with damage to that system, more specifically, from comparisons of aspects of memory processes that are impaired versus intact following hippocampal system damage. As introduced above, the major source of discrepancies among theories of hippocampal function derived from applications of this strategy is that different investigations focus on a particular species and a particular behavioral paradigm. This has led to theoretical positions that cover only a limited domain of the data, consequently distinguishing impaired and spared performance by a particular category of learning materials or response modality within that species and paradigm. An example from the literature on humans is the episodic/semantic distinction that emphasizes the impairment in autobiographical memory prevalent in human amnesics (Schacter & Tulving, 1983). An example from the animal literature is the response perseveration hypothesis that emphasizes the inability to alter prepotent responses prevalent in the performance deficit following hippocampal system damage (Douglas, 1967). Each of these hypotheses has been disproven by specific counterevidence, but the general tendency to focus on a category of learning materials persists. Our working hypothesis, which focuses on a type of representation (relational) and one of its central properties (mnemonic flexibility) marks a departure from this tendency; a major axiom of this hypothesis is that hippocampal memory processing is not material specific and that examples of apparent selectivity are a consequence of the heavy demand some categories of learning put on relational representation. Detailed consideration of another "limited domain" theory receiving considerable current attention will serve as an example of this phenomenon.

The cognitive mapping theory, originally proposed by O'Keefe and Nadel (1978), holds that the hippocampus is selectively involved in learning and memory for places and that learning and memory guided by nonspatial cues is not dependent on the hippocampal system. The major finding strongly supporting this view is that animals with hippocampal system damage are severely and selectively impaired in place learning as opposed to learning guided by "taxons," salient cues contiguous with the reinforcer. The relatively consistent observation of a profound deficit in place learning after hippocampal system damage, as well as evidence of the existence of cells "tuned" to the animals' location in the environment (O'Keefe, 1976; see below), provide impressive and convincing evidence that the hippocampal system is involved in place memory. But accepting the broader conclusion that the role of the hippocampus is limited to place memory is at odds with the wealth of data on human amnesia, a considerable recent literature on nonhuman primates (e.g., Gaffan, 1974; Mishkin, 1978; Zola-Morgan & Squire, 1985), and significant counterevidence in the literature on rodents (e.g., Raffaelle & Olton, 1988; Sutherland & Rudy, 1989; Winocur & Olds, 1978; also see above). Thus the cognitive mapping theory fails to account for the full domain of the literature on functional deficits across species and even within rodents. Moreover, the notion that the hippocampus is solely involved with space is a view much more restrictive than the characterization of cognitive mapping as it was originally proposed by O'Keefe and Nadel (1978).

Consistent with that view, we argue that the comparison of "place cues" versus "taxons" is complicated by the fact that spatial cues are not stimuli in the literal sense, but are the representational consequences of processing positional relations among the same specific visual (or other) stimuli that could serve as adequate taxons in hippocampal-independent learning. A particularly striking demonstration of the characterization of place cues as dependent on positional relations comes from an experiment of O'Keefe and Conway (1980). They found that rats with hippocampal system damage failed to learn the location of reward on a cross-maze guided by multiple extramaze visual stimuli when they were distributed around the maze, but were unimpaired in learning guided by the same stimuli when they were clustered near the reward site, eliminating the need for processing and remembering positional relations among the stimuli. The focus on significant spatial *relations* at the heart of the cognitive mapping theory is, then, consistent with our analysis of the larger literature (see above).

The Hippocampal System and Relational Representation

Demonstrating the validity of a more general view of the importance of relational representation outside place learning requires behavioral assessments of memory employing a nonspatial modality and demonstration that this view can account for the pattern of impaired and spared learning for both nonspatial and spatial materials. We have pursued this strategy, investigating learning capacities in rats with hippocampal system damage on learning identical nonspatial or spatial materials under task variations that encourage or hinder relational processing. Consistent with our hypothesis, we found that rats with hippocampal system damage are impaired on nonspatial learning when the demand for relational representation is high, and that they can succeed at place learning when the demand for relational representation is low.

Odor Discrimination Learning
Our assessment of nonspatial learning exploited the rats' excellent learning and memory capacities in odor discrimination learning. Rats perform at least as well at odor-guided discrimination learning as they do at place learning; they develop odor discrimination learning sets exceedingly rapidly, a capacity previously argued to be only within the repertoire of primates (e.g., Eichenbaum, Otto, Wible, & Piper, 1991; Otto & Eichenbaum, 1991; Slotnick & Katz, 1974). We measured the capacity of intact rats versus rats with disconnection of the hippocampal system via fornix transection (FX) in variations of the odor discrimination learning paradigm, assessing the capacity for relational representation by manipulating the demand for comparison and representation of relations among the same odor cues. We selectively manipulated the demand for stimulus comparison by developing variates of the odor discrimination paradigm that used identical odor cues, but emphasized or hindered comparison between those cues (Eichenbaum, Fagan, Mathews, & Cohen, 1988). In a simultaneous odor discrimination task, two odor cues were presented at the same time and in close spatial juxtaposition; the discriminative response required a selection between equivalent left/right choices (Figure 7.1). Under these training conditions, FX rats were severely and persistently impaired on a series of odor discrimination problems. In striking contrast, in a successive odor discrimination task, odors were presented separately across trials, hindering stimulus comparison, and the response required only completing or discontinuing the stimulus sampling behavior, thus eliminating the response choice. Under these training conditions, FX rats were *superior* to normal rats in acquiring the same series of discrimination problems that they had failed to learn under other task demands (see also Eichenbaum, Fagan, & Cohen, 1986; Otto, Schottler, Staubli, Eichenbaum, & Lynch, 1991; Staubli, Ivy, & Lynch, 1984).

In yet a third variate of the paradigm, odors were presented separately across trials, as in the successive discrimination task, but the response required the same spatial choice as that in the simultaneous discrimination task. Under these training conditions, FX rats were only transiently impaired, despite the same demand for a spatial response as required in simultaneous discrimination. Our interpretation of these findings is that severe impairment, transient impairment, or even facilitation may be observed under different

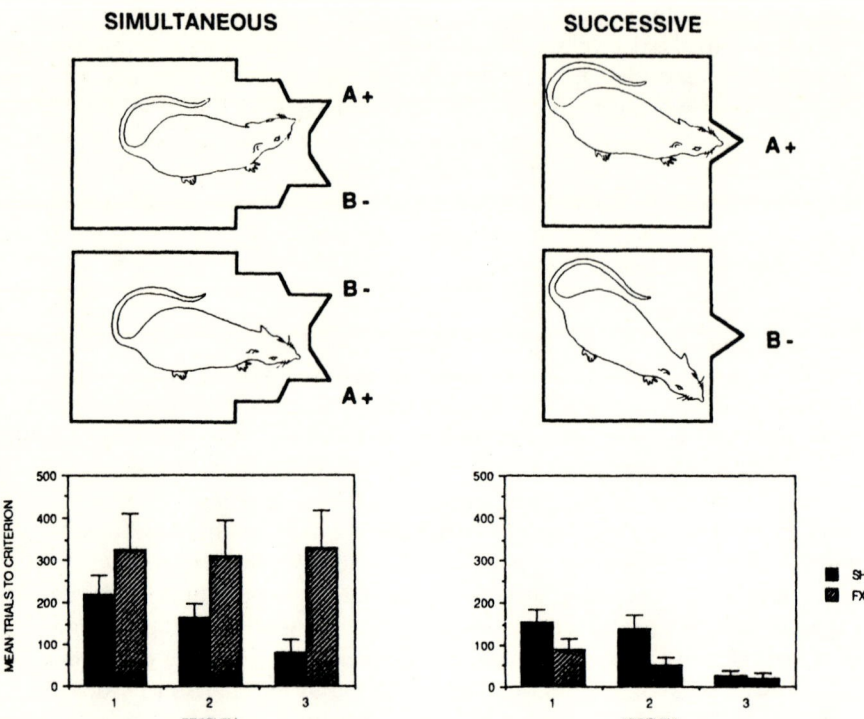

FIGURE 7.1. Assessment of learning on two variates of the odor discrimination paradigm. (Top) Schematic diagrams and trial examples showing both configurations of odor presentation used in each task variate and a rat executing the appropriate response. (Bottom) Performance on these tasks (±SE) by sham-operated rats (SH) and rats with bilateral fimbria/fornix transection (FX). (Taken from Eichenbaum, Fagan, Mathews, & Cohen, 1988)

task demands, even with the identical stimulus materials. Moreover, the differences in performance by FX rats can be related to the demand for stimulus and response comparison. Finally, it is important to note that even in those variates of the paradigm where FX rats failed to learn the odor discrimination, they readily acquired the necessary instrumental procedures that were common across all trials, such as awaiting a signal to begin the trial, performing nose-pokes and discriminative responses, and locating the reward delivery cup.

Place Learning
Can the conclusion that the demand for relational processing determines success or failure in amnesic animals be extended to other learning materials more commonly employed in studies of learning and memory? Might this account even apply to place learning? Perhaps the clearest demonstration of the critical role the hippocampus plays in place learning comes from

experiments using the Morris water maze (Morris, Garrud, Rawlins, & O'Keefe, 1982). The apparatus used in these studies is a large circular swimming pool filled with an opaque water solution and containing an escape platform slightly submerged at a constant locus relative to salient extramaze visual cues. In the standard version of this paradigm, rats are released into the water at different starting points on successive trials. Intact animals rapidly learn the place of the platform, demonstrating their memory in progressively shorter escape latencies. Rats with damage to the hippocampal system fail to learn the escape locus and persist in requiring long escape times even with extended training (Figure 7.2). In contrast, rats with hippocampal system damage learn to escape, as rapidly as normal animals, in another version of the task where the escape platform is made visible above the water surface, providing a nonspatial taxon (Morris et al., 1982).

We postulated that the severe learning deficit observed in rats with hippocampal system damage on the conventional water maze task is due to the emphasis placed on comparisons among the positions of extramaze stimuli and the rat's own position when trials begin from different start locations. Indeed, it is difficult to imagine how the task could be solved without the use of a "map"; such performance would require the rat to disentangle conflicting associations of separate views of the environment seen as it traverses the different trajectories from separate starting loci. To assess the importance of the demand for relational representation in place learning, we eliminated the need to compare views across different starting positions by releasing the rat from the same starting position on each trial (Figure 7.2; Eichenbaum, Stewart, & Morris, 1990). We speculated that these conditions would permit the acquisition of an individual association between a particular place (defined by the same extramaze stimuli as in the conventional, variable start condition), a single swim trajectory, and the reinforcement of escape. We predicted that FX rats would be able to acquire this version of the place learning paradigm.

To diminish the rats' exposure to different views of the environment and swim trajectories, we initially trained all rats to swim from the constant starting point to a visible platform. Both normal and FX rats acquired this task rapidly, although the FX rats were slightly (and significantly) slower (Figure 7.2), foreshadowing the qualitative differences observed in later tests. Then we "faded out" the visibility of the platform over a series of trials, until all animals were swimming directly to the location of the platform guided entirely by extramaze cues. Both groups of rats continued to perform well on most trials.

To confirm that both sets of rats were using the same extramaze cues to guide performance, we applied the standard "transfer" test developed by Morris (1984a) to assess the strength of the place-memory representation. In this test the escape platform was removed and the swimming pattern of the rats is observed for a fixed period, then the amount of time swimming in the quadrant of the pool including the site of the platform versus that

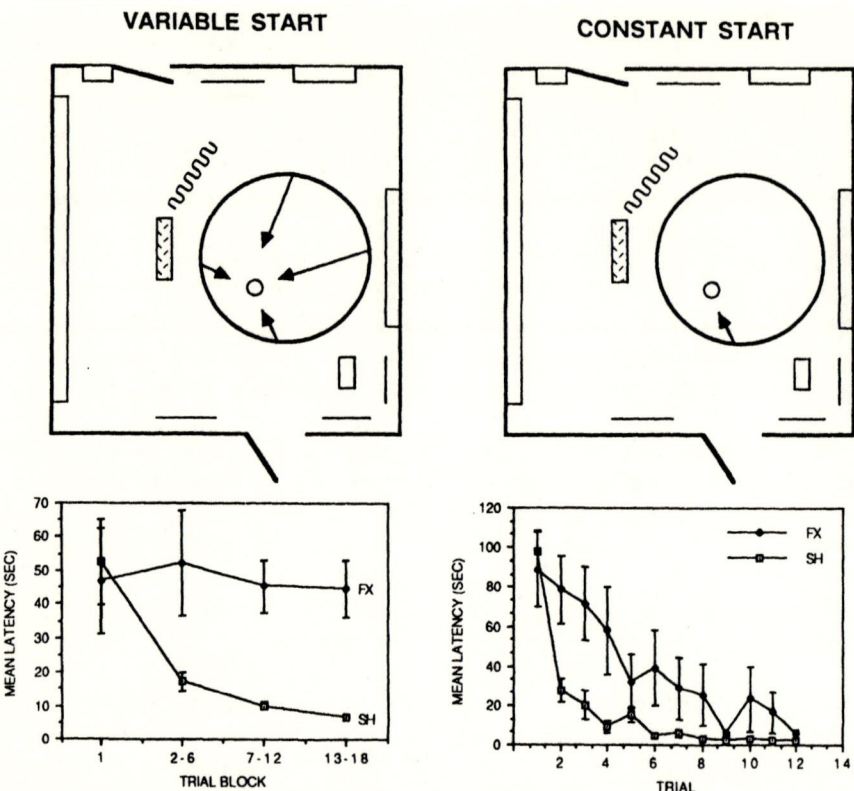

FIGURE 7.2. Assessment of performance on two variates of place learning in the Morris water maze. (Top) Schematic views of the testing room filled with various distal visual stimuli surrounding the swimming pool. Starting points and direct swim routes to the hidden escape platform are indicated by arrows. (Bottom) Acquisition of the Morris water maze task in sham-operated rats (SH) and rats with transection of the fimbria/fornix (FX). Scores are measured in terms of latency to locate the escape platform (±SE). Note that the initial training trials shown for the constant start condition (right) involved a visible escape platform, but both SH and FX animals continued to perform well when the platform was made invisible. (Taken from Eichenbaum, Stewart, & Morris, 1990)

for other quadrants is compared. Scores on this test are sensitive to the rat's perseverance in swimming near the former locus of the platform, and relatively insensitive to the rat's initial trajectory. Both normal and FX rats spent most of the time near the former location of the platform, indicating that they could identify the place of escape by the extramaze cues rather than solely by the approach trajectory.

The Hippocampal System and Mnemonic Flexibility

The key property of relational representation proposed above is the capacity of this sort of memory organization to support the flexible expression of memories in novel situations. A general prediction of this view is that even when amnesic subjects succeed at learning, their representation is abnormally *inflexible*, that it cannot be extended to situations substantially different from repetition of the original learning event.

Odor Discrimination Learning
To assess the importance of mnemonic flexibility in the memory representation of normal rats and rats with hippocampal system damage on odor discrimination learning, we pursued a follow-up experiment based on the simultaneous odor discrimination task (Eichenbaum, Mathews, & Cohen, 1989). Our investigation exploited a surprising variability in the results from that training condition; although FX rats were generally impaired on this task, they succeeded in learning some of the discrimination problems at least as rapidly as normal animals. There are several possible explanations for this variability, including that some problems were "easier," as might be the case if the choice of stimulus odors coincided with innate odor preferences, putting less demand on mnemonic processing, or that FX rats recovered from the effects of the lesion. However, the pattern of impairment was not consistent with either of these explanations.

Another possibility is that FX rats encoded the stimuli present on each trial employing the strategy that was used successfully by them in the successive odor discrimination paradigm. This view would be consistent with our previous findings on tasks using successive odor presentations (see above) and with our views on stimulus encoding in amnesia. However, it would require that the discriminative stimuli be encoded as distinct compounds, each composed of the same pair of odors in a different left–right juxtaposition. For just those problems in which different arrangements of the same odors could be perceived as distinct stimulus compounds, the animals might associate a particular cue with an arbitrary spatial response, as indeed they had done successfully in one of the tasks used in our previous study. To the extent that odor pair compounds made from the same pairs of odors could not be differentiated, discriminative performance would be impossible. We might expect this to be the case with most odor pairs, and, indeed, FX rats usually fail on these problems.

To investigate the stimulus sampling strategies of normal and FX rats and to determine the nature of their representations of odor pairs, we trained yoked pairs of normal and FX rats on a series of simultaneous odor discrimination problems until the FX rat of the pair had acquired two problems within the normal range of scores. Training sometimes required as many as 10 problems, since FX rats failed far more often than they succeeded, replicating our previous findings. In subsequent overtraining on a concurrent discrimination of both problems, we evaluated the stimulus sampling strategies and representation of the odor stimuli in two ways: by measuring their "reaction times" to the stimuli and by testing their odor representations with probe trials composed of novel configurations of the stimuli used on instruction trials.

We determined reaction times by recording the latency between odor onset and response choice. It was expected that FX rats would have shorter reaction times than normal rats, to the extent that they would sample the pair of odors at once (as an odor compound) and that normal rats would require more time to sample each odor separately. This prediction was supported in that each FX rat had a quantitatively shorter average response latency than each normal rat, even though all rats performed consistently at high accuracy and showed the speed-accuracy tradeoff typical of reaction time measures. Furthermore, FX rats also had an abnormal pattern of reaction times (Figure 7.3). Each normal rat had a bimodal distribution of response latencies, and each of the two modes was associated with one of the positions where the S^+ was presented and response executed. This pattern of reaction times suggests that the rat consistently approached and sampled one odor port first, then either performed a nose-poke there, or approached and sampled the other odor port. In contrast, FX rats had a unimodal distribution of response latencies, and the pattern was the same regardless of S^+ position. This pattern is consistent with our prediction that FX rats sample the entire stimulus compound at once, requiring less time to complete the trial. Finally, both the overall finding of reduced reaction

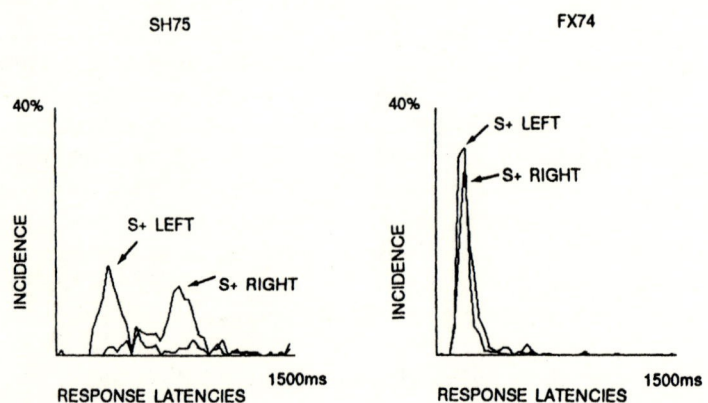

FIGURE 7.3. The distributions of response latencies for a sham-operated rat (SH75) and a rat with a fimbria/fornix transection (FX74) on odor discrimination trials given during overtraining trials where performance was similar for both subjects (87% for SH75 and 84% for FX74). Separate distributions are shown for correct responses when the S^+ odor was presented on the left or on the right. The distribution of response latencies differs for the sham-operated rat, depending on where the S^+ was presented. In contrast, the response latencies of the FX rat had a single mode more rapid than even the early mode of the sham operated rat. (Taken from Eichenbaum et al., 1989)

times and the abnormal pattern of response latencies was also present on problems in which FX rats failed, consistent with our view that FX rats employed the same strategy on all problems.

To investigate the contents of odor representations in normal and FX rats within successfully acquired discrimination problems, we evaluated the responses of rats to probe trials composed of familiar odors presented "mispaired" in combinations not previously experienced. According to our notion of relational representation, normal animals encode all the odor stimuli presented both within and across trials within an organized scheme that would support comparisons among odors not previously experienced together. Conversely, as supported by the findings from the pattern of reaction times, we postulated that FX rats had encoded each left–right arrangement of odor pairs as a compound; this form of representation would not be expected to support recognition of the separate elements within each compound. To test these predictions, we intermixed within a series of trials on two different instruction problems occasional probe trials composed of a mispaired S^+ odor from one problem and the S^- odor from the other (Figure 7.4). Both normal and FX rats continued to perform well on the trials composed of the odor pairings used on instruction trials, demonstrating that the introduction of probe trials did not disrupt their performance on familiar discrimination problems. Normal rats also performed accurately on the probe trials, even when they were first presented. In contrast, FX rats performed at chance levels on the probe trials when they were introduced, as if presented with novel stimuli.

Place Learning

If the property of mnemonic flexibility is to be generalized from our data on odor discrimination learning, we must demonstrate its importance in an account of successful place learning in rats with hippocampal system damage. To assess the capacity for mnemonic flexibility supported by the place representations of normal and FX rats in the constant start condition, we presented them with different types of probe trials, each involving an alteration of the cues or starting points, intermixed within a series of repetitions of the instruction trial. One of our probe tests demonstrated a particularly striking dissociation between the above-described success by FX rats in using the same extramaze cues to identify the place of escape and their inflexibility in novel testing situations, just as had been observed in our experiments on odor discrimination. In this probe test, on every third trial in a series of repeats of the instruction condition, the platform was left in its normal place but the start position was moved to various novel loci (Figure 7.5). When the start position was the same as that used during instruction trials, both normal and FX rats had short escape latencies. On probe trials, normal rats also swam directly to the platform regardless of the starting position. In contrast, FX rats swam out in a variety of directions, requiring more time to escape and sometimes never locating the platform. Thus normal rats could use their representation to navigate from novel

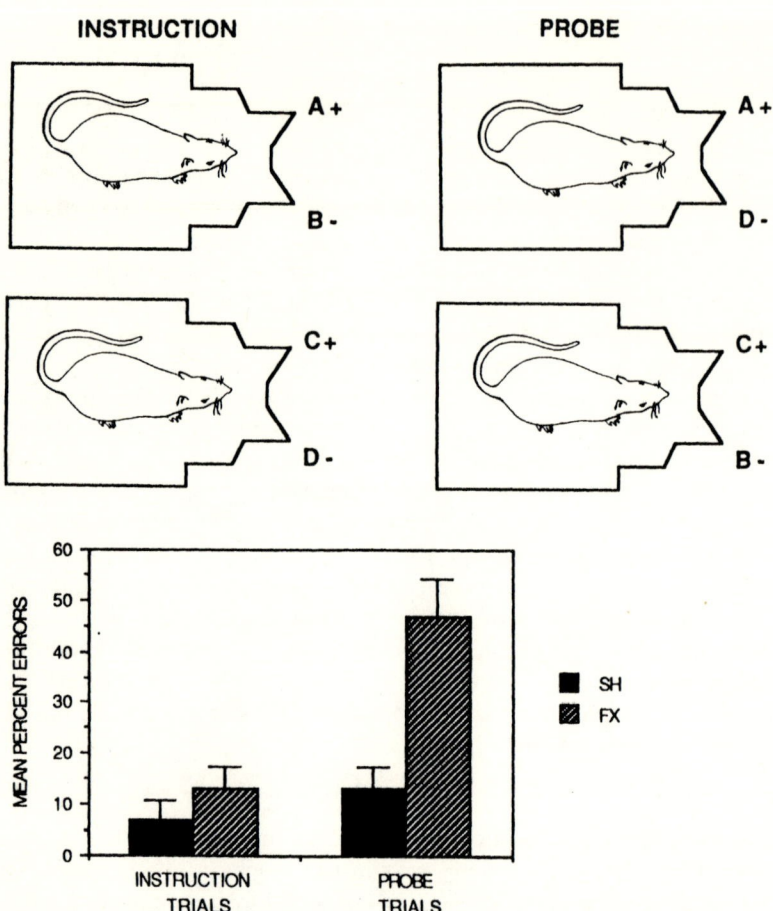

FIGURE 7.4. Assessment of flexible use of odor memory representations in sham-operated rats (SH) and rats with a fimbria/fornix transection (FX). (Top) Schematic diagrams of the odors presented on instruction and probe trials. (Bottom) SH and FX rats perform equivalently well in overtraining on instruction trials. SH rats continue to perform well on probe trials made up of mispairing of odor cues from the instruction trials, but FX rats made as many errors as would be predicted by chance. (Data taken from Eichenbaum, Matthews, & Cohen, 1989)

locations, but FX rats could demonstrate their place memory only in repetitions of the instruction trial.

Combined, these data indicate that in place learning, just as in odor discrimination learning, performance by rats with hippocampal system damage may be either impaired or preserved, depending on the representational demands of the task, even when the same place cues are involved across conditions. Furthermore, as is the case with odor discrimination learning, even when place learning is spared in rats with hippocampal system

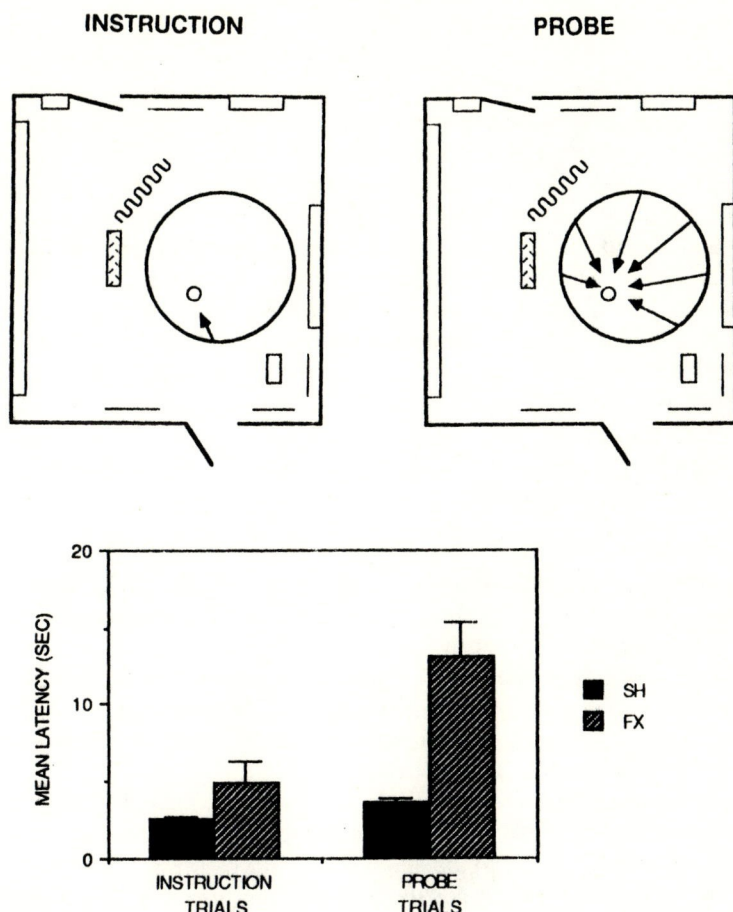

FIGURE 7.5. Assessment of flexible use of place memory in sham-operated rats (SH) and rats with a fimbria/fornix transection (FX). (Top) Schematic diagram of the testing room with Morris water maze. Arrows indicting start positions and direct trajectories to the escape platform on instruction trials and probe trials with novel start positions. (Bottom) SH and FX rats perform equivalently well in overtraining on instruction trials given just before each probe trial. SH rats continue to perform well on probe trials, but FX rats require longer to find the platform from novel start positions. (Taken from Eichenbaum, Stewart, & Morris, 1990)

damage, their memory representation is inflexible; it can be expressed only in repetition of the learning event.

FUNCTIONAL ORGANIZATION OF THE HIPPOCAMPUS

The above-described analyses of abnormal learning and memory in rats with hippocampal system damage provide considerable evidence in favor of the view that this system plays a critical and general role in relational representation and mnemonic flexibility. These studies furthered our understanding about *which* functions depend on the hippocampal system but assessments of the effects of brain damage on learning and memory offer little insight into *how* the hippocampal system performs these functions. In an attempt to address this question more directly, we also performed a parallel series of studies aimed to clarify the functional organization of hippocampal neurons in rats during odor- and place-guided learning. These studies bear on and add to the above-described neuropsychological analyses in two ways. First, analyses based on behavioral physiology will be used to confirm the conclusions of the neuropsychological studies using a different experimental strategy. Second, our findings in these studies will be employed toward an account of how the putative functions of this system are instantiated within hippocampal circuitry. To these ends our electrophysiological analyses were directed at testing the following specific predictions generated by the neuropsychological studies.

1. If the hippocampal participation in learning is not restricted to a specific domain of learning materials, then hippocampal unit activity should reflect the processing of critical nonspatial and spatial cues and events in both kinds of learning tasks.
2. If the hippocampus processes critical relations between items in memory, then the activity of single hippocampal neurons should reflect the processing of conjunctions or combinations of events relevant in both spatial and nonspatial tasks.
3. If the hippocampus participates in a variety of (spatial and nonspatial) memory organizations, then the organization of features encoded within the architecture of the hippocampus should be consistent with a general memory network and unlike the topographic organizations of particular spatial or nonspatial features observed in primary sensory neocortex.

Exploring the Functional Organization of the Hippocampus in Behaving Animals

The details of functional organization in brain structures have been most successfully revealed in neocortical sensory and motor systems. The findings from these studies have been highly valuable both in confirming conclusions from neuropsychological studies about the functional domain of these systems and in generating models of the circuitry that might subserve those functions. We have used these investigations as a point of reference in our attempt to describe the functional organization of the hippocampus.

The parameters that have been employed successfully to define the functional organization of sensory structures are: (a) the sensory receptive fields plus other sensory "features" of the stimuli that trigger neuronal responses, and (b) the topographic organization of feature representation across the spatial extent of the structure. We have the greatest amount of information about functional organization in the primate visual system, suggesting this should provide the best source for comparison. However, the functional organization of visual processing areas varies across processing stages; hence our expectancy for the hippocampus also varies. Thus, for example, the relatively simple trigger features and systematic retinocentric topography of primary visual cortex contrasts with the very complicated and ultraspecific trigger features (e.g. faces) and nontopographic organization of functional properties in inferotemporal cortex (Baylis, Rolls, & Leonard, 1987; Gross, Roche-Miranda, & Bender, 1972; Miyashita & Chang, 1988; Richmond, Optican, Podel, & Spitzer, 1987). Furthermore, unlike earlier stages of visual processing, inferotemporal neurons are relatively unaffected by changes in stimulus size or orientation and greatly affected by attentional and mnemonic variables (c.f. Eichenbaum & Buckingham, 1991). What do we expect to find at an even higher stage of processing in the hippocampus? Our analyses focused on making rather simple-minded comparisons between these general properties of visual cortical areas and analogues of "feature detection" and "topographical organization" in the hippocampus.

"Feature Detection" by Hippocampal Neurons

A reasonable beginning to the consideration of what features of memory tasks are encoded by hippocampal neuronal activity would seem to be the very odor discrimination and place learning tasks that were the focus of earlier sections of this chapter. We have recorded from hippocampal cells in rats performing in the same odor discrimination tasks employed in our lesion experiments (Eichenbaum, Kuperstein, Fagan, & Nagode, 1986b; Otto, Eichenbaum, Wiener, & Wible, 1991; Paul & Eichenbaum, 1989). There are no data on hippocampal unit activity in rats performing the Morris water maze, but we have observed the activity of some of the same cells recorded in our odor tasks in a place task similar in cognitive demands to Olton's radial arm maze task, another spatial memory paradigm for which performance depends critically on hippocampal function (Olton et al., 1979). In addition, there is a wealth of data on the activity of hippocampal neurons in a variety of spatial learning and other open field paradigms. The findings on odor and place tasks will be summarized in turn.

Odor Discrimination Learning

Our analyses focused on putative CA1 principal cells as representative of the final stage of hippocampal processing. In both the simultaneous- and successive-odor discrimination tasks, we identified a population of cells that fired selectively when rats sampled the odors and prepared to make the behavioral response. The activity of the cells was typically time-locked to the ongoing sniffing and hippocampal theta rhythm (Figure 7.6). Some of these cells were activated throughout the stimulus sampling period on all types of trials, beginning to fire on onset of the cues and ceasing to fire abruptly on onset of the response, even though the animal remained in the

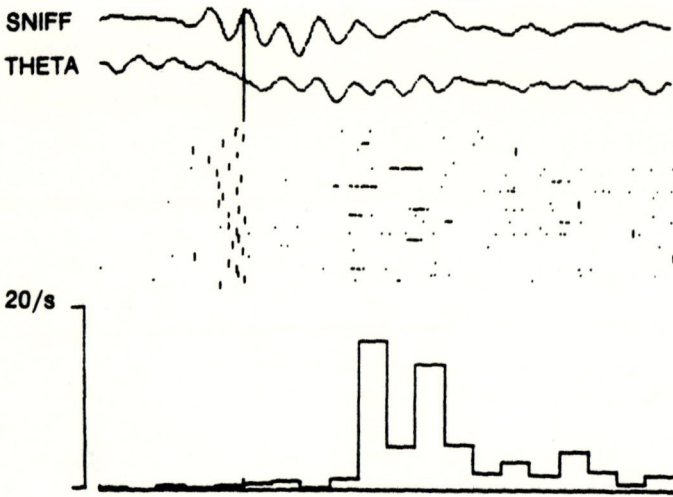

FIGURE 7.6. Raster display and summary histogram of a neuron that fired selectively during odor sampling in the successive odor discrimination task. Unit activity and averaged inhalation cycle (sniff) and hippocampal EEG (theta) are time-locked to the peak of the first sniff after odor onset (tic marks for each trial shown below synchronization line in sniff and theta averages). (From Eichenbaum, Kuperstein, Fagan, & Nagode, 1986)

same location after completing the response (Figure 7.7). Others of this class of cell had a much more selective behavioral correlate of firing; they increased firing dependent on the conjunction of multiple odors presented either in different spatial configurations or temporal sequences. In simultaneous odor discrimination, these cells fired maximally only during sampling of a specific left–right configuration of a particular pair of odors (Figure 7.8A). In successive odor discrimination, these cells fired maximally only during sampling of an S^+ odor preceded by an S^- odor on the previous trial; that is, the firing of these cells was dependent on the sequence of odor presentations (Figure 7.8B). Thus, the activity of a subset of hippocampal output neurons reflects the relevant stimulus relations in each variate of the odor discrimination paradigm, even in variates of the task in which the hippocampal system is not required for performance.

Place Tasks
In several studies it has been shown that hippocampal principal neurons fire selectively when the animal is in a particular place in the environment as rats explore large open fields (cf. O'Keefe, 1976, 1979). An example of the so-called place cell phenomenon taken from our own observations is shown in Figure 7.9. This neuron fired selectively when the rat was approximately at the center of an arena where it performed a place memory task. As others have observed, the activity of place cells, at least in some

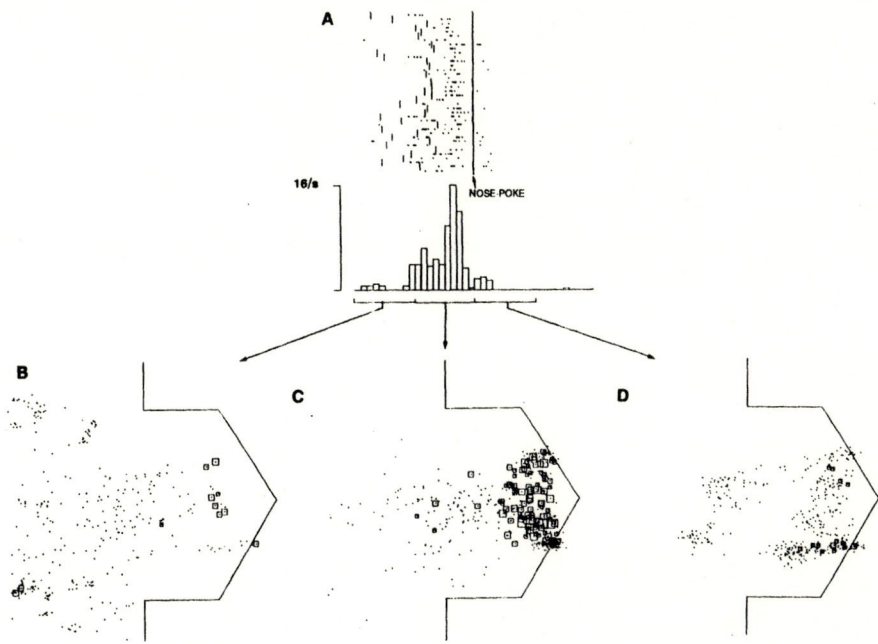

FIGURE 7.7.   Analyses of the activity of a neuron whose firing was synchronized to the nose-poke discriminative response in the simultaneous odor discrimination task. (A) The raster display of this cell indicates maximal firing 200–500 ms prior to the nose-poke (vertical line). Tic marks to the left of the nose-poke indicate odor onset on each trial. (B–D) Spatial analyses show the location of the rat's head (dots) and unit activity (squares of size proportional to firing rate) at 100 ms intervals superimposed on a outline of the cul-de-sac during the 1 s trial periods indicated on the abscissa of the histogram above. (B) The cell begins to fire as the rat approaches the ports. (C) Maximal firing occurs as the rat samples odors before the ports. (D) The cell ceases firing abruptly on the nose-poke to either port. (Taken from Wiener, Paul & Eichenbaum, 1989)

circumstances, is also influenced by aspects of spatial movement, such as the animal's speed, direction, and turning angle, indicating that multiple spatial variables may be encoded in the hippocampus (Eichenbaum & Cohen, 1988).

   What do we make of these observations on the "feature detecting" properties of hippocampal neurons? We can say that these neurons, unlike sensory cells, are not driven passively by simple perceptual features of the stimuli that serve as memory cues in our behavioral paradigms. It would also be an oversimplification to characterize hippocampal neurons simply as multimodal feature detectors, encoding unique items or events as if by a summation of responses to many specific sensory properties across sensory modalities, like polymodal neocortical areas (Baylis et al., 1987; Desimone

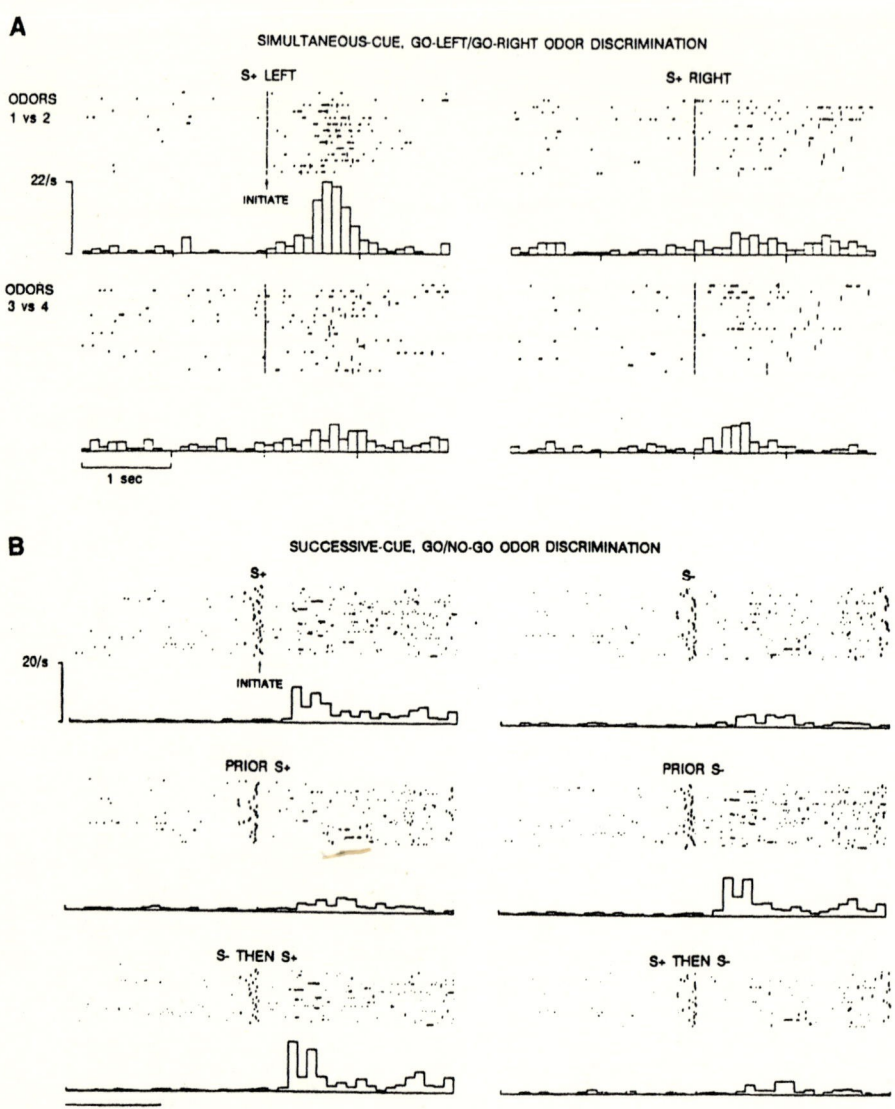

FIGURE 7.8. Raster displays and cumulative histograms of spikes from single hippocampal neurons activated during stimulus sampling during performance of different versions of the odor discrimination paradigm. (A) In simultaneous odor discrimination, unit activity is time-locked to the trial initiation and onset of odor presentation. This cell fires much more during sampling of the particular configuration of odor 1-left and odor-2 right than during sampling of the other configuration of these odors or during sampling of another odor pair (Data taken from Wiener et al., 1989). (B) In successive odor discrimination, unit activity is time-locked to the peak of the first inhalation after odor presentation. This cell fired more during sampling of an S^+ odor than S^-, more if the stimulus on the prior trial was S^- than S^+, most on S^+ trials preceded by S^- trials. (Data taken from Eichenbaum, Kuperstein, Fagan, & Nagode, 1986)

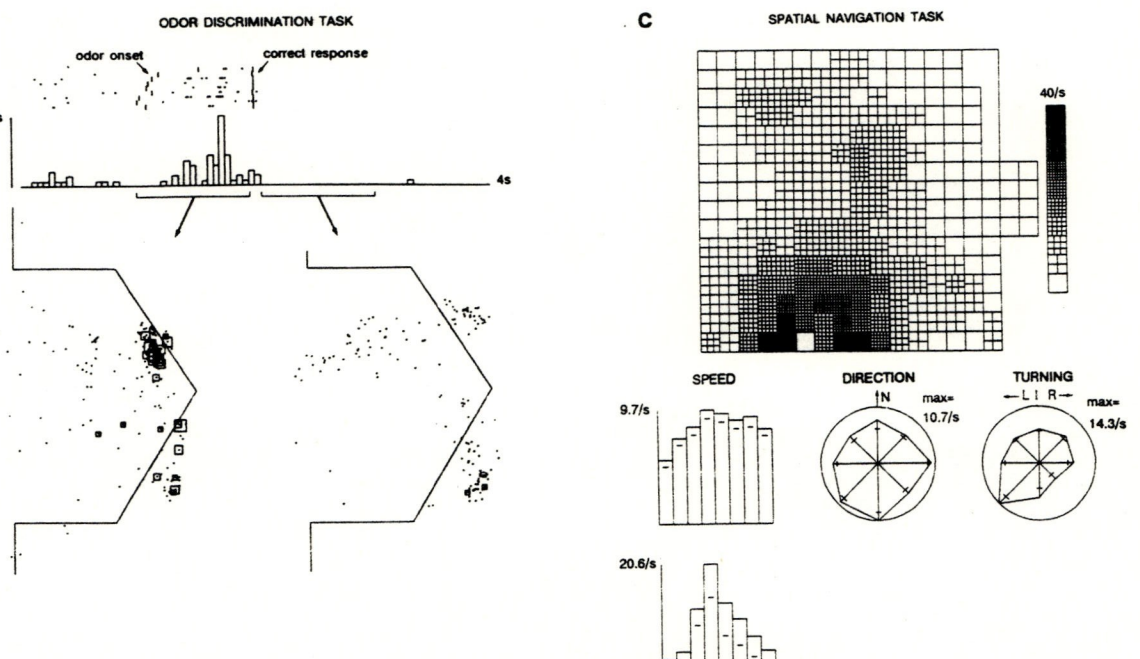

A ODOR DISCRIMINATION TASK

odor onset   correct response

31/s

4s

B

C SPATIAL NAVIGATION TASK

40/s

SPEED   DIRECTION   TURNING
                                  ←L│R→
9.7/s   ↑N   max=   max=
                    10.7/s   14.3/s

20.6/s

32cm/s

FIGURE 7.10. Analyses of spatial and behavioral correlates of a cell recorded in a rat performing the simultaneous odor discrimination (A, B) and performing the place-memory task (C). (A) Raster display and summary histogram of firing time-locked to the discriminative response during presentation of a particular odor configuration. (B) Enlarged schematic view of the odor sampling area showing location of the rat (dots) and firing rate (squares) at 50 ms intervals for 1s periods indicated in (A) . (C) The cell had a distinct place field and was significantly tuned to speed (when the rat was moving in it preferred directions – see lower histogram), direction, and turning angle. (Taken from Eichenbaum & Wiener, 1989)

& Gross, 1979). Nevertheless, some of the characteristics of hippocampal cellular activity may be interpreted by extrapolation from the evidence on progressive stages of unimodal and polymodal sensory processing. Thus, the hippocampus may be viewed as one further stage, what we might call *supramodal* perceptual processing.

Some of the properties of place cells are consistent with this view. Like polymodal cells of association neocortex, place cell properties can be supported by stimuli from multiple sensory modalities (Hill & Best, 1981). Similar to the "enhancement phenomenon" observed in several higher visual processing areas (Robinson, Goldberg, & Stanton, 1978), hippocampal cellular responses are sometimes strongly tied to intended movement as well as sensory input (Berger, Berry, & Thompson, 1986; Eichenbaum, Kuperstein, Fagan, & Nagode, 1986b; Muller & Kubie, 1989; Ranck, 1973; Wiener et al., 1989); these effects may be passed on from neurons in multiple sensory and motor cortical areas afferent to the hippocampal formation (Andersen, 1989; Bruce, Desimone, & Gross, 1981; Funahashi, Bruce, & Goldman-Rakic, 1989; Gnadt & Andersen, 1988; Quintana, Yajeya, & Fuster, 1988).

Furthermore, hippocampal place cells demonstrate ultraspecific sensitivities and stimulus invariances similar to those described for neurons in inferotemporal cortex. Like inferotemporal cells, a maximal response from most hippocampal place cells may require highly specific triggers in the environment (Thompson & Best, 1989). In at least some situations (Bostock, Taube, & Muller, 1988), place cells are not influenced by head orientation, a finding that may be interpreted as an extrapolation of the orientation and size invariance of higher order visual neuron responses (e.g., Gross et al., 1972; Rolls & Baylis, 1986). Indeed, several studies have shown that the place field is determined by where the rat "thinks" it is (Eichenbaum & Cohen, 1988; O'Keefe & Speakman, 1987; Quirk, Muller & Kubie, 1990) even when the appropriate stimuli are unavailable, indicating that current sensory input is not required at all; this phenomenon may be viewed as an extreme of sensory "constancy," and it might be related to the available sensory input in terms of the capacity of neurons in afferent neocortical areas to persist in firing after a critical stimulus has been removed (Baylis & Rolls, 1987; Funahashi et al., 1989; Fuster, in press; Fuster & Alexander, 1971).

There are other ways in which the firing correlates of hippocampal neurons would seem to exceed our ability to characterize them as the ultimate in feature detectors. Even though the sensory–behavioral correlate observed in one behavioral paradigm can be highly specific, the firing correlate of a single hippocampal neuron can change dramatically between behavioral situations. To compare the firing correlates of single hippocampal CA1 neurons across two quite different situations, we recorded from rats successively performing our simultaneous odor discrimination task then our spatial memory task (Wiener et al., 1989). Both tasks were performed by rats in the same behavioral chamber, so that we could determine if spatial or other correlates related to the general environment were maintained across tasks. The activity of individual cells was characterized both in terms of odor-related and behavioral correlates in the odor discrimination task and various spatial correlates in the place-memory task.

We found that many cells had distinct, but unrelated correlates in both tasks. For example, the cell whose analysis is shown in Figure 7.10 fired selectively during the sampling of odor cues in the odor discrimination task and had a place field, and other spatial movement correlates, at a locus distant from the odor sampling area in the spatial memory task. Our analyses of many such cells indicated that each neuron could have a highly specific correlate in both tasks, but there was no obvious relationship between the correlates observed across tasks. Thus, either the functional representation in the hippocampus is "remodeled" across tasks so that individual cells ultimately exhibit highly specific features selective to that particular task, or the fundamental and consistent correlate of each cell reflects the encoding of a higher order variable not specified explicitly in our analyses.

The possibility that functional representation in hippocampus actually changes across tasks has been proposed before to account for unpredictable changes in the place fields of hippocampal cells when a rat is placed in different environments (Muller & Kubie, 1987). "Remapping" (Muller & Kubie, 1987, p. 1951) of an environment occurs when an obstacle for movement, but not perception, is placed in the environment, or when the rat is repeatedly exposed to a novel environment that is very similar to a familiar one (Bostock, Muller, & Kubie, 1986), or even when none of the physical stimuli in the environment are altered, but the reward associations of loci are changed (Breese, Hampson, & Deadwyler, 1989). (Note that these findings argue against the notion that the representation is simply a map of the environment.)

Two explanations for such changes in functional representation come to mind. First, the alterations in neuronal tuning might be consequent to changes in activation level of the divergent inputs each hippocampal neuron receives (Squire, Shimamura, & Amaral, 1989). As the rat switches its attention across different behavioral situations, the proportion of inputs from various sources might change enormously, resulting in unpredictable changes in the behavioral correlate. According to this view, any particular situation would evoke a response that reflects a unique subset of the many inputs a single cell receives. One would expect that a large proportion of the cells would have a significant firing correlate in any situation because of the large variety of inputs but maximal responses would be observed in a few situations that drive a great fraction of those inputs (Thompson & Best, 1989). Second, we might think of the hippocampus as a large-scale massively parallel distributed network in which virtually any item is encoded across a large fraction of the cells (Eichenbaum & Buckingham, 1991; McNaughton & Morris, 1987; Rolls, 1990). According to this view, the pattern of activation in the network (and all of its elements) takes on a different form for each separate representation. These two accounts are not mutually exclusive; they may differ more in perspective than in substance.

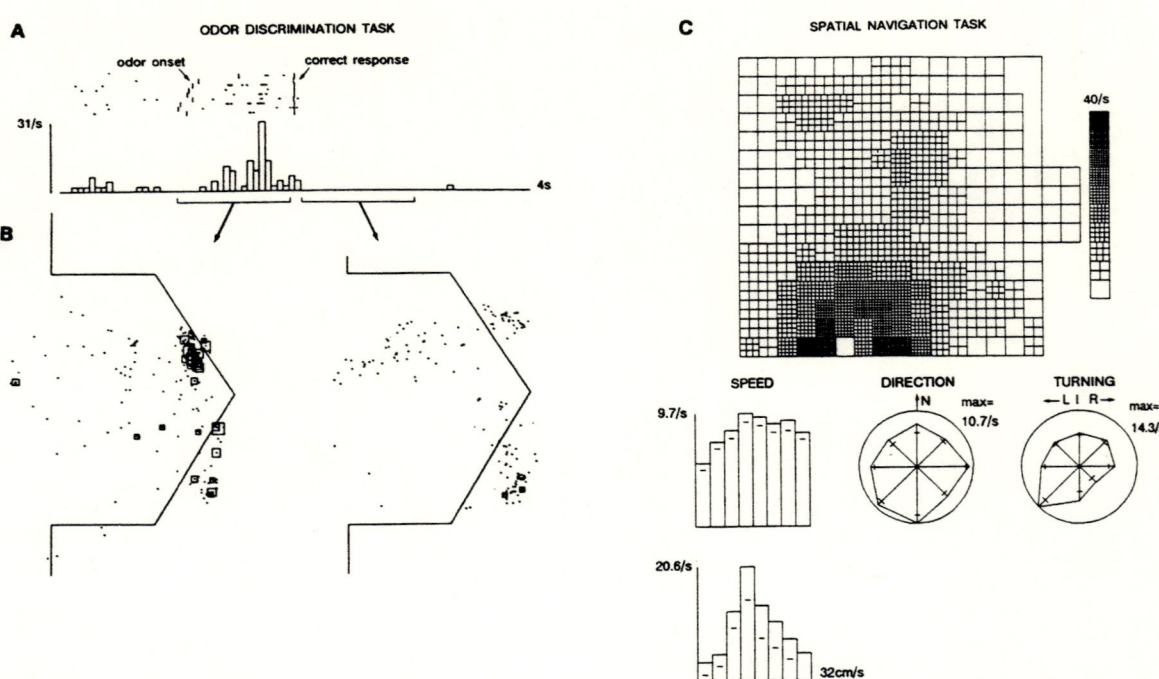

FIGURE 7.10. Analyses of spatial and behavioral correlates of a cell recorded in a rat performing the simultaneous odor discrimination (A, B) and performing the place-memory task (C). (A) Raster display and summary histogram of firing time-locked to the discriminative response during presentation of a particular odor configuration. (B) Enlarged schematic view of the odor sampling area showing location of the rat (dots) and firing rate (squares) at 50 ms intervals for 1s periods indicated in (A). (C) The cell had a distinct place field and was significantly tuned to speed (when the rat was moving in it preferred directions – see lower histogram), direction, and turning angle. (Taken from Eichenbaum & Wiener, 1989)

With regard to the possibility that there is a higher order property captured in the firing of hippocampal neurons, one reasonable candidate would seem to be that hippocampal neurons encode significant *relations* among cues. Our observation of cells whose activity depended on both odor and sniff port location in simultaneous odor discrimination is consistent with our hypothesis that the hippocampus is involved in representing the configurations of multiple cues as choice comparisons are made. These results are similar to reports of hippocampal neurons that are active in relation to specific conjunctions of cues in other paradigms and species; some cells are specifically active in relation to conjunctions of goal box color and position in a spatial delayed response task in rats (Wible et al., 1986), and to conjunctions of two-dimensional patterns and their spatial or temporal positions in visual recognition and delayed response tasks in monkeys (Brown, 1982; Cahusac et al., 1989; Miyashita et al., 1989; Rolls et al., 1989; Watanabe & Niki, 1985; Wilson, Brown & Riches, 1987). In humans, Halgren, Babb, and Crandel (1978) found that hippocampal gyrus cells fired selectively during presentation of words or pictures for which a memory choice had to be made (see also Heit, Smith, & Halgren, 1989).

The observation of cells whose activity depended on both current and previous stimulus valence in successive odor discrimination is consistent with our hypothesis that the hippocampus is involved in representing the relationships between the differential reward-values of stimuli presented across trials (see also Olton, 1986, 1989). These results are similar to Deadwyler and colleagues' observation of "sequential dependencies" of hippocampal unit activity across trials in a tone-cued discrimination (Foster, Christian, Hampson, Campbell, & Deadwyler, 1987). The capacity for hippocampal cellular activity to reflect past events may underlie the persistence of place fields when all the critical cues are removed (O'Keefe and Speakman, 1987; Quirk et al., 1990), and for the locus of the field to be determined by the entry point in an ambiguous environment (Sharp, Kubie, & Muller, 1988).

Finally, in our view, the place cell phenomenon reflects representation of relevant positional (and other) relations among distal stimuli that determine the spatial layout of the environment. This suggestion is supported by the finding that place fields move in concert with rotations of salient visual cues (Miller & Best, 1980; Muller, Kubie, & Rancke, 1987; O'Keefe & Speakman, 1987) and that the place fields of some cells "scale" with enlargement of all features of the environment (Muller & Kubie, 1987). In addition, place fields are disrupted only when a large fraction of the cues for spatial orientation are removed (Hill & Best, 1981; O'Keefe & Conway, 1978); even when a critical cue is removed, the field may be altered only in the dimension associated with that cue (Muller & Kubie, 1987). Thus, one property of hippocampal neuronal activity correlates is preserved across behavioral situations, the representation of relations among critical cues. But so far we have not been able to identify a *constant* relational property that predicts the firing correlates of cells across situations, so it is impossible to say whether a specific relationship is the common "feature" extracted in every situation or whether the relational property changes along with the items represented.

Topographical Organization in the Hippocampus

The assessment of spatial organization of functional properties in sensory neocortex is typically accomplished by recording at adjacent points across the cortical surface, determining the optimal trigger features at each site, and identifying systematic changes in the firing correlate corresponding to electrode position. Surveys of this type have revealed the topographic organization of receptive fields and trigger features in primary sensory and motor cortex. However, this approach is not feasible in the studies on the hippocampus of behaving animals; we instead exploited a capacity for monitoring several neighboring neurons simultaneously as rats performed our behavioral tasks. Recordings from such neuronal ensembles in primary visual cortex would be expected to reveal a group of overlapping receptive fields covering only a small portion of visual space. Our initial exploration of functional organization in the hippocampus asked whether there is an analogous topographical representation of adjacent environmental loci (place fields) across the CA1 cell layer.

We compared the locations of place fields in ensembles of 3–11 neurons recorded simultaneously as rats performed our spatial memory task (Eichenbaum, Wiener, Shapiro, & Cohen, 1989b). In most cells we could identify a place field, but the organization of place fields in neighboring cells was not consistent with that expected from a systematic topographic map of places in the hippocampus. Three major characteristics of individual place cells and their ensemble properties supported this conclusion: (a) as others have observed (Muller et al., 1987; O'Keefe & Speakman, 1987), many individual neurons increased firing when the rat was in separate parts of the environment (see Figure 7.11 [left]); (b) even a small group of cells, including only a tiny fraction of the hippocampal population, had a set of place fields covering up to 75% of the environment, much more than expected in a topographic map; and (c) the place fields of neighboring cells tended to overlap, as would be expected within a small portion of a topographic map, but we often observed multiple "clusters" of place fields recorded from the ensemble scattered throughout the environment in a fashion highly unlike that of a topograpic map.

Examination of two examples illustrates these findings (Figure 7.12). In ensemble A, of seven cells recorded, two each had two separate regions of increased firing, about one-quarter of the environment was covered by these place fields, and each place field fell into one of two clusters in separate regions of the arena. With the exception of the small cluster of place fields in one corner of the arena, this arrangement would have been consistent with the expectation of topographic arrangement. However, in ensemble B, most of the nine cells recorded had multiple place fields and their distribution

RECORDED

SIMULATED

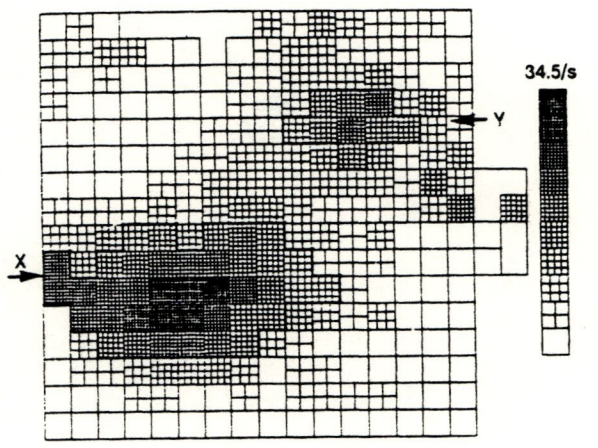

34.5/s

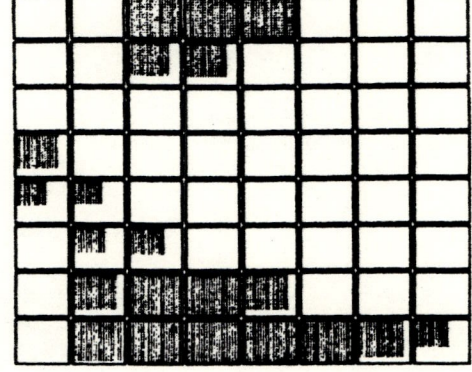

DIRECTION
N↑

SUBFIELD X
max=
19.0/s

SUBFIELD Y
max=
11.8/s

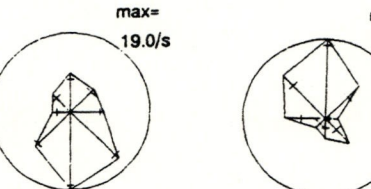

FIGURE 7.11. Dual place fields in recorded and simulated neurons. The recorded cell is one taken from Wiener, Paul, and Eichenbaum (1989). Opposing directional selectivities of the cell for movement through the two parts of the place field (X and Y) is evident in polar diagrams below. The simulated place field is an example of the spatial firing correlate of a hidden unit in the network simulation of Shapiro, Hetherington, Fortin, and Eichenbaum (1990); here the area filled in each pixel corresponds to relative activation level.

PLACE FIELDS   SPATIAL COINCIDENCE   MONTE CARLO DISTRIBUTIONS

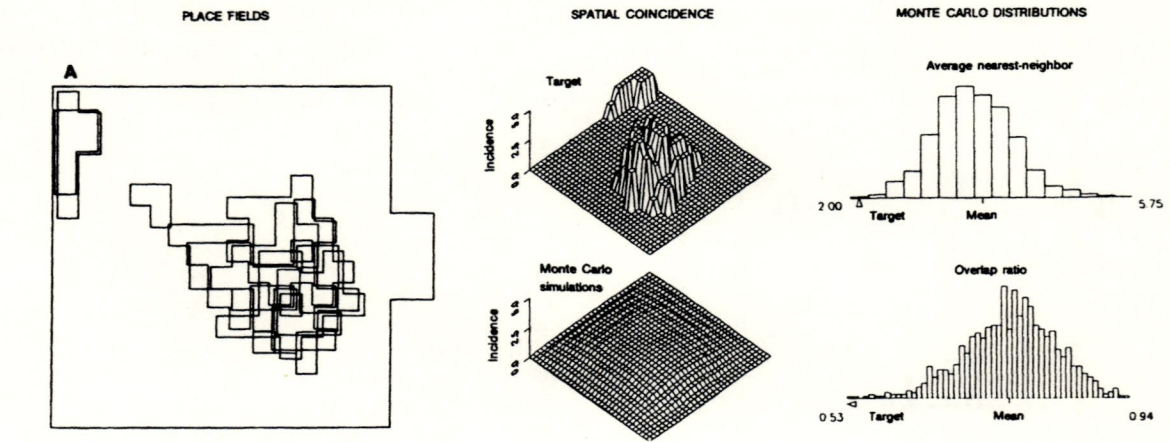

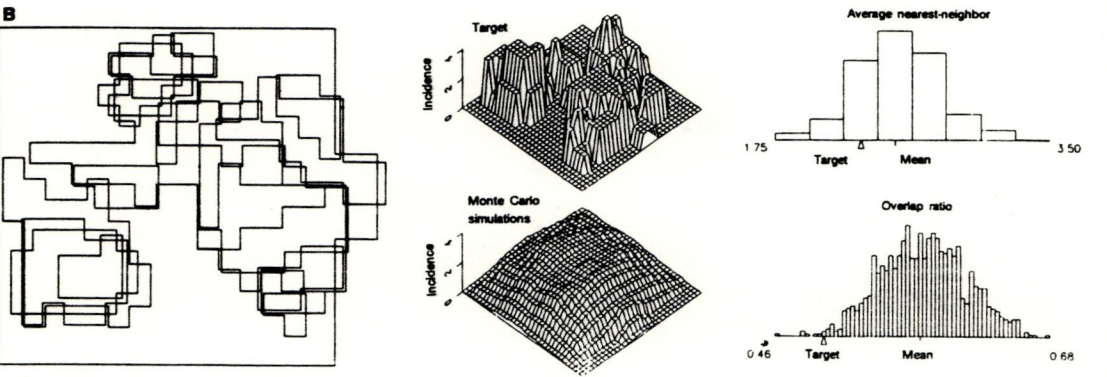

FIGURE 7.12. Analyses of examples of ensemble activity during performance of the spatial memory task. (A and B, left) An outline of the experimental chamber is shown from a top view of the environment; the location of the cul-de-sac where the odor discrimination task is performed is indicated on the right side. The boundaries of the place field of each cell is outlined with overlapping edges of place fields shifted slightly to aid their visualization. (Center). The three-dimensional graphs indicate the spatial coincidence of pixels (i.e., the number of times a given pixel was included in a place field) for both the target recorded ensemble (above) and the average spatial coincidence for the 1000 Monte Carlo runs (below). (Right) The distributions of average nearest-neighbor and overlap ratio for the Monte Carlo runs are shown, with the arrowhead indicating the value of each measure for the target recorded ensemble. The range of the Monte Carlo distribution was determined by the size and number of the place fields used in the simulation: larger and more numerous ensembles were more constrained by the size of the apparatus than were smaller ensembles. The range of each Monte Carlo distribution is noted numerically and illustrated by the width of the bars in the figure. (A) An ensemble of 7 cells had 9 subfields that clustered in two distinct areas of the maze. (B) Nine cells had a total of 16 subfields distributed over 138 pixels, or 52% of the chamber. The measures of place field distribution indicate greater clustering than expected by chance. The average nearest-neighbor proximity was 2.28 pixels, which was in the 9th percentile of the Monte Carlo distribution. The overlap ratio was .49, which was in the 1st percentile for the Monte Carlo distribution.

covered over more than half of the environment, clustering mainly in three regions (right, top, and bottom-left).

The observed pattern of spatial representation in ensembles of neighboring hippocampal neurons indicated the existence of some form of local order, although not one like that of primary sensory neocortex. We compared these findings with three accounts of representation in different neocortical processing areas (Eichenbaum, Wiener, Shapiro, & Cohen, 1989). First, it is possible that the hippocampus contains a nonisomorphic map of space composed of physiologically distinct "patches" corresponding to different regions of space, similar to the representation of visual fields in primate area MT (Maunsell & Van Essen, 1983, 1987). A few of our ensembles had distributions of place fields *less* clustered than expected by chance; these findings may have resulted from our electrode straddling across patches. However, unlike area MT, some of the same cells had fields in different regions of the environment. If the representation of space in the hippocampus is "patchy," the arrangement of patches is more a functional consequence than a reflection of anatomical topography.

Second, it is possible that the hippocampus represents spatial position relative to body orientation. Several investigators have observed that many place cells fire preferentially when the rat faces or moves in a particular direction (see above), as was the case for most cells in our ensembles (Wiener et al., 1989). Indeed, a few cells had dual symmetrical place fields with opposite movement directionalities (see Figure 7.11), consistent with a view that their activity was associated with movement towards certain similarities in the local view of the environment (cf. McNaughton, 1989). Such an encoding of places relative to body orientation could arise from the properties of areas in parietal cortex afferent to the hippocampal system. For example, in part of the inferior parietal area, there are cells with retinotopic visual receptive fields whose response is gated by retinal angle, resulting in representation of places relative to head orientation (Andersen, Essick, & Siegel, 1985).

Third, it is possible that place fields are not so much a reflection of spatial "mapping" as they are representations of independent complex "objects" defined with regard to both positional and nonspatial relations among cues. This view is consistent with the wealth of evidence, described above, that hippocampal neuronal activity reflects many nonspatial features of tasks. It is notable in this context that the representation of relevant visual cues reported for inferotemporal and parahippocampal cortex is also nontopographic. The only organizational quality reported is a tendency of neighboring cells to have similar receptive field shape and trigger features (Desimone & Gross, 1979; Gochin, Miller, Gross, & Gerstein, 1988; Miyashita, this volume, pp. 239–249), similar to our observations in the hippocampus where neighboring cells not only had similar place fields, but also similar spatial movement correlates.

It is reasonable to propose that spatial or other higher order "features" are encoded in distributed representations like those of current interest in computational modeling endeavors (Rumelhart & Zipser, 1986). Therefore one might not expect the elements of a distributed network to have psychologically meaningful correlates. Nevertheless, these were prevalent in the Andersen and Zipser (1990) model of parietal cortex, although examples of elements with more complex behavior (analogous to the observation of single hippocampal neurons with multiple place fields) were observed in both the recorded and simulated cells. Consistent with this notion, topographic representation was not a requisite for successful network simulation of the spatial properties of cells in the parietal cortex, and, indeed, the representation of space in this parietal area is nontopographic. More relevant to our consideration of the hippocampus, the nodes of a distributed network that learned to determine spatial location from the position of an observer relative to multiple distal visual cues, behaved like our ensemble recordings. Most elements had "place fields"; some had single distinct spatial correlates and others had multiple separated place fields (Figure 7.11; Shapiro, Hetherington, Fortin, & Eichenbaum, 1990). Further-more, as in our empirical observations, the spatial representations were distributed across the environment. Future investigations of the ensemble properties of hippocampal neurons in other behavioral paradigms, combined with parallel attempts at computational modeling, may help us understand the nature of functional organization in such nontopographic systems as the hippocampus (Eichenbaum, Otto, Wible, & Piper, 1990). Such endeavors should incorporate unique aspects of hippocampal circuitry such as its multilayered architecture with sequential processing stages, massive associat-ive connectivities, and a gradient topography of functionally qualified inputs at each processing stage (Amaral & Witter, 1989; Eichenbaum & Buckingham, 1991). It is premature to speculate on other substantive aspects of this kind of model. Suffice for it now to suggest that future investigations might be directed at the hypothesis that the architecture of the hippocampus might be ideal for the creation of an organized memory network that supports the properties here described to characterize the declarative expression of experience.

CONCLUSIONS: CHARACTERISTICS OF HIPPOCAMPAL REPRESENTATION IN MEMORY

In this chapter we have offered a summary of our account on the functional role played by the hippocampal system in memory and of the type of representation it supports, together with an outline of some of the empirical work our laboratory has conducted to validate this account. We close with some general principles about the hippcampal system and memory representation, and about the broader body of the empirical results against which the adequacy of this account must be evaluated.

1. *Hippocampal processing is not selective to any particular behavioral paradigm or category of information to be remembered.* After damage to the hippocampal system, either impaired or spared learning can be observed in different variants of the same behavioral paradigm, even when identical learning materials are employed. Within the experiments described here, severe impairment or spared performance were observed in variants of odor discrimination or place learning paradigms guided by the identical odor or place cues, respectively.

   Correspondingly, hippocampal neural activity is not limited to particular features of stimuli or events; it reflects the processing of all types of cues and events significant for learning. The same hippocampal neurons encode relevant features of odor discrimination and spatial memory performance.

2. *The hippocampal system is critical to a relational memory representation. The acquisition of individual associations are supported outside this system.* After damage to the hippocampal system, memory is impaired when the task encourages or demands comparisons among cues and a memory representation based on relations between them. Learning is spared when the task hinders comparison among cues and encourages an individual association between each cue and its reinforcement or response contingency.

   Correspondingly, hippocampal neural activity reflects the critical relations and conjunctions among cues whether or not intact hippocampal function is required for learning. In the experiments presented here, hippocampal neural activity reflected the relevant odor configuration or sequences during olfactory discrimination and the relevant spatial relations and spatially oriented behaviors relevant to performance in the spatial memory task.

3. *Hippocampal representations are concerned with memory for specific items and events in any particular task, not for the procedures by which these memories are acquired.* Even when memory for relations among specific items is severely impaired after hippocampal system damage, the acquisition of task procedures is intact. Within the experiments described here, even when they failed to remember specific odors or places, amnesic rats readily acquire instrumental procedures in both the odor discrimination and place learning tasks. Correspondingly, hippocampal neural activity is related to the configurations of particular items to be remembered, not to simple sensory or motor events.

4. *Hippocampal representations involve the organization of memories and support their flexible use in novel situations.* Even when learning capacity is spared after hippocampal system damage, the acquired associations are inflexible in that they can be revealed only in repetition of the learning event. Within the experiments described here, the representations of normal animals supported the use of odor and place memories in novel situations, but the representation of rats with hippocampal system damage could be revealed only in repetitions of the original learning event.

   Correspondingly, the functional organization of the hippocampus is unlike the topographical representations of primary sensory and motor cortices; its properties are more like those of massively parallel distributed networks that are characterized by the flexibility of their representations.

Acknowledgments: Preparation of this manuscript was supported in part by NIH grant NS26402, and NSF grants BNS-8721157 and BNS-8810095 to H.E.

REFERENCES

Amaral, D.G., & Witter, M. P. (1989). The three-dimensional organization of the hippocampal formation: A review of anatomical data. *Neuroscience, 31*, 571–591.

Andersen, R.A. (1989). Visual and eye movement functions of the posterior parietal cortex. *Annual Review of Neuroscience, 12*, 377–403.

Andersen, J.R. (1990). *Cognitive psychology and its implications*. New York: W. H. Freeman.

Andersen, R. A., Essick, G. K., & Siegel, R. M. (1985). Encoding of spatial location by posterior parietal neurons. *Science, 230*, 456–458.

Andersen, R. A., & Zipser, D. (1990). A network model for learned spatial representation in the posterior parietal cortex. In J. L. McGaugh, N. M. Weinberger, & G. Lynch (Eds.), *Brain organization and memory. Cells, systems, and circuits* (pp. 271–284). New York: Oxford University Press.

Baylis, G. C., & Rolls, E. T. (1987). Responses of neurons in the inferior temporal cortex in short term and serial recognition memory tasks. *Experimental Brain Research, 65*, 614–622.

Baylis, G. C., Rolls, E. T., & Leonard, C. M. (1987). Functional subdivisions of the temporal lobe neocortex. *Journal of Neuroscience, 7*, 330–342.

Berger, T. W., Berry, S. D., & Thompson, R. F. (1986). Role of the hippocampus in classical conditioning of aversive and appetitive behaviors. In R. L. Isaacson & K. H. Pribram (Eds.), *The hippocampus (Vol. 4)*. New York: Plenum Press.

Bostock, E., Muller, R. U., & Kubie, J. L. (1986). Firing fields of hippocampal neurons: A stimulus manipulation that alters place cell mapping of the environment. *Society for Neuroscience Abstracts, 12*, 522.

Bostock, E., Taube, J., & Muller, R. U. (1988). The effects of head orientation on the firing of hippocampal place cells. *Society for Neuroscience Abstracts, 14*, 127.

Breese, C. R., Hampson, R. E., & Deadwyler, S. A. (1989). Hippocampal place cells: Stereotopy and plasticity. *Journal of Neuroscience, 9*, 1097–1111.

Brown, M. W. (1982). Effect of context on the response of single units recorded from the hippocampal region of behaviourally trained monkeys. In C. Ajnone-Marsan & H. Matthies (Eds.), *Neuronal plasticity and memory formation* (pp. 557–573). (IBRO Monograph Series Vol. 9). New York: Raven Press.

Bruce, C., Desimone, R., & Gross, C.G. (1981). Visual properties of neurons in a polysensory area in the superior temporal sulcus of the macaque. *Journal of Neurophysiology, 46*, 369–384.

Bruner, J. S. (1969). Modalities of memory. In G. A. Talland & N. C. Waugh (Eds.), *Pathology of memory* (pp. 253–259). New York: Academic Press.

Cohen, N. J. (1984). Preserved learning capacity in amnesia: Evidence for multiple memory systems. In N. Butters & L. R. Squire (Eds.), *The neuropsychology of memory* (pp. 83–103). New York: Guilford Press.

Cahusac, P. M. B., Miyashita, Y., & Rolls, E.T. (1989). Responses of hippocampal neurons in the monkey related to delayed response and object-place memory tasks. *Behavioural Brain Research, 33*, 229–240.

Cohen, N. J., & Squire, L. R. (1980). Preserved learning and retention of a pattern-analyzing skill in amnesia: Dissociation of knowing how and knowing that. *Science, 210*, 207–210.

Corkin, S. (1968). Acquisition of a motor skill after bilateral medial temporal lobe excision. *Neuropsychologia, 6*, 225–265.

Desimone, R., & Gross, C. G. (1979). Visual areas in the temporal cortex of the macaque. *Brain Research, 178*, 363–380.

Douglas, R. J. (1967). The hippocampus and behavior. *Psychological Bulletin, 67*, 416–442.

Eichenbaum, H., & Buckingham, J. (1991). Studies on hippocampal processing: Experiment, theory, and model. In M. Gabriel and J. Moore (Eds.), *Neurocomputation and learning: foundations of adaptive networks.* (pp. 171–232). Cambridge: M.I.T. Press.

Eichenbaum, H., & Cohen, N. J. (1988). Representation in the hippocampus: What do the neurons code? *Trends in Neuroscience, 11*, 244–248.

Eichenbaum, H., Fagan, A., & Cohen, N. J. (1986). Normal olfactory discrimination learning set and facilitation of reversal learning after combined and separate lesions of the fornix and amygdala in rats: Implications for preserved learning in amnesia. *Journal of Neuroscience, 6*, 1876–1884.

Eichenbaum, H., Fagan, A., Mathews, P., & Cohen, N. J. (1988). Hippocampal system dysfunction and odor discrimination learning in rats: Impairment or facilitation depending on representational demands. *Behavioral Neuroscience, 102*, 331–339.

Eichenbaum, H., Kuperstein, M., Fagan, A., & Nagode, J. (1986). Cue-sampling and goal-approach correlates of hippocampal unit activity in rats performing an odor discrimination task. *Journal of Neuroscience, 7*, 716–732.

Eichenbaum, H., Mathews, P., & Cohen, N. J. (1989). Further studies of hippocampal representation during odor discrimination learning. *Behavioral Neuroscience, 103*, 1207–1216.

Eichenbaum, H., Otto, T., Wible, C., & Piper, J. (1991). Building a model of the hippocampus in olfaction and memory. In J. Davis & H. Eichenbaum (Eds.), *Olfaction as a model system for computational neuroscience.* Cambridge: M.I.T. Press.

Eichenbaum, H., Stewart, C., & Morris, R. G. M. (1990). Hippocampal representation in spatial learning. *Journal of Neuroscience, 10*, 3531–3542.

Eichenbaum, H., Wiener, S. I., Shapiro, M., & Cohen, N. J. (1989). The organization of spatial coding in the hippocampus: A study of neural ensemble activity. *Journal of Neuroscience, 9*, 2764–2775.

Eichenbaum, H., & Wiener, S. I. (1989). Is place the (only) functional correlate? *Psychobiology, 17*, 217–220.

Foster, T. C., Christian, E. P., Hampson, R. E., Campbell, K. A., & Deadwyler, S. A. (1987). Sequential dependencies regulate sensory evoked responses of single units in the rat hippocampus. *Brain Research, 408*, 86–96.

Funahashi, S., Bruce, C. J., & Goldman-Rakic, P. S. (1989). Mnemonic coding of visual space in the monkey's dorsolateral prefrontal cortex. *Journal of Neurophysiology, 61*, 331–349.

Fuster, J. M. (in press). Inferotemporal units in selective visual attention and short-term memory. *Journal of Neurophysiology*.

Fuster, J. M., & Alexander, G. E. (1971). Neuron activity related to short term memory. *Science, 173,* 652–654.

Gabriel, M., Foster, K., Orona, E., Saltwick, S. E., & Stanton, M. (1980). Neuronal activity of cingulate cortex, anteroventral thalamus, and hippocampal formation in discriminative conditioning: Encoding and extraction of the significance of conditional stimuli. *Progress in Psychobiology and Physiological Psychology, 9,* 125–231.

Gaffan, D. (1974). Recognition impaired and association intact in the memory of monkeys after transection of the fornix. *Journal of Comparative and Physiological Psychology, 86,* 1100–1109.

Gochin, P. M., Miller, E. K., Gross, C. G., & Gerstein, G. L. (1988). Circuit properties of inferior temporal cortex in the macaque. *Society for Neuroscience Abstracts, 14,* 11.

Gnadt, J. W., & Andersen, R. A. (1988). Memory related motor planning activity in the posterior parietal cortex of macaque. *Experimental Brain Research, 70,* 216–220.

Graf, P., & Schacter, D. L. (1985). Implicit and explicit memory for new associations in normal and amnesic subjects. *Journal of Experimental Psychology: Learning, Memory, and Cognition, 11,* 501–518.

Graf, P., Squire, L. R., & Mandler, G. (1984). Amnesic patients perform normally on one kind of memory test for previously presented words. *Journal of Experimental Psychology: Learning, Memory, and Cognition, 10,* 164–178.

Gray, J. A. (1979). *The neuropsychology of anxiety.* Oxford: Oxford University Press.

Gray, J. A., & Rawlins, J. N. P. (1986). Comparator and buffer memory: An attempt to integrate two models of hippocampal function. In R. L. Isaacson & K. H. Pribram (Eds.), *The hippocampus* (Vol. 4) (pp. 159–202). New York: Plenum Press.

Gross, C. G., Roche-Miranda, C. E., & Bender, D. B. (1972). Visual properties of neurons in the inferotemporal cortex of the macaque. *Journal of Neurophysiology, 35,* 96–111.

Halgren, E., Babb, T. L., & Crandal, P. H. (1978). Activity of human hippocampal formation and amygdala neurons during memory testing. *Electroencephalography and Clinical Neurophysiology, 45,* 585–601.

Heit, G., Smith, M. E., & Halgren, E. (1988). Neural encoding of individual words and faces by the human hippocampus and amygdala. *Nature, 333,* 773–775.

Hill, A. J., & Best, P. J. (1981). Effects of deafness and blindness on the spatial correlates of hippocampal unit activity in the rat. *Experimental Neurology, 74,* 204–217.

Hirsh, R. (1974). The hippocampus and contextual retrieval of information from memory: A theory. *Behavioral Biology, 12,* 421–444.

Hirsh, R. (1980). The hippocampus, conditional operations and cognition. *Physiological Psychology, 8,* 175–182.

Holland, P. C. (1990). Forms of memory in Pavlovian conditioning. In J. L. McGaugh, N. M. Weinberger, & G. Lynch (Eds.), *Brain organization and memory. Cells, systems, and circuits* (pp. 78–105). New York: Oxford University Press, pp. 78–105.

Johnson, M. K. (1990). Functional forms of memory. In J. L. McGaugh, N. M. Weinberger, & G. Lynch (Eds.), *Brain organization and memory. Cells, systems, and circuits* (pp. 106–136). New York: Oxford University Press.

Kesner, R. P. (1980). An attribute analysis of memory: The role of the hippocampus. *Physiological Psychology, 8,* 189–197.

Kesner, R. P. (1984). The neurobiology of memory: Implicit and explicit assumptions. In J. L. McGaugh, G. Lynch, & N. Weinberger (Eds.), *The Neurobiology of learning and memory* (pp. 111–118). New York: Guildford Press.

Kimble, D. P. (1968). The hippocampus and internal inhibition. *Psychological Bulletin, 70*, 285–295.

Kohonen, T. (1990). Notes on neural computing and associative memory. In J. L. McGaugh, N. M. Weinberger, & G. Lynch (Eds.), *Brain organization and memory. Cells, systems, and circuits* (pp. 323–337). New York: Oxford University Press.

Lynch, G., McGaugh, J. L., & Weinberger, N. M. (Eds.) (1984). *Neurobiology of learning and memory*. New York: Guilford Press.

Mackintosh, N. J. (1985). Varieties of conditioning. In N. M. Weinberger, J. L. McGaugh, & G. Lynch (Eds.), *Memory systems of the brain* (pp. 335–350). New York: Guilford Press.

MacPhail, E. M. (1985). Ecology and intelligence. In N. M. Weinberger, J. L. McGaugh & G. Lynch (Eds.), *Memory systems of the brain* (pp. 279–286). New York: Guilford Press.

Marr, D. (1971). Simple memory: A theory for archicortex. *Philosophical Transactions of the Royal Society, London, B262*, 23–81.

Maunsell, J. H.R., & Van Essen, D. C. (1983). Functional properties of neurons in the middle temporal visual area of the macaque monkey. I. Selectivity for stimulus speed, direction, and orientation. *Journal of Neurophysiology, 49*, 1127–1147.

Maunsell, J. H. R., & Van Essen, D. C. (1987). Topographic organization of the middle temporal visual area in the macaque monkey: Representational biases and the relationship to callosal connections and myeloarchitechtonic boundaries. *Journal of Comparative Neurology, 266*, 535–555.

McGaugh, J. L., Weinberger, N. M., & Lynch, G. (1990). *Brain organization and memory. Cells, systems, and circuits*. New York: Oxford University Press.

McNaughton, B. L. (1989). Neuronal mechanisms for spatial computation and information storage. In L. Nadel, L. A. Cooper, P. Culicover, & R. M. Harnish (Eds.), *Neural connections, mental computation* (pp. 285–350). Cambridge: MIT Press.

McNaughton, B. L., & Morris, R. G. M. (1987). Hippocampal synaptic enhancement and information storage within a distributed memory system. *Trends in Neuroscience, 10*, 408–415.

Miller, V. M., & Best, P. J. (1980). Spatial correlates of hippocampal unit activity are altered by lesions of the fornix and entorhinal cortex. *Brain Research, 194*, 311–323.

Mishkin, M. (1978). Memory in monkeys severely impaired by combined but not separate removal of amygdala and hippocampus. *Nature, 273*, 297–298.

Mishkin, M., Malamut, B., & Bachevalier, J. (1984). Memories and habits: Two neural systems. In J. L. McGaugh, G. Lynch, & N. M. Weinberger (Eds.), *The neurobiology of learning and memory* (pp. 65–77). New York: Guilford Press.

Mishkin, M., & Petri, H. L. (1984). Memories and habits: Some implications for the analysis of learning and retention. In N. Butters & L. R. Squire (Eds.), *The neuropsychology of memory*. New York: Guilford Press.

Miyashita, Y., & Chang, H. S. (1988). Neuronal correlate of pictoral short-term memory in the primate temporal cortex. *Nature, 331*, 68–70.

Miyashita, Y., Rolls, E. T., Cahusac, P. M. B., & Niki, H. (1989). Activity of hippocampal formation neurons in the monkey related to a stimulus-response association task. *Journal of Neurophysiology, 61*, 669–678.

Morris, R. G. M. (1984a). Developments of a water-maze procedure for studying spatial learning in the rat. *Journal of Neuroscience Methods, 11*, 47–60.

Morris, R. G. M. (1984b). Is the distinction between procedural and declarative memory useful with respect to animal models of amnesia. In J. L. McGaugh,

G. Lynch, & N. Weinberger (Eds.), *The neurobiology of learning and memory* (pp. 119–125). New York: Guilford Press.

Morris, R. G. M. (1985). Moving on from modeling amnesia. In N. M. Weinberger, J. L. McGaugh, & G. Lynch (Eds.), *Memory systems of the brain* (pp. 452–462). New York: Guilford Press.

Morris, R. G. M., Garrud, P., Rawlins, J. N. P., & O'Keefe, J. (1982). Place navigation impaired in rats with hippocampal lesions. *Nature, 297,* 681–683.

Morris, R. G. M. (1990). Synaptic plasticity, neural architecture, and forms of memory. In J. L. McGaugh, N. M. Weinberger, & G. Lynch (Eds.), *Brain organization and memory. Cells, systems, and circuits* (pp. 52–77). New York: Oxford University Press.

Moscovitch, M. (1984). The sufficient conditions for demonstrating preserved memory in amnesia. In N. Butters & L.R. Squire (Eds.), *The neuropsychology of memory* (pp. 104–114). New York: Guilford Press.

Muller, R. U., & Kubie, J. L. (1987). The effects of changes in the environment on the spatial firing of hippocampal complex-spike cells. *Journal of Neuroscience, 7,* 1951–1968.

Muller, R. U., & Kubie, J. L. (1989). The firing of hippocampal place predicts the future position of moving rats. *Journal of Neuroscience, 9,* 4101–4110.

Muller, R. U., Kubie, J. L., & Ranck, J. B., Jr (1987). Spatial firing patterns of hippocampal complex spike cells in a fixed environment. *Journal of Neuroscience, 7,* 1935–1950.

Nadel, L., & Wexler, K. (1984). Neurobiology, representations and memory. In J. L. McGaugh, G. Lynch, & N. Weinberger (Eds.), *The neurobiology of learning and memory* (pp. 125–136). New York: Guilford Press.

O'Keefe, J. A. (1976). Place units in the hippocampus of the freely moving rat. *Experimental Neurology, 51,* 78–109.

O'Keefe, J. A. (1979). A review of hippocampal place cells. *Progress in Neurobiology, 13,* 419–439.

O'Keefe, J., & Conway, D. H. (1978). Hippocampal place units in the freely moving rat: Why they fire when they fire. *Experimental Brain Research, 31,* 573–590.

O'Keefe, J., & Conway, D. H. (1980). On the trail of the hippocampal engram. *Physiological Psychology, 2,* 229–238.

O'Keefe, J., & Nadel, L. (1978). *The hippocampus as a cognitive map.* Oxford: Oxford University Press.

O'Keefe, J., & Speakman, A. (1987). Single unit activity in the rat hippocampus during a spatial memory task. *Experimental Brain Research, 68,* 1–27.

Olton, D. S. (1986). Hippocampal function and memory for temporal context. In R. L. Isaacson & K. H. Pribram (Eds.), *The Hippocampus*: (Vol. 4). New York: Plenum Press.

Olton, D. S. (1989). Mnemonic functions of the hippocampus: Single unit analyses in rats. In V. Chan-Palay & Kohler (Eds.), *The hippocampus—new vistas* (pp. 411–424). New York: A. R. Liss.

Olton, D. S., Becker, J. T., & Handlemann, G. E. (1979). Hippocampus, space, and memory. *Brain and Behavioral Sciences, 2,* 313–365.

Otto, T., & Eichenbaum, H. (1991). Olfactory learning and memory in the rat: A "model system" for studies on the neurobiology of memory. In M. Serby & K. Chobor (Eds.), *The science of olfaction.* New York: Springer-Verlag.

Otto, T., Eichenbaum, H., Wiener, S. I., & Wible, C. G. (1991). Learning-related patterns of CA1 spike trains parallel stimulation parameters optimal for inducing hippocampal long term potentiation. *Hippocampus, 1,* 181–192.

Otto, T., Schottler, F., Staubli, U., Eichenbaum, H., & Lynch, G. (1991). The hippocampus and olfactory discrimination learning: Effects of entorhinal cortex lesions on learning-set acquisition and on odor memory in a successive-cue, go/no-go task. *Behavioral Neuroscience, 105,* 111–119.

Quintana, J., Yajeya, J., & Fuster, J. M. (1988). Prefrontal representation of stimulus attributes during delay tasks. I. Unit activity in cross-temporal integration of memory and sensory-motor information. *Brain Research, 474*, 211–221.

Quirk, G. J., Muller, R. U., & Kubie, J. L. (1990). The firing of hippocampal place cells in the dark depends on the rat's recent experience. *Journal of Neuroscience, 10*, 2008–2017.

Raffaelle, K. C., & Olton, D. S. (1988). Hippocampal and amygdaloid involvement in working memory for non-spatial stimuli. *Behavioral Neuroscience, 102*, 349–355.

Ranck, J. B., Jr (1973). Studies on single neurons in the dorsal hippocampal formation and septum in unrestrained rats. *Experimental Neurology, 41*, 461–555.

Rawlins, J. N. P. (1985). Associations across time: The hippocampus as a temporary memory store. *Brain and Behavioral Sciences, 8*, 479–496.

Richmond, B. J., Optican, L. M., Podel, P., & Spitzer, H. (1987). Temporal encoding of two-dimensional patterns by single units in primate inferior temporal cortex. I. Response characteristics. *Journal of Neurophysiology, 57*, 132–146.

Robinson, D. L., Goldberg, M. E., & Stanton, G. B. (1978). Parietal association cortex in the primate: Sensory mechanisms and behavioral modulation. *Journal of Neurophysiology, 41*, 910–932.

Rolls, E. T. (1990). Functions of neuronal networks in the hippocampus and of backprojections in the cerebral cortex in memory. In J. L. McGaugh, N. M. Weinberger, & G. Lynch (Eds.), *Brain organization and memory. Cells, systems, and circuits* (pp. 184–210). New York: Oxford University Press.

Rolls, E. T., & Baylis, G. C. (1986). Size and contrast have only small effects on the responses to faces of neurons in the cortex of the superior temporal sulcus of the monkey. *Experimental Brain Research, 65*, 38–48.

Rolls, E. T., Miyashita, Y., Cahusac, P., Kesner, R. P., Niki, H. D., Feigenbaum, J. D., & Bach, L. (1989). Hippocampal neurons in the monkey with activity related to the place where a stimulus is shown. *Journal of Neuroscience, 9*, 1835–1846.

Rosenzweig, M. R., & Glickman, S. E. (1985). Comparison of learning abilities among species. In N. M. Weinberger, J. L. McGaugh, and G. Lynch (Eds.), *Memory systems of the brain* (pp. 296–310). New York: Guilford Press.

Rumelhart, D., & Zipser, D. (1986). Feature discovery by competitive learning. In D. Rumelhart & J. McClelland (Eds.), *Parallel distributed processing* (Vol. 1). Cambridge, Massachusetts: M.I.T. Press.

Ryle, G. (1949). *The concept of mind*. San Francisco: Hutchinson.

Saunders, R. C., & Weiskrantz, L. (1989). The effects of fornix transection and combined fornix transection, mammillary body lesions and hippocampal ablations on object pair association memory in the rhesus monkey. *Behavioral Brain Research, 35*, 85–94.

Schacter, D. L. (1985). Multiple forms of memory in humans and animals. In N. M. Weinberger, J. L. McGaugh, & G. Lynch (Eds.), *Memory systems of the brain* (pp. 351–380). New York: Guilford Press.

Schacter, D., & Tulving, E. (1983). Memory, amnesia, and the episodic/semantic distinction. In R. L. Isaacson & N. E. Spear (Eds.), *The expression of knowledge*. New York: Plenum Press.

Scoville, W. B., & Milner, B. (1957). Loss of recent memory after bilateral hippocampal lesions. *Journal of Neurology, Neurosurgery, & Psychiatry, 20*, 11–12.

Shapiro, M. L., Hetherington, P. A., Fortin, W. J., & Eichenbaum, H. (1990). A simple PDP model simulates spatial correlates of hippocampal neuronal activity. *Society for Neuroscience Abstracts, 16,* 473.

Sharp, P. E., Kubie, J. L., & Muller, R. U. (1988). Hippocampal place cells can fire differentially in two visually identical locations in a symmetrical chamber. *Society for Neuroscience Abstracts, 14,* 126.

Sherry, D. F., & Schacter, D. L. (1987). The evolution of multiple memory systems. *Psychological Review, 94,* 439–454.

Slotnick, B. M., & Katz, H. M. (1974). Olfactory learning set formation in rats. *Science, 185,* 796–798.

Squire, L. R. (1987). *Memory and brain.* New York: Oxford University Press.

Squire, L. R., Shimamura, A. P., & Amaral, D. G. (1989). Memory and the hippocampus. In J. Byrne & W. Barry (Eds.), *Neural models of plasticity,* New York: Academic Press.

Squire, L. R., & Butters, N. (Eds.) (1984). *Neuropsychology of memory.* New York: Guilford Press.

Staubli, U., Ivy, G., & Lynch, G. (1984). Hippocampal denervation causes rapid forgetting of olfactory information in rats. *Proceedings of the National Academy of Sciences, U.S.A., 81,* 5885–5887.

Sutherland, R. J., Macdonald, R. J., Hill, C. R., & Rudy, J. W. (1989). Damage to the hippocampal formation in rats selectively impairs the ability to learn cue relationships. *Behavioral and Neural Biology, 52,* 331–356.

Sutherland, R. J., & Rudy, J. W. (1989). Configural association theory: The role of the hippocampal formation in learning, memory, and amnesia. *Psychobiology, 17,* 129–144.

Thomas, G. J., & Gash, D. M. (1986). Differential effects of posterior septal lesions on dispositional and representational memory. *Behavioral Neuroscience, 100,* 712–719.

Thompson, L. T., & Best, P. J. (1989). Place cells and silent cells in the hippocampus of freely-behaving rats. *Journal of Neuroscience, 9,* 2382–2390.

Warrington, E. K., & Weiskrantz, L. (1968). New method for testing long-term retention with special reference to amnesic patients. *Nature, 217,* 972–974.

Watanabe, T., & Niki, H. (1985). Hippocampal unit activity and delayed response in the monkey. *Brain Research, 325,* 241–254.

Weinberger, N. M., McGaugh, J. L., & Lynch, G. (Eds.) (1985). *Memory systems of the brain.* New York: Guilford Press.

Weiskrantz, L. (1985). On issues and theories of the human amnesic syndrome. In N. M. Weinberger, J. L. McGaugh, & G. Lynch (Eds.), *Memory systems of the brain* (pp. 380–418). New York: Guilford Press.

Wiener, S. I., Paul, C. A., & Eichenbaum, H. (1989). Spatial and behavioral correlates of hippocampal neuronal activity. *Journal of Neuroscience, 9,* 2737–2763.

Weiskrantz, L. (1982). Comparative aspects of studies of amnesia. *Philosophical Transactions of the Royal Society, London, B298,* 97–109.

Wible, C. G., Findling, R. L., Shapiro, M., Lang, E. J., Crane, S., & Olton, D. S. (1986). Mnemonic correlates of unit activity in the hippocampus. *Brain Research, 399,* 97–110.

Wilson, F. A. W., Brown, M. W., & Riches, I. P. (1987). Neuronal activity in the inferomedial temporal cortex compared with that in the hippocampal formation: Implications for amnesia of medial temporal lobe origin. In C. D. Woody (Ed.), *Cellular mechanisms of conditioning and behavioral plasticity.* New York: Plenum.

Winocur, G. (1980). The hippocampus and cue utilization. *Physiological Psychology, 8,* 280–288.

Winocur, G., & Olds, J. (1978). Effects of context manipulation on memory and reversal learning in rats with hippocampal lesions. *Journal of Comparative and Physiological Psychology, 92*, 312–321.

Zipser, D., & Andersen, R. A. (1988). A back propagation programmed network that simulates response properties of a subset of posterior parietal neurons. *Nature, 331*, 679–684.

Zola-Morgan, S., & Squire, L. R. (1984). Preserved learning in monkeys with medial temporal lesions: Sparing of motor and cognitive skills. *Journal of Neuroscience, 4*, 1072–1085.

Zola-Morgan, S., & Squire, L. R. (1985). Medial temporal lesions in monkeys impair memory on a variety of tasks sensitive to human amnesia. *Behavioral Neuroscience, 99*, 22–34.

8

Systems and Synapses of Emotional Memory

JOSEPH E. LEDOUX

One of the great challenges, and promises, of modern neuroscience is to understand the neural basis of memory. Recent work emphasizes that memory is a multifaceted psychological process and that the neuroanatomical organization of memory is correspondingly diverse and complex (e.g., Mishkin, 1982; Squire, 1987; Thompson, 1986; Weinberger, McGaugh & Lynch, 1985). Thus, brain lesions that eliminate the ability to remember certain kinds of information leave intact the ability to remember other things. This is dramatically illustrated by a classic case from the human amnesia literature reported by Claparede (1911). The patient, suffering with anterograde amnesia, was unable to recall the details of events experienced only moments earlier. Once, Claparede concealed a pin in his hand and stuck the patient. Henceforth, the patient refused to shake Claparede's hand but could not provide any explanation for her avoidance behavior. The injury to the patient's brain seriously compromised her ability to consciously recollect life's experiences but her ability to store information about the affective significance of the same experiences and respond adaptively on the basis of the stored information was preserved. Conscious recollections, sometimes referred to as declarative memories (Squire, 1987), are often treated as the sine qua non of memory. However, conscious recollections are only one aspect of memory. We will not understand "memory" until its many facets have been elucidated.

Although it is impossible to truly know, it seems likely that the spared ability in Claparede's patient represents an instance of Pavlovian defensive conditioning, whereby an innocuous stimulus (the sight of Claparede's hand) came to be associated with an aversive event (the pin prick). The innocuous stimulus thereby acquired aversive properties and was subsequently avoided.

Memories established through Pavlovian defensive or fear conditioning are acquired rapidly (Hall & Pearce, 1979; Mackintosh, 1983) and last for long, perhaps indefinite, periods of time (Jacobs & Nadel, 1985; LeDoux, Xaguraris, & Romanski, 1989). This form of learning is ubiquitous in the animal kingdom (Thorpe, 1963) and is particularly well suited for neurobiological analysis (Hawkins, Clark, & Kandel, 1987; Kandel & Spencer, 1968; Thompson, 1986). To the extent that the cellular mechanisms underlying Pavlovian conditioning are preserved across species (Alkon, 1984; Hawkins & Kandel, 1984), progress in elucidating the mechanisms of defensive conditioning in animals may foster advances in understanding how the human brain processes and stores information about the emotional significance of stimuli. This is especially important since Pavlovian aversive conditioning may play a major role in human emotional disorders, especially (but not exclusively) anxiety, phobic, and stress disorders (Davis, Hitchcock, & Rosen, 1987; Eysenck, 1979; Gray, 1982; LeDoux, 1987; Reiser, 1984). While fear conditioning may not be the only mechanism through which emotional memories are formed, it is certainly an important one.

NEUROANATOMY OF FEAR CONDITIONING

Evidence for the localization of fear processes in the brain was first obtained by Brown and Schafer (1888) and later confirmed by Kluver and Bucy (1937). These investigators observed that large lesions of the temporal lobe made monkeys tame in the presence of previously feared stimuli. Weiskrantz (1956) determined that the taming effect could be produced by lesions restricted to the amygdala. Disconnection of the visual association cortex from the amygdala produces taming to visual but not somatosensory stimuli, indicating that specific sensory pathways activate the amygdala to produce fear responses (Downer, 1961; Horel & Keating, 1969). Amygdala lesions also produce taming in cats (Ursin & Divac, 1975), rats (Blanchard & Blanchard, 1972), dogs (Fonberg, 1972), and birds (Phillips, 1964). Particularly relevant, though, is the observation that amygdala lesions interfere with the establishment of learned fear responses to novel stimuli (Blanchard & Blanchard, 1972; Cohen, 1980; Davis et al., 1987; Goddard, 1964; Kapp, Pascoe, & Bixler, 1984; LeDoux, 1987). The amygdala is thus critically involved in fear processes, including fear learning.

One advance in thinking about the brain mechanisms of behavior has been a shift in emphasis away from localized centers and toward anatomical systems. While the discovery that the amygdala plays a role in fear and fear learning is extremely important, it is also essential to ask how the amygdala fits into the larger system that mediates fear. For a given fear response, what are the structures afferent to and efferent to the amygdala? Since the amygdala is a heterogeneous brain region, it is necessary to know something about its internal organization in the mediation of fear responses as well. Does the entire amygdala contribute to fear or are only select subnuclei involved?

Considerable evidence now points to the central nucleus of the amygdala as a critical link in fear pathways. Lesions of the central nucleus prevent the conditioning of fear responses to sensory cues in several species (Davis et al., 1987; Gentile, Jarrel, Teich, McCabe, & Schneiderman, 1986; Iwata,

LeDoux, Meeley, Arneric, & Reis, 1986; Kapp et al., 1984). Unit activity recorded in the central amygdala is modified by explicit pairing of the conditioned stimulus (CS) and unconditioned stimulus (US) but not by unpaired presentations (Pascoe & Kapp, 1985). The central nucleus projects to brain stem areas involved in autonomic and somatomotor response control (e.g., Schwaber, Kapp, Higgins, & Rapp, 1982) and electrical or chemical stimulation of the central nucleus elicits autonomic and behavioral fear responses (Iwata, Chida, & LeDoux, 1987; Kapp et al., 1984). Lesions of the lateral hypothalamic and central gray areas, two efferent targets of the central amygdala, interfere separately with autonomic and somatomotor conditioned fear responses (Iwata, LeDoux, & Reis, 1986; LeDoux, Iwata, Cicchetti, & Reis, 1988; Powell & Levine-Bryce, 1989; Smith, Astley, Devito, Stein, & Walsh, 1980), suggesting that these lesions disrupt response control, rather than fear learning, mechanisms. The central nucleus of the amygdala is afferent to both structures and may be the final site of response-independent processing in the fear conditioning pathway.

Recent studies have also begun to characterize the afferent pathways to the amygdala underlying fear learning. For an auditory CS, the afferent pathway to the amygdala must be an output (either a direct or an indirect one) of structures in the auditory system. Lesions of the auditory cortex do not interfere with the conditioning of fear responses to acoustic stimuli paired with footshock, but lesions of the auditory thalamocortical relay station (the medial geniculate body) or the auditory midbrain station (the inferior colliculus) do interfere with conditioning (LeDoux, Sakaguchi, & Reis, 1984). These data suggest that the acoustic CS is transmitted through the auditory system to the medial geniculate body and from there to some region other than the auditory cortex. Anatomical tracing studies demonstrate that the medial geniculate body, in addition to projecting to the auditory cortex, also sends efferents to the amygdala (LeDoux, Ruggiero, & Reis, 1985; Ottersen & Ben-Ari, 1979; Turner & Herkenham, 1981; Veening, 1978). One of the amygdaloid targets of the thalamic projection is the central nucleus. The central nucleus might thus be the primary amygdaloid region involved in fear learning, serving as the direct interface between sensory (acoustic thalamus) and motor (lateral hypothalamic area and midbrain central gray area) systems in the fear conditioning circuitry. However, careful analysis of the organization of the cells of origin of the thalamoamygdala projections with respect to the thalamic projection field of the inferior colliculus suggests otherwise (LeDoux, Farb, & Ruggiero, 1990). The central amygdala receives its thalamic inputs from a region displaced medially from the medial geniculate body (MGB) and outside the projection of the inferior colliculus. In contrast, the lateral nucleus of the amygdala receives projections from the medial division of MGB and the underlying posterior intralaminar nucleus (PIN), both of which are within the collicular projection field. Furthermore, the lateral nucleus projects to the central nucleus (Krettek & Price, 1978) and lesions of the lateral nucleus interfere with fear conditioning (LeDoux, Cicchetti, Xagoraris, & Romanski,

1990). The lateral, not the central, amygdaloid nucleus thus appears to be the sensory interface of the amygdala.

These various observations allow a first approximation of the structures and pathways underlying fear conditioning from sensory to motor neurons. The circuitry involves transmission of inputs through the auditory system to the acoustic thalamus and from there to the lateral amygdala and then to the central amygdala. Efferent to the central amygdala, the pathway bifurcates, with projections to the lateral hypothalamus mediating autonomic conditioned responses and projections to the central gray region mediating somatomotor conditioned responses. These latter structures project to brain stem areas involved in autonomic and somatomotor response control, thereby suggesting an input–output description of the through-processing circuit at the level of brain nuclei and pathways. However, other brain areas certainly also contribute, possibly modulating activity in the through-processing circuit.

As described, the auditory cortex is not part of the conditioning circuitry, probably reflecting the fact that most of the studies performed have used simple (undiscriminated) stimuli. However, unit activity is modified in the auditory cortex during aversive conditioning (Weinberger, Hopkins, & Diamond, 1984) and differential aversive conditioning is disrupted by ablation of the auditory cortex (Jarrell, Gentile, Romanski, McCabe, & Schneiderman, 1987). As the sensory processing demands of the task are increased beyond the limits of thalamic neurons, the cortical system and corticoamygdala projections become involved. The corticoamygdala and thalamoamygdala projections converge in the lateral amygdala (LeDoux, Farb, & Romanski, in press), suggesting that the monosynaptic arrival of inputs in the amygdala from the acoustic thalamus might influence the processing of inputs arriving later over multisynaptic corticoamygdala pathways (LeDoux, 1986).

The circuits identified are responsible for the transmission and coding of the CS and the execution and control of the conditioned responses (CR). These circuits thus constitute the CS–CR pathways for fear conditioning. Little is known at present about other, equally important circuits. Two critical pieces of information are needed. First, how does the US elicit autonomic and somatic unconditioned responses (URs). This is a question about the US–UR circuit and should be addressable using the same strategies that have been used to identify the CS–CR circuits. Second, how does the US modify the processing of the CS? This is a completely different question from the first. For example, the elicitation of autonomic changes by an aversive US is mediated by a brain stem reflex circuit, the somatosympathetic reflex arc, whereas the modification of CS processing most likely takes place in the forebrain areas of the CS–CR pathway. Thus, the US processing circuits that elicit URs are not the US processing circuits that modify the processing of the CS. Modifications in CS processing during conditioning most likely occur by the convergence of inputs from US transmission systems with neurons in the CS pathway. The exact locus or loci and the nature of the modifications are important issues for future research.

SYNAPTIC PLASTICITY AND FEAR CONDITIONING

The neural modifications underlying learning probably involve synapses (Eccles, 1987; Hawkins et al., 1987; Hebb, 1949; Kandel & Spencer, 1986; Konorski, 1948; Lynch & Baudry, 1984; Squire, 1987; Thompson, 1986). A major obstacle to the study of the synaptic basis of learning, particularly in complex nervous systems, is the identification of the brain area or areas containing the critical synapses. Having identified the CS–CR pathway, a set of circuits that are likely to contain the modified synapses in fear conditioning, we can now begin to ask where in the circuits do neural modifications occur during conditioning.

Unit recording studies have shown that neurons in the medial MGB (a region that projects to the lateral amygdala) exhibit learning-induced changes in activity during classical conditioning (Disterhoft & Stuart, 1976; Gabriel, Slatwick, & Miller, 1976; Ryugo & Weinberger, 1978), as do neurons in the lateral (Le Gal, La Salle & Ben-Ari, 1981) and central amygdala (Pascoe & Kapp, 1985), and in the lateral hypothalamic region (Linseman & Olds, 1973; Ono, Nakamura, Nishijo, Tamura, & Tabuchi, 1986). Structures all along the conditioning circuit, from sensory-related to motor-related areas, thus exhibit physiological plasticity (learning-induced changes in neural activity) during conditioning. While at first this would seem to be hopelessly complex, knowledge of the circuit organization within which these changes take place suggests that each locus of change has a role in the overall learning process. Plasticity that takes place in structures afferent to the amygdala (e.g., acoustic or visual thalamic and cortical areas) is likely to be relatively "sensory specific" and plasticity observed in structures efferent to the amygdala (e.g., lateral hypothalamus or central gray) is likely to be relatively "motor specific." Sensory-specific modifications probably facilitate the subsequent selection and processing of the CS while motor-specific modifications facilitate the execution of the CR. In contrast, modifications in the amygdala may represent universal, integrative changes in neural activity that are present regardless of the sensory modality of the CS or the motor modality of the CR.

If the foregoing analysis is correct, the modification of sensory-specific inputs within the amygdala during learning is an important step in the establishment of emotional memories. Recent studies demonstrating that pathways transmitting sensory inputs to the amygdala from the thalamus (Clugnet & LeDoux, 1990) and cortex (Chapman & Brown, 1988) are highly plastic are therefore of special interest. These studies show that high-frequency stimulation applied to thalamic or cortical input pathways to amygdala induces long-lasting changes in synaptic efficacy, often described as long-term potentiation (LTP), in the amygdala.

LTP has been proposed as a candidate cellular mechanism of memory (Bliss & Lynch, 1988; Brown, 1989; Eccles, Ganong, Kairiss, Keenan, & Kelso, 1987; Lynch & Baudry, 1984; Thompson, 1986). LTP is rapidly established and long lasting; furthermore, and of special significance, LTP exhibits "associativity." That is, plasticity can be induced using two temporally overlapping inputs, neither of which is sufficient alone to modify the synapses. In this paradigm, the second input must come while the postsynaptic cell is still depolarized from the first input, making LTP at least superficially similar to forward classical conditioning (Brown et al., 1989). LTP may therefore be particularly suitable as a candidate mechanism for associative emotional memories established through classical conditioning.

LTP has been most extensively studied in the hippocampus (Bliss & Lynch, 1988; Brown et al., 1989; Lynch & Baudry, 1984; Teyler & DiScenna, 1987), where it can be produced in several different circuits. In some of these circuits, the changes in synaptic efficacy are induced by glutamate acting at N-methyl-D-aspartate (NMDA) receptors (Collingridge, Kehl, & McLennan, 1983; Cotman, Monaghan, & Ganong, 1988; Wigström & Gustafsson, 1986). NMDA receptor mechanisms seem also to function "associatively." The first input releases the excitatory amino acid transmitter, glutamate, which binds to postsynaptic non-NMDA receptors. This depolarizes the postsynaptic neuron and releases a magnesium block on the channel, allowing calcium to enter the postsynaptic cell. If other inputs to the postsynaptic cell arrive during this state, NMDA receptors are activated.

Excitatory amino acid receptor mechanisms may also contribute to synaptic plasticity in the thalamoamygdala system. The cells of origin of the thalamoamygdala projection are immunoreactive for glutamate (Farb, LeDoux, & Milner, 1989), as are terminals in the amygdala that originate in the thalamus (Farb & LeDoux, 1990). Furthermore, blockade of excitatory amino acid transmission prevents thalamic stimulation from evoking unit activity changes in the lateral amygdala amygdala (Clugnet, LeDoux, Morrison, & Reis, 1988). Moreover, excitatory amino acid receptors (both NMDA and non-NMDA receptors) are highly concentrated in the lateral amygdala (Greenamyre, Young, & Penney, 1984; Halpain, Wieczorek, & Rainbow, 1984; Monaghan & Cotman, 1985). While it has not yet been shown that glutamate and NMDA receptors mediate amygdala LTP, recent studies have shown that blockade of NMDA receptors in the amygdala prevents the establishment of conditioned emotional memories (Miserendino, Sananes, Melia, & Davis, 1990). While the determination of whether the changes in synaptic efficacy seen in the amygdala involve the same fundamental mechanisms as seen in hippocampus will have to await the outcome of future studies, the evidence to date suggests that at least some overlap may exist.

Results of Golgi studies indicate that the lateral amygdala contains two classes of neurons distinguished by the presence of spines (McDonald, 1982; Millhouse & DeOlmos, 1983). The spiny cells (Type 1) predominate, are pyramidal in shape, and are mostly relay or projection neurons. Spine-free cells (Type 2) tend to be smaller neurons with dense local axonal arborizations that appear to make synapses with spiny dendrites of Type 1 cells and are likely to be local circuit or interneurons. Since the thalamoamygdala projection mainly terminates on spines (Farb, LeDoux, & Milner, 1989;

Le Doux, Farb, & Milner, 1990), we can conclude that Golgi Type 1 neurons are the input cells. Since the Type 1 neurons are projection (as opposed to local circuit) neurons, the input–output transform within the lateral amygdala may be accomplished by these neurons. However, it seems likely that this transform is modified by local circuit processes.

Excitatory-evoked responses in the lateral amygdala are usually short lasting and followed by a period of inhibition (Clugnet, LeDoux, & Morrison, 1990; Le Gal La Salle & Ben-Ari, 1981), possibly regulated by GABA-mediated long-duration inhibitory post-synaptic potential (IPSPs) (Takagi & Yamamoto, 1981). Inhibition may be via recurrent collaterals such that excitation of projection cells by afferent input excites local GABA interneurons that then inhibit further firing of the projection neurons (Le Gal La Salle & Ben-Ari, 1981). GABA interneurons (Golgi Type 2 cells) thus appear to regulate the through-processing by projection neurons (Golgi Type 1 cells).

Sustained transmission of sensory input through the lateral amygdala, as in fear processing, may require either the shutdown of local GABA neurons by extrinsic inhibitory inputs or by an increase in the net excitatory input to the projection neurons. Extrinsic afferents from neurons processing the US could accomplish this.

Extrinsic afferents to the lateral amygdala from areas other than acoustic regions of thalamus and cortex are poorly characterized. Immunocytochemical and receptor binding studies indicate that the lateral amygdala receives projections from dopaminergic, serotonergic, cholinergic, and several peptidergic systems (Carlsen & Heimer, 1986; Fallon, 1981; Roberts et al., 1981). Relay of US inputs to the lateral amygdala could be through these projections, some of which may contact neurons in the CS pathway.

The lateral amygdala also contains a high concentration of benzodiazepine receptors (Niehoff & Kuhar, 1983; Young & Kuhar, 1980). Benzodiazepine receptors are closely linked with the GABA receptor complex and appear to exert their anxiolytic actions by enhancing GABA transmission (Costa & Guidotti, 1979). It is thus significant that microinjection of benzodiazepines directly into the lateral amygdala has anxiolytic effects (Scheel-Kruger & Petersen, 1982). If fear conditioning involves a release of lateral amygdala projection neurons from inhibition, benzodiazepine-mediated relief of the fear evoked by conditioned stimuli might involve a reinstatement of inhibition of lateral amygdala projection neurons by enhancement of GABA transmission.

The foregoing observations suggest several hypotheses about the cellular mechanisms of fear conditioning. Sensory transmission to the lateral amygdala from the medial geniculate body is mediated by an excitatory amino acid transmitter, possibly glutamate (Glu). Binding of Glu (released presynaptically from acoustic projections) to postsynaptic, non-NMDA (kainate/quisqualate) receptors located on lateral amygdala projection neurons results in a brief, initial excitation followed by a prolonged inhibition. The inhibition is generated by collaterals of the projection neurons that terminate locally on GABA interneurons that in turn synapse back on the projection neurons. Part of the cellular machinery of fear learning involves an associative LTP-like sustained excitation of lateral amygdala projection neurons. This is achieved by convergence of afferents from US pathways that override the inhibition of lateral amygdala projection neurons by either (a) directly inhibiting the activity of GABA interneurons, (b) increasing the net excitatory postsynaptic inputs to projection neurons, or (c) facilitating presynaptic transmitter release. Increased excitation (depolarization) of the postsynaptic neurons might then open the NMDA channel and stabilize and strengthen the synapses involved. Reduction of the learned salience of feared stimuli by benzodiazepines may involve an override, by enhancement of GABA inhibition, of the strengthened excitatory synapses. These hypotheses are largely untested but are empirically based. It seems highly likely that they will, for the most part, be confirmed by future studies. If so, we will have taken a major step towards a cellular understanding of fear conditioning and of the way in which the brain forms at least one class of emotional memory.

REFERENCES

Alkon, D. L. (1984). Calcium-mediated reduction of ionic currents: a biophysical memory trace. *Science, 226,* 1037–1045.

Blanchard, D. C., & Blanchard, R. J. (1972). Innate and conditioned reactions to threat in rats with amygdaloid lesions. *Journal of Comparative Physiology and Psychology, 81,* 281–290.

Bliss, T. V. P., & Lynch, M. A. (1988). In P. W. Landfield & S. Deadwyler (Eds.), *Long-term potentiation: from biophysics to behavior* (pp. 3–72). New York: Alan R. Liss.

Brown, S., & Schafer, A. (1888). An investigation into the functions of the occipital and temporal lobes of the monkey's brain. *Philosophical Transctions of the Royal Society, London, B179,* 303–327.

Brown, T. H., Ganong, A. H., Kairiss, E. W., Kennan, C. L., & Kelso, S. R. (1989). Long-term potentiation in two synaptic systems of the hippocampal brain slice. In J. H. Byrne & W. O. Berry (Eds.), *Neural models of plasticity,* (pp. 266–306). San Diego: Academic Press.

Carlsen, J., & Heimer, L. (1986). A correlated light and electron microscopic immunocytochemical study of cholinergic terminals and neurons in the rat amygdaloid body with special emphasis on the basolateral amygdaloid nucleus. *Journal of Comparative Neurology, 244,* 121–136.

Chapman, P.F., & Brown, T. H. (1988). Long-term potentiation in amygdala brain slices. *Society for Neuroscience Abstracts, 14,* 566–566.

Claparede, E. (1911). Recognition and "me-ness". Reprinted in D. Rapaport (Ed.), *Organization and pathology of thought (1951)* (pp. 58–75). New York: Columbia University Press.

Clugnet, M. C., & LeDoux, J. E. (1990). Synaptic plasticity in fear conditioning circuits: Induction of LTP in the lateral nucleus of the amygdala by stimulation of the medial geniculate body. *Journal of Neuroscience, 10.*

Clugnet, M. C., LeDoux, J.E., and Morrison, S. F. (1990). Unit responses evoked in the amygdala and striatum by electrical stimulation of the medial geniculate body. *Journal of Neuroscience, 10,* 1055–1061.

Clugnet, M. C., LeDoux, J. E., Morrison, S. F., and Reis, D. J. (1988). Short latency orthodromic action potentials evoked in the amygdala and caudate-putamen by stimulation of the medial geniculate body. *Society for Neuroscience Abstracts, 14*, 1227–1227.

Cohen, D. H. (1980). The functional neuroanatomy of a conditioned response. In R. F. Thompson, L. H. Hicks, & B. Shvyrkov (Eds.), *Neural mechanisms of goal-directed behavior and learning* (pp. 283–302). New York: Academic Press.

Collingridge, G. L., Kehl, S. J., & McLennan, H. (1983). Excitatory amino acids in synaptic transmission in the Schaffer collateral-commissural pathway of the rat hippocampus. *Journal of Physiology, 334*, 33–46.

Costa, E., & Guidotti, A. (1979). Molecular mechanisms in the receptor action of benzodiazepines. *Annual Review of Pharmacology and Toxicology, 19*, 531–545.

Cotman, C. W., Monaghan, D.T., & Ganong, A. H. (1988). Excitatory amino acid neurotransmission: NMDA receptors and Hebb-type synaptic plasticity. *Annual Review of Neuroscience, 11*, 61–80.

Davis, M., Hitchcock, J. M., & Rosen, J. B. (1987). Anxiety and the amygdala: Pharmacological and anatomical analysis of the fear-potentiated startle paradigm. In G. H. Bower (Ed.), *The psychology of learning and motivation*. San Diego: Academic Press.

Disterhoft, J., & Stuart, D. (1976). Trial sequence of changed unit activity in auditory system of alert rat during conditioned response acquisition and extinction. *Journal of Neurophysiology, 39*, 266–281.

LeDoux, J. E., Farb, C., Ruggiero, D. A. (1990). Topographic organization of neurons in the acoustic thalamus that project to the amygdala. *Journal of Neuroscience, 10*, 1043–1054.

Downer, J. D. C. (1961). Changes in visual gnostic function and emotional behavior following unilateral temporal lobe damage in the "split-brain" monkey. *Nature, 191*, 50–51.

Eccles, J.C. (1987). Mechanisms of learning in complex neural systems. In F. Plum (Ed.), *Handbook of physiology: section 1. The nervous system: Vol. 5. Higher functions of the brain* (pp. 137–167). Bethesda: American Physiological Society.

Eysenck, H. J. (1979). The conditioning model of neurosis. *Behavioral and Brain Sciences, 2*, 155–199.

Fallon, J. H. (1981). Histochemical characterization of dopaminergic, noradrenergic and serotonergic projections to the amygdala. In Y. Ben-Ari (Ed.), *The amygdaloid complex* (pp. 175–183). New York: Elsevier/North-Holland Biomedical Press.

Fallon, J. H., & Ben-Ari, Y. (1981). Chairmen's comments. In Y. Ben-Ari (Ed.), *The amygdaloid complex* (pp. 151–162). New York: Elsevier/North-Holland Biomedical Press.

Farb, C. R., and LeDoux, J. E. (1990). Glutamate is present in presynaptic terminals of thalam-amygdala projections. *Society for Neuroscience Abstracts, 16*, 607–607.

Farb, C. F., LeDoux, J.E., & Milner, T. A. (1989). Glutamate is present in medial geniculate body neurons that project to lateral amygdala and in lateral amygdala presynaptic terminals. *Society for Neuroscience Abstracts, 15*, 890–899.

Fonberg, E. (1972). Control of emotional behavior through the hypothalamus and amygdaloid complex. In D. Hill (Ed.), *Physiology, emotion, and psychosomatic illness* (pp. 131–162). Amsterdam: Elsevier.

Gabriel, M., Slatwick, S. E., & Miller, J. D. (1976). Multiple unit activity of the rabbit medial geniculate nucleus in conditioning, extinction, and reversal. *Physiological Psychology, 4*, 124–134.

Gentile, C. G., Jarrel, T. W., Teich, A., McCabe, P. M., & Schneiderman, N. (1986). The role of amygdaloid central nucleus in the retention of differential Pavlovian conditioning of bradycardia in rabbits. *Behavioral Brain Research, 20*, 263–273.

Goddard, G. (1964). Functions of the amygdala. *Psychological Review, 62*, 89–109.

Gray, J. A. (1982). *The neuropsychology of anxiety*. Oxford: Clarendon.

Greenamyre, J. T., Young, A. B., & Penney, J. B. (1984). Quantitative autoradiographic distribution of L-[3H]-glutamate binding sites in rat central nervous system. *Journal of Neuroscience, 4*, 2133–2144.

Hall, G., & Pearce, J. M. (1979). Latent inhibition of a CS during CS–US pairings. *Journal of Experimental Psychology: Animal Behavior Processes, 5*, 31–42.

Halpain, S., Wieczorek, C. M., & Rainbow, T. C. (1984). Localization of L-glutamate receptors in rat brain by quantitative autoradiography. *Journal of Neuroscience, 4*, 2247–2258.

Hawkins, R. D., Clark, G. A., & Kandel, E. R. (1987). Cell biological studies of learning in simple vertebrate and invertebrate systems. In F. Plum (Ed.), *Handbook of physiology: Section 1. The nervous system: Vol. V. Higher functions of the brain* (pp. 25–83). Bethesda: American Physiological Society.

Hawkins, R. D., & Kandel, E. R. (1984). Is there a cell-biological alphabet for simple forms of learning? *Psychological review, 91*, 375–391.

Hebb, D. O. (1949). *The organization of behavior*. New York: John Wiley.

Horel, J. A., & Keating, E. G. (1969). Partial Kluver-Bucy syndrome produced by cortical disconnection. *Brain Research, 16*, 281–284.

Iwata, J., Chida, K., & LeDoux, J.E. (1987). Cardiovascular responses elicited by stimulation of neurons in the central amygdaloid nucleus in awake but not anesthetized rats resemble conditioned emotional responses. *Brain Research, 418*, 183–188.

Iwata, J., LeDoux, J. E., Meeley, M. P., Arneric, S., & Reis, D. J. (1986). Intrinsic neurons in the amygdaloid field projected to by the medial geniculate body mediate emotional responses conditioned to acoustic stimuli. *Brain Research, 383*, 195–214.

Iwata, J., LeDoux, J. E., & Reis, D. J. (1986). Destruction of intrinsic neurons in the lateral hypothalamus disrupts cardiovascular but not behavioral conditioned emotional responses. *Brain Research, 368*, 161–166.

Jacobs, W. J., & Nadel, L. (1985). Stress-induced recovery of fears and phobias. *Psychological Review, 92*, 512–531.

Jarrell, T. W., Gentile, C. G., Romanski, L. M., McCabe, P. M., & Schneiderman, N. (1987). Involvement of cortical and thalamic auditory regions in retention of differential bradycardia conditioning to acoustic conditioned stimuli in rabbits. *Brain Research, 412*, 285–294.

Kandel, E. R., & Spencer, W. A. (1968). Cellular neurophysiological approaches to the study of learning. *Physiological Review, 48*, 65–134.

Kapp, B. S., Pascoe, J. P., & Bixler, M. A. (1984). The amygdala: A neuroanatomical systems approach to its contributions to aversive conditioning. In N. Buttlers & L.R. Squire (Eds.), *Neuropsychology of memory*. New York: Guilford.

Kluver, H., & Bucy, P. C. (1937). "Psychic blindness" and other symptoms following bilateral temporal lobectomy in rhesus monkeys. *American Journal of Physiology, 119*, 352–353.

Konorski, J. (1948). *Conditioned reflexes and neuron organization*. Cambridge: Cambridge University Press.

Krettek, J. E., & Price, J. L. (1978). Amygdaloid projections to subcortical structures within the basal forebrain and brainstem in the rat and cat. *Journal of Comparative Neurology, 178*, 225–254.

Le Gal La Salle, G., & Ben-Ari, Y. (1981). Unit activity in the amygdaloid complex: A review. In Y. Ben-Ari (Ed.), *The amygdaloid complex* (pp. 227–237). New York: Elsevier/North-Holland Biomedical Press.

LeDoux, J.E. (1986). Sensory systems and emotion. *Integrative Psychiatry. 4*, 237–248.

LeDoux, J. E. (1987). Emotion. In F. Plum (Ed.), *Handbook of physiology: 1. The nervous system: Vol. V. Higher functions of the brain* (pp. 419–460). Bethesda: American Physiological Society.

LeDoux, J. E., Cicchetti, P., Xagoraris, A., & Romanski, L.R. (1990). The lateral amygdaloid nucleus: Sensory interface of the amygdala in fear conditioning. *Journal of Neuroscience, 10*, 1062–1069.

LeDoux, J. E., Iwata, J., Cicchetti, P., & Reis, D. J. (1988). Different projections of the central amygdaloid nucleus mediate autonomic and behavioral correlates of conditioned fear. *Journal of Neuroscience, 8*, 2517–2529.

LeDoux, J. E., Ruggiero, D. A., Forest, R., Stornett, R., & Reis, D. J. (1987). Topographic organization of convergent projections to the thalamus from the inferior colliculus and spinal cord in the rat. *Journal of Comparative Neurology, 264*, 123–146.

LeDoux, J. E., Ruggiero, D.A., & Reis, D. J. (1985). Projections to the subcortical forebrain from anatomically defined regions of the medial geniculate body in the rat. *Journal of Comparative Neurology, 242*, 182–313.

LeDoux, J. E., Sakaguchi, A., & Reis, D. J. (1984). Subcortical efferent projections of the medial geniculate nucleus mediate emotional responses conditioned to acoustic stimuli. *Journal of Neuroscience, 4*, 683–698.

LeDoux, J. E., Xagoraris, A., & Romanski, L. M. (1989). Indelibility of subcortical emotional memories. *Journal of Cognitive Neuroscience, 1*, 238–243.

LeDoux, J. E., Farb, C. R., & Milner, T. A. (1991). Ultrastructure and synaptic associations of auditory thalamo-amygdala projections in the rat. *Experimental Brain Research, 85*, 577–586.

LeDoux, J. E., Farb, C. R., & Romanski, L. R. (in press). Convergent projections to the amygdala from auditory processing areas of the thalamus and cortex. *Neurosci. Lett.*

Linseman, M., & Olds, J. (1973). Activity changes in rat hypothalamus, preoptic area, and striatum associated with Pavlovian conditioning. *Journal of Neurophysiology, 36*, 1038–1050.

Lynch, G., & Baudry, M. (1984). The biochemistry of memory: A new and specific hypothesis. *Science, 224*, 1057–1063.

Mackintosh, N. J. (1983). *Conditioning and associative learning.* Oxford: Oxford University Press.

McDonald, A. J. (1982). Neurons of the lateral and basolateral amygdaloid nuclei: a golgi study in the rat. *Journal of Comparative Neurology, 212*, 293–312.

Millhouse, O. E., & DeOlmos, J. (1983). Neuronal configurations in lateral and basolateral amygdala. *Neuroscience, 10*, 1269–1300.

Miserendino, M. J. D., Sananes, C. B., Melia, K. R., & Davis, M. (1990). Blocking of acquisition but not expression of conditioned fear-potentiated startle by NMDA antagonists in the amygdala. *Nature, 345*, 716–718.

Mishkin, M. (1982). A memory system in the monkey. *Philosophical Transactions of the Royal Society, London, B298*, 85–95.

Monaghan, D.T., & Cotman, C. W. (1985). Distribution of N-methyl-D-aspartate-sensitive L-[3H]glutamate-binding sites in rat brain. *Journal of Neuroscience, 5*, 2909–2919.

Niehoff, D. L., & Kuhar, M. J. (1983). Benzodiazepine receptors: Localization in rat amygdala. *Journal of Neuroscience, 3*, 2091–2097.

Ono, T., Nakamura, K., Nishijo, H., Tamura, R., & Tabuchi, E. (1988). Lateral hypothalamus and amygdala involvement in rat learning behavior. *70*, 123–126.

Ono, T., Nishijo, H., Nakamura, K., Tamura, R., & Tabuchi, E. (1988). Role of amygdala and hypothalamic neurons in emotion and behavior. In *Biowarning System in the Brain*, H. Takagi, Y. Oomura, M. Ito and M. Otsuka (Eds.), pp. 309–331. Tokyo: University of Tokyo Press.

Ottersen, O. P., & Ben-Ari, Y. (1979). Afferent connections to the amygdaloid complex of the rat and cat: Projections from the thalamus. *Journal of Comparative Neurology, 187*, 401–424.

Pascoe, J. P., & Kapp, B. S. (1985). Electrophysiological characteristics of amygdaloid central nucleus neurons during Pavlovian fear conditioning in the rabbit. *Behavioral Brain Research, 16*, 117–133.

Phillips, R. E. (1964). "Wildness" in the Mallard duck: Effects of brain lesions and stimulation on "escape behavior" and reproduction. *Journal of Comparative Neurology, 122*, 139–155.

Powell, D. A., & Levine-Bryce, D. (1989). Conditioned bradycardia in the rabbit: Effects of knife cuts and ibotenic acid lesions in the lateral hypothalamus. *Experimental Brain Research, 76*, 103–121.

Reiser, R. (1984). *Mind, brain, and body.* New York: Basic Books.

Roberts, G. W., Polak, J. M., & Crow, T. J. (1981). The peptidergic circuitry of the amygdaloid complex. In Y. Ben-Ari (Ed.), *The amygdaloid complex* (pp. 185–195). New York: Elsevier/North-Holland Biomedical Press.

Ryugo, D. K., & Weinberger, N. M. (1978). Differential plasticity of morphologically distinct neuron populations in the medial geniculate body of the cat during classical conditioning. *Behavioral and Neural Biology, 22*, 275–301.

Scheel-Kruger, J., & Petersen, E. N. (1982). Anticonflict effect of the benzodiazepines mediated by GABAergic mechanism in the amygdala. *European Journal of Pharmacology, 82*, 115–116.

Schwaber, J. S., Kapp, B. S., Higgins, G. A., & Rapp, P. R. (1982). Amygdaloid and basal forebrain direct connections with the nucleus of the solitary tract and the dorsal motor nucleus. *Journal of Neuroscience, 2*, 1424–1438.

Smith, O. A., Astley, C. A., Devito, J. L., Stein, J. M., & Walsh, R. E. (1980). Functional analysis of hypothalamic control of the cardiovascular responses accompanying emotional behavior. *Federation Proceedings, 29*, 2487–2494.

Squire, L. R. (1987). Memory: Neural organization and behavior. In F. Plum (Ed.), *Handbook of physiology: Section 1. The nervous system: Vol. V. Higher functions of the brain* (pp. 295–371). Bethesda: American Physiological Society.

Takagi, M., & Yamamoto, C. (1981). The long lasting inhibition recorded in vitro from the lateral nucleus of the amygdala. *Brain Research, 206*, 474–478.

Teyler, T. J., & DiScenna, P. (1987). Long-term potentiation. *Annual Review of Neuroscience, 10*, 131–161.

Thompson, R. F. (1986). The neurobiology of learning and memory. *Science, 233*, 941–947.

Thorpe, W. H. (1963). *Learning and instinct in animals.* London: Methuen.

Turner, B., & Herkenham, N. (1981). An autoradiographic study of thalamo-amygdaloid connections in the rat. *Anatomical Record, 199*, 260A.

Ursin, H., & Divac, I. (1975). Emotional behavior in feral cats with ablation of prefrontal cortex and subsequent lesions in amygdala. *Journal of Comparative and Physiological Psychology, 88*, 36–39.

Veening, J. G. (1978). Subcortical afferents of the amygdaloid complex in the rat: An HRP study. *Neuroscience Letters, 8*, 197–202.

Weinberger, N. M., Hopkins, W., & Diamond, D. M. (1984). Physiological plasticity of single neurons in auditory cortex of the cat during acquisition of the pupillary conditioned response: I Primary field (A1). *Behavioral Neuroscience, 98*, 171–188.

Weinberger, N. M., McGaugh, J. L., & Lynch, G. (1985). *Memory systems of the brain: Animal and human cognitive processes.* New York: Guilford Press.

Weiskrantz, L. (1956). Behavioral changes associated with ablation of the amygdaloid complex in monkeys. *Journal of Comparative and Physiological Psychology, 49*, 381–391.

Young, W. S., & Kuhar, M. J. (1980). Radiohistochemical localization of benzodiazepine receptors in rat brain. *Journal of Pharmacology and Experimental Therapeutics, 212*, 337–346.

9

Alterations of the Functional Organization of Primary Somatosensory Cortex Following Intracortical Microstimulation or Behavioral Training

GREGG H. RECANZONE
MICHAEL M. MERZENICH

A number of different electrophysiological strategies have been employed to elucidate the governing principles of neocortical function. One useful approach has been to record from cortical neurons in awake or anesthetized animals, parametrically defining the specific stimuli that best activate the sampled neurons. These studies have led to an understanding of the functionally effective projections to the cortex at that time in the life of an adult animal.

A second approach has been to study the distributed, specific responses of cortical neurons at different times in the life of an animal, with some experimental manipulation that alters this aspect of functional organization introduced between the two samples. One model system that has yielded a large body of data on this issue in the past decade is the lemniscal somatosensory system terminating in the "primary" somatosensory cortical fields. In these studies, the topographic representations within "primary" somatosensory (SI) cortical fields, or "maps" of the skin surface, have been shown to be altered over time following denervation of restricted skin areas (Calford & Tweedale, 1988; Franck, 1980; Kalaska & Pomeranz, 1979; Merzenich et al., 1983a, b, 1984; Rasmusson, 1982; Wall & Cusick, 1984), by shuffling the peripheral inputs after nerve transection (Allard, Clark, Grajski, & Merzenich, 1988), digit syndactyly (Allard, Clark, Jenkins, & Merzenich, in press; Clark, Allard, Jenkins, & Merzenich, 1988), island pedicle transfers (Clark, Allard, Jenkins, & Merzenich, 1986; Merzenich, Recanzone, Jenkins, Allard, & Nudo, 1988), restricted cortical lesions (Doetsch, Johnston, & Hannan, 1990; Jenkins & Merzenich, 1987), and following extensive mechanical stimulation or differential use (Jenkins,

Merzenich, Ochs, Allard, & Guic-Robles, 1990; Yun & Merzenich, 1987). The above studies have been conducted in a wide variety of mammalian species including the New World owl and squirrel monkey, as well as the rat, cat, raccoon, and flying fox. This demonstration of changes in distributed neural responses ("representational topography") induced by peripheral or cerebral manipulation of inputs or by behavioral training, is not restricted to primary somatosensory cortical fields, as examples in other cortical areas have recently been documented, including motor cortex (Merzenich et al., 1988; Merzenich, Recanzone, & Jenkins, in press; Sanes, Suner, & Donoghue, 1990); auditory cortex (Robertson & Irvine, 1989), second somatosensory cortex (SII) (Pons, Garraghty, & Mishkin, 1988), and in primary visual cortex (Kaas et al., 1990).

A second line of research has been to study the response properties of single neurons or small groups of neurons before, during and/or immediately after a specific behavioral manipulation. This behavioral manipulation usually pairs a limited set of stimuli to a positive or negative reinforcement in a classical or operant conditioning paradigm. These manipulations have shown, in several different cortical areas and species, that the response properties of the neurons can be altered as a function of the behavioral contingencies imposed on the stimulus (Buchhalter, Brons, & Woody, 1978; Disterhoft & Olds, 1972; Disterhoft & Stuart, 1976; Kitzes, Farley, & Starr, 1978; Kraus & Disterhoft, 1982; Olds, Disterhoft, Segal, Kornblith, & Hirsch, 1972; Oleson, Ashe, & Weinberger, 1975; Woody, Knispel, Crow, & Black-Cleworth, 1976; see also Miyashita, 1988; Miyashita & Chang, 1988). A recent example is a change in the frequency tuning profiles of auditory cortical neurons in awake cats when the presentation of a specific frequency was paired with a negative reinforcing stimulus in a classical conditioning paradigm (Diamond & Weinberger, 1986, 1989). With conditioning, some neurons changed their response properties to respond to the presentation of the conditioned tone. This effect was not seen when the tone and the aversive stimulus were not temporally paired, and was reversed by an extinction schedule. The dependence of a behavioral relevance to the stimulus as a requisite condition to change the neuronal response properties is a consistent finding across cortical areas and species (see references cited above).

One feature that all these studies have in common is that the numbers of neurons and cortical locations at which such effects are observed is very high. Although these studies have not specifically addressed the issue of the distributed spatial "representations" of these responses, the high proportion of affected neurons that respond to behaviorally important stimuli strongly suggests that the cortical areas representing these important stimuli are increased following behavioral training.

The primary somatosensory cortical fields as a model system has an experimental advantage in that it is straightforward to determine the spatial location of the skin necessary to evoke a neural response. If the representation of that skin location is altered as the result of a peripheral or central manipulation or as the consequence of behavioral training, one can conclude that the effective input to that location in the brain has been altered over a measurable spatial distance. An assumption inherent in all studies of the cerebral cortex through use of such "mapping" techniques is that the principles of cortical organization elucidated by these studies apply to all other areas in the cortex (see Merzenich et al., 1988, in press). If this is the case, the governing principles of dynamic functional cortical organization in the "simple" primary sensory cortex can be studied in order to gain insight into the general functions of the cerebral cortex, and how its operations can account for higher cognitive functions such as learning, memory, language, and abstract thought.

PROPOSED MECHANISMS OF FUNCTIONAL CORTICAL REORGANIZATION

Mechanisms proposed to account for the topographic reorganization described in the cerebral cortex are based primarily on changes in the efficacies of already present inputs, usually through a Hebbian-synapse type of mechanism (see Edelman, 1987; Edelman & Mountcastle, 1978; Merzenich et al., 1988, in press; Singer, 1990; von der Malsburg & Singer, 1988; but see also Calford & Tweedale, 1988; Killackey, 1990). At the same time it is acknowledged that representational changes may also involve highly localized morphological changes: for example, new synapse formation or local dendritic or spine changes. Indeed, a number of studies indicate that local changes, but not afferent arbor changes, are generated in behaviorally engaged sectors of the neocortex (e.g., Connor & Diamond, 1982; Greenough, Larson, & Withers, 1985; Withers & Greenough, 1989).

Studies over the past decade have provided a wealth of data on the anatomical divergence of input from the ventrobasal thalmus to SI cortex, and this divergence appears to be sufficient to account for the topographic changes observed experimentally. Tracing of single thalamocortical afferents either through intracellular injection of horseradish peroxidase (HRP) or Golgi stains have shown that the arborization of the terminals projecting to area 3b in monkeys or its homologue in cats extend over a range from several hundred microns to several millimeters (Garraghty, Pons, Sur, & Kaas, 1989; Garraghty & Sur, 1990; Jones, 1975a; Landry & Deschenes, 1981). Afferents with multiple branches, in which each branch had dense terminations over an area of several hundred microns, have been observed in all studies. Similar techniques addressing the extent of the dendritic spread of individual neurons in cortex have shown that pyramidal and spiny stellate cells in layers III–IV, where the thalamic afferents terminate, have dendritic spreads of 300–500 μm (Jones, 1975b; Schwark & Jones, 1989).

Small injections of tracers into the ventrobasal thamalus or SI, which label many neurons at the injection site, suggest an even greater divergence of thalamic inputs in the cortex. Studies in which the receptive fields of neurons at the injection site are defined suggest that label restricted to the representation of one or two digits in the thalamus projects to an area several millimeters in width in the cortex, which represents three to five digits (Cusick & Gould, 1990; Jones & Friedman, 1982; Jones, Friedman, & Hendry, 1982; Lin, Merzenich, Sur, & Kaas, 1979; Mayner & Kaas, 1986).

Physiological techniques used to address the same issue are consistent with this anatomical evidence (Snow, Nudo, Rivers, Jenkins, & Merzenich, 1988; Zarzecki & Wiggin, 1982). Pharmacological manipulations of GABA-ergic inhibition have shown that cortical neurons receive input from a large skin area. Iontophoretic application of GABA antagonists result in 4–10-fold increases of the receptive field size in cat SI (Alloway, Rosenthal, & Burton, 1989; Batuer, Alexandrov, & Scheynikov, 1982; Hicks & Dykes, 1984) but not in the thalamus (6/48 cells increased; Hicks, Metherate, Landry, & Dykes, 1986). These changes occur of the order of seconds and are reversible. Similar receptive field enlargements follow several hours of electrical stimulation of a peripheral cutaneous nerve (Recanzone, Allard, Jenkins, & Merzenich, 1990). Finally, labeling metabolic activity as a result of cutaneous stimulation in the adult cat shows an almost twofold increase in the cortical area activated by cutaneous stimulation in the presence of the GABA antagonist bicuculline (Juliano, Whitsel, Tommerkahl, & Cheema, 1989). All these results are consistent with the notion that there is sufficient anatomical divergence from the thalamus to the cortex to account for the experimentally or behaviorally induced changes in topographic representations. It should be emphasized again that the existence of sufficient divergence of thalamocortical inputs is, of course, not conclusive evidence that some local sprouting or morphological alteration of thalamic afferents, cortical dendrites, or dendritic spines does not occur.

It is necessary to account for the fact that a cortical neuron, although receiving inputs from a large skin region, responds to only a limited subset of those inputs. One likely mechanism to account for this is that specific synapses are strengthened or weakened in a Hebbian fashion (Hebb, 1949). These synapses are thought to increase in efficacy by the temporal coactivation of pre- and postsynaptic elements. A number of studies have shown that the response properties of particular neurons can be altered by temporally pairing the activity of neurons with either a previously subthreshold neuronal input, with a specific sensory stimulus, or with the application of pharmacological agents (cited above, see also Bindman, Murphy, & Pockett, 1988; Delacour, Houcine, & Talbi, 1987; Frégnac, Shulz, Thorpe, & Bienenstock, 1988; Iriki, Pavlides, Keller, & Asanuma, 1989; Metherate, Tremblay, & Dykes, 1987; Sakamoto, Porter, & Asanuma, 1987). These studies lend support to the conclusion that such mechanisms are plausible, as they already exist within the cortex.

The long-term changes in synaptic efficacy that occur after a relatively brief period of temporal coactivation of the pre- and postsynaptic neurons have been hypothesized to be the result of immediate short-term changes, for example by protein phosphorylation through a second messenger system, followed by a longer term modification, perhaps including morphological changes of the pre- and postsynaptic elements themselves (e.g., Baranyi, Szente, & Woody, 1988). These temporally based mechanisms of synaptic strengthening are precisely the type necessary to account for changes in the response properties of cortical neurons following the variety of surgical and behavioral modifications described above.

An important anatomical feature when considering this synaptic mechanism in the cerebral cortex is that cortical neurons are not only functionally connected with the thalamic afferents, but also to neighboring neurons, and to neurons projecting from other cortical areas. If the rules governing synaptic efficacy are effective not only for the thalamocortical synapse, but also for corticocortical synapses, the potential to shape networks of functionally interconnected neurons by behavior also exists. These potential "aggregates," or "groups" or "assemblies" have been postulated to be the functional unit of the cerebral cortex (see Edelman, 1978, 1987; Merzenich et al., 1988, in press; Singer, 1990; von der Malsburg & Singer, 1988). By this view individual cortical neurons are members of a specific unit, the membership of a neuron is dependent on the competitive interactions between the influence of the neurons' own unit and the neighboring units. There is by necessity some interaction between these functional units that shape the specific topographic relationship of the response properties of neurons within a unit. The resulting receptive field defined electrophysiologically is the product of the competition between the excitatory inputs from the thalamic afferents and the local cortical neurons with the inhibitory influence from the surrounding cortical neurons. These interactions then form the foundation of response selectivities and the topographic representations observed in primary sensory cortex.

What is the evidence that these types of corticothalamic and corticocortical interactions form the foundation of cortical function? High-density mapping studies have shown a robust topography within the representation of the skin surface. Plasticity studies are all consistent with changes in the response properties of cortical neurons being dependent on the temporal coactivation of inputs to the skin (see Merzenich et al., 1988, in press). Neural network models incorporating these principles have replicated the experimental findings noted above (Grajski & Merzenich, 1990; Pearson, Finkel, & Edelman, 1987). Inactivation of the postsynaptic neuron prevents normal ocular dominance plasticity in striate cortex (Reiter & Stryker, 1988; see also Frégnac et al., 1988). These experimental and modeling findings are consistent with the hypotheses presented above, but are not conclusive. There has been no clear evidence to date on the horizontal extents of these "groups" or "units" in the cortex, or that neurons shift their response properties to become "members" of a different unit. The following is a presentation of two results from our studies that provide further evidence that there are experimentally and behaviorally alterable functional interconnections between neurons in the adult cerebral cortex.

ACUTE ALTERATION OF COUPLED CORTICAL NEURON GROUPS

The effects of temporally synchronous excitation of all elements in a local region of the primary somatosensory cortical field was investigated using intracortical microstimulation (ICMS) (Recanzone, Merzenich, & Dinse, submitted). In these experiments, a normal adult rat or owl monkey was anesthetized with barbiturate and the distributed responses in a small region of the primary somatosensory cortex was mapped in detail. The experimental procedure was to make multiple microelectrode penetrations roughly normal to the cortical surface and perpendicular to each other into the middle cortical layers. In each electrode penetration the cutaneous receptive field of the recorded neurons was defined by exploring the skin surface with fine probes. Following derivation of an initial "map," the microelectrode was inserted at a location roughly in the center of the mapped region and microstimulated using the current parameters: 3–5 μA biphasic pulses; 300 p.p.s. rate; 40 ms duration. Bursts were presented once per second for 2–6 h. These stimulation parameters have been estimated to excite neurons over a horizontal cortical distance of less than 100 μm (Stoney, Asanuma, & Thompson, 1968). Thus, over this limited cortical area, neurons were strongly temporally coactivated for several hours. We then remapped the same cortical area as before, making every effort to reintroduce the microelectrode into some of the same cortical locations as in the previously defined map. If cortical organization is influenced by the competitive cortical network interactions as described above, this experimental paradigm could be expected to result in a change in the neuron membership of the group centered at the stimulation site.

Some of the results of two typical experiments in this series are shown diagramatically in Figure 9.1. Examples of receptive fields defined in the pre-ICMS condition are shown in A for the trunk representation of a representative rat (left) and the hand representation of a representative owl monkey (right). The receptive field at the location of the ICMS electrode is shown as shaded for both cases, and its location on the body is shown in C. Receptive fields defined following 6 h of ICMS in the rat and after 4 h of conditioning stimulation in the monkey are shown in part B of the figure. It is clear that a large proportion of these receptive fields *now* represent the same skin surface that was originally represented at the location of the ICMS electrode. An important feature of this experiment is that in every case, the sizes and the locations of the receptive fields at the ICMS location were not significantly altered. However, the area of cortical tissue that came to represent this same restricted segment of skin was greatly enlarged.

The area effected by this stimulation is shown for two different examples in Figure 9.2. In this figure, each cortical penetration location is represented by either a circle or square. The fill pattern of the symbol represents the amount of overlap, measured as the area of the receptive field that is continuous with the ICMS location receptive field divided by the total area

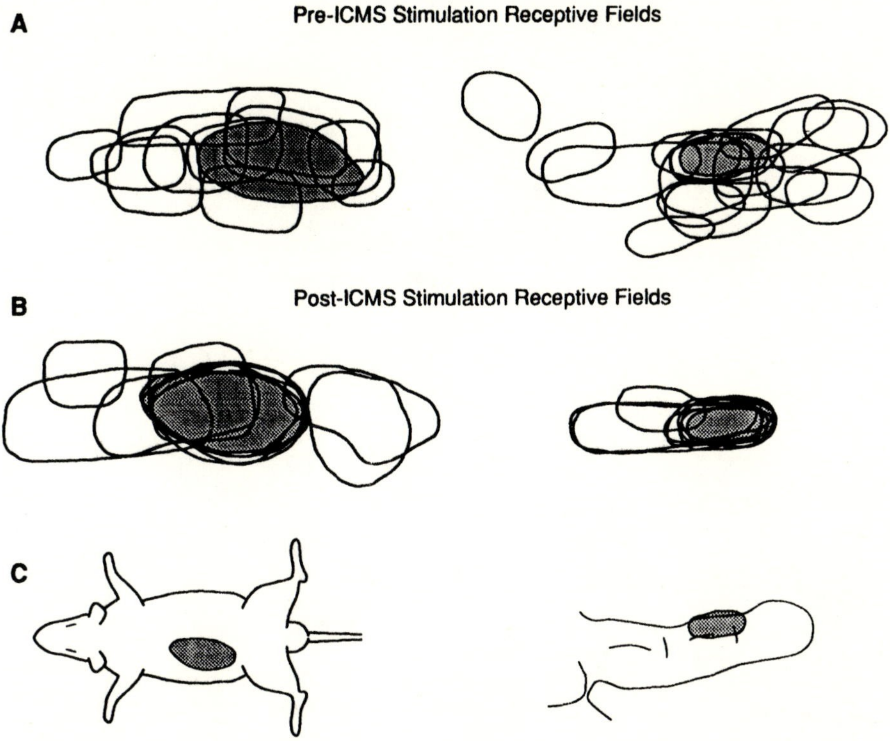

A   Pre-ICMS Stimulation Receptive Fields

B   Post-ICMS Stimulation Receptive Fields

C

FIGURE 9.1. Cortical receptive fields defined prior to (A) and following (B) low-level, high-frequency intracortical microstimulation (ICMS) at a single site in SI. The stippled area shows the receptive field defined at the ICMS location. Receptive fields were located on the trunk of the rat, and on the ulnar aspect of the middle phalange of digit 5 of the monkey in these representative examples (C). ICMS was applied for 6 h in the rat (left) and for 4 h in the owl monkey (right), with dramatic changes in the receptive fields recorded from neurons sampled in this same cortical zone. (Figure is adapted from Recanzone, Merzenich, & Dinse, 1991a)

of that receptive field. This overlap is divided into four categories as shown in the legend. In these representative examples the amount of overlap of receptive fields between two cortical locations is very small in the pre-ICMS condition (top panel). This percentage overlap increases for both the squirrel monkey hand representation and the rat forepaw representation (bottom panel). This is indicated by the large area of filled squares, which represent overlap of over 85% of the ICMS receptive field.

This expansion of representation of a restricted skin region is not seen in the absence of ICMS, with all other factors of the experimental paradigm being equal. It should also be noted that the representation was always asymmetric about the ICMS location. The distance at which a cortical location could represent the ICMS site could be several hundred microns in one direction, and there could be only limited or no overlap at a location

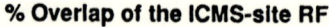

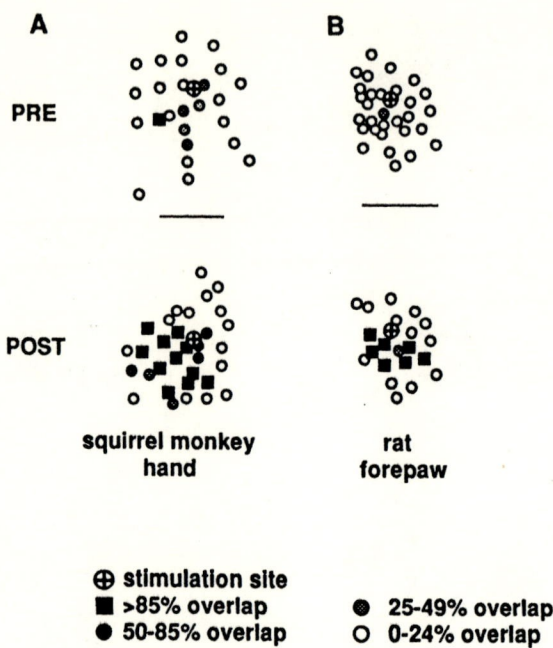

% Overlap of the ICMS-site RF

FIGURE 9.2.   Cortical microelectrode penetration locations before (top) and after (bottom) ICMS in the hand representation of a squirrel monkey (A) and the forepaw representation of a rat (B). The open circle with crosses denotes the ICMS site. Solid squares denote receptive fields that overlap the ICMS site receptive field by more than 85%. The other solid symbols represent percentage overlaps as indicated in the legend. Bar represents 500 μm in both A and B. (Adapted from Recanzone, Merzenich, & Dinse, 1991a)

less than 100 μm away in the other direction. An additional feature to note is that a cortical location adjacent to one that had changed receptive fields could be seemingly unaffected by the ICMS, as locations with percentage overlaps of greater than 85% could be within 100 μm of locations with no overlap. Finally, the absolute size of the receptive fields was not significantly changed by the ICMS. Although some receptive fields increased in size as the percentage overlaps increased, at a roughly equal number of cortical locations the receptive field size decreased.

The results of this experiment, in which cortical neurons over a significant horizontal extent come to represent identical or nearly identical inputs, is predicted by models of competitive interactions between functional cortical groups. The ICMS stimulus presumably creates a relatively localized synchronization of activity around the electrode tip. This would result in all local neurons being simultaneously depolarized by the stimulating current, followed by depolarization of their functionally connected neighbors. This synchronized input would presumably result in the recruitment of neighboring neurons into the functional unit or group located at the ICMS site. As the neuronal group enlarges, it could then influence more distant neurons.

DISTRIBUTED CHANGES INDUCED BY TRAINING A MONKEY IN A BEHAVIORAL TASK ENGAGING A SMALL SKIN LOCUS

In a second approach to these issues, a restricted region of the cerebral cortex was excited through its natural input pathways by presenting a specific tactile stimulus to an invariant location on the skin. We have recently accomplished this by behaviorally training adult owl monkeys to discriminate the frequency of a tactile stimulus presented to a very restricted, invariant location on a single digit. The animals' task was to maintain contact with the stimulus probe through the presentation of 650 ms bursts of 20 Hz sinusoidal stimulation, and to break contact with the probe on detection of an increase in the stimulus frequency. Monkeys trained at this task progressively improved in performance. This improvement was initially rapid and was generalized to adjacent, untrained digits. Following this rapid component, there was further, more gradual improvement in performance that was limited to the trained digit. Ultimately, these animals could detect a difference in frequency of approximately 2 Hz above the 20 Hz standard on the trained digit, as compared with a difference of about 4 Hz on an adjacent, untrained digit (Recanzone, Hradek, Jenkins, & Merzenich, submitted).

These animals were then anesthetized and the functional organization of the hand surface representation was studied in detail in both the contralateral and ipsilateral SI cortical fields (Recanzone, Merzenich, Jenkins, Grajski, & Dinse, submitted). Receptive fields were defined at several hundred microelectrode penetrations as described above, and the data analyzed with respect to (a) the representation of the skin trained in the task that improved performance with training; (b) the representation of the same stimuli on an adjacent digit, whose behavioral thresholds were measured to be greater than those of the trained digit; and (c) of the corresponding skin locations on the contralateral, untrained hand. A representative example of one such monkey is shown in Figure 9.3. In this figure, the area bounding the microelectrode penetration locations with receptive fields representing the skin stimulated during the task on the trained digit is shown as dark stippling, and those areas bounding the representation of the corresponding skin on the adjacent, untrained digit are shown as lighter stippling. The cortical representation of the trained digit shows a dramatic increase in the representation of the stimulated skin as opposed to the adjacent unstimulated, untrained skin. This also holds true when the comparison is made between these representations and those of the corresponding skin of the contralateral hemispheres. These observations were consistent with those recorded in

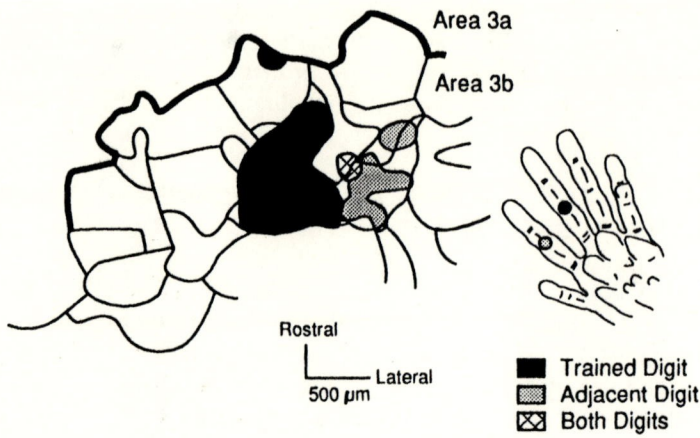

FIGURE 9.3. Area of representation in somatosensory cortical area 3b of two restricted skin segments in an adult owl monkey trained in the tactile frequency discrimination task. The heavy line marks the physiologically defined area 3a–area 3b border. Thinner lines denote the representation of different hand segments (unlabeled). The area of cortex with receptive fields including the skin area stimulated in the behavioral task is shown as dark stippling (Digit 3, inset). The area representing a corresponding site on an adjacent, untrained digit is shown as light stippling (Digit 2,inset). The cross-hatched area represents the location of one large receptive field that included both skin sites. (Adapted from Recanzone, Merzenich, Jenkins, Grajski, & Dinse, 1991c)

three other trained monkeys, for which equivalent maps of distributed responses were obtained (Recanzone, Merzenich, Jenkins, Grajski, & Dinse, submitted).

An interesting observation was that the increase in the representation of the stimulated skin was not accompanied by an increase in the overall representation of the entire digit. When the area of representation of all of the glabrous skin of each digit was measured, there was no obvious difference between the area representing the trained digit and any other digit of that monkey. A second interesting observation was that the increase in the cortical representation of the restricted skin region stimulated in the behavioral task was accompanied by an increase in receptive field size. All receptive fields defined in these two representations are shown in Figure 9.4. The receptive fields on the trained digit, D3 of the left hand, showed both an increase in size when compared with the receptive fields on other portions of the two hands, and also a tendency to accumulate over the behaviorally engaged skin locus (black circle). This was a common observation in animals trained in this tactile frequency discrimination task.

The receptive fields representing the trained skin showed a high degree of overlap over a much greater cortical distance that was seen in the contralateral hemisphere. Receptive field overlap, as measured by using six

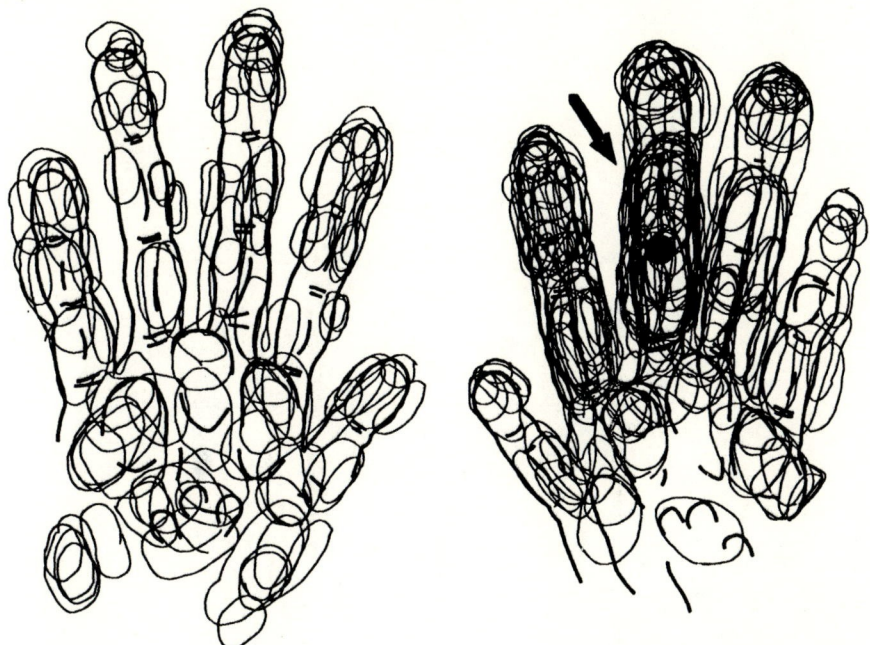

Untrained Hand   **Trained Hand**

FIGURE 9.4.   All receptive fields defined in cortical area 3b representing the trained hand (right) and the untrained hand (left) of the monkey whose representational data are shown in Figure 9.3. The black circle denotes the area of skin stimulated in the behavioral task. The arrow indicates the large number of receptive fields that include this region of skin. The population of receptive fields defined on the trained digit was statistically significantly larger that the receptive fields defined on any other digit (two-tailed *t*-test, $p < .01$). (Adapted from Recanzone, Merzenich, Jenkins, Grajski, & Dinse, 1991c)

to eight standard receptive fields by which all other receptive fields on the same digit are compared, is plotted as a function of horizontal distance between the cortical locations for a representative example in Figure 9.5. Part A shows this function for the cortical representation of the digit trained in the behavioral task. The overlap of receptive fields can be nearly 100% at cortical distances of several hundred microns on this trained digit. This is in contrast to the function derived in normal owl monkeys, which drops off to zero overlap with cortical distances of approximately 600 μm in a roughly linear function (Sur, Merzenich, & Kaas, 1980). This function holds true in the owl monkey regardless of the body surface investigated. A more normal function of percentage overlap with cortical distance is seen for the contralateral, untrained hemisphere (part B). The overlap is clearly much less for the representation of this unstimulated and untrained digit.

The cortical location in which receptive field overlap was high was found to be predominantly located for the representation of the stimulated skin.

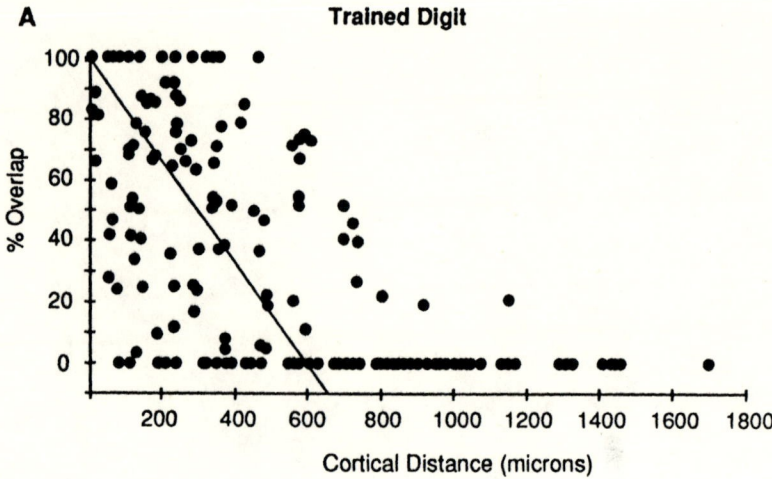

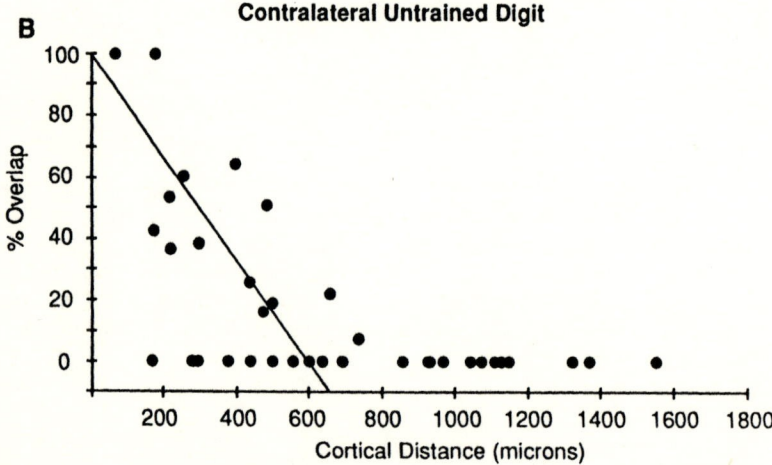

FIGURE 9.5. Percentage of receptive field overlap of two cortical locations as a function of the distance between them. Receptive field overlap was defined with reference to one of seven different standard receptive fields for all cortical locations representing the trained digit (A) and the corresponding digit on the contralateral, untrained hand (B). A hypothetical linear function in which overlap drops to zero at 600 μm distance (see Sur, Merzenich, & Kaas, 1980) is also shown. Receptive fields with no overlap at small cortical distances usually reflected receptive fields separated in the radial–ulnar dimension. (Adapted from Recanzone, Merzenich, Jenkins, Grajski, & Dinse, 1991c)

A clear demonstration of this is seen by plotting the percentage overlap as a function of cortical distance with respect to a single receptive field that was roughly centered on the stimulation site. If the cortical distance is plotted as a function of the rostrocaudal location relative to this receptive field, a plot such as that shown in Figure 9.6 is generated. The percentage overlap of receptive fields relative to one representing the trained skin area is very high, extending rostrally for several hundred microns. In contrast, a receptive field at the corresponding location on the untrained digit had an overlap with distance function characteristic of that of a normal animal.

These results show again that an area of cortex representing a small region of skin can expand across a significant horizontal extent. This expansion of the representation was brought about by training the animal to attend to and discriminate the temporal features of a tactile stimulus. This tactile stimulus was presented to a very restricted spot on a single digit, and this same region of skin could now drive neurons throughout this expanded representational area. The increase in the representation of the skin region, the expansion of the receptive field size, and the clustering of receptive fields at a restricted location are all within the realm of prediction of cortical network models based on changes of synaptic efficacy via coincident input. By these models, the synchronous input from the invariant skin location stimulated behaviorally is predicted to strengthen the synapses specifically representing the stimulated skin. The neighboring cortical neurons that initially represented some portion of the stimulated skin would thus be activated simultaneously, thereby strengthening all local-circuit synapses of this group or cluster of neurons. The tighter coupling of these neighboring neurons is then imagined to result in the group of neurons firing to any stimulus sufficient to fire one or some small subset of neurons. Thus, the synapses that initially excited any significant subset of the group could now fire all neurons of the group, resulting in the large and constant receptive field size. As this large group of cortical neurons representing the stimulated skin expanded, the neurons that initially represented skin removed from the stimulation site could presumably still retain most of their original synaptic efficacies and therefore represent the same, unstimulated skin area. This could then account for the constant area of representation of the entire digit, and put constraints on the total area of representation of the stimulated skin.

The above model predicts that if the skin stimulation site was not restricted to a single location, but was instead positioned at different locations across the skin, these particular changes in topography and receptive field size would not result, because in that case each stimulated skin site would be an effective competitor when those inputs are translated throughout the cortical network. A study of frequency discrimination in the macaque, in which tactile stimuli were presented to different locations on the skin, did not report differences in receptive field sizes (Mountcastle, Steinmetz, & Romo, 1990).

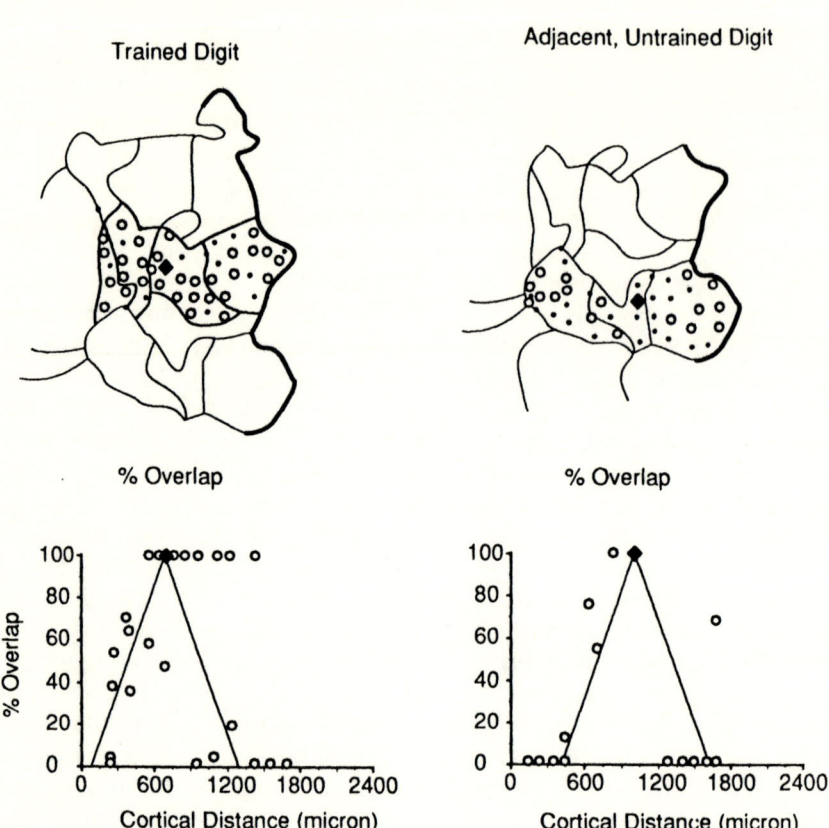

FIGURE 9.6. Percentage overlap of receptive fields as a function of cortical location. In the top panel the representation of the trained digit (left) and an adjacent, untrained digit (right) are shown, using the conventions as in Figure 9.3. The solid diamond denotes the cortical location of the reference receptive field. The open symbols represent the cortical location of the receptive fields used in this analysis. Small dots represent other cortical locations with receptive fields on the extreme ulnar or radial aspects of the digit, and were not used in this analysis. The percentage overlap by cortical distance function is shown in the bottom panels. Cortical distance is measured only in the rostro–caudal axis. The x-axis is scaled to this dimension. Points that overlap by greater than 50% are shown as a single point for clarity of view. (Adapted from Recanzone, Merzenich, Jenkins, Grajski, & Dinse, 1991c)

EVIDENCE OF COUPLING OF NEURONS IN THE TEMPORAL DOMAIN

The hypothesis that these cortical neurons are indeed functionally coupled is supported by the temporal response properties of these neurons to stimulation of the skin at the same skin location tested behaviorally. At many cortical locations in which receptive field data were derived, the responses of neurons at these locations to sinusoidal tactile stimulation was also tested. This stimulus was tested regardless of where the receptive field was at each cortical location. This resulted in many locations giving no responses or only onset responses to the tactile stimulation. Neurons at many locations did respond to each cycle of the stimulus presented to this invariant skin location. In these cases, the neural response was plotted as a function of time relative to the most recent zero-cross of the stimulus (a cycle histogram). When all cycle histograms for stimulation of the trained digit were combined for all cortical locations that gave a response to each stimulus cycle, and plotted, the resulting "population cycle histogram" showed a very crisp response to each stimulus cycle. This result is shown for the response to stimulation of the trained digit (top) and to stimulation of the untrained, adjacent digit (bottom) in Figure 9.7. The response to stimulation of the trained digit was sharp and had a very rapid rising phase to the beginning portion of each stimulus waveform. If the neural response was not tightly locked in time—that is, if the neurons over this enlarged cortical area were not tightly coupled functionally—the cycle histogram would be expected to be much broader.

Coupling of neurons across the network has been examined before and after intracortical microstimulation resulting in cortical group enlargement (see Dinse, Recanzone, & Merzenich, 1990). Both the strengths of non-stimulus-driven discharge correlation and the distances over which response correlations were recorded were altered by this stimulation. Neurons all across the topographically reorganized cortical zone showed evidence of coupling after the conditioning ICMS stimulation, while coupling was initially evident on only a very local neural network scale.

These studies have provided us with a new paradigm in which to test the hypotheses and models of cortical organization (Edelman, 1987; Edelman & Mountcastle, 1978; Merzenich, 1988, in press; von der Malsburg & Singer, 1988). A key feature of the described behavioral experiments that distinguishes them from those of previous investigators is that the behaviorally relevant stimulus was presented to a constant, invariant location on the skin. Thus the afferent inputs were restricted to a limited cortical region and resulted in an expansion of the representation of that input. This expansion is consistent with predictions of the competitive, coincidence-based models of cortical organization proposed above: that is, cortical neurons over a significant horizontal extent came to be tightly coupled and responded to nearly identical stimulation. This functional coupling was also evident in the very high resolution of the temporal responses to the behaviorally relevant sinusoidal stimuli. In spite of the distance between these cortical locations and despite the laborious process of sampling suprathreshold temporal responses at each individual cortical location, the responses to each stimulus cycle were very tightly locked in time. The temporal coincidence of the cortical responses over this broad area was always greater than that for stimuli presented to the adjacent, untrained

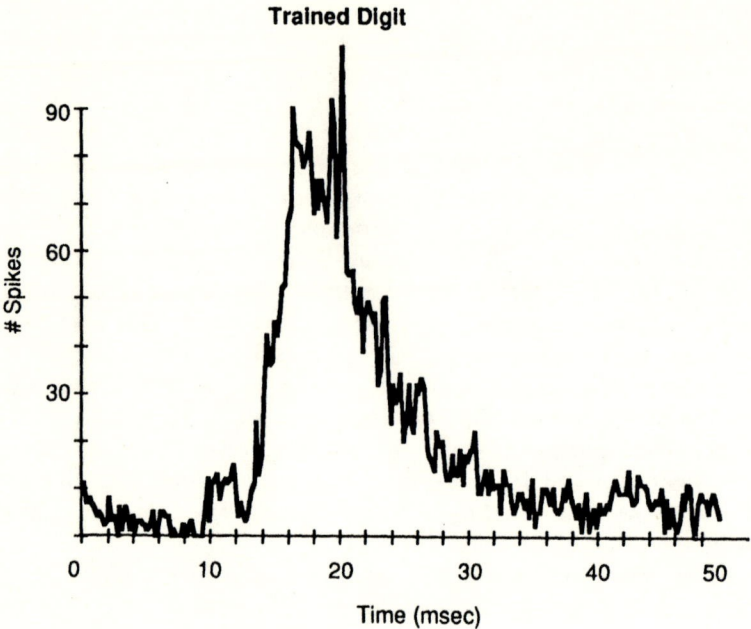

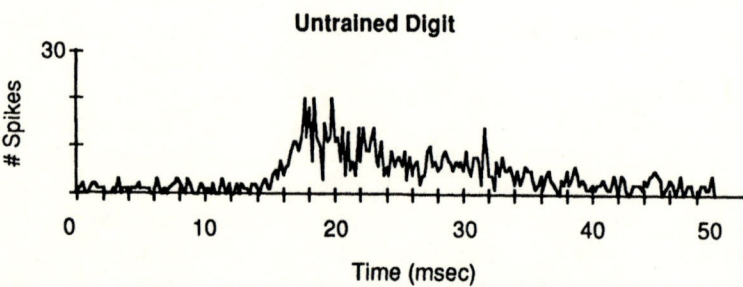

FIGURE 9.7. Population cycle histogram of the response to 20 Hz sinusoidal stimulation of the skin trained in the behavioral task (top) and of the corresponding skin location on the adjacent, untrained digit (bottom). Cycle histograms were constructed from all cortical locations that gave a frequency following response to stimulation at that skin location. Histograms are plotted in milliseconds relative to the immediately preceding zero-cross of the tactile stimulus. Binwidth is 200 μs. (Adapted from Recanzone, Merzenich, & Schreiner, submitted)

digit represented over a relatively smaller cortical area. This implies that during presentation of the behavioral stimulus a large cortical area was simultaneously active. This observation is consistent with the formation of an essentially single module or positively coupled group of neurons that covered a large cortical area.

In retrospect, it is surprising that more investigators have not attempted to determine whether or how distributed cortical network cell assemblies might be perturbed by simple local stimulation. In fact, they are dramatically perturbed, again in ways consistent with the interpretation that the cortical cell assemblies are themselves shaped and continually remodelled by our experiences.

The results presented herein, although not conclusive evidence, are nonetheless consistent with models of functional cortical organization based on competitive interactions of cortical neurons and coincidence of inputs. These results also further confirm the proposition that the functional organization of the cortex is alterable throughout life, and that this organization reflects the behavioral capacities of the animal (Recanzone, Merzenich, & Schreiner, submitted). The demonstration of the alterability of the distributed response properties has profound implications for other cortical areas, and thus other behaviors and perceptions, if the phenomenon and principles outlined here are generalizable to other areas of the neocortex.

Acknowledgments: The authors would like to thank W. M. Jenkins, H. R. Dinse, C. E. Schreiner, and G.T. Hradek for their intellectual and technical support in the experiments described in this report. This work was supported by NIH Grants NS-10414 and GM-07449 and the Coleman Fund.

REFERENCES

Allard, T. T., Clark, S. A., Grajski, K. A., & Merzenich, M. M. (1988). Plasticity in primary somatosensory cortex after digital nerve section and regeneration in adult owl monkey. *Society for Neuroscience Abstracts, 14* (2), 844.

Allard, T. T., Clark, S. A., Jenkins, W. M., & Merzenich, M. M. (in press). Reorganization of somatosensory area 3b representation in adult owl monkeys following digital syndactyly. *Journal of Neurophysiology*.

Alloway, K. D., Rosenthal, P., & Burton, H. (1989). Quantitative measurements of receptive field changes during antagonism of GABAergic transmission in primary somatosensory cortex of cats. *Experimental Brain Research, 78*, 514–532.

Baranyi, A., Szente, M. B., & Woody, C. D. (1988). Activation of protein kinase C induces long-term changes of postsynaptic currents in neocortical neurons. *Brain Research, 440*, 341–347.

Batuev, A. S., Alexandrov, A. A., & Scheynikov, N. A. (1982). Picrotoxin action on the receptive fields of the cat sensorimotor cortex neurons. *Journal of Neuroscience Research, 7*, 49–55.

Bindman, L. J., Murphy, K. P. S. J., & Pockett, S. (1988). Postsynaptic control of the induction of long-term changes in efficacy of transmission at neocortical synapses in slices of rat brain. *Journal of Neurophysiology, 60*, 1053–1065.

Buchalter, J., Brons, J., & Woody, C. (1978). Changes in cortical neuronal excitability after presentations of a compound auditory stimulus. *Brain Research, 156*, 162–167.

Calford, M. B., & Tweedale, R. (1988). Immediate and chronic changes in responses of somatosensory cortex in adult flying-fox after digit amputation. *Nature, 332*, 446–448.

Clark, S. A., Allard, T. T., Jenkins, W. M., & Merzenich, M. M. (1986). Cortical map reorganization following neurovascular island skin transfers on the hands of adult owl monkeys. *Society for Neuroscience Abstracts, 12* (1), 391.

Clark, S. A., Allard, T., Jenkins, W. M., & Merzenich, M. M. (1988). Syndactyly results in the emergence of double digit receptive fields in somatosensory cortex in adult owl monkeys. *Nature, 332,* 444–445.

Connor, J. R., & Diamond, M. C. (1982). A comparison of dendritic spine number and type on pyramidal neurons of the visual cortex of old adult rats from social or isolated environments. *Journal of Comparative Neurology, 210,* 99–106.

Cusick, C. G., & Gould, H. J. III (1990). Connections between area 3b of the somatosensory cortex and subdivisions of the ventroposterior nuclear complex and the anterior pulvinar nucleus in squirrel monkeys. *Journal of Comparative Neurology, 292,* 83–102.

Delacour, J., Houcine, O., & Talbi, B. (1987). "Learned" changes in the responses of the rat barrel field neurons. *Neuroscience, 23* (1), 63–71.

Diamond, D. M., & Weinberger, N. M. (1986). Classical-conditioning rapidly induces specific changes in frequency receptive fields of single neurons in secondary and ventral ectosylvian auditory cortical fields. *Brain Research, 372,* 357–360.

Diamond, D. M., & Weinberger, N. M. (1989). Role of context in the expression of learning-induced plasticity of single neurons in auditory cortex. *Behavioral Neuroscience, 103* (3), 471–494.

Dinse, H. R., Recanzone, G. H., & Merzenich, M. M. (1990). Direct observation of neural assemblies during neocortical representational reorganization. In R. Eckmitler, G. Hartmann, & G. Hauske (Eds.), *Parallel processing in neural systems and computers* (pp. 65–70). North Holland: Elsevier Science Publishers.

Disterhoft, J. F., & Olds, J. (1972). Differential development of conditioned unit changes in thalamus and cortex of rat. *Journal of Neurophysiology, 35,* 665–679.

Disterhoft, J. F., & Stuart, D. K. (1976). Trial sequence of changed unit activity in auditory system of alert rat during conditioned response acquisition and extinction. *Journal of Neurophysiology, 39,* 266–281.

Doetsch, G. S., Johnston, K. W., & Hannan, C. J. (1990). Physiological changes in the somatosensory forepaw cerebral cortex of adult raccoons following lesions of a single cortical digit representation. *Experimental Neurobiology, 108,* 162–175.

Edelman, G. M., & Mountcastle, V. B. (1978). *The mindful brain: Cortical organization and the group-selective theory of higher brain function.* Cambridge: MIT Press.

Edelman, G. M. (1987). *Neuronal Darwinism: The theory of neuronal group selection.* New York: Basic Books.

Franck, J. I. (1980). Functional reorganization of cat somatic sensory-motor cortex (SmI) after selective dorsal root rhizotomies. *Brain Research, 186,* 458–462.

Frégnac, Y., Shulz, D., Thorpe, S., & Bienenstock, E. (1988). A cellular analogue of visual cortical plasticity. *Nature, 333,* 367–370.

Garraghty, P. E., Pons, T. P., Sur, M., & Kaas, J. H. (1989). The arbors of axon terminations in middle cortical layers of somatosensory area 3b in owl monkeys. *Somatosensory and Motor Research, 6* (4), 401–411.

Garraghty, P. E., & Sur, M. (1990). Morphology of single intracellularly stained axons terminating in area 3b of macaque monkeys. *Journal of Comparative Neurology, 294,* 583–593.

Grajski, K. A., & Merzenich, M. M. (1990). Hebb-type dynamics is sufficient to account for the inverse magnification rule in cortical somatotopy. *Neural Computation, 2*, 74–81.

Greenough, W. T., Larson, J. R., & Withers, G. S. (1985). Effects of unilateral and bilateral training in a reaching task on dendritic branching of neurons in the rat motor-sensory forelimb cortex. *Behavioral and Neurological Biology, 44*, 301–304.

Hebb, D. O. (1949). *The organization of behavior: A neuropsychological theory.* New York: Wiley.

Hicks, T. P., & Dykes, R. W. (1984). Receptive field size for certain neurons in primary somatosensory cortex is determined by GABA-mediated intracortical inhibition. *Brain Research, 274*, 160–164.

Hicks, T. P., Metherate, R., Landry, P., & Dykes, R. W. (1986). Bicuculline induced alterations of response properties in functionally identified ventroposterior thalamic neurons. *Experimental Brain Research, 63*, 248–264.

Iriki, A., Pavlides, C., Keller, A., & Asanuma, H. (1989). Long-term potentiation in the motor cortex. *Science, 245*, 1385–1387.

Jenkins, W. M., & Merzenich, M. M. (1987). Reorganization of neocortical representations after brain injury: A neurophysiological model of the bases of recovery from stroke. *Progress in Brain Research, 71*, 249–266.

Jenkins, W. M., Merzenich, M. M., Ochs, M., Allard, T. T., & Guic-Robles, E. (1990). Functional reorganisation of primary somatosensory cortex in adult owl monkeys after behaviorally controlled tactile stimulation. *Journal of Neurophysiology, 63* (1), 82–104.

Jones, E. G. (1975a). Lamination and differential distribution of thalamic afferents within the sensory-motor cortex of the squirrel monkey. *Journal of Comparative Neurology, 160*, 167–204.

Jones, E. G. (1975b). Varieties and distribution of non-pyramidal cells in the somatosensory cortex of the squirrel monkey. *Journal of Comparative Neurology, 160*, 205–268.

Jones, E. G., & Friedman, D. P. (1982). Projection pattern of functional components of thalamic ventrobasal complex on monkey somatosensory cortex. *Journal of Neurophysiology, 48* (2), 521–544.

Jones, E. G., Friedman, D. P., & Hendry, S. H. C. (1982). Thalamic basis of place- and modality-specific columns in monkey somatosensory cortex: a correlative anatomical and physiological study. *Journal of Neurophysiology, 48* (2), 545–568.

Juliano, S. L., Whitsel, B. L., Tommerkahl, M., & Cheema, S. S. (1989). Determinants of patchy metabolic labeling in the somatosensory cortex of cats: A possible role for intrinsic inhibitory circuitry. *Journal of Neuroscience, 9* (1), 1–12.

Kaas, J. H., Krubitzer, L. A., Chino, Y. M., Langston, A. L., Polley, E. H., & Blair, N. (1990). Reorganization of retinotopic cortical maps in adult mammals after lesions of the retina. *Science, 228*, 229–231.

Kalaska, J., & Pomeranz, B. (1979). Chronic paw denervation causes an age-dependent appearance of novel responses from forearm in "paw cortex" of kittens and adult cats. *Journal of Neurophysiology, 42* (2), 618–633.

Killackey, H. P. (1990). Static and dynamic aspects of cortical somatotopy: a critical evaluation. *Journal of Cognitive Neuroscience, 1* (1), 1–11.

Kitzes, L. M., Farley, G. R., & Starr, A. (1978). Modulation of auditory cortex unit activity during the performance of a conditioned response. *Experimental Neurology, 62*, 678–697.

Kraus, N., & Disterhoft, J. F. (1982). Response plasticity of single neurons in rabbit auditory association cortex during tone-signalled learning. *Brain Research, 246*, 205–215.

Landry, P., & Deschenes, M. (1981). Intracortical arborizations and receptive fields of identified ventrobasal thalamocortical afferents to the primary somatic sensory cortex in the cat. *Journal of Comparative Neurology, 199*, 354–371.

Lin, C. S., Merzenich, M. M., Sur, M., & Kaas, J. H. (1979). Connections of areas 3b and 1 of the parietal somatosensory strip with the ventroposterior nucleus in the owl monkey (*Aotus trivirgatus*). *Journal of Comparative Neurology, 185* (2), 355–371.

Mayner, L., & Kaas, J. H. (1986). Thalamic projections from electrophysiologically defined sites of body surface representations in areas 3b and 1 of somatosensory cortex of cebus monkeys. *Somatosensory and Motor Research, 4* (1), 13–29.

Merzenich, M. M., Kaas, J. H., Wall, J. T., Nelson, R. J., Sur, M., & Felleman, D. J. (1983a). Topographic reorganization of somatosensory cortical areas 3b and 1 in adult monkeys following restricted deafferentation. *Neuroscience, 10*, 33–55.

Merzenich, M. M., Kaas, J. H., Wall, J.T., Sur, M., Nelson, R. J., & Felleman, D. J. (1983b). Progression of change following median nerve section in the cortical representation of the hand in areas 3b and 1 in adult owl and squirrel monkeys. *Neuroscience, 10*, 639–665.

Merzenich, M. M., Nelson, R. J., Stryker, M. P., Cynader, M. S., Shoppmann, A., & Zook, J. M. (1984). Somatosensory cortical map changes following digital amputation in adult monkey. *Journal of Comparative Neurology, 224*, 591–605.

Merzenich, M. M., Recanzone, G. H., & Jenkins, W. M. (in press). How the brain functionally rewires itself. In M. Buchsbaum, W. E. Bunney, & R. Haier (Eds.), *Neural and artificial parallel computations*. New York: MIT Press.

Merzenich, M. M., Recanzone, G. H., Jenkins, W. M., Allard, T. T., & Nudo, R. J. (1988). Cortical representational plasticity. In T. P. Rakic & W. Singer (Eds.), *Neurobiology of neocortex* (pp. 41–67). New York: John Wiley.

Metherate, R., Tremblay, N., & Dykes, R. W. (1987). Acetylcholine permits long-term enhancement of neuronal responsiveness in cat primary somatosensory cortex. *Neuroscience, 22* (1), 75–81.

Miyashita, Y. (1988). Neural correlate of visual associative long-term memory in the primate temporal cortex. *Nature, 335*, 817–820.

Miyashita, Y., & Chang, H. S. Neural correlate of pictorial short term memory in the primate temporal cortex. *Nature, 331*, 68–70.

Mountcastle, V. B., Steinmetz, M. A., & Romo, R. (1990). Frequency discrimination in the sense of flutter: Psychophysical measurements correlated with postcentral events in behaving monkeys. *Journal of Neuroscience, 10* (9), 3032–3044.

Olds, J., Disterhoft, J. F., Segal, M., Kornblith, C. L., & Hirsh, R. (1972). Learning centers of rat brain mapped by measuring latencies of conditioned unit responses. *Journal of Neurophysiology, 35*, 202–219.

Oleson, T. D., Ashe, J. H., & Weinberger, N. M. (1975). Modification of auditory and somatosensory system activity during pupillary conditioning in the paralyzed cat. *Journal of Neurophysiology, 38*, 1114–1139.

Pearson, J. C., Finkel, L. H., & Edelman, G. M. (1987). Plasticity organization of adult cerebral cortical maps: A computer simulation based on neuronal group selection. *Journal of Neuroscience, 7*, 4209–4333.

Pons, T. P., Garraghty, P. E., & Mishkin, M. (1988). Lesion-induced plasticity in the second somatosensory cortex of adult macaques. *Proceedings of the National Academy of Sciences, U.S.A., 85*, 5279–5281.

Rasmusson, D. D. (1982). Reorganization of raccoon somatosensory cortex following removal of the fifth digit. *Journal of Comparative Neurology, 205*, 313–326.

Recanzone, G. H., Allard, T. T., Jenkins, W. M., & Merzenich, M. M. (1990). Receptive field changes induced by peripheral nerve stimulation in SI of adult cats. *Journal of Neurophysiology, 63*, 1213–1225.

Recanzone, G. H., Hradek, G. T., Jenkins, W. M., & Merzenich, M. M. (1991b). Progressive improvement in discriminative abilities in adult owl monkeys performing a tactile frequency discrimination task. *Journal of Neurophysiology* (in press).

Recanzone, G. H., Merzenich, M. M., & Dinse, H. R. (1991a). Expansion of the cortical representation of a restricted skin field in primary somatosensory cortex following intracortical microstimulation. *Cerebral Cortex* (in press).

Recanzone, G. H., Merzenich, M. M., Jenkins, W. M., Grajski, K. A., & Dinse, H. R. (1991c). Topographic reorganization of the hand representation in cortical area 3b of owl monkeys trained in a frequency discrimination task. *Journal of Neurophysiology* (in press).

Recanzone, G. H., Merzenich, M. M., & Schreiner, C. E. (submitted). Changes in the distributed temporal response properties of SI cortical neurons reflect improvements in performance on a temporally-based tactile discrimination task. *Journal of Neurophysiology.*

Reiter, H. O., & Stryker, M. P. (1988). Neural plasticity without post-synaptic action potentials: Less active inputs become dominate when kitten visual cortical cells are pharmacologically inhibited. *Proceedings of the National Academy of Sciences, U.S.A., 85* (10), 3623–3627.

Robertson, D., & Irvine, D. R. F. (1989). Plasticity of frequency organization in auditory cortex of guinea pigs with partial unilateral deafness. *Journal of Comparative Neurology, 282*, 456–471.

Sakamoto, T., Porter, L. L., & Asanuma, H. (1987). Long-lasting potentiation of synaptic potentials in the motor cortex produced by stimulation of the sensory cortex in the cat: A basis of motor learning. *Brain Research, 413*, 360–364.

Sanes, J. N., Suner, S., & Donoghue, J. P. (1990). Dynamic organization of primary motor cortex output to target muscles in adult rats. I. Long-term patterns of reorganization following motor or mixed peripheral nerve lesions. *Experimental Brain Research, 79*, 479–491.

Schwark, H. D., & Jones, E. G. (1989). The distribution of intrinsic cortical axons in area 3b of cat primary somatosensory cortex. *Experimental Brain Research, 78*, 501–513.

Singer, W. (1990). Search for coherence: A basic principle of cortical self-organization. *Concepts in Neuroscience, 1* (1), 1–26.

Snow, P. J., Nudo, R. J., Rivers, W., Jenkins, W. M., & Merzenich, M. M. (1988). Somatotopically inappropriate projections from thalamocortical neurons to the SI cortex of the cat demonstrated by the use of intracortical microstimulation. *Somatosensory Research, 5*, 349–372.

Stoney, S. D. Jr., Thompson, W. D., & Asanuma, H. (1968). Excitation of pyramidal tract cells by intracortical microstimulation: Effective extent of stimulating current. *Journal of Neurophysiology, 31*, 659–669.

Sur, M., Merzenich, M. M., & Kaas, J. H. (1980). Magnification, receptive fields area, and "hypercolumn" size in areas 3b and 1 of somatosensory cortex in owl monkeys. *Journal of Neurophysiology, 44*, 295–311.

von der Malsburg, C., & Singer, W. (1988). Principles of cortical network organization. In T. P. Rakic & W. Singer (Eds.), *Neurobiology of neocortex* (pp. 69–99). New York: John Wiley.

Wall, J. T., & Cusick, C. G. (1984). Cutaneous responsiveness in primary somatosensory (S-I) hindpaw cortex before and after partial hindpaw deafferentation in adult rats. *Journal of Neuroscience, 4*, 1499–1515.

Withers, G. S., & Greenough, W. T. (1989). Reach training selectively alters dendritic branching in subpopulations of layer II–III pyramids in rat motor-somatosensory forelimb cortex. *Neuropsychologia, 27* (1), 61–69.

Woody, C. D., Knispel, J. D., Crow, T. J., & Black-Cleworth, P. A. (1976). Activity and excitability to electrical current of cortical auditory receptive neurons of awake cats as affected by stimulus association. *Journal of Neurophysiology, 39*, 1045–1061.

Yun, J. T., Merzenich, M. M., & Woodruff, T. (1987). Alteration of functional representations of vibrissae in the barrel field of adult rats. *Society for Neuroscience Abstracts, 13* (3), 1596.

Zarzecki, P., & Wiggin, D. M. (1982). Convergence of sensory inputs upon projection neurons of somatosensory cortex. *Experimental Brain Research, 48*, 28–42.

10

Localization of Primal Long-Term Memory in the Primate Temporal Cortex

YASUSHI MIYASHITA
KUNIYOSHI SAKAI
SEI-ICHI HIGUCHI
NAOHIKO MASUI

LONG-TERM MEMORY: STAGES WITH DISTINGUISHABLE LOCALIZATIONS

Memory has stages. The distinction between short- and long-term memory has been supported not only by their capacity, optimal code, and time parameters but also by the double dissociation of neuropsychological deficits (Milner, Corkin, & Teuber, 1968; Warrington, 1982). Long-term memory itself has been claimed to have at least two components: one is the recently acquired, labile memory that can be readily disrupted by head injury, as retrograde amnesia demonstrates clinically (Russell, 1971). The other is the remote, fully consolidated memory (Squire, Slater, & Chace, 1975). Drug applications selectively depress or facilitate the labile component (McGaugh & Herz, 1972).

Bilateral damage to the medial temporal region, which includes the hippocampus, amygdala, and adjacent cortex, accompanied a short-span retrograde amnesia (Milner et al., 1968). Bilateral lesions of the hippocampal CA1 field (case R.B.) produced little retrograde amnesia, although the possibility remains that the patients could have suffered some retrograde amnesia for a period of a few years prior to their surgery (Zola-Morgan, Squire, & Amaral, 1986). In monkeys, effects of hippocampal lesion (including the entorhinal and parahippocampal cortex) were tested on the retention of 100 object-discrimination problems learned 2, 4, 8, 12, and 16 weeks before surgery (Zola-Morgan & Squire, 1990). The monkeys were severely impaired at remembering recently learned objects, but they remembered objects learned long ago as well as normal monkeys did.

These data suggest the possibility that the labile component of long-term memory is localized in the hippocampus and/or adjacent cortex, or is strongly influenced by these structures. Possible contributions of the hippocampal neural circuits have been examined previously (Miyashita, Roll, Cahusac, Niki, & Feigenbaum, 1989; Cahusac, Rolls, Miyashita, & Niki, in press). In this chapter, we propose a hypothesis that the anterior ventral temporal cortex contains a group of neurons that encodes one component of the visual associative long-term memory. The neurons are first of all characterized by (a) the code of recently learned visual–visual association (Miyashita, 1988a), and by (b) limited spatial distribution along the border between area 35 and area TE (Miyashita, in press). This area is tightly connected with the hippocampus via the entorhinal cortex (area 28) and via area 35 (Insausti, Amaral, & Cowan, 1987) or directly with the CA1 field (Suzuki & Amaral, 1990). We propose to name the mnemonic code on these neurons *primal long-term memory (Primal LTM)*. Recording the activities of these neurons (*primal LTM neurons*) in monkeys that learn and perform visual memory tasks will give vivid concrete shape to the presumed multiple representation of LTM, complementary to that obtained by neuropsychological observations.

PRIMAL LONG-TERM MEMORY

Figure 10.1 represents a hypothetical structure of the visual memory system of the primate. The physical properties of a visual object (such as its size, color, texture, and shape) are analyzed in the multiple subdivisions of the prestriate-posterior temporal complex (Mishkin, 1982; Zeki & Shipp, 1988). The anterior part of the inferior temporal cortex (AIT), especially area TE, synthesizes the analyzed attributes into a unique configuration and forms a central image of the object (Gross, 1972; Mishkin, 1982).

The primal LTM neurons are presumed to receive synthesized perceptual images of the object from this part of the AIT, since the neurons' activity is highly selective for coded pictorial information and is independent of the physical attributes such as size, orientation, color, or position of the object (Miyashita & Chang, 1988; see below). The region where the primal LTM neurons are located indeed receives afferent projections from more lateral part of AIT (Van Hoesen & Pandya, 1975).

Since localization of the primal LTM neurons is limited to a region not far from the rhinal sulcus, it is likely that the LTM system has another group of neurons to store the remote, fully consolidated long-term memory. Columnar organization of the primal LTM neurons seems to support the idea. By systematic electrophysiological mapping, the primal LTM neurons were found to cluster along the direction perpendicular to the cortical surface (Miyashita, in press, and to be published), forming a column-like

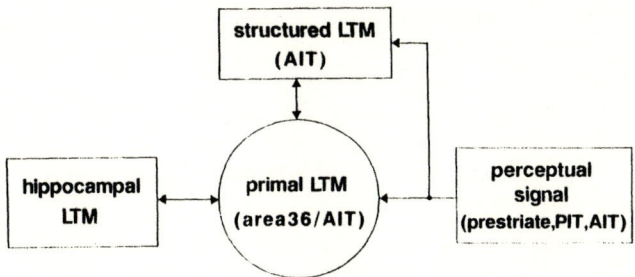

FIGURE 10.1. A hypothesis: the primal LTM and related visual memory systems of the primate.

organization. However, when we simultaneously recorded activities of two adjacent neurons in the column with a single microelectrode, both of which were selective to learned fractal patterns, their optimal pictures were not common at all (Miyashita, to be published). Thus, the primal LTM neurons were incompletely structured from the viewpoint of the functional columnar organization. By contrast, shape-selective neurons in the lateral surface of the TE (Fujita, Cheng, & Tanaka, 1990; Saito, Tanaka, Fukumoto, & Fukada, 1987), as well as the face neurons in the superior temporal sulcus (Perrett et al., 1984; Perrett, Mistlin, & Chitty, 1987), seem to form a cluster with common optimal pictures. For this reason, we named the latter stage of LTM "structured LTM" in Figure 10.1. In the following, we describe evidence supporting the brief sketch given above, and examine some detailed properties of the primal LTM, obtained by unit recording in monkeys that learned and performed visual memory tasks.

BEHAVIORAL TASK AND RECORDING OF NEURAL ACTIVITIES

In a trial of our visual memory task (delayed matching-to-sample task), sample and match stimuli were successively presented on a video monitor, each for 0.2 s at a 16 s delay interval. Three adult monkeys (*Macaca fuscata*) were trained to memorize the sample stimulus during a delay period and then to decide whether the match stimulus was the same as the sample. A correct response was rewarded with fruit juice. A set of 97 color patterns was generated by a fractal algorithm with a 32-bit seed of random numbers (Miyashita, 1988b); the set was repeatedly used during an overtraining session ("learned stimuli") in a fixed sequence according to an arbitrary attached number (serial position number, SPN). While extracellular discharges of a neuron were recorded, a sample stimulus was selected not only from the 97 learned patterns but also from a new set of 97 patterns ("new stimuli"). Different sets of new stimuli were created for each neuron using the same algorithm but a different seed. The learned stimuli and new stimuli were used at random, independent of the SPNs.

SELECTIVITY OF NEURAL DISCHARGES IS ACQUIRED THROUGH LEARNING

A few of the 97 learned stimuli reproducibly activated a particular neuron in the anterior ventral temporal cortex during the sample period and/or during the delay period of the task. The optimal picture differed from cell to cell, and the entire population of optimal pictures for the tested cells covered a substantial part of the repertory of the pictorial stimuli (Miyashita, Cho, & Mori, 1987).

Intuition told us that learning but not genetic determinants had formed the stimulus selectivity of these neurons, since (a) the optimal stimuli were computer-generated artificial patterns (fractal patterns), which the monkeys would rarely have seen in their life before the experiments; and (b) the responsive neurons were not scattered randomly in the temporal cortex but formed a high density cluster in a limited area related to the hippocampus.

We obtained several lines of experimental evidence supporting our intuition. First we compared the discharge selectivity of a neuron for two different sets of the fractal stimuli: the learned stimuli that the monkeys stored in their long-term memory through the training sessions and the new stimuli that they had never seen before the recording session. Figure 10.2 shows the results. A few of the 97 learned stimuli were effective in activating high-frequency sustained delay discharges in a cell (Figure 10.2a). By

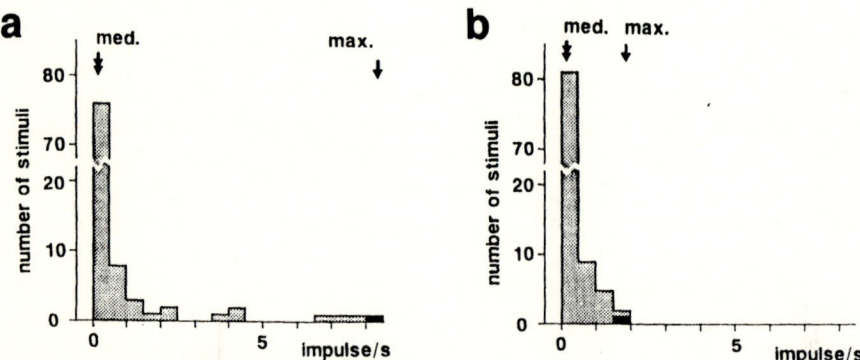

FIGURE 10.2. Selectivity of neural discharges of a cell to the "learned" and "new" stimuli. (a) Frequency distribution of the average firing rate measured during the delay period following 97 "learned" sample pictures. (↓ max.) (↓ med.) Maximum and median values in the distribution. (b) Similar illustration to (a) but "new" pictures are used as sample stimuli in the same cell.

contrast, the 97 new patterns produced only weak delay responses. The distribution of the delay discharge rate to the new stimuli (Figure 10.2b) lacked the small population of high-frequency responses (> 2 impulses), which characterized the distribution to the learned stimuli (Figure 10.2a).

Of the 206 neurons recorded in the anterior ventral temporal cortex of the overtrained monkeys, 57 neurons exhibited shape-selective delay discharges, and 17 of the 57 cells were successfully tested with both learned and new stimuli. In these 17 cells, the maximum delay discharge for learned stimuli (e.g., the arrow in Figure 10.2a) was always larger than that for new stimuli (e.g., the arrow in Figure 10.2b), and the difference was highly significant ($p < .001$, Wilcoxon test). When the selectivity of a neuron to a set of 97 patterns was represented by the sharpness of the response distribution, the kurtosis of the distribution (Snedecor & Cochran, 1980), the selectivity to the learned patterns was almost always (15/17) higher than that to the new patterns ($p < .005$). In spite of the presence of a few effective pictures in the learned stimuli, there was no difference between the median responses to the learned and new stimuli (e.g., the double arrows in Figures 10.2a and 10.2b) for the 17 cells ($p > .5$). These results suggest that the sharpness of the response selectivity of these neurons to the learned patterns was formed throughout the course of training.

ACQUIRED SELECTIVITY REPRESENTS THE ASSOCIATION AMONG MEMORIZED OBJECTS

In human long-term memory, ideas and concepts become associated through learning. We ask whether the neurons with acquired selectivity can code such associations. To be more specific, is it possible that training determines not only how sharply the effective learned patterns are represented in each neuron (as shown above) but also which patterns are conjointly chosen as the few optimal stimuli? We first examined the geometric similarity of the optimal stimuli of a cell, and found that the stimuli were often completely different, as seen in Figure 10.3 for six cells, suggesting a nongeometric criterion in choosing these patterns as the optimal stimuli of a cell. I then examined the effect of a fixed-order presentation of the patterns during the training session according to an arbitrarily assigned SPN. If the consecutively presented patterns tended to be associated together, and if the association was fixed in the choice of effective patterns for a cell, we could expect to find the effective patterns correlated with the SPN, in spite of a random presentation of the stimuli during the unit-recording session.

Figure 10.4 shows the results. The effective responses to the learned stimuli indeed cluster along the SPNs and the clustering was not due to an artifact in the testing procedure because the responses simultaneously obtained from the new stimuli were not clustered. In the 17 cells that were tested with both learned and new stimuli, the responses to the learned stimuli were significantly correlated (Figure 10.4, ●) in the nearest neighbor

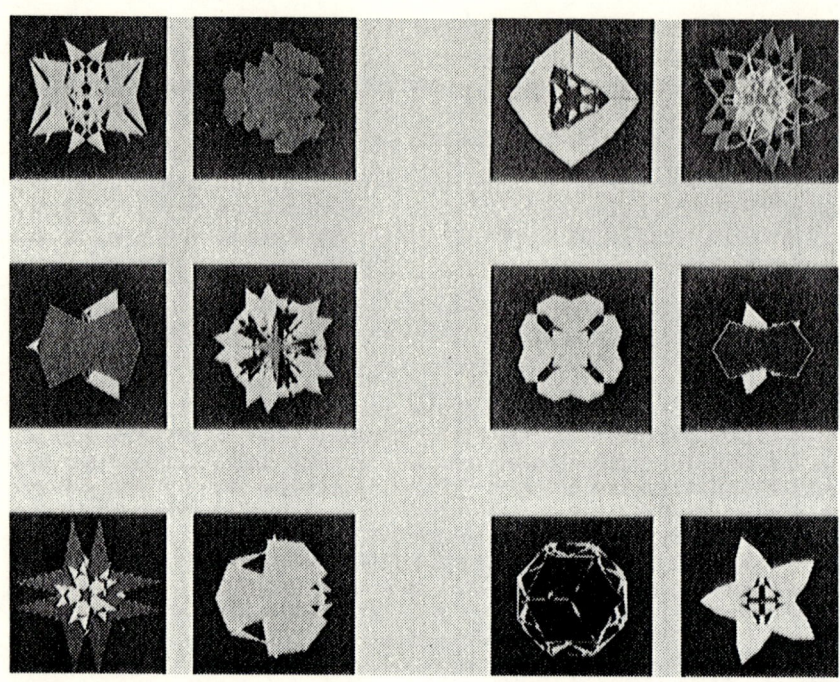

FIGURE 10.3.   Fractal patterns that produced the strongest and second strongest delay discharges in learned stimuli for six different cells. Note that the two optimal stimuli for a neuron have no similarities in their geometric patterns. See the original color pictures in Miyashita (1988a).

of the SPNs, as compared with the responses to the new stimuli (O) ($p < .01$, Kolmogorov-Smirnov test). The 57 cells tested by the learned stimuli exhibited similar correlated responses along the SPN (▲). The nearest-neighbor correlation for the learned stimuli differed from cell to cell, and was significant ($p < .05$) in 28 of the 57 cells according to Kendall's correlation test (Snedecor & Cochran, 1980), while that for the new stimuli was not significant in any of the 17 cells. Thus, we conclude that these neurons are a good candidate for one of the visual associative LTM stores (i.e., the primal LTM).

It is interesting to ask how many times the monkey should see and/or memorize the fractal pattern that eventually develop the neural representation of the stimulus–stimulus associations. Unfortunately no direct answer is available from the experimental procedure described above, because two factors were confounded in the training: one was to learn the rule of the delayed matching-to-sample task, and the other to learn the association. We roughly estimate the upper limit to be about a few hundred trials

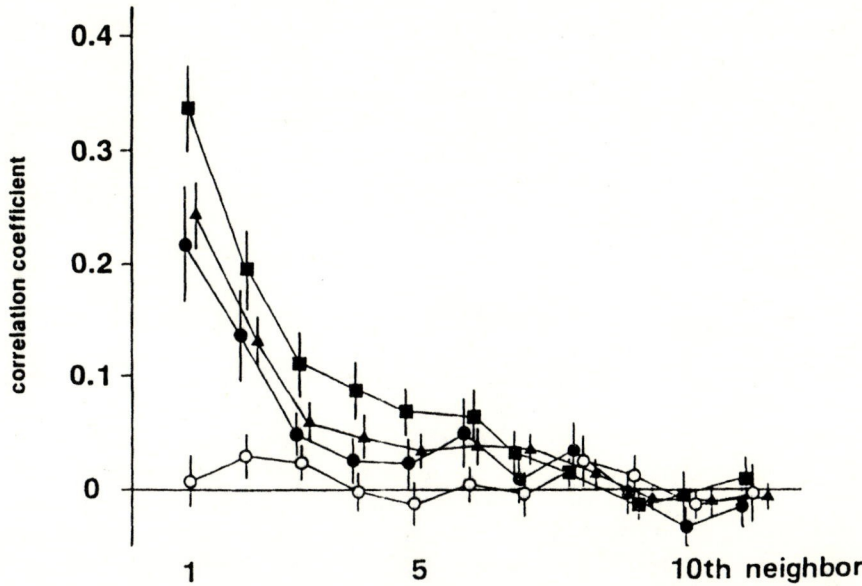

FIGURE 10.4. Stimulus–stimulus association between the learned fractal patterns. Ordinate, autocorrelations of the delay discharge rate along the SPN of the stimuli. (●, ○) Average autocorrelogram for the learned and new stimuli in the 17 cells. (▲) Learned stimuli in the 57 cells. (■) Learned stimuli in the 28 cells for which the nearest-neighbor correlation along the SPN was significant ($p<.05$) according to Kendall's test. Error bars, standard errors. $p<.001$, $p<.01$, $p<.05$, according to the Kolmogorov-Smirnov test in comparison with the value for new stimuli.

(500 trials/day/100 patterns × 30 days). In order to estimate the lower limit we have developed a new association task, the result of which is to be published soon (Sakai & Miyashita, 1991).

CATEGORIZED PERCEPT OF A PICTURE IS MEMORIZED

The anterior ventral temporal cortex has been designated as the last link from the visual system to the hippocampus (Insausti et al., 1987; Suzuki & Amaral, 1990; Van Hoesen & Pandya, 1975; Yukie & Iwai, 1988). Thus the primal LTM neurons would receive final-stage information in serial visual processing along occipitotemporal cortices (Figure 10.1). Indeed the primal LTM neurons encode highly abstract pictorial properties of the stimulus, as demonstrated by the following analyses of triggering features of the delay responses (Miyashita and Chang, 1988). Sample pictures were manipulated in three different ways: (a) the stimulus size was reduced by one half, (b) the stimuli were rotated by 90° in a clockwise direction, and (c) colored stimuli were transformed into monochrome by referring to a pseudocolor look-up table. Figure 10.5 illustrates the responses of a neuron that consistently fired during the delay after one particular picture but not after others, irrespective of stimulus size (Figure 10.5b), orientation (Figure 10.5c), or color (Figure 10.5d). Similar tolerance of responses was observed in a majority of the tested delay neurons: to size (16/19), to orientation (5/7), to color-monochrome (15/20), and to position (8/13). In other neurons, manipulation of the most effective stimulus reduced or abolished the thereby-evoked delay discharge.

MEMORY DISORDER AND THE PRIMAL LONG-TERM MEMORY

The primal LTM neurons were most frequently found along the border between the areas TE and 35. Interestingly, this strip-like area overlaps with the "PR/PH area" of Zola-Morgan, Squire, Amaral, and Suzuki, (1989). They found that monkeys with PR/PH lesions were as impaired or more impaired on delayed non-matching-to-sample tasks than the comparison group of monkeys with H^+A^+ lesions (which includes the hippocampal formation, amydala, and adjacent cortex). They argued that "the more severe impairment associated with the PR/PH lesion indicates that the perirhinal cortex itself must contribute significantly to memory functions" (Zola-Morgan et al., pp. 4368). The memory disorder found in the PR/PH monkeys may result, at least in part, from the loss of the primal LTM neurons, whose unique properties are reviewed in this chapter.

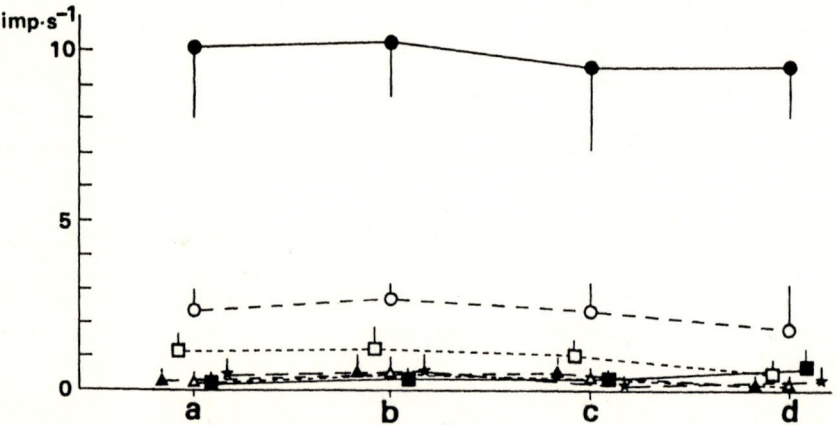

FIGURE 10.5. Response tolerance under stimulus transformation in size, orientation, or color. (a) Control responses; (b), (c), and (d) show the effects of stimulus size reduction by half, stimulus rotation by 90° in a clockwise direction, and color-to-monochrome transformation. Ordinate, average delay spike frequencies as a function of stimulus transformation. Responses to seven different sample pictures are plotted with different symbols. Error bars indicate standard deviations for 4–15 trials.

Closer inspection of the spatial distribution of the primal LTM neurons allows us further elaborations of these statements. For example, area 35 seems to contain much fewer primal LTM neurons than area 36, which suggests differential functional roles of areas 35 and 36. This may be related to the results of the behavioral experiments by Murray and Mishkin (1986), designed to remove "rhinal cortex" (defined as "the perirhinal cortex, which occupies the lateral bank of the rhinal sulcus," "the prorhinal cortex, which occupies the medial bank of the rhinal sulcus," and the entorhinal cortex) in combination with the hippocampus or amygdala. It is interesting to examine whether these "rhinal" lesions were limited to area 35 and spared area 36, because they described "adding a rhinal cortical removal to hippocampectomy yields little, if any, additional impairment in recognition" (Murray and Mishkin, pp. 1991). The border between areas TF or 36 and the laterally adjacent area TE is not defined sharply, as Suzuki and Amaral (1990) pointed out. The differential functional roles of these areas are also to be clarified by further studies of the primal LTM neurons.

CONCLUSIONS

In this chapter, we proposed a hypothesis that the anterior ventral temporal cortex contains a group of neurons that encode one component of the LTM, the primal LTM (Figure 10.1). Highly abstract visual information is inputted to the primal LTM through the occipitotemporal visual cortices. Bidirectional communication with the hippocampal system may play a key role in forming the associative organization of the memory code in the primal LTM rather than the organization along geometrical similarity.

Interestingly, the dorsolateral part of temporal cortex, which contains neurons selectively responsive to particular visual patterns, was reported to have column-like structures (Fujita et al., 1990; Perrett et al., 1984, 1987). However, common preference to a geometrically similar object characterized vertical clustering of cells in these reports; for example, in the bank of superior temporal sulcus (mainly area TPO), cells responding to the frontal faces and to the profile faces formed distinct vertical clumps (Perrett et al., 1987). The primal LTM neurons also form a cluster, but closely adjacent neurons do not have common optimal patterns (Miyashita, to be published), which suggests a primitive, incompletely structured organization of the primal LTM. The structured LTM (Figure 10.1) of faces, for example, may be stored in area TPO. The general pertinence of the distinction between the primal LTM and structured LTM should be examined in future research.

In the present stages of investigation, it is not clear whether the primal LTM described here is identical with the labile component of LTM, which can be revealed in retrograde amnesia or with application of drugs after learning. Since a hippocampal neuron can encode a newly formed association (Cahusac et al., in press; Miyashita, Roll, Cahusac, Niki, & Feigenbaum, 1989a), it is urgent to compare it with the primal LTM and to assess their susceptibilities to electric shock and/or convulsant drugs. It will be possible to confirm or reject the present hypothesis on the primal LTM (Figure 10.1) by an appropriate combination of neuropsychological and electrophysiological experiments.

Acknowledgment: This work was supported by a grant from the Japanese Ministry of Education, Science and Culture (02102008).

REFERENCES

Cahusac, P. M. B., Rolls, E. T., Miyashita, Y., & Niki, H. (in press). Modification of the responses of hippocampal neurons in the monkey during the learning of a conditional spatial response task.

Gross, C. G. (1972). Visual functions of inferotemporal cortex. In R. Jung (Ed.), *Handbook of sensory physiology* (Vol. VIII/3B) (pp. 451–482). Berlin: Springer-Verlag.

Fujita, I., Cheng, K., & Tanaka, K. (1990). Stimulus selectivity of inferior temporal cortex neurons: Simultaneous recording from adjacent cells. *Society for Neuroscience Abstracts, 16*, 1220.

Herzog, A. G., & Van Hoesen, G. W. (1976). Temporal neocortical afferent connections to the amygdala in the rhesus monkey. *Brain Research, 115*, 57–69.

Horel, J. A., & Pytko, D. E. (1982). Behavioral effects of local cooling in temporal lobe of monkeys. *Journal of Neurophysiology, 47*, 11–22.

Insausti, R., Amaral, D. G., & Cowan, W. M. (1987). The entorhinal cortex of the monkey: II. Cortical afferents. *Journal of Comparative Neurology, 264*, 356–395.

Jones, E. G., & Powell, T. P. S. (1970). An anatomical study of converging sensory pathways with in the cerebral cortex of the monkey. *Brain, 93*, 793–820.

McGaugh, J. L., & Herz, M. J. (1972). *Memory consolidation*. San Francisco: Albion.

Milner, B. (1968). Visual recognition and recall after right temporal-lobe excision in man. *Neuropsychologia, 6*, 191–209.

Milner, B., Corkin, S., & Teuber, H. L. (1968). Further analysis of the hippocampal amnesic syndrome: 14-year follow-up study of H.M. *Neuropsychologia, 6*, 215–234.

Mishkin, M. (1982). A memory system in the monkey. *Philosophical Transactions of the Royal Society, London, B, B298*, 85–95.

Miyashita, Y. (1988a). Neuronal correlate of visual associative long-term memory in the primate temporal cortex. *Nature, 335*, 817–820.

Miyashita, Y. (1988b). Neuronal representation of pictorial working memory in the primate temporal cortex. In M. A. Arbib & S. Amari (Eds.), *Dynamic interactions in neural networks: Models and data* (pp. 183–192). Berlin: Springer-Verlag.

Miyashita, Y. (1991). Primal long-term memory in the primate temporal cortex: Linkage between visual perception and memory. In A. Gorea (Ed.), *Representation of Vision*, (pp. 141–152). Montrouge: John Libbey Eurotext.

Miyashita, Y., & Chang, H. S. (1988). Neuronal correlate of pictorial short-term memory in the primate temporal cortex. *Nature, 331*, 68–70.

Miyashita, Y., Cho, K., & Mori, K. (1987). Selective pictorial information is retained by neurons in the ventral temporal cortex of the monkey during the delay period of a matching-to-sample task. *Society for Neuroscience Abstracts, 13*, 608.

Miyashita, Y., Roll, E. T., Cahusac, P. M. B., Niki, H., & Feigenbaum, J. D. (1989). Activity of hippocampal neurons in the monkey related to a stimulus–response association task. *Journal of Neurophysiology, 61*, 669–678.

Murray, E. A., & Mishkin, M. (1986). Visual recognition in monkeys following rhinal cortical ablations combined with either amygdalectomy or hippocampectomy. *Journal of Neuroscience, 6*, 1991–2003.

Perrett, D. I., Mistlin, A. J., & Chitty, A. J. (1987). Visual neurones responsive to faces. *Trends in Neuroscience, 10*, 358–364.

Perrett, D. I., Smith, P. A. J., Potter, D. D., Mistlin, A. J., Head, A. S., Milner, A. D., & Jeeves, M. A. (1984). Neurones responsive to faces in the temporal cortex: Studies of functional organization, sensitivity to identity and relation to perception. *Human Neurobiology, 3*, 197–208.

Russel, W. R. (1971). *The traumatic amnesia*. London: Oxford University Press.

Saito, H., Tanaka, K., Fukumoto, M., & Fukada, Y. (1987). The inferior temporal cortex of the macaque monkey: II. The level of complexity in the integration of pattern information. *Society for Neuroscience Abstracts, 13*, 628.

Sakai, K., & Miyashita, Y. (1991). Neural organization for the long-term memory of paired associates. *Nature* (in press).

Snedecor, G. W., & Cochran, W.G. (1980). *Statistical method*. Iowa University Press.

Squire, L.R., Slater, P. C., & Chace, P. M. (1975). Retrograde amnesia: Temporal gradient in very long term following electroconvulsive therapy. *Science, 187*, 77–79.

Suzuki, W. A., & Amaral, D. G. (1990). Cortical inputs to the CA1 field of the monkey hippocampus originate from the perirhinal and parahippocampal cortex but not from area TE. *Neuroscience Letters, 115*, 43–48.

Van Hoesen, G. W., & Pandya, D. N. (1975). Some connections of the entorhinal (area 28) and perirhinal (area 35) cortices of the rhesus monkey. I. Temporal lobe afferents. *Brain Research, 95*, 1–24.

Warrington, E. K. (1982). The double dissociation of short- and long-term memory deficits. In L. S. Cermak (Ed.), *Human memory and amnesia*. Hillsdale: Lawrence Erlbaum Associates.

Yukie, M., & Iwai, E. (1988). Direct projections from the ventral TE area of the inferotemporal cortex to hippocampal field CA1 in the monkey. *Neuroscience Letters, 88*, 6–10.

Zeki, S., & Shipp, S. (1988). The functional logic of cortical connections. *Nature, 335*, 311–317.

Zola-Morgan, S., & Squire, L. R. (1990). The primate hippocampal formation: Evidence for a time-limited role in memory storage. *Science, 250*, 288–290.

Zola-Morgan, S., Squire, L. R., & Amaral, D.G. (1986). Human amnesia and the medial temporal region: Enduring memory impairment following a bilateral lesion limited to field CA1 of the hippocampus. *Journal of Neuroscience, 6*, 2950–2967.

Zola-Morgan, S., Squire, L. R., Amaral, D. G., & Suzuki, W. A. (1989). Lesions of perirhinal and parahippocampal cortex that spare the amygdala and hippocampal formation produce severe memory impairment. *Journal of Neuroscience, 9*, 4355–4370.

11

Mnemonic Functions of the Cholinergic Septohippocampal System

DAVID S. OLTON
BENNET S. GIVENS
ALICJA L. MARKOWSKA
MATTHEW SHAPIRO
STEPHANIE GOLSKI

Many lines of evidence suggest that the cholinergic projection from the medial septal area (MSA) to the hippocampus has an important role in mnemonic processing. Anatomically, these neurons project to areas that have fundamental roles in memory, the hippocampus and temporal cortex. Neurochemically, the system contains acetylcholine (ACh), a neurotransmitter that has been closely linked to mnemonic functions. Clinically, pathology in the MSA is correlated with amnesia, and many attempts to improve impaired mnemonic function focus on compounds that alter the cholinergic system. Experimentally, neurotoxic lesions of the basal forebrain cholinergic system (BFCS) produce impairments in tasks that involve recent memory, and the pattern of impairments suggests that one of the psychological processes disrupted by these lesions is memory.

A simplified diagram (Figure 11.1) of some of the important characteristics of the septohippocampal system has two functions in the context of this chapter. First, it summarizes the neuroanatomical and neurochemical connections that form the basis for these experiments. Second, it provides a convenient means of organizing the experimental strategies to investigate the mnemonic functions of the septohippocampal system. Each of these points will be discussed in turn, and then the relevant experiments will be summarized.

The MSA is composed of the medial septal nucleus and the vertical limb of the diagonal band of Broca. Cholinergic and GABAergic receptors on MSA neurons have complementary effects. The cholinergic afferents are

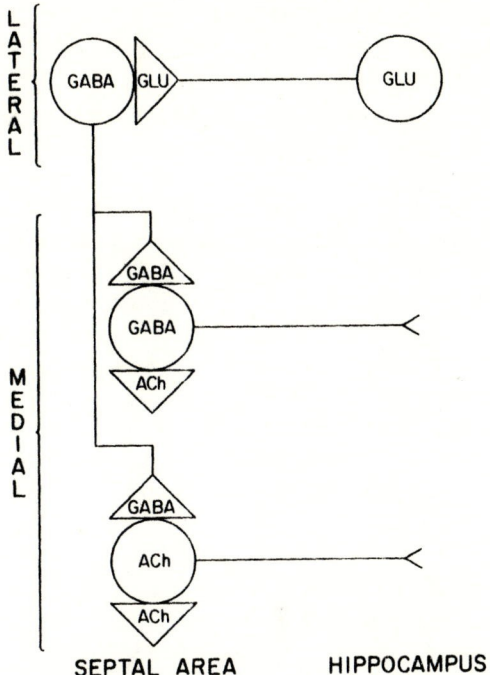

FIGURE 11.1.   A simplied diagram of some relevant neuronal connections in the septohippocampal system. For further explanation, see text.

excitatory, while the GABAergic afferents are inhibitory. Cholinergic agonists (carbachol, oxotremorine) stimulate the neurons, while cholinergic antagonists (scopolamine) block excitation. In a complementary fashion, GABAergic agonists (muscimol) produce inhibition and GABAergic antagonists (Bicuculine) block this inhibition (Leranth & Frotscher, 1989; Segal, 1986).

Direct microinfusion of drugs into the MSA can alter the activity of MSA cholinergic neurons, which in turn influence hippocampal function. Excitation of MSA neurons increases the amount of ACh released in the hippocampus, and increases the power of the theta frequency. Inhibition of these MSA neurons has a complementary effect, decreasing the amount of ACh released and decreasing the power of theta. To the extent that mnemonic processing in the hippocampus depends on the electrophysiological and neurochemical processes controlled by MSA neurons, intraseptal infusion (ISI) of compounds that alter these septohippocampal processes should also alter memory. The first set of experiments investigates several specific predictions that are obvious consequences from this conceptual framework.

The second set of experiments investigates the terminals of the septohippocampal system, and the effects of behavior on high affinity choline uptake (HACU). HACU is a useful measure of the activity of cholinergic neurons because it reflects the number of sites that are actively transporting choline across the membrane, which in turn reflects the amount of ACh recently released in the synaptic cleft. More action potentials produce more ACh, which increases HACU. If specific mnemonic processes engage the cholinergic system, then performance in tasks that require these mnemonic processes should increase HACU.

The third set of experiments examines the extent to which cholinergic stimulation of the hippocampus can be effective in the absence of anatomical connections between the septum and hippocampus. The fornix was transected, destroying septohippocampal and hippocamposeptal connections. Fetal basal forebrain tissue was implanted in the hippocampus. Both behavioral and electrophysiological measures of the influence of the graft were obtained. If cholinergic stimulation of the hippocampus in the absence of septohippocampal afferents can have beneficial effects, implants of basal forebrain tissue should reduce the electrophysiological and behavioral abnormalities produced by the fornix transection.

RECENT MEMORY AND HIPPOCAMPAL THETA ARE ALTERED BY INTRASEPTAL INFUSIONS

Inhibition of MSA Neurons Impairs Recent Memory

To infuse substances into the MSA, a guide cannula was implanted so that its tip was just dorsal to the MSA. To measure theta, bipolar electrodes were placed so that their tips were in the dentate hilus of the hippocampus. To assess recent memory, rats were trained to perform spatial alternation in a T-maze. For the first, forced trial, one arm of the maze was blocked, and the rat entered the available arm to obtain reinforcement. For all subsequent, choice trials, both arms were available, but reinforcement was present only in the arm not entered during the previous trial. Consequently, in order to determine the arm that was correct on any given trial, the rat had to remember the arm that was entered on the immediately preceding trial. Each test session had 20 choice trials. All rats were trained until they had a stable and high level of choice accuracy, about 18 correct responses in the 20 trials of a session (Givens & Olton, 1990).

Both theta and recent memory were assessed three times each test day: (a) before the infusion to obtain a normal baseline; (b) 10 min after the infusion, when the substance should have a substantial effect; and (c) 90 min after the infusion, when the effects of the substance should have disappeared. The substances and doses infused were:

1. Tetracaine: 2, 5, 10 μg
2. Scopolamine: 3, 15, 30 μg
3. Muscimol: 15, 30 ng
4. Carbachol: 0.5 μg

Both muscimol and scopolamine, 10 min after the infusion, reduced the power of theta and choice accuracy in a dose-dependent fashion. Muscimol (30 ng) reduced the power of theta from more than 700 mv^2 to less than 200 mv^2 and choice accuracy from 18 to 14. Scopolamine (15 μg) had a similar effect, reducing the power of theta to less than 200 mv^2 and choice accuracy to 14. For all doses of all compounds, the magnitude of reduction in theta and the magnitude of the reduction in choice accuracy were strongly correlated. More data are necessary, of course, to determine the extent to which this correlation reflects a causal relation, and the extent to which the mechanisms responsible for the change in theta are the same as those responsible for the change in choice accuracy.

These data confirm the predictions based on the neuroanatomical and neurochemical characteristics of the septohippocampal system. Direct inhibition of cholinergic MSA neurons by the GABAergic agonist, muscimol, disrupted hippocampal electrophysiology and impaired recent memory. Blockade of endogenous cholinergic excitation of these MSA neurons by the cholinergic antagonist, scopolamine, produced similar effects. These two sets of experiments provide converging operations that the cholinergic neurons in the MSA have important electrophysiological and functional consequences in the hippocampus (Gray & McNaughton, 1983).

Carbachol, a cholinergic agonist, did not have a significant complementary effect. Although it did increase the power of theta and choice accuracy, these increases were slight and statistically insignificant. Several factors may be responsible for this failure. (a) In these young rats, the baseline for theta and choice accuracy was high. Consequently, little room was available for improvement, which might have limited the ability to detect significant improvements. (b) Only one dose of carbachol was tested. This dose might not have been optimal to produce improvement. (c) These rats and their brains may have been performing optimally so that no intervention could produce an improvement.

Stimulation of MSA Cholinergic Neurons Improves Recent Memory in Aged Rats

The relative merits of these three explanations were assessed in the experiment described here. Aged rats, 24 months old, as well as young rats, 4 months old, were subjects. A dose–response curve for oxotremorine, 2, 5, and 10 μg, was obtained. The task was continuous spatial alternation in a T-maze, as described previously. The intertrial interval for both the old rats and the young rats was adjusted so that the baseline level of choice accuracy for each rat was less than 80%. The predictions for each of the three explanations outlined above are obvious. (a) If the baseline level of choice accuracy is the most important variable, oxotremorine should improve choice accuracy in both young and aged rats because they both have reduced levels of choice accuracy. (b) If the dose of carbachol was not appropriate, the dose–response curve used here should find some dose that is effective.

(c) If performance in the young rats was at its best, oxotremorine should have beneficial effects in the aged rats but not in the young rats.

The preliminary data are clear. At 15 min after the infusion, oxotremorine had a significant dose–response effect in aged rats, improving choice accuracy, but not in young rats. The two lower doses of oxotremorine, 2 μg and 5 μg, improved choice accuracy by 22% and 14%, respectively. The higher dose, 10 μg, impaired choice accuracy by 24%. In the young rats, all three doses of oxotremorine had only slight effects, and none of them produced a substantial increase in choice accuracy.

The improvement in choice accuracy in aged rats has several implications. First, it demonstrates that although these neurons were not functioning at their best, they were still capable of being influenced by afferent connections, and these in turn could have substantial functional consequences. Thus, the septohippocampal system in the aged rats must be capable of mediating more accurate recent memory than it actually does. Second, this successful enhancement of performance with a cholinergic agonist provides some support for the attempt to alleviate amnesia with cholinergic therapies, and suggests that direct intracranial interventions may have advantages over systemic interventions because they can directly influence the relevant brain region while minimizing undesirable side-effects resulting from the substance's effects elsewhere in the brain or in the peripheral nervous system. Third, it shows that direct tonic activation of the basal forebrain cholinergic system can be an effective therapeutic intervention in spite of the obvious problems inherent in an approach that provides noncontingent neural stimulation (Sarter, Bruno, & Dudchenko, 1990). The increase in the power of hippocampal theta suggests that the ISI of oxotremorine enhanced the action of the septal pacemaking cells (Stewart & Fox, 1990).

The failure of oxotremorine to improve choice accuracy in the young rats must be due to the fact that the rat's brain was functioning optimally, at least in this task. Both a decreased baseline of performance and a dose–response analysis did not improve choice accuracy.

Inhibition of MSA Cholinergic Neurons Impairs Nonspatial Recent Memory

The extent to which the hippocampus is selectively involved in spatial as distinguished from nonspatial mnemonic functions has received considerable debate (O'Keefe & Nadel, 1978; Rawlins, 1985). Some descriptions of hippocampal function emphasize a primary role in spatial functions, others emphasize its role in certain types of mnemonic processing irrespective of the type of material that is to be remembered. The experimental evidence on this point is also complicated, with data supporting both views. Consequently, determining whether the manipulations described above affect performance in a nonspatial recent memory task is important to assess the extent to which these septohippocampal systems are selectively involved in processing certain types of material to be remembered. (See Barnes, 1988, for a review of lesion experiments, and Olton, 1989b for a review of single unit recording experiments.)

A test of recent memory for nonspatial stimuli was conducted in an operant box using a continuous delayed conditional discrimination task. The discriminative stimuli were a light and a tone. One stimulus was presented on each trial. Two levers were available. If the stimulus presented for the current trial was different from the stimulus presented for the previous trial (nonmatch trial), one lever was correct. If the stimulus presented for the current trial was the same as that presented for the previous trial (match trial), the other lever was correct. Because the two discriminative stimuli were located in a central position in the operant box, spatial location could not be used to indicate the nature of the stimulus on the previous trial. Choice accuracy in this type of procedure is impaired by systemic injections of the cholinergic antagonist, scopolamine (Spencer, Pontecorvo, & Heise, 1985).

This task also provides the opportunity to obtain extensive temporal information. In the present experiment, each test session was 90 min long. During baseline performance, with no drugs infused, all measures of performance were stable throughout this test.

Data are currently available following muscimol (30 ng). Within 10 min, this infusion reduced choice accuracy at all delays to a level only slightly greater than that expected by chance. During the next 30 min, choice accuracy at the shortest intertrial interval (ITI), which was 2.5 s, increased to almost 80%, but it remained at this level for an extended period of time. Only during the last 20 min of the session did choice accuracy at this delay begin to reach baseline levels. Choice accuracy at the middle (10 s) and long (20 s) ITIs remained depressed throughout testing. Although some recovery took place during the 90 min, choice accuracy remained at approximately 70%. These results indicate a profound and enduring impairment of choice accuracy as a result of GABAergic inhibition of MSA neurons.

Other measures of performance were stable. Responses during the ITI were never reinforced and were always inappropriate. These were increased only slightly during the first 20 min following muscimol. Each stimulus provided the opportunity to obtain a reinforcement, and some response was always appropriate after every stimulus. However, response omissions occasionally occurred, especially if the previous response was reinforced and the current ITI was short. Muscimol had no effect on the number of response omissions. Consequently, nonmnemonic aspects of performance were generally unaffected by the infusion; whatever effects did occur were transient, whereas the impairments in choice accuracy were enduring.

This dissociation of the effects of muscimol on mnemonic and nonmnemonic aspects of performance suggest that the infusion had a primary influence on recent memory, rather than on some other psychological process (motivation, perception, etc.). However, this interpretation is slightly complicated by the pattern of results obtained with the three delays. An interaction of an intervention with the length of the delay is often taken as a prerequisite to indicate that the intervention had a primary effect on memory processing rather than on some other psychological process. At the end of the test session, such an interaction was present, with choice accuracy at the shortest delay near normal levels, while choice accuracy at the longer delay was still impaired. However, at the beginning of the test session, such a dissociation did not occur; choice accuracy at all delays was reduced to approximately the level expected by chance.

The fact that muscimol impaired choice accuracy at all delays immediately following the infusion, but only at the longer delays at the end of the test session, leads to two alternative explanations of the initial effects of muscimol. (a) These may have been due to a nonmnemonic influence, with muscimol having nonmnemonic as well as mnemonic effects at that time. (b) Alternatively, muscimol may have been having only mnemonic effects even at the start of the test session, but these were so extensive that they impaired choice accuracy even with the shortest ITI. Choosing between these two alternatives is difficult. The fact that other nonmnemonic measures of performance (the number of ITI responses and the number of omissions) were normal while choice accuracy was substantially depressed, even at the shortest delay, suggests that the effects of muscimol at the short delay were most likely due to impairments of mnemonic function.

This continuum of the effects of muscimol emphasizes the importance of parametric manipulations to evaluate dichotomous dissociations of types of memory. Although some theories of hippocampal memory have assessed their predictions by manipulating task demand in tasks that measure one type of memory, none of them has made systematic manipulations of task demand in tasks that represent each type of memory process. Systematic parametric manipulations of each type of task demand are necessary to evaluate the validity of any dissociation, and the absence of this information severely compromises any theory (Olton, 1989a).

In any case, the pattern of results at the end of the test session provides strong evidence that inhibition of MSA cholinergic neurons has a deleterious influence on recent memory even when this memory is for nonspatial information. Together with the results from the spatial alternation task in the T-maze, these data provide strong converging operations to indicate that modulation of these cholinergic MSA neurons can have a profound effect on both spatial and nonspatial recent memory, producing impairments when this cholinergic activity is decreased, and at least in some cases producing improvements when this cholinergic activity is increased.

HIGH AFFINITY CHOLINE UPTAKE IN HIPPOCAMPUS

If the MSA cholinergic neurons are active during recent memory, then HACU in the hippocampus should be increased by performance in tasks that require recent memory (Antonelli, Beani, Pedata, & Pepeu, 1981;

Atweh, Simon, & Kuhar, 1976; Burgel & Rommelspacher, 1978). If hippocampal HACU is increased by performance in recent memory tasks, an additional question concerns the specificity of this relationship. Is recent memory the only kind of memory that engages the septohippocampal cholinergic system, increasing hippocampal HACU, or can other kinds of memory have this same effect?

The logic for the experimental design is similar to that used in positron emission tomographic (PET) scanning, conditioning, and other experiments designed to determine the extent to which any neurobiological process is selectively involved with certain kinds of associative processes. The present experiment included four groups. A Cage Group remained in the cage for the entire experiment. A Recent Memory Group was trained on a spatial alternation task on a radial arm maze. Performance in this task included three components of interest: (a) recent memory was required in order to determine which arm should be chosen; (b) reference memory was required in order to learn the general rules and procedures of the task; and (c) movement through the maze was required to obtain reinforcement. The next two groups were designed to assess the extent to which reference memory and movement through the maze increased hippocampal HACU in the recent memory procedure. The Reference Memory Group was given a left–right spatial discrimination in a T-maze. Like the recent memory task, this reference memory task required rats to learn a spatial discrimination. However, because the arm that was correct was the same for each trial, recent memory was not required. If only recent memory, but not reference memory, activates the cholinergic septohippocampal system, hippocampal HACU should not be increased in this group. If, however, the septohippocampal cholinergic system is engaged even by tasks that do not require recent memory, then hippocampal HACU might be increased in this group. A final group, the Treadmill Group, was included to control for the possibility that movement itself might increase hippocampal HACU. These rats walked on a treadmill for the same period of time that the rats in the two discrimination tasks performed the respective discriminations (Wenk, Hepler, & Olton, 1984).

The results were clear. The Treadmill Group had hippocampal HACU almost identical to that in the Cage Group, indicating that movement itself did not engage the septohippocampal system. The two memory groups had similar and highly elevated hippocampal HACU, indicating that both types of discriminations engaged the septohippocampal cholinergic system.

The fact that performance in the recent memory test on the radial arm maze raised hippocampal HACU is important because it provides converging evidence that the septohippocampal cholinergic system is important for accurate performance in tasks that require recent memory. The experiments described in the first part of this chapter indicate that direct manipulation of the septohippocampal system can affect recent memory. HACU experiments indicate that performance in recent memory tasks can engage this same system. The temporal parameters of this engagement remain to be demonstrated. Relatively few trials can produce significant increases in hippocampal HACU, and these increases can persist for an extended period of time after the end of testing. More parametric studies are necessary to determine the temporal parameters and their functional significance (Toumane, Durkin, Marighetto, Galey, & Jaffard, 1988; Toumane, Durkin, Marighetto, & Jafford, 1989).

One other result of these experiments is relevant to functional analyses of the basal forebrain cholinergic system. Performance in the two memory discriminations described above, which increased HACU in the hippocampus, did not increase HACU in the frontal cortex. The frontal cortex receives innervation from a different part of the basal forebrain cholinergic system, the nucleus basalis magnocellularis. The dissociation between the effects of behavior on HACU in the hippocampus and in the frontal cortex indicates that these neuroanatomically distinct portions of the basal forebrain cholinergic system are associated with different psychological functions (Olton & Wenk, 1987; Olton, 1990; Olton, Markowska, Voytko, et al., in press; Olton, Wenk, & Markowska, in press).

INTRAHIPPOCAMPAL IMPLANTS OF BASAL FOREBRAIN CHOLINERGIC TISSUE

The present experiments were designed to determine the extent to which a direct intervention in the hippocampus can have beneficial effects on electrophysiology and behavior even in the absence of the reciprocal septohippocampal connections through the fornix. Transection of the fornix, which severs these reciprocal connections, produces severe impairments in spatial recent memory and alters the characteristics of place fields recorded from hippocampal neurons. Fetal basal forebrain tissue, implanted into the hippocampus, can reduce the behavioral impairments produced by these lesions. Electrophysiological analyses of the characteristics of place units can help determine the extent to which the behavioral improvements produced by the grafts are due to reorganization or restoration of the neuronal circuitry in the hippocampus (Shapiro et al., 1989).

Complex spike cells in the hippocampus of normal rats have distinctive place fields, areas in the environment in which the rate of activity is markedly increased. Extramaze distal stimuli, rather than intramaze proximal stimuli, are the discriminative stimuli for these place fields. Fornix lesions alter the characteristics of place fields; although hippocampal neurons still have elevated activity in certain locations, the discriminative stimuli identifying these locations are intramaze, proximal stimuli rather than extramaze, distal ones.

If implants of basal forebrain tissue in the hippocampus restore normal electrophysiological activity, then they should shift the kinds of discriminative stimuli influencing place fields, reducing the effectiveness of intramaze proximal stimuli and increasing the effectiveness of extramaze distal stimuli.

If these implants reorganize hippocampal circuitry, then some other pattern of results should occur.

For this experiment, the fornix was completely transected. A suspension of fetal basal forebrain tissue was implanted into the hippocampus. Approximately 6 months later, each rat was tested in a place discrimination in a Morris Water Maze. Rats that showed substantial behavioral recovery as a result of the implant had electrodes placed in the hippocampus to record the place fields of single units. Each rat was tested on a radial arm maze. Each unit with a place field was tested with the maze in two positions. In the normal position, the arms of the maze were in the standard position used for training. In the rotated position, the arms of the maze were rotated 90° to move the intramaze stimuli to a new position relative to extramaze stimuli. The correlation between the pattern of unit activity in the normal position and the rotated position was calculated. Place stability, which indicates control by extramaze stimuli, was defined as the correlation of unit activity in each spatial location in the room. Maze stability, which indicates control by intramaze cues, was defined as the correlation of unit activity in each spatial location on the arms.

Normal rats had place fields with high place stability and low maze stability, indicating control by extramaze distal stimuli. Fornix lesions changed the discriminative stimuli controlling the place fields; maze stability was high, and place stability was low. The implants produced a substantial, but incomplete, normalization of the stimuli controlling the place fields, increasing place stability and decreasing maze stability as compared with rats with fornix lesions and no implants.

The significant normalization of place field activity indicates that the influence of the basal forebrain system can have beneficial effects on hippocampal function even in the absence of direct septohippocampal and hippocamposeptal fibers. These data suggest that tonic stimulation of hippocampal neurons by the implanted basal forebrain cholinergic neurons can have beneficial effects, and are consistent with the results of many other experiments demonstrating that neural grafts can improve behavior (Nilsson, Shapiro, Gage, Olton, & Bjorklund, 1987).

The absence of complete normalization requires further investigation, and has at least two classes of explanation. The first is technical. The implants may not have been optimally effective, and the partial recovery may reflect a partially effective implant. If such is the case, better technology should produce more significant recovery. The second class of explanations is neural. The failure to obtain complete restoration of place fields and complete behavioral recovery may reflect important functions normally carried out by the septohippocampal and hippocamposeptal fibers. The loss of information from the MSA neurons to the hippocampus, and feedback from the hippocampus to these neurons, may both have significant functional consequences, and no intervention may be able to produce complete normalization in their absence.

An important component of this analysis was the explicit test for the class of discriminative stimuli determining the place field. Relatively normal place fields in a consistent environment remained following fornix lesions or inactivation of septal neurons. Only when the classes of discriminative stimuli were manipulated independently did the abnormalities in the place fields appear. Because spatial environments typically provide many relevant redundant strategies to guide correct responding, eliminating the redundancy in specially designed probe tests is critical to interpret the empirical data (Leonard & McNaughton, 1990; Miller & Best, 1980; Mizumori, Barnes, & McNaughton, 1990; O'Keefe & Conway, 1978; O'Keefe & Nadel, 1988; Olton & Markowska, in press; Roitblatt, 1982).

SPECIFICITY: NEUROANATOMY, NEUROCHEMISTRY, AND PSYCHOLOGY

The behavioral effects of a neurotransmitter differ depending on the area of the brain in which the neurotransmitter is active. For example, consider the effects of intracranial infusions of neuropeptide Y on the retention of foot-shock avoidance in a T-maze. In the MSA, it improved retention; in the amygdala, it impaired retention; in the thalamus or caudate, it had no effect (Flood, Baker, Hernandez, & Morley, 1989). Similar dissociations occur within the basal forebrain cholinergic system. As described earlier, the MSA projects to the hippocampus and posterior cortex, whereas the nucleus basalis magnocellularis (NBM) projects to the frontal cortex and other cortical areas. As might be expected by the different theoretical descriptions of the psychological functions of the frontal cortex and hippocampus, lesions of the MSA and NBM had substantially different behavioral effects in tests of divided attention and recent memory. The divided attention task assessed the ability to respond appropriately to two stimuli at the same time. The recent memory task assessed the ability to remember the duration of a previously presented stimulus. Neurotoxic lesions of cells in the MSA and NBM produced a double dissociation in these two tasks. MSA lesions disrupted recent memory, but not divided attention. NBM lesions disrupted divided attention, but not recent memory. These, and other dissociations following lesions of the NBM and MSA, indicate that the psychological consequences of disrupting cholinergic activity in the brain depend on the neuroanatomical area in which this disruption takes place (Meck, Church, Wenk, & Olton, 1987; Olton, Wenk, Church, & Meck, 1988; Olton, Wenk, & Markowska, in press).

Likewise, the behavioral effects of activity in a specific neuroanatomical area depend on the neurotransmitter that is active, reflecting the afferent input to those cells. When infused into the MSA, muscimol, a GABA agonist, and oxotremorine, a cholinergic agonist, had opposite effects on performance in recent memory tasks, as described earlier. When infused into the amygdala, posttrial infusions of neuropeptide Y and substance P impaired retention of inhibitory avoidance, whereas naloxone, an opiate antagonist, improved retention (Brioni, Nagahara, & McGaugh, 1989; Gallagher, Fanelli, & Bostock, 1985; Huston & Stabuli, 1979).

This three-fold specificity of neuroanatomy, neurochemistry, and psychology is important for both basic science and clinical applications. Because psychological functions are influenced by the action of a specific neurotransmitter in a specific brain area, any attempt to describe the functional organization of the brain must consider all three of these variables simultaneously. The activity of some neurotransmitters systems (cholinergic, GABAergic, opioid) in some brain areas (MSA, NBM, amygdala) are important for mnemonic associations in some types of tasks (place discrimination, spatial alternation, inhibitory avoidance). However, a systematic analysis of all possible combinations is required to indicate the extent to which certain combinations of neurotransmitters and neuroanatomical areas are involved in specific types of mnemonic associations. This type of analysis can be assisted markedly by two components in the experimental design. The first is a parametric manipulation of task difficulty (Olton, 1989a). The second is a functional equating of dosages of different substances on the basis of their effects on electrophysiology and neurochemistry (see pages 263–264).

This three-fold specificity may have an important impact on the way in which we conceptualize localization of function. For example, the "cholinergic hypothesis" of memory function has a long history (see Bartus, Reginald, Pontecorvo, & Flicker, 1985 for review). Although numerous articles have discussed the relative merits of this hypothesis, the view expressed here suggests that the basic hypothesis itself must be stated more succinctly in order to be evaluated accurately. Cholinergic activity in different neuroanatomical areas may be critical for different kinds of psychological processes. For example, consider the following possibilities: frontal cortex, divided attention; striatum, motor responding; brain stem, arousal.

In describing the functions of the parasympathetic system, Koizummi and Brooks (1974) wrote:

> [There is probably not] a physiologic rationale for the discharge of the parasympathetic system as a whole. Simultaneous dilation of the pupil, salivation, slowing of the heart, increased activity of the gut, defecation, urination, and erection of the penis have no sensible function . . . . The components of the parasympathetic system behave independently, participating in specific reflexes or well-integrated reactions.

Analogously, there may not be a psychological rationale for the discharge of the entire cholinergic system in the brain. A more profitable approach might be to add neuroanatomical specificity to the cholinergic hypothesis, describing the psychological functions that may be mediated by its activity in different areas of the brain. This chapter reports data that are consistent with a more specific cholinergic hypothesis stating that the septohippocampal cholinergic system is critical for recent, working memory. This specific cholinergic hypothesis makes two predictions. (a) Disruption of septohippocampal cholinergic transmission will impair recent memory in individuals that have normal recent memory if the task demand is sufficient. (b) Enhancement of septohippocampal cholinergic function in individuals with impaired memory will improve memory if the septohippocampal dysfunction is responsible for the memory impairment, and the rest of the brain functions well enough to allow the improved mnemonic function to be expressed. Most of the data reported in this chapter are consistent with this more specific version of the cholinergic hypothesis. Other predictions that are concurrently specific for neuroanatomy, neurochemistry, and psychology should be helpful to determine the extent to which the approach advocated here can be successful.

This three-fold specificity is also important for clinical issues. In humans, cognitive impairments and neuropathological signs are often limited. Consequently, the ideal intervention is a "magic bullet", one that goes directly to the targeted pathology and alleviates the associated psychological impairment. The problem with nonspecific interventions is that they may alter neural activity in unimpaired systems, interfering with their function and producing undesirable side-effects. In this shooting analogy, the nonspecific intervention is like a shotgun. Although one pellet may hit the target, other pellets may stray to unintended locations, causing unwanted havoc. The disrupting side-effects in nonspecific treatments may mask the beneficial effects that would have been detected if a more specific intervention had been used, rejecting an intervention that is potentially beneficial.

The skeptic might argue that although the goal of site-specific drug delivery is reasonable in animal experiments, it may never be appropriate for therapeutic treatment in humans. Such a perspective is unduly pessimistic. Many novel approaches are being pursued in the attempt to obtain site-specific delivery of drugs in humans, and both mechanical and neurochemical strategies provide promising options (Harbaugh, 1989). For example, adding an appropriate substance to a cholinergic compound might produce differential affinity for cholinergic receptors in a specific brain area, or specific subtypes of cholinergic receptor. As usual, necessity might be the parent of invention. If future laboratory experiments continue to indicate the importance of the three-fold specificity described above, more effort might be applied to developing techniques for the appropriate interventions.

If the psychological effects of a neurotransmitter depend on the neuroanatomical location in which that neurotransmitter is active, interpreting the psychological effects of systemically injected compounds can be very difficult. For example, muscimol in the MSA produced relatively selective changes in mnemonic parameters of task performance in the continuous delayed conditional discrimination task described in this chapter, but in the NBM, it had a strong effect on many nonmnemonic aspects of performance in a visual discrimination task (Dudchencko & Sarter, in press). A wide spectrum of effects following systemic injections of scopolamine may be due to independent actions in different brain areas (Spencer, Pontecorvo, & Heise, 1985). Because the criteria for distinguishing mnemonic from nonmnemonic effects require strong dissociations, intracranial infusions may be the only reasonable means to determine the extent to which the actions of a specific neurotransmitter can have a selective effect on mnemonic processes.

THE NEWS: GOOD, BAD, AND FORTHCOMING

The good news is that these experiments indicate a consistent role of the septohippocampal cholinergic system in memory processing. Changing the activity of MSA cholinergic neurons altered hippocampal electrophysiology, neurochemistry, and behavior in recent memory tasks. Performance in tasks that require recent memory engaged the septohippocampal cholinergic system as indicated by changes in HACU. These converging data give strong support to the idea that the septohippocampal cholinergic system is required for recent memory, and provide the basis to pursue a number of important questions about the details of this function.

The bad news, as usual, takes longer to tell than the good news. Although the ISIs described here did affect cholinergic neurons, they also affected GABAergic neurons that project to the hippocampus. Although the basal forebrain grafts that were placed in the hippocampus contained cholinergic neurons, they also contained noncholinergic neurons. In both cases, noncholinergic neurons may have been responsible for the mnemonic effects, and the role of these noncholinergic neurons in the results reported here must be determined. Intraseptal infusion of substances that selectively influence different populations of neurons, and microdialysis of neurotransmitters in the hippocampus, can both be effective tools to approach this issue.

The lack of a mnemonic effect of an ISI of beta-endorphin in a test of recent memory on the radial arm maze is puzzling. Opioid peptides alter cholinergic activity in the septohippocampal system (see Gallager, Fanelli, & Bostock, 1985, for a review). However, an ISI of beta-endorphin (1 mg) did not reduce choice accuracy in the standard test procedure in a familiar room (Bostock, Gallagher, & King, 1988). Only a single dose of beta-endorphin was used in this experiment. Consequently, larger doses might have produced the expected behavioral impairment. However, this same dose did impair choice accuracy in a related experimental procedure: acquisition of the same task in an unfamiliar room.

This lack of a behavioral effect of beta-endorphin on choice accuracy in the test of recent memory in a familiar spatial environment is especially surprising in light of the fact that decreased hippocampal cholinergic function usually impairs recent spatial memory, but is difficult to interpret without further information. The critical experiment is one obtaining a dose–response curve for a GABAergic agonist, a cholinergic antagonist, and an opioid agonist, equating the three substances for their effects on theta and cholinergic activity in the hippocampus. If disruption of theta and hippocampal cholinergic activity are markers for a common mechanism that is necessary for recent memory, then doses of all three substances, when equated for their electrophysiological and neurochemical effects, should produce equivalent mnemonic impairments. If, however, the opioid peptides alter septohippocampal function through a mechanism independent of the cholinergic/GABAergic one that is necessary for recent memory, then recent memory may not be impaired by a dose of beta-endorphin that reduces hippocampal theta and hippocampal HACU to levels that are associated with impairments produced by muscimol and scopolamine. The same line of reasoning can be used to examine the effects of the complementary substances, a GABAergic antagonist, a cholinergic agonist, and an opioid antagonist, such as naloxone.

The HACU data also have some problems. Hippocampal HACU was increased in a reference memory task that didn't require the hippocampus for normal performance (Wenk et al., 1984). Hippocampal HACU was decreased following performance in a place discrimination in the Morris water maze (Decker, Pelleymounter, & Gallagher, 1988). Carefully designed tasks that encompass a variety of stimulus dimensions and associative processes are required in order to determine the interaction of variables that alter cholinergic activity in the septohippocampal system.

The dose–response curves from different experimental procedures have varied substantially, and reconciliation of these differences requires insight and care. Recent memory in the continuous alternation task in the T-maze and in the operant continuous discrimination was severely impaired by an ISI of 30 mg (0.34 nmol) muscimol. However, a much larger dose (0.75 nmol, 84 mg) had little effect when given at the beginning of the delay interval in a recent memory test on a radial arm maze (Chrobak, Stackman, & Walsh, 1989), and 0.5 nmol (57 mg) had no effect in a place of discrimination task in the Morris water maze (Brioni, Decker, Gamboa, Izquierdo, & McGaugh, 1990). Higher doses of muscimol did impair performance in both of these tasks, suggesting that the septohippocampal system is indeed involved in this performance. However, the differences in the dose–response curves are striking and require resolution.

The absent news is still substantial. The septohippocampal cholinergic system does not exist in isolation, but in complicated circuits that involve feedback from the hippocampus and the lateral septum. These additional neuronal circuits must influence the way in which the septohippocampal cholinergic system functions, and must be incorporated into any neuronal model. Noncholinergic transmitters, particularly in the amygdala, influence memory. Do these influences occur through the septohippocampal system, or do they have an independent mechanism of action (Decker & McGaugh, 1991)? Within the basal forebrain cholinergic system, are the functions of the neurons in the NBM directly related to memory, or do they alter behavior in mnemonic tasks because of nonmnemonic influences? Most of the information required to address these issues can be readily obtained through appropriate experiments, infusing different substances into different brain areas, and measuring their neurochemical, electrophysiological, and behavioral effects (Malthe-Sorenssen, Cheney, & Costa, 1978; Nagel & Huston, 1988; Staubli & Huston, 1980).

Although much is known about the neurobiological mechanisms within the hippocampus, these mechanisms must still be linked to mnemonic processes. Many alternatives are possible, and the theta rhythm may be a critical component. The large theta rhythm dominates hippocampal EEG when a rat is actively exploring its environment (Bland, 1986), and increases the specificity of place fields, increasing the ratio of activity in the place field to activity outside of it (Kubie, Muller, & Fox, 1985). The normalization of place field activity following intrahippocampal grafts of fetal basal forebrain tissue may have resulted from the restoration of theta activity (Buszaki, Gage, Czopf, & Bjorklund, 1987; Shapiro et al., 1989). Long-term potentiation, an important neural mechanism for synaptic plasticity in the hippocampus, is optimal with stimulation at the theta frequency (Larson, Wong, & Lynch, 1986). The evoked response of hippocampal neurons, which are involved in the plasticity associated with long-term potentiation, is influenced by the cholinergic system (Bilkey & Goddard, 1985; Mizumori, McNaughton, & Barnes, 1989). If neurochemically altered theta has effects similar to naturally occurring theta, then alterations in theta produced by an ISI might have profound effects on neural plasticity and mnemonic processing. One advantage of the hippocampus is the extensive body of literature describing its electrophysiology, neurochemistry, and anatomy. Consequently, relating the results obtained here from ISIs to those of other investigations of hippocampal plasticity should be an obtainable goal.

A fundamental question about the cholinergic system concerns the extent to which it functions as a neuromodulator or as a substrate of specific mnemonic associations. A primary role as a neuromodulator is suggested by the consistent improvement in performance produced by an ISI of a direct cholinergic agonist, oxotremorine, and by transplants of fetal tissue from the basal forebrain cholinergic system. Both of these interventions increase cholinergic activity in the hippocampus, but neither of them should enhance the signal processing capabilities of the cholinergic system because both of them produce noncontingent stimulation of hippocampal neurons (Sarter, Bruno, & Dudchenko, 1990). A strong test of this hypothesis would be to infuse a cholinergic agonist directly into the hippocampus. If the cholinergic system does function as a neuromodulator, this view has many significant implications. First, the behavioral effects of chronic stimulation of the MSA may be mediated by phasic changes in the hippocampal theta activity, which is produced by the pacemaker system in the septum (Steward & Fox, 1990). Second, the ability of the hippocampus to mediate mnemonic associations must depend on cholinergic activation, but the mnemonic associations themselves must be made through noncholinergic systems because direct septohippocampal afferents are not necessary for improved memory following intrahippocampal grafts. Third, for therapeutic intervention, a neuromodulatory role makes treatment much easier because chronic stimulation of cholinergic neurons can have beneficial mnemonic effects.

Acknowledgments: D.S.O. thanks the faculty and staff of the Center for Neurobiology of Learning and Memory for their hospitality and the invitation to participate in this Conference, and A. Dürr for preparing the manuscript. B.S.G. was supported by NRSA #NS8616.

REFERENCES

Antonelli, T., Beani, F., Pedata, F., & Pepeu, G. (1981). Changes in synaptosomae high affinity choline uptake following electrical stimulation of guinea pig cortical slices: Effect of atropine and physostigmine. *British Journal of Pharmacology, 74*, 525–531.

Atweh, S., Simon, J. R., & Kuhar, M. J. (1976). Utilization of sodium-dependent high affinity choline uptake in vitro as a measure of the activity of the cholinergic neurons in vivo. *Life Science, 17*, 1535–1544.

Barnes, C. A. (1988). Spatial learning and memory processes: The search for their neurobiological mechanisms in the rat. *Trends in Neuroscience, 11*(4), 163–169.

Bartus, R. T., Reginald, L. D., Pontecorvo, M. J., & Flicker, C. (1985). The cholinergic hypothesis: A historical overview, current perspective, and future directions. In D. S. Olton, E. Gamzu, & S. Corkin (Eds.), *Memory dysfunctions: An integration of animal and human research from preclinical and clinical perspectives* (pp. 332–358). New York: The New York Academy of Sciences.

Bilkey, D. K., & Goddard, G. V. (1985). Medial septal facilitation of hippocampal granule cell activity is mediated by inhibition of inhibitory interneurons. *Brain Research, 361*, 99–106.

Bland, B. H. (1986). The physiology and pharmacology of hippocampal formation theta rhythms. *Progress in Neurobiology, 26*, 1–54.

Bostock, E., Gallagher, M., & King, R. A. (1988). Effects of opioid microinjections into the medial septal area on spatial memory in rats. *Behavioral Neuroscience, 102*, 643–652.

Brioni, J. D., Decker, M. W., Gamboa, L. P., Izquierdo, I., & McGaugh, J. L. (1990). Muscimol injections in the medial septum impair spatial learning. *Brain Research, 522*, 227–234.

Brioni, J. D., Nagahara, A. H., & McGaugh, J. L. (1989). Involvement of the amygdala GABAergic system in the modulation of memory storage. *Brain Research, 487*, 105–112.

Burgel, P., & Rommelspacher, H. (1978). Changes in high affinity choline uptake in behavioral experiments. *Life Sciences, 23*, 2423–2428.

Buszaki, G., Gage, F. H., Czopf, J., & Bjorklund, A. (1987). Restoration of rhythmic slow activity (0) in the subcortically denervated hippocampus by fetal CNS transplants. *Brain Research, 400*, 334–347.

Chrobak, J. J., Stackman, R. W., & Walsh, T. J. (1989). Intraseptal administration of muscimol produces dose–dependent memory impairments in the rat. *Behavioral and Neural Biology, 52*, 357–369.

Decker, M. W., & McGaugh, J. L. (1991). The role of interactions between the cholinergic system and other neuromodulatory systems in learning and memory. *Synapse, 7,* 151–168.

Decker, M. W., Pelleymounter, M. A., & Gallagher, M. (1988). Effects of training on a spatial memory task on high affinity choline uptake in hippocampus and cortex in young adult and aged rats. *Journal of Neuroscience, 8*(1), 90–99.

Dudchenko, P., & Sarter, M. (in press). GABAergic control of basal forebrain cholinergic neurons and memory. *Behavioural Brain Research.*

Flood, J. F., Baker, M. L., Hernandez, E. N., & Morley, J. E. (1989). Modulation of memory processing by neuropeptide Y varies with brain injection site. *Brain Research, 503,* 73–82.

Gallagher, M., Fanelli, R. J., & Bostock, E. (1985). Opioid peptides: Their position among other neuroregulators of memory. In J. L. McGaugh (Ed.), *Contemporary psychology: Biological processes and theoretical issues* (pp. 69–93). North Holland: Elsevier Science Publishers B.V.

Givens, B. S., & Olton, D. S. (1990). Cholinergic and GABAergic modulation of medial septal area: Effect on working memory. *Behavioral Neuroscience, 104,* 849–855.

Gray, J. A., & McNaughton, N. (1983). Comparison between the behavioural effects of septal and hippocampal lesions: A review. *Neuroscience and Biobehavioral Reviews, 7,* 119–188.

Harbaugh, R. E. (1989). Novel CNS-directed drug delivery systems in Alzheimer's disease and other neurological disorders. *Neurobiology of Aging, 10,* 623–629.

Huston, J. P., & Staubli, U. (1979). Rapid communication: Post-trial injection of substance P into lateral hypothalamus and amygdala, respectively, facilitates and impairs learning. *Behavioral and Neural Biology, 27,* 244–248.

Kirk, R. C., White, K. G., & McNaughton, N. (1988). Low dose scopolamine affects discriminability but not rate of forgetting in delayed conditional discrimination. *Psychopharmacology, 96,* 541–546.

Koizumi, K., & Brooks, C. (1974). The autonomic nervous system and its role in controlling visceral activities. In V. B. Mountcastle (Ed.), *Medical physiology* (Vol. 1) (pp. 783–812). St Louis: C. V. Mosby.

Kubie, J. L., Muller, R. U., & Fox, S. E. (1985). Firing fields of hippocampal place fields: Interim report. In G. Buzsaki & C. H. Vanderwolf (Eds.), *Electrical activity of the archicortex* (pp. 221–231). Budapest: Akademial Kiado.

Larson, J. L., Wong, D., & Lynch, G. (1986). Patterned stimulation at the theta frequency is optimal for the induction of hippocampal long-term potentiation. *Brain Research, 368,* 347–350.

Leonard, B., & McNaughton, B. L. (1990). Spatial representation in the rat: Conceptual, behavioral, and neurophysiological perspectives. In R. P. Kesner & D. S. Olton (Eds.), *Neurobiology of comparative cognition* (pp. 363–421). Hillsdale, New Jersey: Lawrence Erlbaum.

Leranth, C., & Frotscher, M. (1989). Organization of the septal region in the rat brain: Cholinergic–GABAergic interconnections and the termination of hippocampo-septal fibers. *Journal of Comparative Neurology, 289,* 304–314.

Malthe-Sorenssen, D., Cheney, D. L., & Costa, E. (1978). Modulation of acetylcholine metabolism in the hippocampal cholinergic pathway by intraseptally injected substance P. *Journal of Pharmacology and Experimental Therapeutics, 206,* 21–28.

Meck, W. H., Church, R. M., Wenk, G. L., & Olton, D. S. (1987). Nucleus basalis magnocellularis and medial septal area lesions differentially impair temporal memory. *Journal of Neuroscience, 7*(11), 3505–3511.

Miller, V. M., & Best, P. J. (1980). Spatial correlates of hippocampal unit activity are altered by lesions of the fornix and entorhinal cortex. *Brain Research, 194*, 311–323.

Mizumori, S. J. Y., Barnes, C. A., & McNaughton, B. L. (1990). Behavioral correlates of theta-on and theta-off cells recorded from the hippocampus of mature young and aged rats. *Experimental Brain Research, 80*, 365–373.

Mizumori, S. J. Y., McNaughton, B. L., & Barnes, C. A. (1989). A comparison of supramammillary and medial septal influences on hippocampal field potentials and single-unit activity. *Journal of Neurophysiology, 61*(1), 15–31.

Nagel, J. A., & Huston, J. P. (1988). Enhanced inhibitory avoidance learning produced by post-trial injections of substance P into the basal forebrain. *Behavioral and Neural Biology, 49*, 374–385.

Nilsson, O. G., Shapiro, M. L., Gage, F. H., Olton, D. S., & Bjorklund, A. (1987). Spatial learning and memory following fimbria-fornix transection and grafting of fetal septal neurons to the hippocampus. *Experimental Brain Research, 67*, 195–215.

O'Keefe, J., & Conway, D. H. (1978). Hippocampal place units in the freely moving rat; why they fire when they fire. *Experimental Brain Research, 31*, 573–590.

Olton, D. S., & Wenk, G. L. (1987). Dementia: Animal models of the cognitive impairments produced by degeneration of the basal forebrain cholinergic system. In H. Y. Meltzer (Ed.), *Psychopharmacology: The third generation of progress* (pp. 941–953). New York: Raven Press.

Olton, D. S. (1989a). Dimensional mnemonics. In G. H. Bower (Ed.), *The psychology of learning and memory* (pp. 1–23). San Diego: Academic Press.

Olton, D. S. (1989b). Mnemonic functions of the hippocampus: Single unit analyses in rats. In Victoria Chan-Palay & Christer Kohler (Eds.), *The hippocampus: New vistas* (pp. 411–424). New York: Alan R. Liss.

Olton, D. S. (1990). Dementia: Animal models of the cognitive impairments following damage to the basal forebrain cholinergic system. *Brain Research Bulletin, 25*, 499–502.

Olton, D. S., Markowska, A. L., Voytko, M. L., Givens, B., Gorman, L., & Wenk, G. L. (in press). Basal forebrain cholinergic system: A functional analysis. In T. C. Napier, P. W. Kalivas, & I. Hanin (Eds.), *The basal forebrain: Anatomy to function*. New York: Plenum Press.

Olton, D. S., Wenk, G. L., Church, R. M., & Meck, W. H. (1988). Attention and the frontal cortex as examined by simultaneous temporal processing. *Neuropsychologia, 26*, 307–318.

Olton, D. S., Wenk, G. L., & Markowska, A. M. (1991). Basal forebrain, memory, and attention. In R. Richardson (Ed.), *Activation to acquisition: Functional aspects of the basal forebrain* (pp. 247–262). Boston: Birkhauser.

Olton, D. S., & Markowska, A. L. (in press). Mazes. In F. Von Harren (Ed.), *Methods in behavioral pharmacology*. Amsterdam: Elsevier.

Rawlins, J. N. P. (1985). Associations across time: The hippocampus as a temporal memory store. *Behavioral and Brain Sciences, 8*, 479–497.

Roitblat, H. L. (1982). The meaning of representation in animal memory. *Behavioral and Brain Sciences, 5*, 353–372.

Sarter, M., Bruno,, J. P., & Dudchenko, P. (1990). Activating the damaged basal forebrain cholinergic system: Tonic stimulation versus signal amplification. *Psychopharmacology, 101*, 1–17.

Segal, M. (1986). Properties of rat medial septal neurones recorded in vitro. *Journal of Physiology, 379*, 309–330.

Shapiro, M. L., Simon, D. K., Olton, D. S., Gage, F. H. III, Nilsson, O. G., & Bjorklund, A. (1989). Intrahippocampal grafts of fetal basal forebrain tissue influence the place-correlates of complex spike units in the hippocampus of behaving rats with fimbria-fornix lesions. *IRBO Neuroscience, 32*, 1–18.

Spencer, D. G., Pontecorvo, M., & Heise, G. A. (1985). Central cholinergic involvement in working memory: Effects of scopolamine on continuous nonmatching and discrimination performance in the rat. *Behavioral Neuroscience, 99*(6), 1049–1065.

Staubli, U., & Huston, J. P. (1980). Facilitation of learning by post-trial injection of substance P into the medial septal nucleus. *Behavioural Brain Research, 1*, 245–255.

Stewart, M., & Fox, S. E. (1990). Do septal neurons pace the hippocampal theta rhythm? *Trends in Neuroscience, 13*, 163–168.

Toumane, A., Durkin, T., Marighetto, A., Galey, D., & Jaffard, R. (1988). Differential hippocampal and cortical cholinergic activation during the acquisition, retention, reversal and extinction of a spatial discrimination in an 8-arm radial maze by mice. *Behavioral Brain Research, 30*, 225–234.

Toumane, A., Durkin, T., Marighetto, A., & Jaffard, R. (1989). The durations of hippocampal and cortical cholinergic activation induced by spatial discrimination testing of mice in an eight-arm radial maze decrease as a function of acquisition. *Behavioral and Neural Biology, 52*, 279–284.

Wenk, G. L., Helper, D., & Olton, D. S. (1984). Behavior alters the uptake of (^{3}H)-choline into acetylcholinergic neurons of the nucleus basalis magnocellularis and medial septal area. *Behavioral Brain Research, 13*, 129–138.

III

Locus of Cellular Change

12

The Anatomy of Long-Term Sensitization in *Aplysia*: Morphological Insights into Learning and Memory

CRAIG H. BAILEY
MARY CHEN

Among the most difficult and profound problems facing both neurobiology and psychology is an understanding of the mechanisms that underlie learning and memory. Since the initial proposals of Ramón y Cajal and others at the turn of the century, it has seemed almost axiomatic that learning must be expressed as a change in synaptic function and form (Cajal, 1894; Lugaro, 1899; Tanzi, 1893). However, prior to the last few decades there was little direct evidence to either support this hypothesis or to indicate precisely what aspects of synaptic change might be important for information storage.

In recent years, the cellular specificity of several favorable higher invertebrates has proven useful for the analysis of behavioral problems and has enhanced our knowledge about the synaptic loci and mechanisms that are involved in the acquisition and retention of various elementary forms of learning and memory (Alkon, 1984; Byrne, 1987; Kandel & Schwartz, 1982). In this chapter we describe how a simple defensive behavior, the gill- and siphon-withdrawal reflex of the marine mollusc *Aplysia californica,* can be used as a model system for examining the contribution of individual synapses to the learning process. In particular, we will focus on a specific set of identified synapses to review morphological studies of learning and to explore the functional relationship between synaptic structure and the enduring changes in synaptic effectiveness that underlie long-term memory.

STRUCTURE OF THE CENTRAL NERVOUS SYSTEM SYNAPSE IN *APLYSIA*: ORGANIZATION OF THE PRESYNAPTIC ACTIVE ZONE

Synapses in the central nervous system of *Aplysia* are most often found at small varicose expansions that occur along or at the end of fine neurites

(Bailey, Thompson, Castellucci, & Kandel, 1979). These axonal specializations can take the form of relatively symmetrical bead-like varicosities, more eccentrically placed swellings, expansions that occur at some, but not all branch points and terminal club-like endings. A typical synaptic contact in this mollusc consists of a single presynaptic component—which is almost always a vesicle-containing varicosity and a single postsynaptic component that is most often a small, spinelike element (Bailey et al., 1979; Coggeshall, 1967: Tremblay, Colonnier, & McLennon, 1979). Only a restricted portion of both the pre- and postsynaptic elements is structurally modified for synaptic transmission. These focal regions of membrane specialization and vesicle accumulation appear analogous to the active zones that have been most fully characterized at peripheral synapses (Couteaux & Pecot-Dechavassine, 1970; Heuser et al., 1979) and which are now thought to be a common feature of central synapses in a variety of species. As is the case in other animals, the active zone at *Aplysia* synapses consists of a presynaptic component that is thought to facilitate the positioning of synaptic vesicles prior to their fusion and subsequent exocytotic release and a postsynaptic component that is modified for the reception of this chemical information.

Figure 12.1 illustrates the appearance of a synaptic junction in *Aplysia* following conventional fixation with glutaraldehyde and osmium tetroxide. The presynaptic terminal contains a population of small electron-lucent synaptic vesicles which converge on a patch of specialized membrane. Lying above the vesicle domain, and to some extent coextensive with it, are elements of the cytoskeleton. The axoplasm contiguous to the presynaptic active zone contains an amorphous electron-dense material that surrounds synaptic vesicles and adheres to the cytoplasmic leaflet of the plasma membrane. Depending on the method of tissue preparation, this can occur as either a sparse mat of fine filaments that occasionally links synaptic vesicles with each other and with the presynaptic membrane or, in some instances, as more focal patches of electron-dense material that take the form of small, truncated dense projections (Figure 12.2). All of these observations on *Aplysia* central synapses are in general agreement with a large body of previous work on a variety of vertebrate and invertebrate synapses (Gray, 1959; King, 1976; Muller & McMahan, 1976; Palay, 1958; Pfenninger, Sandri, Akert, & Eugster, 1969; Vrensen & Nunes Cardozo, 1981; for a review see Peters, Palay, & Webster, 1976)

Landis, Hall, Weinstein and Reese (1988) have recently exploited the technical advantages of rapid freezing and shallow freeze etching to study this filamentous organization of the presynaptic active zone in detail. By examining excitatory synapses in the mammalian cerebellar cortex, they have found that the axoplasm in the presynaptic terminal appears as a specialized compartment of the neuronal cytoplasm containing several distinct components. Synaptic vesicles cluster in the axoplasm in the vicinity of the synaptic junction and are surrounded by a complex meshwork of fine filaments. One set of filaments has molecular dimensions and an immunoreactive distribution similar to Synapsin I and appears to interconnect

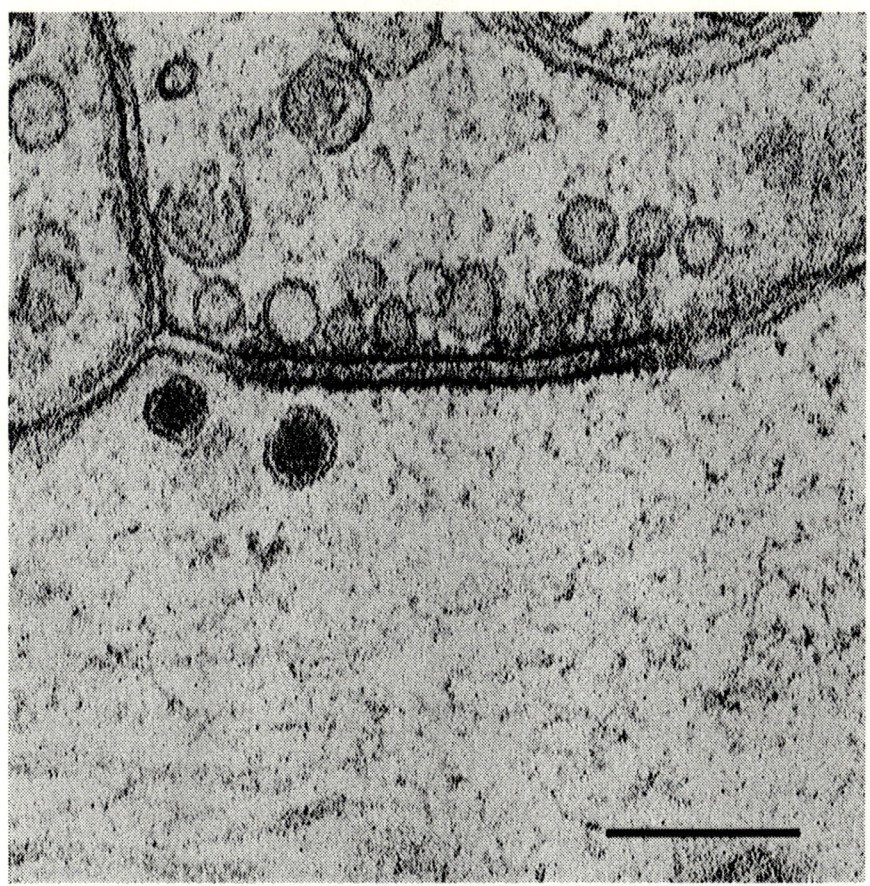

FIGURE 12.1. Synaptic junction in *Aplysia*. When appropriately visualized, the active zone at *Aplysia* synapses is characterized by rigidly parallel pre- and postsynaptic membranes that bound a widened synaptic cleft containing some form of electron-dense material. Small lucent vesicles are preferentially found clustered along these specialized sites and varying amounts of electron-dense material is attached to the cytoplasmic leaflet of both pre- and postsynaptic membranes. Scale = 0.25 μm. (From Bailey, Kandel, & Chen, 1981)

adjacent vesicles as well as link individual vesicles with larger filaments that extend inward from the presynaptic membrane. This relationship suggests a presynaptic protein meshwork that may serve to concentrate vesicles at the active zone and perhaps modulate their availability for exocytotic release. By contrast, the axoplasm that is not occupied by synaptic vesicles and which is further removed from the active zone, has completely different appearance and includes actin microfilaments, neurofilaments, microtubules, and clathrin assemblies.

A useful approach for the visualization of synaptic junctions and one that

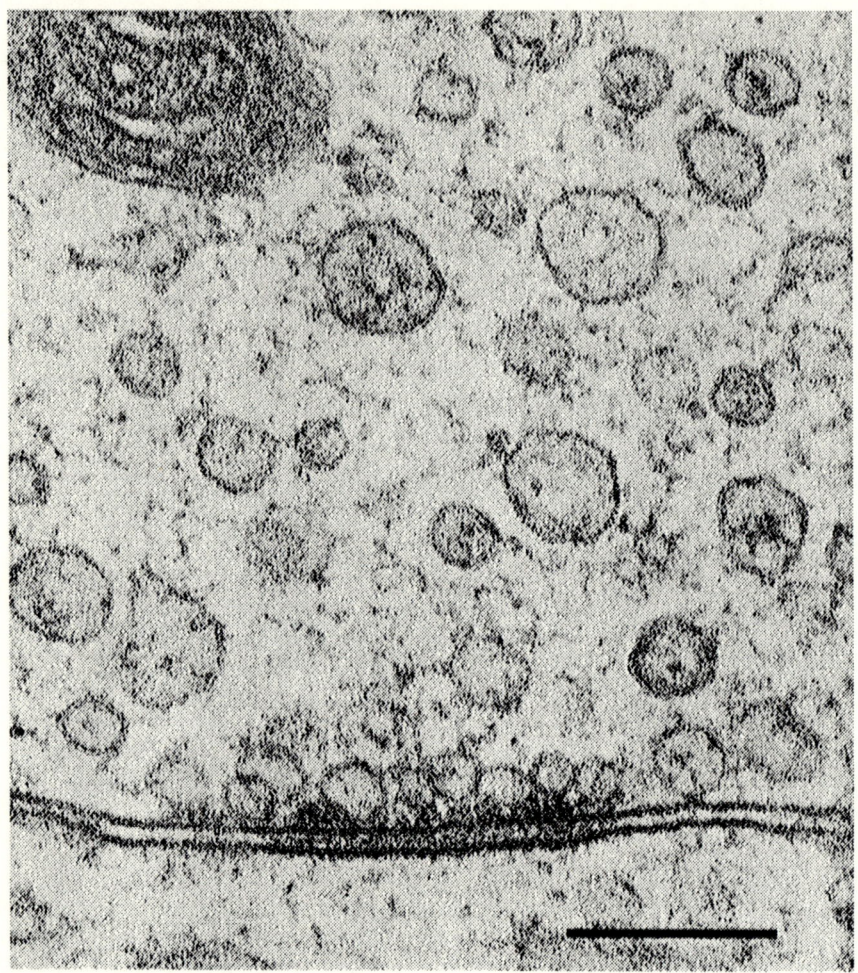

FIGURE 12.2.   Presynaptic specialization at *Aplysia* synapses. Presynaptic densities often take the form of small, truncated, dense projections that appear flattened against the presynaptic membrane. Scale = 0.25 µm. (From Bailey, Kandel, & Chen, 1981)

provides a somewhat different view of presynaptic organization is the use of cytochemical techniques such as ethanolic phosphotungstic acid (Bloom & Aghajanian, 1968), or bismuth–iodine impregnation followed by uranyl acetate and lead (Pfenninger et al., 1969). The paramembranous components of the active zone can be isolated and studied in detail with these selective staining techniques. Using such approaches, the presynaptic specialization at *Aplysia* synapses can be seen to consist of a series of small, truncated dense projections that probably represent a condensed form of the filamentous material present near the active zone membrane in conventionally fixed material (Bailey, Kandel, & Chen, 1981). En face views at the level of the presynaptic membrane reveal oval-shaped plaques that vary in size. Within these areas, discrete dense projections can exist in a regular hexagonal lattice suggesting some similarities to the coherent networks described for the presynaptic grid in vertebrates (Figure 12.3). By contrast, the postsynaptic specialization at the majority of *Aplysia* synapses is much less developed and appears as a fairly continuous, electron-dense sheet.

Based on these morphological studies, the central synapses of *Aplysia* appear to have clearly differentiated transmitter release sites whose organization can be similar to that described in other species. Our next goal was to determine what effect, if any, long-term memory might have on the structure of these specialized regions of the synapse.

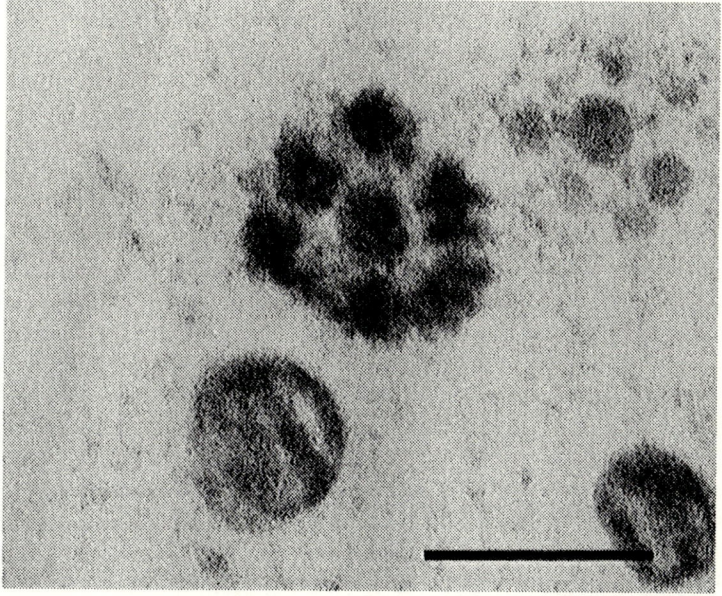

FIGURE 12.3. Three-dimensional organization of the presynaptic active zone at *Aplysia* synapses. Selective staining techniques such as E-PTA can reveal in detail the paramembranous components of the active zone. This en face view of the presynaptic area—a section taken parallel to the synaptic cleft and viewed from above—reveals a precise hexagonal array of discrete dense projections. This organization is similar to the presynaptic grid described in some vertebrate synapses. Scale = 0.25 µm. (From Bailey, Kandel, & Chen, 1981)

THE MEMORY FOR LONG-TERM SENSITIZATION IN *APLYSIA* HAS A SPECIFIC SYNAPTIC LOCUS

Learning and memory are probably universal features of the nervous system and most animals appear to be capable of at least elementary forms of learning (Thorpe, 1956). Many simple forms of learning first described in mammals, such as habituation, sensitization, and classical conditioning, have now been shown to be formally similar in a number of invertebrates. This observation suggests that the mechanisms that underlie the learning process may share common features across species (Kandel, 1976).

In recent years, this realization has encouraged the use of several higher invertebrate preparations where the advantages of a tractable central nervous system and identified neurons have facilitated the study of learning and memory at the cellular and molecular level. One such model system has been the gill- and siphon-withdrawal reflex of *Aplysia*. In *Aplysia*, as is the case in other molluscs, the mantle cavity, a respiratory chamber housing the gill, is covered by a protective sheet, the mantle shelf, that terminates in a fleshy spout, the siphon. When the siphon or mantle shelf is stimulated by light touch, the siphon, mantle shelf, and underlying gill all contract vigorously and withdraw into the mantle cavity. This reflex is analogous to vertebrate defensive escape and withdrawal responses and like them can be modified by several types of nonassociative and associative learning. Two elementary forms of nonassociative learning in *Aplysia* are habituation and sensitization, each capable of giving rise to a short-term memory lasting minutes to hours (Carew, Castellucci, & Kandel, 1971; Pinsker, Kupfermann, Castellucci, & Kandel, 1970) and a long-term memory that persists for several weeks (Carew, Pinsker, & Kandel, 1972; Frost, Castellucci, Hawkins, & Kandel, 1985; Pinsker, Hening, Carew, & Kandel, 1973).

Habituation is the most elementary and ubiquitous form of nonassociative learning by which an animal learns about the properties of a single, innocuous stimulus. When a weak tactile stimulus is first presented to the siphon in *Aplysia*, the animal will initially respond with a brisk withdrawal of the gill and siphon, but with repeated stimulation, the animal learns to ignore the stimulus and gives a progressively weaker response to it because it has lost novelty or importance.

Sensitization is a slightly more complex form of nonassociative learning by which an animal learns about the properties of a single, noxious stimulus. The animal learns to strengthen its defensive reflexes and to respond vigorously to a variety of previously neutral or indifferent stimuli after it has been exposed to a potentially threatening or noxious stimulus. A single strong stimulus applied to the head or tail of the animal produces short-term sensitization that lasts for several minutes to greater than 1 h (Pinsker et al., 1970). Repeated training trials result in a memory that can persist from days to weeks (Frost et al., 1985; Pinsker et al., 1973). Whereas habituation requires that the animal learns to ignore a particular stimulus because its consequences are innocuous or trivial, sensitization requires the animal to learn to attend to that stimulus because it is potentially accompanied by painful or dangerous consequences.

Among the many advantages of the invertebrate brain for analyzing the mechanisms that underlie learning and memory is a greatly reduced cell number and the presence of large, invariant, identified nerve cells. In *Aplysia*, for example, certain elementary behaviors that can be modified by learning may use fewer than 100 cells. This neural parsimony makes it possible to delineate in detail the wiring diagram of the behavior and thus to pinpoint the contribution of individual nerve cells to the behavior in which they participate. Using behavioral and cell biological techniques, Eric Kandel and his colleagues have exploited this reductionist approach to analyze the neuronal circuit responsible for the gill- and siphon-withdrawal reflex. A particularly well studied component of this reflex is the monosynaptic connection between mechanoreceptor sensory neurons that innervate the siphon skin and motor neurons that supply the gill and the siphon. There are six motor cells to the gill, which receive information from the siphon skin by means of 24 sensory neurons and several excitatory and inhibitory interneurons. Stimulating the skin activates the sensory neurons, which make direct connections to the interneurons and to the motor cells; the motor cells connect directly to muscle, causing contraction.

The simplicity of the monosynaptic component of the reflex has allowed reduction of the analysis of the memory for both habituation and sensitization to the cellular and molecular levels. Several aspects of the biophysical and biochemical mechanisms that underlie both habituation and sensitization are understood and involve changes in synaptic effectiveness produced by modulation of the calcium current at this critical locus: the synapses made by the identified mechanoreceptor sensory neurons onto their follower cells. Short-term habituation results from a homosynaptic depression in the number of transmitter quanta released per impulse from sensory neuron terminals (Castellucci & Kandel, 1974) and is due to a reduced Ca^{2+} influx (Klein & Kandel, 1980). Short-term sensitization is produced when a noxious stimulus is applied to the neck or tail of *Aplysia*. This activates facilitating neurons that act in a heterosynaptic fashion by releasing their transmitter onto the presynaptic terminals of the sensory neuron to enhance transmitter release. Based on extensive electrophysiological, voltage clamp, patch clamp, and biochemical experiments, the Kandel group has suggested a very specific molecular model for the presynaptic facilitation that underlies sensitization (Kandel & Schwartz, 1982). According to this model, serotonin, and other transmitters released by the facilitatory neurons, activate a transmitter-sensitive adenylate cyclase in the membrane of the presynaptic terminals of the sensory neurons that increases the cyclic AMP content within the terminals. Cyclic AMP then activates a protein kinase that phosphorylates a family of substrate proteins. One of these is a K^+ channel protein or a protein that is associated with it (Shuster, Camardo, Siegelbaum, & Kandel,

1985). The phosphorylation reduces the K^+ current that normally contributes significantly to the repolarization of the action potential. Reduction of this K^+ current prolongs the action potential and allows more Ca^{2+} to flow into the terminals and more transmitter is released (Castellucci et al., 1980; Klein & Kandel, 1978; Siegelbaum, Camardo, & Kandel, 1982). In addition, protein phosphorylation modulates the buffering of Ca^{2+} within the cell, which in turn can increase the amount of transmitter available for release (Hochner, Klein, Schacher, & Kandel, 1986). Biophysical studies have indicated that the same synaptic loci are involved in the storage of the long-term memories for both habituation and sensitization and are reflected by a prolonged alteration in the strength of the sensory-to-follower cell connection following long-term training (Castellucci, Carew, & Kandel, 1978; Frost et al., 1985).

MORPHOLOGICAL ASPECTS OF SYNAPTIC PLASTICITY IN *APLYSIA*: AN ANATOMICAL BASIS FOR LEARNING AND MEMORY

Although several aspects of the biophysical and biochemical changes are now particularly well understood, less is known about the morphological mechanisms that underlie habituation and sensitization and the role that structural alterations at identified sensory neuron synapses may play in mediating the transition of their short-term form to one of longer duration. Toward this end, we have developed a variety of cell marking and quantitative techniques for studying the morphological basis of synaptic transmission, with the idea of relating synaptic structure to behavior. Since the short- and long-term forms of habituation and sensitization in *Aplysia* share a common locus of plasticity—the synapses between identified sensory neurons and follower cells—this simple behavioral system offers a unique opportunity to explore the structural basis of both forms of learning and memory with a realistic hope of comparing them at the mechanistic level (Bailey & Kandel, 1985). For example, one can begin to consider a family of related questions that are central to the study of learning: How does the short-term form of memory relate to the long-term form? What are the mechanisms of memory storage? Can they be specified in morphological and molecular terms? Do they reflect different processes or progressive modifications using extensions of the same mechanism?

We have begun to address these issues and their structural corollaries by examining the nature, extent, and time course of the morphological changes at identified sensory neuron synapses that underlie short- and long-term memory. We have identified the presynaptic terminals of sensory neurons by the intrasomatic injection of horseradish peroxidase (HRP) as originally described by Muller and McMahan (1976). With this technique, labeled sensory neuron profiles are easily distinguished from unlabeled neighboring elements while maintaining excellent overall preservation and good cellular spacing. Moreover, there is no obvious disruption of normal spatial relationships within the injected terminal. We have combined this selective labeling technique with the analysis of serial sections. With this approach it is possible to quantitatively study complete reconstructions of unequivocally labeled identified synapses from both control modified and behaviorally modified animals.

We shall begin by reviewing our initial ultrastructural studies of learning where we examined the effects of long-term training on the morphology of the active zone at identified sensory neuron synapses (Bailey & Chen, 1983). Three groups of animals were used in this study: control (untrained animals) and animals trained for either long-term habituation or sensitization (Carew et al., 1972; Pinsker et al., 1973). The behavioral memory for both tasks is retained for several weeks. To examine in detail the fine structure of the synaptic terminals of injected cells, a total of 14 sensory neurons from 6 animals was analyzed through a blind procedure. We completely reconstructed over 300 sensory neuron synapses, a task that required the collection of nearly 5,000 thin sections and the quantitative analysis of over 12,000 HRP-labeled profiles.

We first examined the incidence of active zones at sensory neuron varicosities of control and experimental animals (Figure 12.4). Two aspects of this survey proved surprising. The first was that only 41% of the varicosities in control animals had an active zone. At the time this observation seemed somewhat puzzling; however, in the context of what is now known about silent but recruitable synapses, it seems less so (Atwood, Dixon, & Wojtowicz, 1989; Atwood & Govind, 1990; Redman, 1990). The second was that long-term behavioral training actually modulated the frequency of active zones, decreasing them to 12% in habituated animals and increasing them to 65% in sensitized animals.

A parallel trend was observed when we examined the total surface membrane area of completely reconstructed sensory neuron active zones and the total number of vesicles associated with each release site in the three behavioral groups. These values were smaller in habituated animals compared with controls and larger in sensitized animals.

Our results indicated that clear morphological changes could accompany long-term memory in *Aplysia* and demonstrated, for the first time, that these alterations could be detected at the level of those identified synapses that were known to be critically involved in the behavior. In addition, this study provided experimental support for a fundamental notion—that active zones might be plastic rather than immutable components of the synapse and in particular that these specialized sites could be modified by learning and memory. In an attempt to delineate the limits of this synaptic remodeling that accompanied long-term memory, we exploited a slightly different experimental approach.

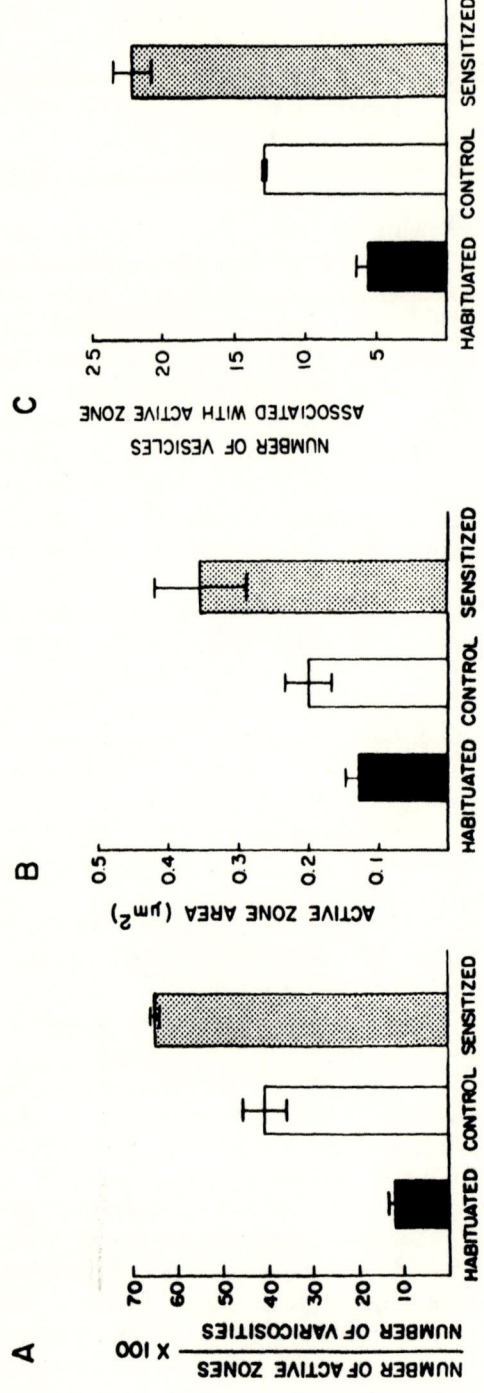

FIGURE 12.4. Effects of long-term memory on active zone morphology at identified sensory neuron synapses. (A) Incidence of active zones; (B) active zone area; (C) vesicle complement. Each bar represents the mean score of two animals ± SEM in each behavioral group. (Data taken from Bailey & Chen, 1983; figure from Bailey & Kandel, 1985)

LONG-TERM SENSITIZATION IS ACCOMPANIED BY AN INCREASE IN THE NUMBER OF SENSORY NEURON SYNAPSES

An additional possibility that we could not rule out at the time of our initial ultrastructural study was that long-term behavioral modifications might also produce a change in the number of varicosities per sensory neuron. To address this question directly, we have quantitatively analyzed the total axonal arbor of single HRP-labeled sensory neurons from control and long-term habituated and sensitized animals (Bailey & Chen, 1988a). The results of this study examining the effects of long-term memory on synapse number are illustrated in Figure 12.5 and reveal a trend similar to that described above for active zone morphology but expressed here in an even more dramatic and global fashion since it appears to involve a modulation of the total synaptic field of each sensory neuron. Sensory neurons from control animals had on average 1300 varicose expansions per sensory neuron. This number was reduced to approximately 840 varicosities per sensory neuron in long-term habituated animals and increased to 2700 in long-term sensitized animals. Figure 12.6 illustrates the positive correlation between these changes in the total number of varicosities per sensory neuron and long-term training. The statistical correlation between these structural changes and the differences in the degree of behavioral efficacy exposed by two different experimental manipulations supports the notion that changes in the number of sensory neuron varicosities may contribute to the persistent synaptic plasticity that underlies both long-term habituation and sensitization.

In addition to changes in the total number of presynaptic varicosities, sensory neurons from long-term sensitized animals demonstrate additional evidence of growth, that is, they display enlarged neuropil arbors (Figure 12.7). Quantitative analysis of completely reconstructed cells indicates that the total linear extent of the central axonal tree of sensory neurons from sensitized animals is 2.7 times greater than that from controls.

In an attempt to determine which of these anatomical changes at sensory neuron synapses are required for the onset of long-term sensitization and which are necessary for its maintenance, we have examined the temporal relationship between each class of morphological alteration and the behavioral duration of the memory (Bailey & Chen, 1989a and b). Toward this end we have quantitated differences in the total number of varicosities and their active zone morphology in single-HRP labeled sensory neurons taken from both control and long-term sensitized animals but now examined at different intervals following the completion of the training protocol (Figure 12.8). Our results suggest that not all of the structural changes last as long as the memory. The increases in both the size and vesicle complement of sensory neuron active zones, present 24–48 h following the completion of training do not persist as long as the behavioral signs of long-term sensitization and are back to control levels when tested 1 week later (Figure 12.9). These data indicate that insofar as modulation of active zone size and associated vesicles is one of the structural mechanisms underlying long-term sensitiz-

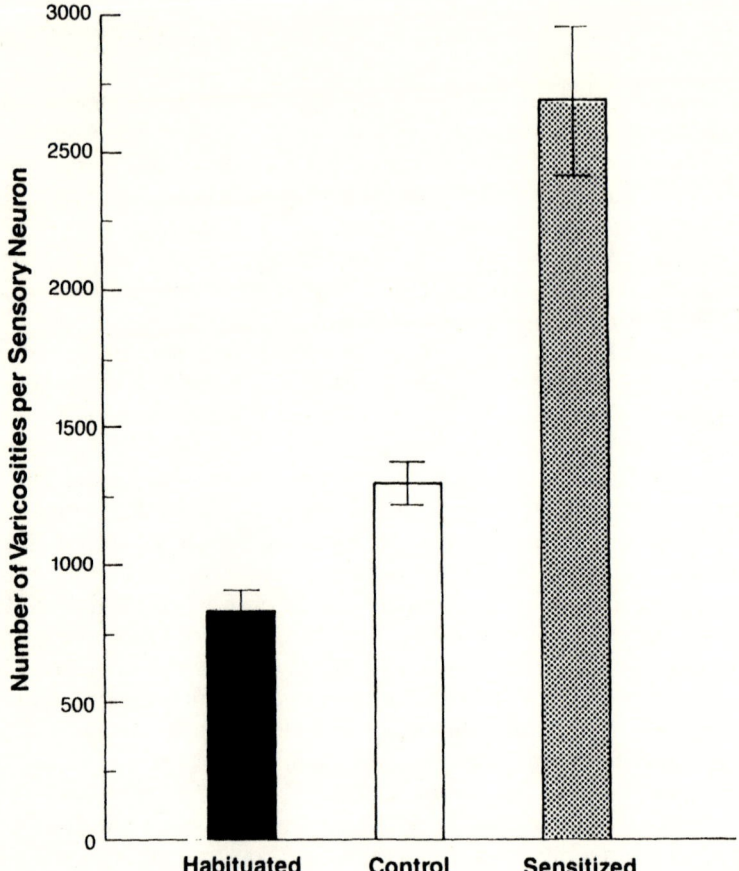

FIGURE 12.5.   Effects of long-term memory on synapse number. The total number of varicosities per sensory neuron in control and long-term behaviorally modified animals is shown. Each bar represents the mean ± SEM. Control groups from both experiments were not significantly different from one another and have been combined (1306 ± 82 varicosities, mean ± SEM, $n = 16$). The total number of varicosities per sensory neuron from each group was as follows: for long-term habituation animals, 836 ± 675 varicosities (mean ± SEM, $n = 10$), and for their controls, 1291 ± 138 varicosities (mean ± SEM, $n = 8$); and for long-term sensitized animals, 2697 ± 277 variocities (mean ± SEM, $n = 10$), and for their controls, 1320 ± 99 varicosities (mean ± SEM, $n = 8$). The mean number of varicosities for long-term habituated animals is significantly less than the mean for their controls ($t = 3.05$, $p < .01$), and the mean for long-term sensitized animals is significantly larger than the mean for their controls ($t = 4.25$, $p < .01$). (From Bailey & Chen, 1988a)

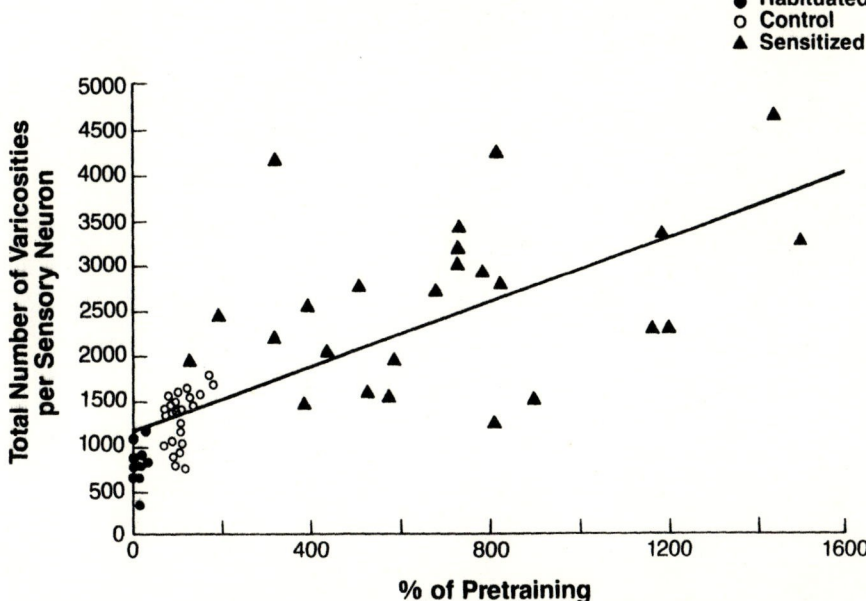

FIGURE 12.6. Correlation between changes in varicosity number and long-term memory. Data points represent animals trained for long-term habituation, long-term sensitization, and untrained (control) animals. Structural changes (total number of varicosities per sensory neuron) are plotted against changes in behavioral efficacy. The responses of each 10 trial session, 24–48 h following the completion of training, has been summed and expressed as a single median score compared with each animal's own pretraining score (Spearman's rank correlative coefficient 0.825, $p < .001$). (From Bailey & Chen, 1989a)

ation, it is associated with the acquisition and initial phases of stabilization of the long-term process and not to its persistence. By contrast, we have found that the duration of changes in varicosity and active zone number are the most enduring and that both persist unchanged for at least 1 week and are only partially reversed at the end of 3 weeks (Figure 12.10). The relative permanence of these changes in varicosity and active zone number and their similarity in duration to the behavioral time course of the memory suggest that an alteration in the number of sensory neuron synapses is the most likely of the structural candidates to contribute to the retention of long-term sensitization.

Additional support for this notion of synapse number changes during long-term memory comes from a recent study examining the effects of long-term sensitization on the structure of an identified postsynaptic target of the sensory neuron, the gill motor neuron L7 (Bailey & Chen, 1988b). This sensory to L7 connection is probably the most fully characterized synapse for the cellular changes that underlie both short- and long-term sensitization. By quantitatively analyzing serial sections of HRP-labeled L7 processes, we were able to determine the effects of long-term training on the organization

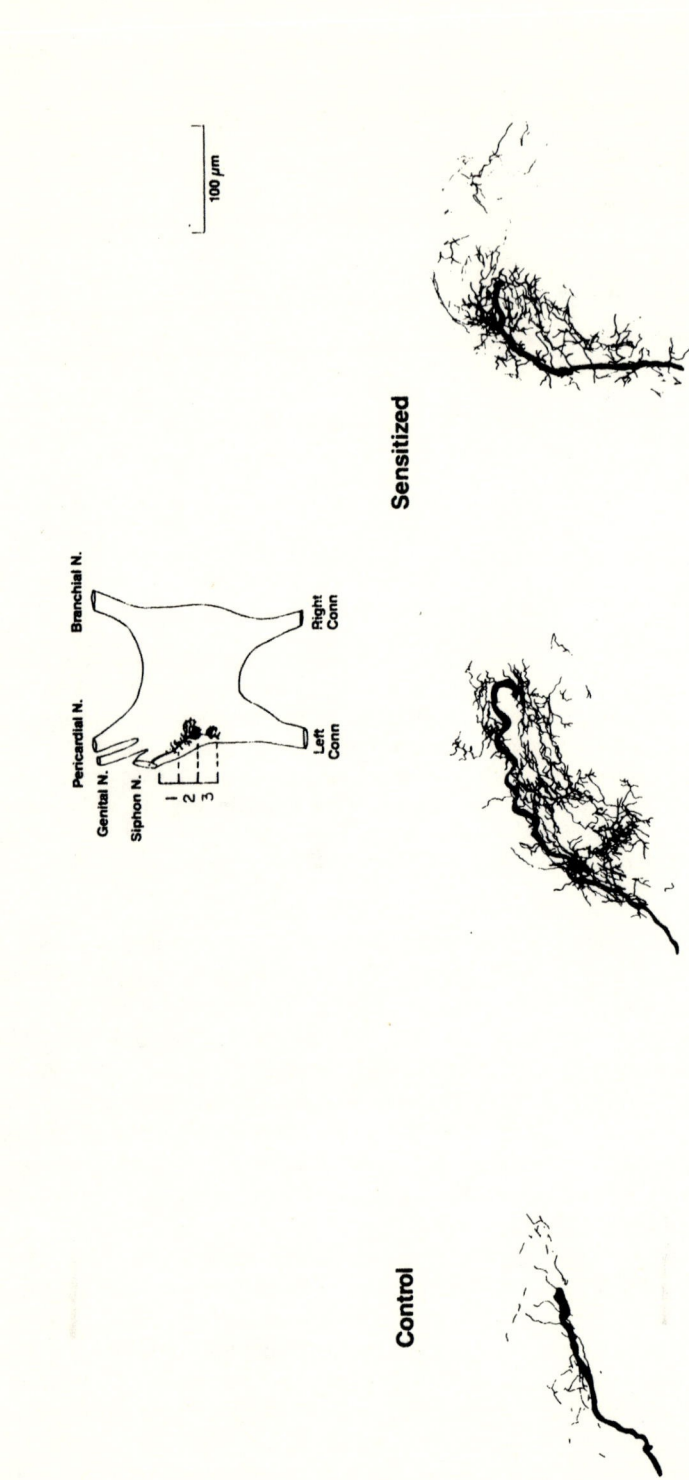

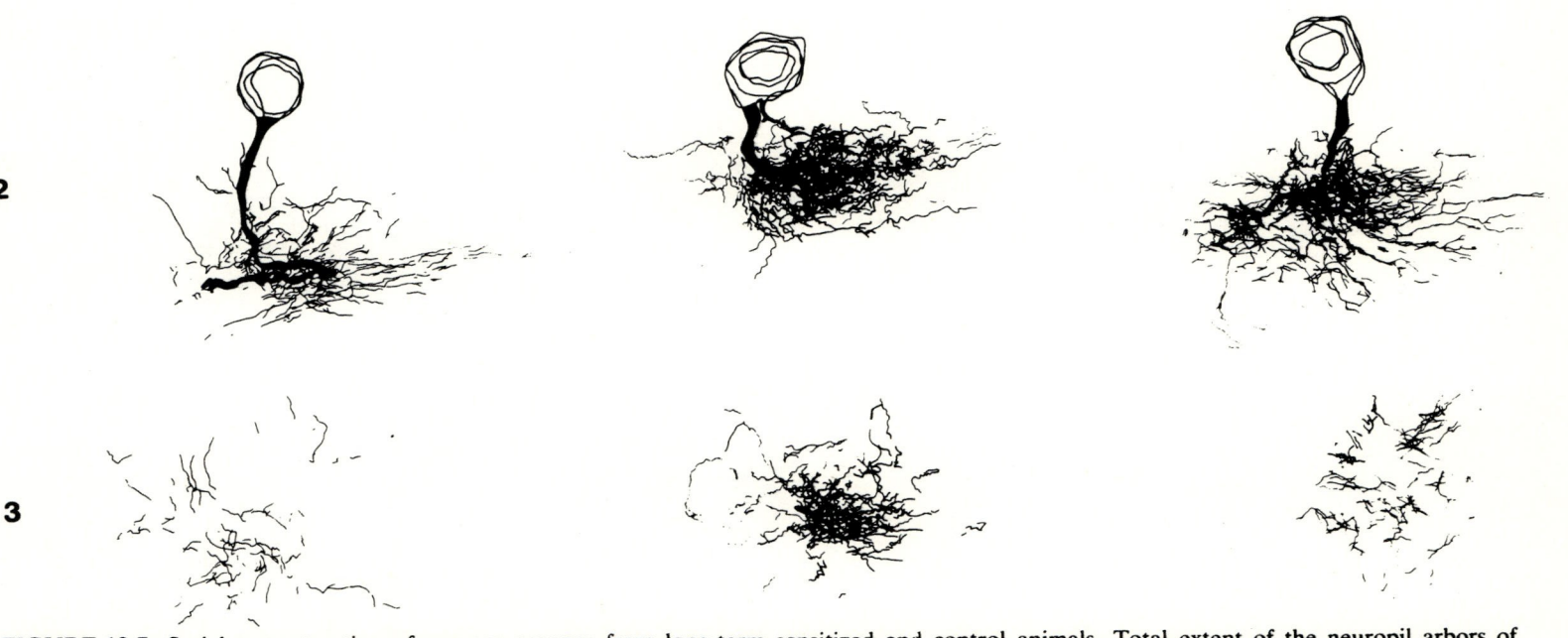

FIGURE 12.7. Serial reconstruction of sensory neurons from long-term sensitized and control animals. Total extent of the neuropil arbors of sensory neurons from one control and two long-term sensitized animals are shown. In each case the rostral (row 3) to caudal (row 1) extent of the arbor is divided roughly into thirds. Each panel was produced by the superimposition of camera-lucida tracings of all HRP-labeled processes present in 17 consecutive slab-thick sections and represents a linear segment through the ganglion of ~ 340 μm. For each composite, ventral is up, dorsal is down, lateral is to the left, and medial is to the right. By examining images across each row (rows 1,2, and 3), the viewer is comparing similar regions of each sensory neuron. In all cases, the arbor of long-term sensitized cells is markedly increased compared with the control. Quantitative estimates indicate that the total neuropil arbor of sensory neurons from long-term sensitized animals is 2.7 times greater in extent (22,254 ± 2415 μm; mean ± SEM, $n = 6$) than that from control animals (8415 ± 1640 μm; mean ± SEM, $n = 3$; $t = 3.746$; $p < .01$, two-tailed test). Siphon N., Genital N., etc., are various peripheral nerves of the abdominal ganglion; Left and Right Conn are left and right connectives, fiber tracts connecting the abdominal ganglion with other ganglia. (From Bailey & Chen, 1988a)

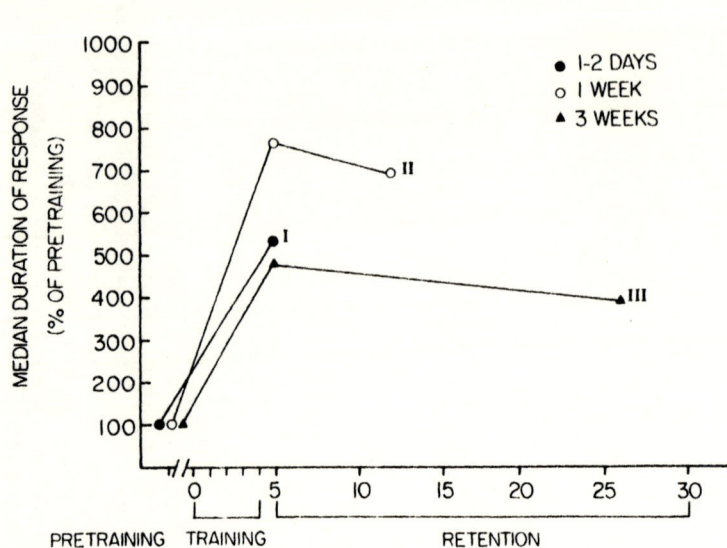

FIGURE 12.8. Behavioral time course of long-term sensitization. Retention of sensitization was tested at different intervals following the completion of 4 days of long-term training. Behavioral performance of animals in each group was estimated by comparing their behavioral scores with their pretraining scores. This was achieved by summing the responses for each daily session (10 trial block, intertrial interval 30 s) and expressing each as a single score compared with their own pretraining score. Animals in behavioral experiments were examined at 1–2 days (*I*, 529 ± 121 SEM, *n* = 6), 1 week (II, 700 ± 173, *n* = 4), and 3 weeks (III, 414 ±86, *n* = 5) following training and the structure of sensory neuron synapses in each group analyzed. (From Bailey & Chen, 1989a)

of the dendritic arbor of L7 and in particular on the extent of the synaptic input it receives. Our study revealed an increase in the frequency, size, and vesicle complement of presynaptic contact onto L7 processes in sensitized compared with control animals. Altogether these data suggest a striking increase in the percentage of the surface area of L7 that is occupied by synaptic contact following long-term training (Figure 12.11). The results from this study are consistent with our earlier observations that long-term sensitization produces an increase in the number of synapses that sensory neurons make on their follower cells and support the hypothesis of synapse formation as a mechanism underlying long-term memory. Detection of these increases following independent examination of both pre- and postsynaptic halves of the sensory to L7 connection strengthen the evidence that these morphological alterations can occur at the same synaptic loci where functional changes have been described following long-term sensitization and provide additional support for the notion that these changes share at least some specificity to the learning experience.

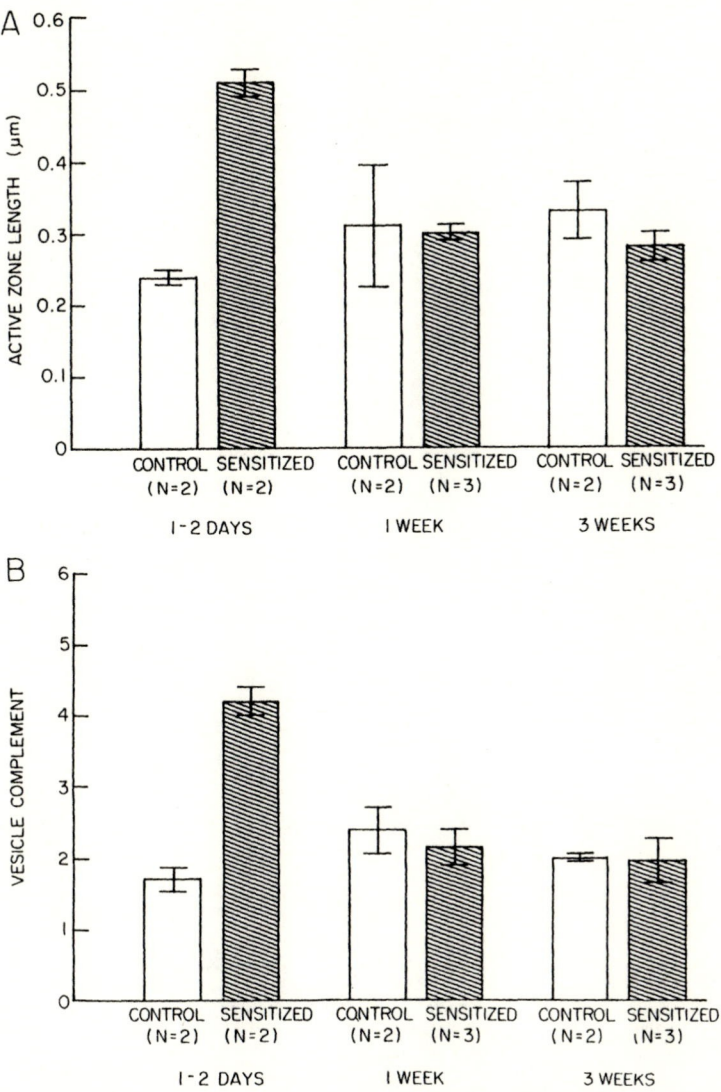

FIGURE 12.9. Transient structural changes at sensory neuron synapses during long-term sensitization. (A) Duration of changes in active zone size; (B) duration of changes in the vesicle complement of active zones. Unlike the changes in varicosity and active zone number, the increases in active zone size and associated vesicles per neuron peak at 1–2 days following the completion of training and then return to control levels at 1 week and 3 weeks, making them unlikely candidates to contribute to the maintenance of long-term sensitization. Each bar represents the mean ± SEM. (From Bailey & Chen, 1989a)

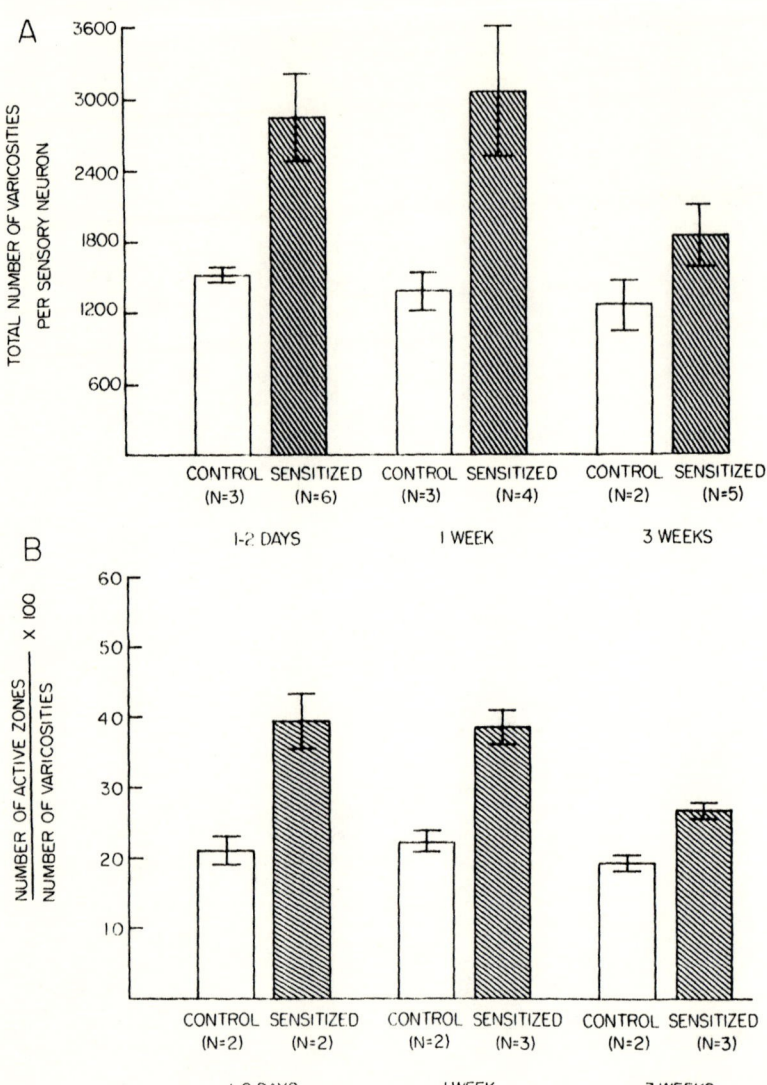

FIGURE 12.10. Enduring structural changes at sensory neuron synapses during long-term sensitization. (A) Duration of changes in the total number of varicosities per sensory neuron. (B) Duration of changes in the incidence of sensory neuron active zones. To determine which class of alterations in the functional architecture of identified sensory neuron synapses might underlie long-term sensitization, we have compared their duration to the persistence of the memory. By examining the structure of sensory neuron synapses at different intervals following the completion of training (1–2 days, 1 week, and 3 weeks) we have found that only the duration of changes in the number of varicosities and their active zones parallels the behavioral time course for the retention of long-term sensitization. Each bar represents the mean ± SEM. (From Bailey & Chen, 1989a)

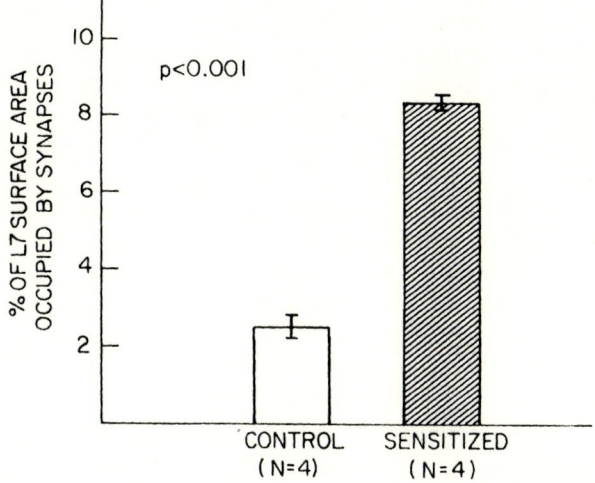

FIGURE 12.11. Percentage of the surface area of L7 that is occupied by presynaptic contacts in control and long-term sensitized animals. Long-term training increases both the frequency and size of presynaptic contacts onto L7 with a resultant increase in the percentage of L7's receptive surface that is occupied by synaptic contact. Each bar represents the mean ± SEM. (From Bailey & Chen, 1988b)

THE NATURE OF LONG-TERM MEMORY: A MORPHOLOGICAL PERSPECTIVE

During the last decade, it has become increasingly apparent that the mature central nervous system of both vertebrates and invertebrates is endowed with a remarkable capacity for structural plasticity. This striking ability to modify its anatomical circuitry can occur with normal functioning (Purves & Voyvodic, 1985) or with learning (Greenough & Bailey, 1988). Thus, changes in environmental complexity, social structure, or training in the intact animal (Bailey & Chen, 1983; Bailey & Chen, 1988a; Bennett, Diamond, Krech, & Rosenzweig, 1964; Greenough, Juraska, & Volkmar, 1979; Greenough & Volkmar, 1973; Stewart, 1990; Turner & Greenough, 1985;Vrensen & Nunes Cardozo, 1981) as well as electrical stimulation in vitro (Bailey & Chen, 1988c; Chang & Greenough, 1984) and in vivo (Fifkova & van Harreveld, 1977; Lee, Schottler, Oliver, & Lynch 1980; Lnenicka, Atwood, & Marin, 1986) have been shown to alter both the number of synapses and their structure. Determining the relevance of this synaptic remodeling within a neuronal circuit to the information encoded and processed during a specific behavioral modification is not a trivial issue. In fact, the functional role such structural changes may play during learning and memory has been a question central to the modern study of behavior but one that has been difficult to address in the more complex nervous systems of vertebrates where the contribution of individual synapses to the learning process is not yet well defined.

To bridge this gap, the more tractable nervous systems of several higher invertebrates have proven useful for the cellular and molecular analysis of learning. One such model system, the gill- and siphon-withdrawal reflex in *Aplysia*, has been particularly advantageous for examining the specific synaptic loci and mechanisms that underlie learning and memory. This reflex undergoes two simple types of nonassociative learning, habituation and sensitization, both of which can exist in a short-term form lasting minutes to hours and a long-term form that persists for more than 3 weeks. Since aspects of the memory for both habituation and sensitization can be trapped at specific synaptic locus—the connections between identified mechanoreceptor sensory neurons and their target cells—we have been able to analyze in a set of identified neurons that are causally related to the behavior, the mechanisms underlying the acquisition and retention of a long-term memory trace.

Our results indicate that learning in *Aplysia* produces morphological as well as functional changes at specific synaptic loci. Long-term memory (lasting several weeks) is accompanied by a family of alterations at identified sensory neuron synapses. These changes reflect structurally detectable modifications at two different levels of synaptic organization: (a) alterations in focal regions of membrane specialization—the number, size, and vesicle complement of sensory neuron active zones are larger in sensitized animals than controls, and smaller in habituated animals; and (b) a parallel but more pronounced and global trend involving modulation of the total number of presynaptic varicosities per sensory neuron. By examining animals at different intervals following the completion of training, we have been able to compare directly the duration of these structural changes at sensory neuron synapses with the persistence of memory. This approach has allowed us to distinguish between transient and more permanent effects and thereby to determine which class of structural alterations at the synapse might underlie long-term memory rather than being a stage in its development or a byproduct of its formation. Quantitative analysis of the time course over which these anatomical changes occur during long-term sensitization has demonstrated that only alterations in the number of sensory neuron synapses persist in parallel with the behavioral retention of the memory. These results directly link a change in synaptic structure to a long-lasting behavioral memory. Moreover, these findings indicate that individual presynaptic varicosities and their active zones are not immutable components of the nervous system and suggest that even relatively simple learning experiences such as the acquisition of habituation and sensitization can modulate aspects of synaptic strucure to alter the functional expression of neural connections. Such morphological changes could represent an anatomical substrate for memory consolidation.

In contrast to these extensive anatomical changes following long-term training, the morphological correlates of short-term memory in *Aplysia* (lasting minutes to hours rather than days to weeks) are far less pronounced and are restricted to shifts in the proximity of synaptic vesicle populations contiguous to sensory neuron active zones (Bailey & Chen, 1988c). Altogether these studies begin to suggest a clear difference in the sequelae of structural events that may underlie memories of differing durations. The transient durations of short-term memories probably involve the covalent modification of pre-existing proteins (proteins that turn over slowly) and, at least in *Aplysia*, are accompanied by modest structural rearrangements in the vicinity of the active zone such as the translocation of synaptic vesicles near the release site. The mechanisms underlying the more prolonged durations of long-term memories are probably dependent on new macromolecular synthesis and are accompanied by more substantial and potentially more enduring structural alterations that are reflected by changes in both the number of synaptic contacts and their active zone morphology.

Each mechanoreceptor sensory neuron in *Aplysia* appears to possess a marked capacity for behaviorally relevant structural plasticity that is differentially expressed depending on the type of long-term training it receives (Figure 12.12). The persistent depression that accompanies long-term habituation is reflected not only by a decrease in the total number of synaptic varicosities but also by a reduction in the incidence and extent of their active zones. In contrast, the morphological changes that accompany long-term facilitation in *Aplysia* appear to involve an element of long-lasting growth resulting in a doubling in the total number of varicosities, an enlarged neuropil arbor, and an increase in the incidence of active zones. The nature and extent of these structural alterations at sensory neuron synapses are consistent with both the known behavioral efficacy of long-term habituation and sensitization in *Aplysia* (Carew et al.,1972; Pinsker et al., 1973) as well as with the results of physiological studies indicating a prolonged alteration in the strength of sensory-to-follower cell connections following long-term training (Castellucci et al., 1978; Frost et al., 1985).

The changes in the structure of transmitter release sites that we have observed at CNS synapses in *Aplysia* during learning and memory are consistent in many respects with the alterations in active zone morphology reported at the neuromuscular junction following various forms of experimental manipulation (Atwood et al., 1989; Atwood & Govind, 1990; Atwood & Marin, 1983; Chiang & Govind, 1986; Herrera, Grinnell, & Wolowski, 1985; Rheuben, 1985; Walrond & Reese, 1985). These peripheral synapses provide a remarkable diversity of performance and are particularly accessible for morphometric comparison. Correlative studies of both invertebrate and vertebrate neuromuscular junctions now seem to indicate that changes in specific aspects of active zone structure may be critical indicators of changes in synaptic efficacy (for reviews see Atwood & Wojtowicz, 1986; Atwood & Lnenicka, 1986).

Finally, the increases in synapse number following long-term sensitization in *Aplysia* share striking similarities with reports in the vertebrate brain of alterations in the number and/or pattern of synaptic connections following

LONG - TERM HABITUATION

CONTROL

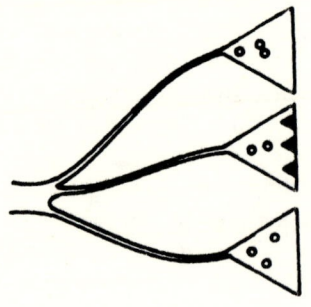

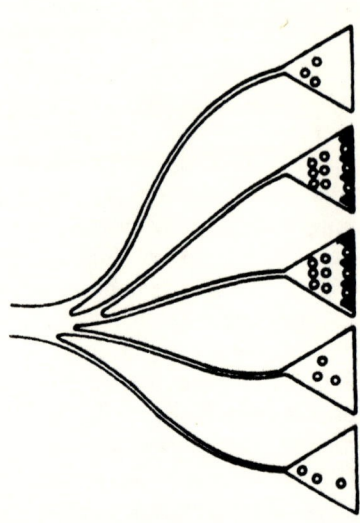

LONG - TERM SENSITIZATION

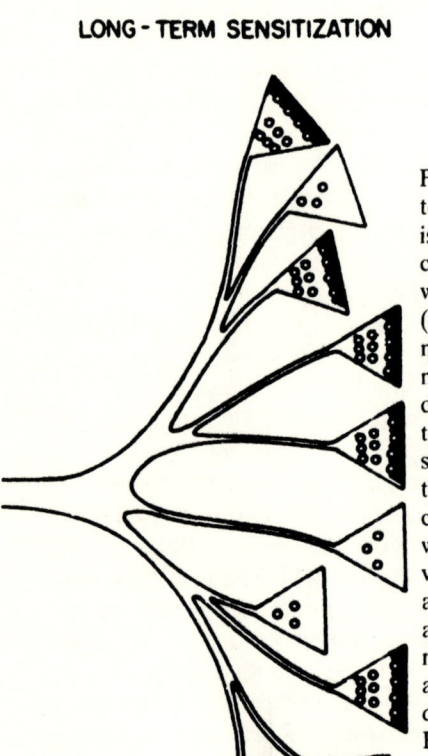

FIGURE 12.12. Morphological basis of long-term memory in *Aplysia*. Long-term memory is accompanied by a family of structural changes at identified sensory neuron synapses, which include a remodeling of the active zone (solid triangles) and modulation of the total number of presynaptic varicosities per sensory neuron. These morphological changes can be differentially expressed depending on which type of long-term training (habituation or sensitization) is employed. Habituation leads to a decrease in the number, size, and vesicle complement of sensory neuron active zones as well as a reduction in the total number of varicosities. By contrast, sensitization involves a near doubling in the number of varicosities as well as an increase in active zone morphology. Only the changes in active zone and varicosity number seem to persist for the duration of the behavioral memory. (From Bailey & Chen, 1988a)

environmental manipulation and training (for reviews see Greenough, 1984; Greenough & Chang, 1985). Although the specific role that these structural changes at the synapse may play in learning and memory is still not known, the increased convergence of behavioral, molecular, and morphological approaches has begun to suggest some mechanistic candidates. One important clue comes from the results of studies in both vertebrates and invertebrates, which indicate that the consolidation of long-term memory is likely to depend on new protein and RNA synthesis (Davis & Squire, 1984; Montarolo et al., 1986). In order to appreciate fully how these newly synthesized proteins might contribute to the stabilization of a long-term memory trace, one is forced to consider the ample body of evidence that now associates structural changes in synapses with learning. For example, in *Aplysia* at least some of the newly synthesized proteins induced during the training for long-term sensitization presumably must lead not only to functional alterations but must also contribute to the potentially more enduring structural changes—growth of synaptic contacts—that occur in the sensory neurons.

In an attempt to determine the specific gene products that underlie the acquisition of long-term sensitization, Barzilai, Kennedy, Sweatt, and Kandel (1989) have studied the incorporation of labeled amino acids (^{35}S-methionine) into proteins in the sensory neurons. They have found that long-term training initiates a large increase in overall protein synthesis. Moreover, beyond these overall effects, long-term training also produces a set of changes in specific proteins that could be resolved on two-dimensional gels. These changes include rapid and transient alterations in the expression of 15 proteins, perhaps suggestiing the possibility of a gene cascade, as well as a sustained increase in the expression of two proteins that persists for the maintenance phase of the long-term memory (Castellucci, Kennedy, Kandel & Goelet, 1988). The structural changes at sensory neuron synapses are likely to require the increased expression of a substantial number of such late effector proteins (Kandel, 1989).

Some additional insights into the nature of the signaling mechanisms that may underlie these structural changes have come from two recent studies in *Aplysia*. The first is work by Glanzman, Kandel, and Schacher (1990) using dissociated cell cocultures of sensory neurons and the gill motor neuron L7. They have found that repeated exposure to the facilitating transmitter serotonin produces a long-term enhancement in the amplitude or the sensory-to-motor cell excitatory postsynaptic potential (EPSP) as well as a long-lasting increase in the number of sensory neuron varicosities. Moreover, this increase in varicosity number depends on the presence of the motor cell. Sensory neurons that are plated alone do not exhibit long-lasting growth in response to serotonin suggesting a role for the postsynaptic neuron in these structural changes. A second macromolecular candidate for the structural changes in sensory neurons seen following long-term training comes from the studies of Nazif, Byrne, and Cleary (1989). They have shown that the injection of cyclic AMP into pleural sensory neurons is sufficient to mimic the increase in varicosity number and enlarged neuropil arbor that accompany long-term sensitization. Combined results of both of these studies begin to clarify the nature of the cytoplasmic signals that are involved in the flow of information from membrane receptors to the genome during learning and clearly implicate a role for serotonin and the cyclic AMP cascade in the structural changes that accompany long-term sensitization. These studies have recently been extended by the Kandel group, which now reports that learning-related structural changes in *Aplysia* are also accompanied by transmitter mediated changes in cell adhesion molecules (see Bailey, Chen, Keller, & Kaudel, 1991).

Whatever the underlying molecular mechanisms turn out to be, the increasing body of anatomical evidence, emanating initially from studies on mammalian development and more recently embodying results from studies on nonmammalian vertebrates as well as higher invertebrates, strongly suggests a role for synaptic structural plasticity during learning and memory. The morphological correspondence between the invertebrate and vertebrate studies indicates that learning may resemble a process of neuronal growth and differentiation across a broad segment of the animal kingdom and suggests that experience-dependent synapse formation may be a highly conserved feature accompanying long-lasting behavioral memory.

Acknowledgments: This work was supported by Grant MH37134 from the National Institutes of Health, GM32099 from the National Institutes of Health and the McKnight Endowment Fund for Neuroscience.

REFERENCES

Alkon, D.L. (1984). Calcium-mediated reduction of ionic currents: A biophysical memory trace. *Science, 226,* 1037–1045.

Atwood, H.L., Dixon, D., & Wojtowicz, J.H. (1989). Rapid introduction of long-lasting synaptic changes at crustacean neuromuscular junctions. *Journal of Neurobiology, 20,* 373–385.

Atwood, H.L., & Govind, C.K. (1990). Activity-dependent and age-dependent recruitment and regulation of synapses in identified crustacean neurons. *Journal of Experimental Biology, 153,* 105–127.

Atwood,H.L., & Lnenicka, G.A. (1986). Structure and function in synapses: Emerging correlations. *Trends in Neuroscience, 9,* 248–250.

Atwood, H.L., & Marin, L. (1983). Ultrastructure of synapses with different transmitter-releasing characteristics on motor axon terminals of a crab, *Hyas areneas. Cell and Tissue Research, 231,* 103–115.

Atwood, H.L., & Wojtowicz, J.M. (1986). Short-term and long-term plasticity and physiological differentiation of crustacean motor systems. *International Review of Neurobiology, 28,* 275–362.

Bailey, C.H., & Chen, M. (1983). Morphological basis of long-term habituation and sensitization in *Aplysia. Science, 220,* 91–93.

Bailey, C.H., & Chen, M. (1988a). Long-term memory in *Aplysia* modulates the total number of varicosities of single identified sensory neurons. *Proceedings of the National Academy of Sciences, U.S.A., 85*, 2373–2377.

Bailey, C.H., & Chen, M. (1988b). Long-term sensitization in *Aplysia* increases the number of presynaptic contacts onto the identified gill motor neuron L7. *Proceedings of the National Academy of Sciences, U.S.A., 85*, 9356–9359.

Bailey, C.H., & Chen, M. (1988c). Morphological basis of short-term habituation in *Aplysia. Journal of Neuroscience, 8*, 2452–2459.

Bailey, C.H., & Chen, M. (1989a). Time course of structural changes at identified sensory neuron synapses during long-term sensitization in *Aplysia. Journal of Neuroscience, 9*(5), 1774–1780.

Bailey, C.H., & Chen, M. (1989b). Onset of structural changes at identified sensory neuron synapses and the acquisitions of long-term sensitization in *Aplysia*. Society for Neuroscience Abstracts, *15*, 1285.

Bailey, C.H., Chen, M., Keller, F., & Kandel, E. K. (1991). Early steps in learning-related synaptic growth: 5-HT induces endocytic activation and internalization of N-CAM related cell adhesion molecules in *Aplysia*. Society for Neuroscience Abstracts, *17* (in press).

Bailey, C.H., & Kandel, E.R. (1985). Molecular approaches to the study of short- and long-term memory. In C.W. Coen (Ed.), *Functions of the Brain* (pp. 98–129). New York: Clarendon Press.

Bailey, C.H., Kandel, P., & Chen, M. (1981). The active zone at *Aplysia* synapses: Organization of presynaptic dense projection. *Journal of Neurophysiology, 46*, 356–368.

Bailey, C.H., Thompson, E.B., Castellucci, V.F., & Kandel, E.R. (1979). Ultrastructure of the synapses of sensory neurons that mediate the gill-withdrawal reflex in *Aplysia. Journal of Neurocytology, 8*, 415–444.

Barzilai, A., Kennedy, T.E., Sweatt, J.D., & Kandel, E.R. (1989). 5-HT modulates protein synthesis and the expression of specific proteins during long-term facilitation in *Aplysia* sensory neurons. *Neuron, 2*, 1577–1586.

Bennett, E.L., Diamond, M.C., Krech, D., & Rosenzweig, M.R. (1964). Chemical and anatomical plasticity of brain. *Science, 146*, 610–619.

Bloom, F.E., & Aghajanian, G.K. (1968). Fine structural and cytochemical analysis of the staining of synaptic junctions with phosphotungstic acid. *Journal of Ultrastructural Research, 22*, 361–375.

Byrne, J.H. (1987). Cellular analysis of associative leaning. *Physiological Review, 67*, 329–439.

Cajal, S.R. (1894). La fine structure des centres nerveux. *Proceedings of the Royal Society, London, 55*, 444–468.

Carew, T.J., Castellucci, V.F., & Kandel, E.R. (1971). An analysis of dishabituation and sensitization of the gill-withdrawal reflex in *Aplysia. International Journal of Neuroscience, 2*, 79–98.

Carew, T.J., Pinsker, H.M., & Kandel, E.R. (1972). Long-term habituation of a defensive withdrawal reflex in *Aplysia. Science, 175*, 451–454.

Castellucci, V.F., Carew, T.J., & Kandel, E.R. (1978). Cellular analysis of long-term habituation of the gill-withdrawal reflex of *Aplysia californica. Science, 202*, 1306–1308.

Castellucci, V.F., & Kandel, E.R. (1974). A quantal analysis of the synaptic depression underlying habituation of the gill-withdrawal reflex in *Aplysia. Proceedings of the National Academy of Sciences, U.S.A., 71*, 5004–5008.

Castellucci, V.F., Kandel, E.R., Schwartz, J.H., Wilson, F.D., Nairn, A.C., & Greengard, P. (1980). Intracellular injection of the catalytic subunit of cyclic AMP-dependent protein kinase simulates facilitation of transmitter release underlying behavioral sensitization in *Aplysia. Proceedings of the National Academy of Sciences, U.S.A., 77*, 7492–7496.

Castellucci, V.F., Kennedy, T.E., Kandel, E.R., & Goelet, P. (1988). A quantitative analysis of 2-D gels identifies proteins in which labeling is increased following long-term sensitization in *Aplysia*. *Neuron, 1*, 321–328.

Chang, F.F., & Greenough, W.T. (1984). Transient and enduring morphological correlates of synaptic activity and efficacy change in the rat hippocampal slice. *Brain Research, 309*, 35–46.

Chiang, R.G., & Govind, C.K. (1986). Reorganization of synaptic ultrastructure at facilitated lobster neuromuscular terminals. *Journal of Neurocytology, 15*, 63–74.

Coggeshall, R.E. (1967). A light and electron microscope study of the abdominal ganglion of *Aplysia californica*. *Journal of Neurophysiology, 30*, 1263–1287.

Couteaux, R., & Pecot-Dechavassine, M. (1970). Vesicules synaptiques et poches au niveau des zones actives de la jonction neuromusculaire. *C.R. Hebd. Séances Acad.Sci. Sér. D. Sci.–Nat., 271*, 2346–2349.

Davis, H.P., & Squire, L.R. (1984). Protein synthesis and memory: A review. *Psychological Bulletin, 96*, 518–559.

Fifkova, E., & van Harreveld, A. (1977). Long-lasting morphological changes in dendritic spines of dentate granular cells following stimulation of the entorhinal area. *Journal of Neurocytology, 6*, 211–230.

Frost, W.N., Castellucci, V.F., Hawkins, R.D., & Kandel, E.R. (1985). Monosynaptic connections made by the sensory neurons of the gill- and siphon-withdrawal reflex in *Aplysia* participate in the storage of long-term memory for sensitization. *Proceedings of the National Academy of Sciences, U.S.A., 82*, 8266–269.

Glanzman, D.L., Kandel, E.R., & Schacher, S. (1990). Target-dependent structural changes accompanying long-term synaptic facilitation in *Aplysia* neurons. *Science. 249*, 799–802.

Gray, E.G. (1959). Axosomatic and axodendritic synapses of the cerebral cortex: An electron microscopic study. *Journal of Anatomy, 83*, 420–433.

Greenough, W.T. (1984). Structural correlates of information storage in the mammalian brain: A review and hypothesis. *Trends in Neuroscience, 7*, 229–233.

Greenough, W.T., & Bailey, C.H. (1988). The anatomy of memory: Convergence of results across a diversity of tests. *Trends in Neuroscience, 11*, 142–147.

Greenough, W.T., & Chang, R.-L.F. (1985). Synaptic structural correlates of information storage in mammalian nervous systems. In C.W. Cotman (Ed.), *Synaptic plasticity* (pp. 335–372). New York: Guilford Press.

Greenough, W.T., Juraska, J.M., & Volkmar, F.R. (1979). Maze training effects on dendritic branching in occipital cortex of adult rats. *Behavioral and Neural Biology, 26*, 287–297.

Greenough, W.T., & Volkmar, F.R. (1973). Pattern of dendritic branching in occipital cortex of rats reared in complex environments. *Experimental Neurology, 40*, 491–504.

Herrera, A.A., Grinnell, A.P., & Wolowske, B. (1985). Ultrastructural correlates of naturally occurring differences in transmitter release efficacy in frog motor nerve terminals. *Journal of Neurocytology, 14*, 193–202.

Heuser, J.E., Reese, T.S., Dennis, M.J., Jan, Y., Jan, L., & Evans, L. (1979). Synaptic vesicle exocytosis captured by quick freezing and correlated with quantal transmitter release. *Journal of Cell Biology, 81*, 275–300.

Hochner, B., Klein, M., Schacher, S., & Kandel, E.R. (1986). Additional components in the cellular mechanism of presynaptic facilitation contributes to behavioral dishabituation in *Aplysia*. *Proceedings of the National Academy of Sciences, U.S.A., 83*, 8794–8798.

Kandel, E.R. (1976). *Cellular basis of behavior: An introdction to behavioral neurobiology*. San Francisco: W.H. Freeman.

Kandel, E.R. (1989). Genes, nerve cells and the remembrance of things past. *Journal of Neuropsychiatry, 1*, 103–125.

Kandel, E.R., & Schwartz, J.H. (1982). Molecular biology of an elementary form of learning: Modulation of transmitter release by cyclic AMP. *Science, 218*, 433–443.

King, D.G. (1976). Organization of crustacean neuropil. I. Patterns of synaptic connections in lobster stomatogastric ganglion. *Journal of Neurocytology, 5*, 207–237.

Klein, M., & Kandel, E.R. (1978). Presynaptic modulation of voltage-dependent Ca^{++} current: Mechanism for behavioral sensitization in *Aplysia californica*. *Proceedings of the National Academy of Sciences, U.S.A., 75*(7), 3512–3516.

Klein, M., & Kandel, E.R. (1980). Mechanism of calcium current modulation underlying presynaptic facilitation and behavioral sensitization in *Aplysia*. *Proceedings of the National Academy of Sciences, U.S.A., 77*, 6912–6916.

Landis, D.M.D., Hall, A.K., Weinstein, L.A., & Reese, T.S. (1988). The organization of cytoplasm at the presynaptic active zone of a central nervous system synapse. *Neuron, 1*, 201–209.

Lee, K.S., Schottler, F., Oliver, M., Lynch, G. (1980). Brief bursts of high frequency stimulation produce two types of structural change in rat hippocampus. *Journal of Neurophysiology, 44*, 247–258.

Lnenicka, G.A., Atwood, H.L., & Marin, L. (1986). Morphological transformation of synaptic terminals of a phasic motor neuron by long-term stimulation. *Journal of Neuroscience, 6*, 2252–2258.

Lugaro, E. (1989). I recenti progressi dell' anatomia del sistema nervoso in rapporto alla psicologia ed alla psichiatria. *Riv. Patol. Nerv. Ment. tIV fasc.* 11–12.

Montarolo, P.G., Goelet, P., Castellucci, V.F., Morgan, J., Kandel, E.R., & Schacher, S. (1986). A critical period of macromolecular synthesis in long-term heterosynaptic facilitation in *Aplysia*. *Science, 234*, 1249–1254.

Muller, K.J., & McMahan, U.J. (1976). The shapes of sensory and motor neurons and the distribution of their synapses in ganglia of the leech: A study using intracellular injection of horseradish peroxidase. *Proceedings of the Royal Society, London, B194*, 481–499.

Nazif, F., Byrne, J.H., & Cleary, L.J. (1989). Intracellular injection of cAMP produces a long-term (24 hr) increase in the number of varicosities in pleural sensory neurons of *Aplysia*. *Society for Neuroscience Abstracts, 15*, 1283.

Palay, S.L. (1958). The morphology of synapses in the central nervous system. *Experimental Cell Research, 5*, 275–293.

Peters, A., Palay, S.L., & Webster, H.deF. (1976). *The fine structure of the nervous system. The neurons and supporting cells*. Philadelphia: Saunders.

Pfenninger, K., Sandri, C., Akert, K., & Eugster, C.H. (1969). Contribution to the problem of structural organization of the presynaptic area. *Brain Research, 12*, 10–18.

Pinsker, H.M., Hening, W.A., Carew, T.J., & Kandel, E.R. (1973). Long-term sensitization of a defensive withdrawal reflex in *Aplysia*. *Science, 182*, 1039–1042.

Pinsker, H.M., Kupfermann, I., Castellucci, V.F., & Kandel, E.R. (1970). Habituation and dishabituation of the gill-withdrawal reflex in *Aplysia*. *Science, 167*, 1740–1742.

Purves, D., & Voyvodic, J.T.(1987). Imaging mammalian nerve cells and their connections over time in living animals. *Trends in Neuroscience, 10*, 398–404.

Redman, S. (1990). Quantal analysis of synaptic potentials in neurons of the central nervous system. *Physiological Review, 70*(1), 165–198.

Rheuben, M.D. (1985). Quantitative comparison of the structural features of slow and fast neuromuscular junctions in *Manduca*. *Journal of Neuroscience, 5*, 1704–1716.

Shuster, M.J., Camardo, J.S., Siegelbaum, S.A., & Kandel, E.R. (1985). Cyclic-AMP-dependent protein kinase closes the serotonin-sensitive K^+ channels of *Aplysia* sensory neurons in cell-free membrane patches. *Nature, 313,* 392–395.

Siegelbaum, S.A., Camardo, J.S., & Kandel, E.R. (1982). Serotonin and cyclic AMP close single K^+ channels in *Aplysia* sensory neurons. *Nature, 299,* 413–417.

Stewart, M.G. (1990). Morphological correlates of long-term memory in the chick forebrain consequent on passive avoidance learning. In L.R. Squire & E. Lindenlaub (Ed.), *23rd Symposia Medicum Hoechst—The biology of memory* (pp. 193–215). Stuttgart: F.K. Shattauer.

Tanzi, E. (1893). I fatti e le induzioni nell' odierna istologia del sistema nervosa. *Riv. Sper. Freniatr. Med. Leg. Alienazioni Ment., 19,* 419–472.

Thorpe, W.H. (1956). *Learning and instincts in animals.* Cambridge, Massachusetts: Harvard University Press.

Turner A.M., & Greenough, W.T. (1985). Differential rearing effects on rat visual cortex synapses. I. Synaptic and neuronal density and synapses per neuron. *Brain Research, 329,* 195–203.

Tremblay, J.P., Colonnier, M., & McLennan, H. (1979). An electron microscopic study of synaptic contacts in the abdominal ganglion of *Aplysia californica. Journal of Comparative Neurology, 188,* 367–396.

Vrensen, G., & Nunes Cardozo, J. (1981). Changes in size and shape of synaptic connections after visual training: An ultrastructural approach of synaptic plasticity. *Brain Research, 218,* 79–97.

Walrond, J.P., & Reese, T.S. (1985). Structure of axon terminals and active zones at synapses on lizard twitch and tonic muscle fibers. *Journal of Neuroscience, 5,* 1118–1131.

13

Activity-Dependent Neuronal Gene Expression: A Potential Memory Mechanism?

CHRISTINE M. GALL
JULIE C. LAUTERBORN

One of the long-held tenets of memory research is that information storage entails new or specialized protein synthesis. This view is primarily supported by studies demonstrating that inhibition of protein or RNA synthesis disrupts the formation of some types of memory (Davis & Squire, 1984) but not all (see Staubli, Faraday, & Lynch, 1985, for a recent report). One might envisage a number of possible roles for gene expression in learning and memory. The most typically discussed is that patterns of physiological activity alter gene expression in critical neurons with the affected gene products contributing directly to the synaptic changes that encode memory. It is possible, however, that newly synthesized proteins promote memory formation without contributing in a direct fashion to the "memory trace." For example, levels of gene expression might be set (or modulated) in a nonspecific fashion, reflecting such things as transient shifts in arousal, and the expression products might increase or decrease the probability that nongenomic plasticities will occur. Alternatively, activity patterns acting over days or weeks could set levels of particular gene products that affect the firing thresholds or other nonlinear properties of individual cells and thereby affect network computational properties. A lack of information on the relationship between neuronal activity and gene expression has made it difficult to evaluate ideas of these types or develop more formal hypotheses about the role of protein synthesis in the acquisition and consolidation of memory.

With the recent advent and popular use of molecular biological techniques in neuroscience research, this situation has begun to change. This chapter is concerned with certain results collected with these methods and in particular focuses on three questions that are of critical importance to any argument relating gene expression to learning and memory. First, does physiological activity up- or down-regulate the expression of specific neuronal genes in the adult brain? Animals learn cues that are present for fractions of seconds and that generate electrical patterns in brain circuitries that are unlikely to last much longer than that. Whether or not such brief periods of even very intense physiological activity could affect gene transcription is a question of primary importance. Second, if physiological events do influence expression, which genes are involved and over what time course? The identity of gene products that increase or decrease following activity should provide clues as to the nature of the changes likely to emerge from physiologically induced changes in expression. Obvious examples would be mRNAs encoding for neurotransmitters or their receptors. Establishing the time courses for such effects is also important because it might allow for correlations between biochemistry and specific temporal attributes of memory. Third, are there regional variations in altered gene expression? Neurobehavioral research has linked particular brain regions (e.g., amygdala, hippocampus, frontal cortex) with specific types of memory or memory operations. Regional differences could therefore be indicative of the type of role gene regulation might play in learning and memory.

Although there are now examples of alterations in neuronal content of particular mRNAs or proteins in response to "normal" levels of physiological activity, the more numerous studies of the effects of experimentally induced seizures and direct electrical stimulation have been particularly fruitful in providing answers to the above questions. As will be described in the following pages, work with these paradigms has demonstrated that neuronal activity induces an orderly cascade of changes in gene expression including alterations in the abundance of mRNAs for transcriptional activation factors, neuromodulatory peptides, the nerve growth factor (NGF)-like neurotrophic factors, and at least one major neurotransmitter receptor. Moreover, these studies have allowed us to characterize differences in the threshold and temporal parameters of changes in the expression of different genes within the same neurons. This information provides a basis for future studies of genomic responses to normal levels and patterns of physiological activity and has identified gene products that may be of critical importance to learning and memory.

SEIZURE- AND STIMULATION-INDUCED CHANGES IN GENE EXPRESSION

Immediate-Early Genes

The most rapid genomic response to activity is an increase in the expression of immediate-early genes including, most notably, c-*fos*. These genes are designated "immediate and early" because they can be induced very rapidly by cell surface events (e.g., depolarization or stimulation of cell surface receptors) via second messengers but without the necessity of intervening protein synthesis (Sheng & Greenberg, 1990). Hence, a criterion generally used to classify a change in gene expression as an immediate-early gene (IEG) response is the capability to induce the changes in mRNA synthesis in the presence of protein synthesis inhibition. There is particular interest in IEG responses because these genes encode known and putative transcription activation factors that bind particular regions of the DNA and influence (facilitate or repress) the transcription of other genes (Curran & Morgan, 1987; Morgan and Curran, 1989). Hence, the IEG products act as "tertiary" messengers whereby cell surface events regulate the expression of other, phenotype specific, genes. Work with tissue culture has demonstrated that in the sympathetic neuron-like phaeochromocytoma PC12 cell, depolarization or nicotinic receptor activation can stimulate an increase in levels of c-*fos* mRNA within 5 min of activation in a calcium-dependent manner (Greenberg, Ziff, & Greene, 1986; Morgan & Curran, 1986). It was therefore not entirely surprising when it was discovered that seizure activity could stimulate large and rapid increases in the expression of c-*fos* mRNA in neurons in the mammalian forebrain (Morgan, Cohen, Hempstead, & Curran, 1987; White & Gall, 1987). Since that time a large number of studies have demonstrated that seizures, induced in a variety of paradigms, cause large but transient increases in the expression of a number of the IEGs, including c-*fos*, c-*jun* and NGFI-A (a.k.a. Tis 8, *zif*/268) (Daval, Nakjima, Gleiter, Post, & Marangos, 1989; Dragunow & Robertson, 1987; Saffen et al., 1988).

The IEGs c-*fos* and c-*jun* encode the Fos and Jun proteins, respectively. The evolving story of Fos and Jun action has come to serve as the prototype for the expected IEG function and demonstrate the pertinence of IEGs to the regulation of other patterns of gene expression. It has now been demonstrated that the Fos and Jun proteins form a DNA-binding heterodimer, which, in turn, binds to the AP-1 (activating protein-1) binding site within the 5' (or promotor) region of target genes. The AP-1 consensus sequence has now been identified in the 5' flanking region of genes encoding preproenkephalin (Van Nguyen, Kobierski, Comb, & Hyman, 1990) and nerve growth factor (Hengerer et al., 1990) among others. It is thought that binding of the Fos–Jun complex to the AP-1 site either directly facilitates transcription or renders the gene "inducible" by other conditions such as elevated levels of cyclic AMP (Van Nguyen et al., 1990). Beyond this, both Fos and Jun participate in the formation of a variety of other DNA-binding dimers (e.g., with fos-related antigens (FRAs) and cAMP response element binding proteins (CREBs); Macgregor, Abate, & Curran, 1990) that are likely to have different specificities of action in regard to both the genes influenced and to the direction of change that binding has on transcription. Moreover, the different IEG products that participate in transcriptional control have different half-lives and latencies to induction; hence, different collections of these proteins will be represented at different poststimulus intervals (Morgan & Curran, 1989; Sonnenberg, Macgregor-Leon, Curran, & Morgan, 1989). As such, one finds an elevation of the Fos/Jun, AP-1, heterodimer (and stimulation of target genes) at short poststimulus latencies but greater abundance of the FRA/Jun heterodimer or the Jun/Jun homodimer at later invertals (and the stimulation, or suppression, of different groups of genes). Thus, with the activity-induced increases in the expression of just a few IEG products it is possible to activate a variety of different changes in gene expression that exhibit different temporal characteristics. This is important to keep in mind as one considers the cellular mechanisms that might coordinate the various different changes in gene expression that occur within individual neurons following epileptiform activity.

As mentioned above, we have found studies of the effects of seizure activity have illuminated basic principals that govern the regulation of neuronal expression of IEGs and genes that encode neuropeptides, growth factors, and transmitter receptors in adult brain. We have studied the influence of seizure activity in the regulation of the IEGs and other phenotype-specific genes primarily using two different experimental seizure paradigms. The first entails the placement of a focal electrolytic lesion in the hilus of one dentate gyrus in anesthetized rat (Gall, Pico, & Lauterborn, 1988). This leads to a period of recurrent seizure activity, with numerous full electrographic seizure discharges of hippocampal neurons and behavioral seizures of the limbic kindling type, which begins 1.5–2 h following the lesion and continues for 8–10 h. In this hilus lesion (HL) paradigm, the great majority of seizure discharges occur during the first 3 h of seizure activity (i.e., from 2 to 5 h postlesion). From the appearance of coordinated behavioral seizures it is clear that seizures radiate to the neocortex with this treatment. Second, we have studied the effects of individual epileptiform afterdischarges of hippocampal neurons to characterize the time course for changes in gene expression and to begin evaluating the threshold for stimulation-induced effects. In this paradigm, the perforant path is stimulated at 10 Hz until an individual afterdischarge of 25–40 s duration is initiated within hippocampus; this is the limit of epileptiform activity in these rats. In all studies to be described, changes in levels of a particular mRNA species were evaluated by quantitative autoradiographic detection of in situ hybridization of ^{35}S-labeled cRNA probes (complementary to the naturally occurring mRNA sequences) with corroboration by either Northern blot or S1 nuclease protection analysis. Moreover, in each instance, analyses of mRNA levels in a variety of control rats (i.e., (a) sham surgical controls; (b) lesioned rats with seizures blocked by sodium pentobarbital; and (c) rats with electrolytic hilus lesions placed with platinum iridium wire which does not induce seizures; Campbell, Bank, & Milgram, 1984) have verified that changes in gene expression to be described are due to physiological activity as opposed to other potentially confounding effects of treatment.

In untreated rats, c-*fos* mRNA levels are very low in the forebrain; hybridization to c-*fos* mRNA is sparse and only lightly labels neurons in neocortex, olfactory cortex, and, more lighly still, a few cells in the hippocampus. In contrast, by 3 and 6 h following a hilus lesion it appears that virtually all neurons in the hippocampal formation are densely labeled by the cRNA probe (Figure 13.1). In addition, hybridization is strikingly

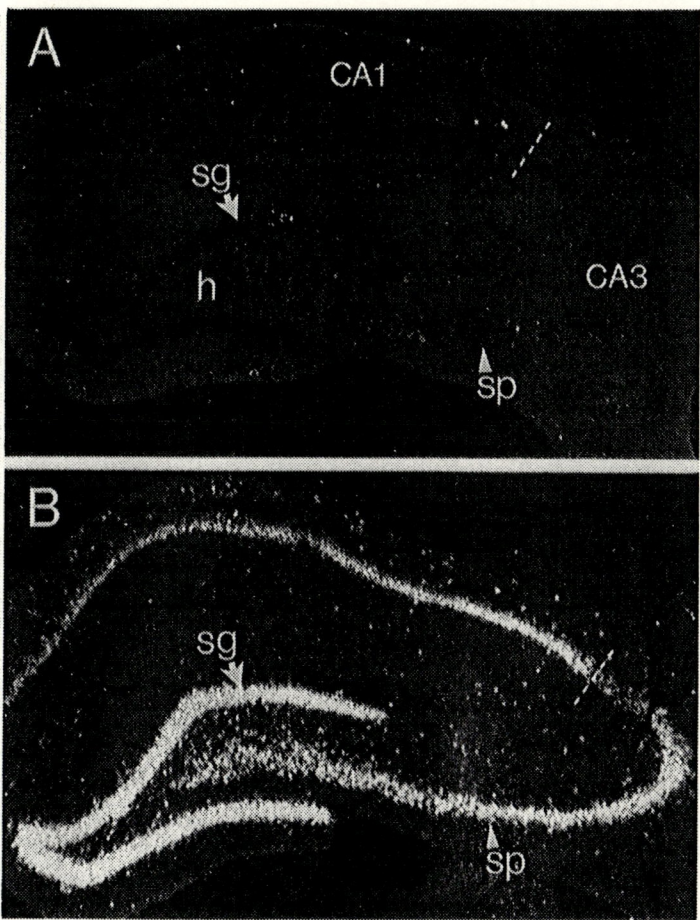

FIGURE 13.1. Dark-field photomicrographs showing the localization of in situ hybridization to c-*fos* mRNA (autoradiographic label seen as white) in sections through hippocampus of an untreated rat (A) and a paired rat sacrificed 3 h following a seizure-producing hilus lesion (B). In the experimental tissue, increased hybridization to c-*fos* mRNA densely labels stratum granulosum (sg), stratum pyramidale (sp) of regions CA3 through CA1, and neurons scattered outside of these principal cell layers (h, dentate gyrus hilus).

elevated in the neocortex, all major relays in the olfactory telencephalon (olfactory, cortex and tubercle, amygdaloid complex, anterior olfactory nucleus, granule cell layer of olfactory bulb), and more modestly in the nucleus accumbens (Gall, Lauterborn, Isackson, & White, 1990). There is no obvious evidence for phenotypic specificity in this response; it appears that hybridization is increased in all cells activated by the seizure episode.

Studies of the effects of individual afterdischarges have demonstrated that these activity-dependent increases in IEG expression are extremely rapid

(Gall, Lauterborn, & Isackson, 1990). As early as 10 min following one discharge of 25–40 s duration, hybridization to both c-*fos* and Tis 8 mRNA is more than doubled in the dentate gyrus granule cells bilaterally (Gall, Lauterborn, & Isackson, 1990; Shin, McNamara, Morgan, Curran, & Cohen, 1990). Hybridization reaches maximal density by 30 min after the discharge, then declines significantly by 1 h following stimulation. Hence, like the stimulation of IEG expression in cultured neurons, in vivo adult neurons respond within minutes to this extremely brief burst of stimulation with a rapid and rapidly transient increase in the expression of the IEGs.

Studies of the effects of subseizure afferent stimulation have demonstrated that a common threshold for stimulation is not shared for the different IEGs. For example, with subseizure high-frequency stimulation of the perforant path, sufficient to induce long-term potentiation (LTP) in the dentate gyrus granule cells, mRNA for the IEG *zif*/268 is dramatically increased within the ipsilateral dentate gyrus granule cells (Cole, Saffen, Baraban, & Worley, 1989; Wisden et al., 1990). Levels of c-*fos* mRNA was less reliably increased in the same group of rats. Treatment with the N-methyl-D-aspartate (NMDA) channel blocker MK-801 did suppress the increase in mRNA expression thereby indicating NMDA mechanisms might be critical to induction in these paradigms (Cole et al., 1989). However, although high-frequency stimulation of the sort which induces LTP was more effective than lower frequency stimulation in *zif*/268 induction, on an individual animal basis two separate groups have found no reliable correlation between *zif*/268 (Cole et al., 1989), or c-*fos* (Dragunow et al., 1989) induction and the expression of LTP. These results demonstrate that subseizure activation is sufficient for induction of some IEGs and therefore presumably also increases the production of specific transcription activation factors, but that the full battery of activation factors is not necessarily increased in any given case. Although NMDA receptors seem to be involved, these studies have not found an association between IEG induction and the appearance of LTP.

Neuroactive Peptides

Activity-dependent changes in the expression of neuroactive peptides have been studied in a number of laboratories (for reviews see Gall, Lauterborn, Isackson, & White, 1990; Gall & White, 1989). In general, it has been found that recurrent seizures stimulate changes in the expression of certain neuropeptides but the relationships of the various peptides to seizure activity can be remarkably different, including instances of differential regulation of colocalized gene products. This is illustrated by the changing patterns of neuropeptide expression in hippocampal neurons following hilus lesion-induced recurrent seizure activity.

The expression of neuropeptides enkephalin, dynorphin, and neuropeptide Y (NPY) have been studied at both the mRNA and protein level within the hippocampal formation. Both enkephalin and dynorphin are normally expressed by the dentate gyrus granule cells (Gall, Brecha, Karten, & Chang, 1981; McGinty, Henriksen, Goldstein, Terenius, & Bloom, 1983) whereas NPY (as detected by the presence of NPY mRNA or NPY immunoreactivity) is expressed by scattered, probable local circuit, neurons outside the principal cell layers (Köhler, Eriksson, Davies, & Chan-Palay, 1986). In the granule cell layer of untreated rats, hybridization to preproenkephalin mRNA is sprase and of variable density whereas hybridization to preprodynorphin mRNA is moderately dense and appears to label virtually all neurons in the layer. During the approximately 10 h period of recurrent seizures induced by hilus lesion, hybridization to both ot these mRNA species becomes progressively more dense within the granule cell layer. This is illustrated by data from one experiment shown in Figure 13.2 in which the density of hybridization to preprodynorphin and preproenkephalin mRNA in the granule cells increased to 6- and 10-fold control levels by 12 h postlesion, respectively. However, preproenkephalin mRNA continues to increase and remains elevated through 48 h postlesion; at these intervals virtually all neurons in the granule cell layer appear to be autoradiographically labeled by the preproenkephalin cRNA (Figure 13.3B). During this same period, dynorphin expression by the granule cells becomes severely depressed; hybridization to preprodynorphin mRNA within stratum granulosum declines to control levels by 24 h following the hilus lesion and declines further to several fold below control densities by 48–96 h postlesion.

The differential influence of seizure activity on these codistributed opioids is also evident at the protein level. During the period of seizures (1.5 to about 10 h after the hilus lesion), immunoreactivities for both enkephalin and dynorphin are depleted from the mossy fiber axons of the granule cells

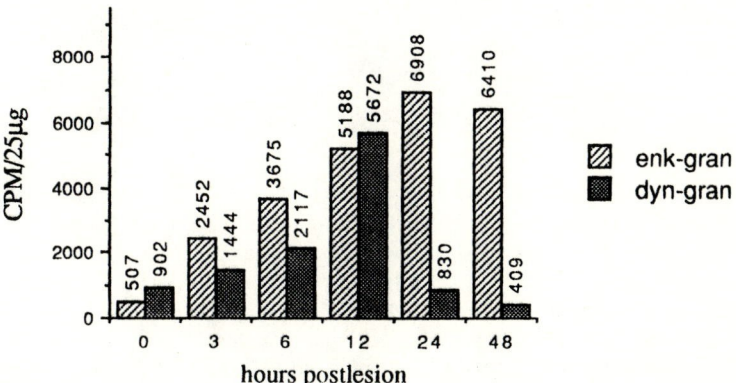

FIGURE 13.2. Bar graph showing differential changes in the density of in situ hybridization to mRNAs for preproenkephalin (euk) and preprodynorphin (dyn) in stratum granulosum at various time points following a seizure-producing hilus lesion. Each bar represents the mean density measurement for one rat; all tissue was processed in one experiment and values are expressed relative to the same paired control.

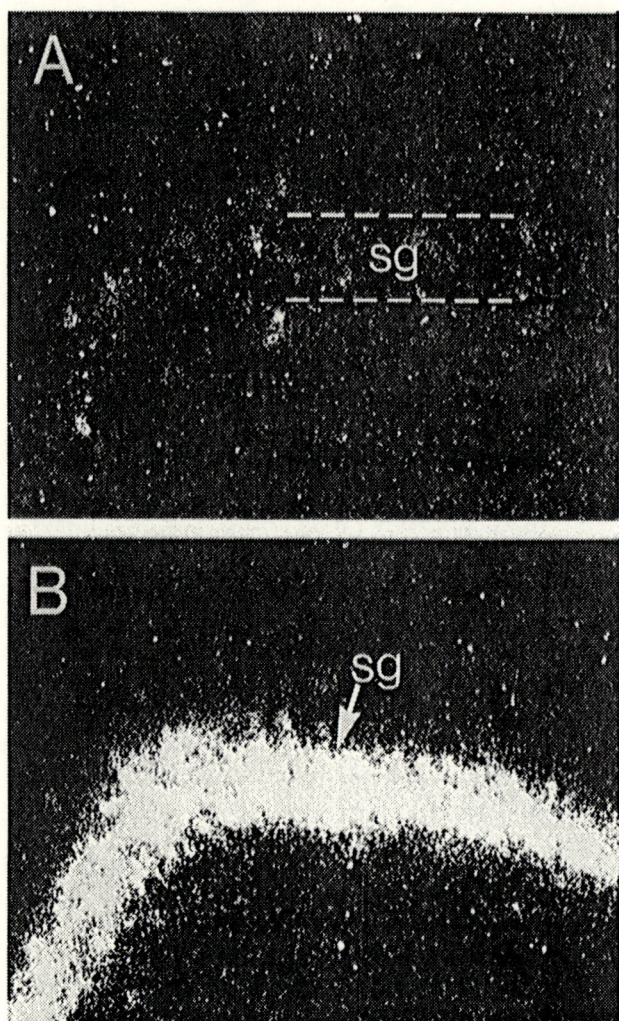

FIGURE 13.3.   Dark-field photomicrographs illustrating the autoradiographic local-ization of in situ hybridization to preproenkephalin mRNA (A,B) and preproNPY mRNA (C,D) in tissue sections through hippocampus of an untreated rat (A,C) and a paired rat sacrificed 24 h (B,D) following a seizure-producing hilus lesion (HL). As seen at high magnification in (A) and (B), hybridization to preproenkephalin mRNA is very light in dentate gyrus stratum granulosum (sg) of the untreated rat (A) but dramatically increased in this layer following the HL. The low-magnification photomicrographs of (C) and (D) show the novel appearance of hybridization to preproNPY mRNA within stratum granulosum (open arrow) and stratum pyramidale (sp) of region CA1 following HL-induced seizures.

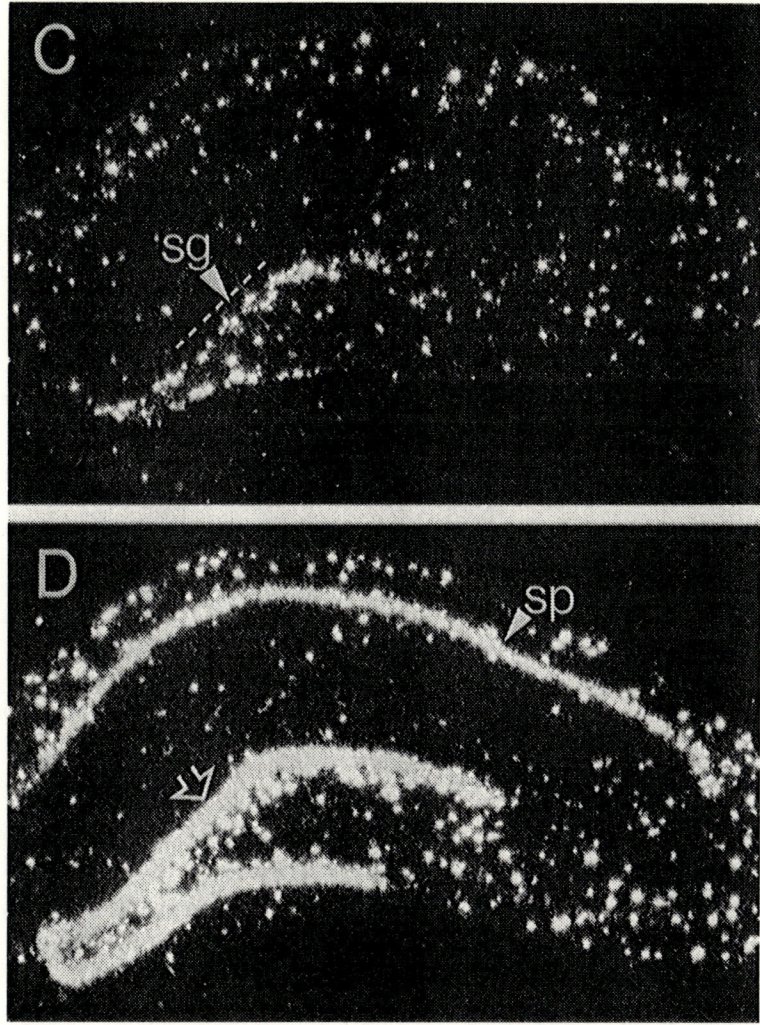

(Gall et al., 1988). Enkephalin immunoreactivity returns to control levels in these axons by about 1 day postlesion and continues to increase to several fold higher than seen in control rats for the period of 2 to about 10 days postlesion. In vivo radiolabeling studies have determined that, during the period of heightened preproenkephalin mRNA content (from 18 to 24 h postlesion) the transport of newly synthesized enkephalin peptide to the mossy fiber terminal field is 14-fold greater than measured in paired controls (White, Gall, & McKelvy, 1987). In contrast, following the initial depletion, dynorphin immunoreactivity remains depressed in this terminal field for at least 1 week following the seizure episode (Gall, 1988).

These changes in levels of enkephalin and dynorphin production by the granule cells demonstrate that an episode of extreme activity can differentially alter the expression of colocalized messenger molecules. This suggests the possibility that periods of extreme, or possibly patterned, physiological activity might also influence the relative proportion of coreleased neuromodulators for a period of days to weeks following the initial event. The influence of seizures on NPY further reinforces this impression. As mentioned above, in the normal rat NPY is produced by probable local circuit neurons within hippocampus. It was therefore surprizing to detect expression of high levels of preproNPY (ppNPY) mRNA in both the majority of granule cells and CA1 pyramidal cells following hilus lesion-induced seizures (Figure 13.3C, D). These effects emerge rather late relative to changes in enkephalin and dynorphin expression. PreproNPY mRNA only becomes detectable within stratum granulosum by about 10 h postlesion and within CA1 stratum pyramidale by 17 h postlesion. Like seizure-induced changes in enkephalin mRNA, levels of ppNPY mRNA continue to increase beyond these time points to reach maximal levels of about 1 day postlesion. Thus, seizures stimulate high levels of ppNPY mRNA expression in populations of neurons that do not normally contain detectable levels of this mRNA species and these increases become evident *after* the termination of the seizure episode.

Our findings on seizure-induced changes in opioid peptide expression are in good agreement with results from other laboratories using different recurrent seizure paradigms (i.e., repeated electroconvulsive shock, chemical, or electrical kindling) or intense electrical stimulation of hippocampus, although with the selection of time points in these studies the rapidly transient increase in dynorphin mRNA was not detected in some instances (Douglass, Grimes, Shook, Lee, & Hong, 1991; Kanamatsu et al., 1986; McGinty et al., 1986; Morris, Feasely, Bruggencate, Herz, & Höllt, 1988). Moreover, our observation of the novel appearance of ppNPY mRNA within the granule cells following seizures is consistent with reports that seizures induce the new appearance of NPY immunoreactivity within the granule cell mossy fiber axons (Marksteiner, Ortler, Bellmann, & Sperk, 1990).

As will be discussed, these results demonstrate that recurrent seizures alter the expression of mRNAs for neuropeptides within a subset of the forebrain neurons that increase c-*fos* mRNA in response to the same stimulation. However, studies of the effects of individual hippocampal afterdischarges demonstrate that the thresholds for IEG and neuropeptide stimulation differ. It will be remembered that one afterdischarge of hippocampal neurons stimulates large increases in c-*fos* and Tis 8 (a.k.a., NGFI-A) mRNA levels within the dentate gyrus granule cells. In contrast, we have found that in these same cells, levels of preproenkephalin mRNA are not perturbed by one afterdischarge but are increased by six such afterdischarges induced at 2.5 min intervals. Thus, although Fos protein may play a role in the regulation of preproenkephalin transcription, increased c-*fos* expression alone is not sufficient to activate increased expression of the preproenkephalin gene. This conclusion is consistent with the studies of

Van Nguyen et al. (1990), which demonstrate that depolarization-induced calcium influx, which presumably increases both IEG expression and AP-1 binding, has little effect on preproenkephalin transcription. However, they find calcium influx is synergistic with elevated levels of cAMP in stimulating *large* increases in the production of preproenkephalin mRNA. Thus, for at least this one neuropeptide, a convergence of conditions is required to increase expression. As will be described below, these threshold conditions distinguish the regulation of preproenkephalin mRNA from that of the NGF-like growth factors and makes differential activation of these genes possible under some conditions.

Glutamate Receptors

The recent characterization of DNA sequences encoding putative subunits of the non-NMDA glutamate receptor have made it possible to evaluate the cellular localization and to test for activity-dependent regulation of these genes in brain. The possible modulation of glutamate receptor expression by activity could have tremendous importance to theories of the ceullar mechanisms of memory formation. Glutamate is thought to be the major excitatory neurotransmitter in forebrain. There is good evidence that in hippocampus all intrinsic excitatory pathways as well as innervation from the entorhinal cortex act through glutamate-based transmission. Moreover, in region CA1, the expression of LTP by the Schaffer/commissural afferents has been demonstrated to reflect primarily a change in responses mediated by the non-NMDA glutamate receptor (Muller, Joly, & Lynch, 1988).

We have examined the effects of hilus lesion-induced seizures on the abundance of mRNA for the glutamate receptor subunit designated GluR1 (originally considered to be a putative kainate receptor but now recognized as a glutamate receptor subunit with alpha-amino-3-hydroxy-5-methyl-4-isoxazolepropionate (AMPA) subclass properties) (Boulter et al., 1990; Hollmann, O'Shea-Greenfield, Rogers, & Heinemann, 1989). Recurrent seizure activity caused a dramatic *reduction* in hybridization in GluR1 mRNA in the dentate gyrus granule cells and superficial cortex, which appeared approximately 20 h after seizure onset and was maximal in stratum granulosum, with hybridization decreased to 20% of control values, 24–30 h postlesion (Figure 13.4). Hybridization returned to control levels in these neurons 48 h postlesion. These changes in mRNA content have been corroborated by Northern blot analysis (Gall, Sumikawa, & Lynch, 1990).

These data demonstrate that mRNA for at least one major glutamate receptor subunit is down-regulated by extreme physiological activity and suggest the possibility that glutamate receptors as a class may be regulated by activity within the normal physiological range. However, before we can begin to appreciate the importance of activity-dependent changes in glutamate receptor expression, more information is needed. First, it is critical that we define the threshold conditions necessary to influence expression. Second, it will be equally important to determine if the other non-NMDA glutamate

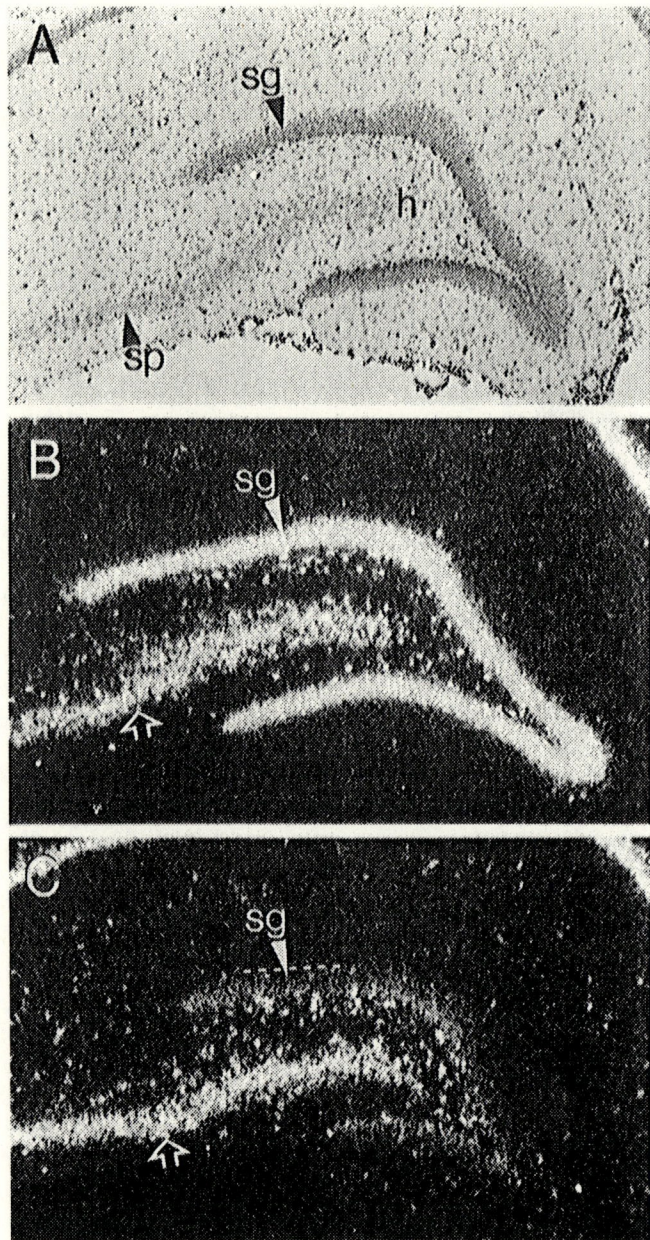

FIGURE 13.4. Low-magnification photomicrographs showing (A) Nissl-stained cell layers and (B, C) the autoradiographic labeling of in situ hybridization to GluR1 mRNA in sections through the dentate gyrus of an untreated rat (B) and a rat sacrificed 24 h following a hilus lesion (C) (dark-field illumination). (A) and (C) show the same tissue section as viewed with bright-field and dark-field illumination, respectively. Note the large seizure-induced decrease in hybridization within stratum granulosum (sg). The open arrow indicates stratum pyramidale (sp) of region CA3 (h, dentate gyrus hilus).

receptor subunits also respond to activity and, if so, whether there is coordinate regulation of the different subunit genes. Current studies by Heinemann and colleagues indicate that although the different receptor subunits each confer glutamate responsivity, differences in the ratio by which the subunits are expressed profoundly influence the physiological properties of the glutamate receptor complex (Boulter et al., 1990). Thus, selective activity-dependent changes in subunit expression could effect reversible cell-wide changes in the physiological properties of non-NMDA glutamate receptors independent of a change in the total number of receptor complexes (or binding sites).

NGF-like Neurotrophic Factors

Following, just slightly, behind stimulated increases in c-*fos* mRNA content, seizures effect a very rapid change in the abundance of mRNAs for NGF and related neurotrophic factors in brain. As the best characterized trophic factor, NGF has for years served as the prototype for theories of central trophic interactions (see Whittemore & Seiger, 1987, for a review). Evidence suggests that NGF, produced by forebrain neurons, is critical for the survival and expression of differentiated phenotypic characteristics of basal forebrain cholinergic cells. Moreover, even in the adult, NGF application has been demonstrated to influence the biosynthetic activities, and possibly the further morphological elaboration, of these neurons (Hefti, 1986; Higgins, Sookyong, Chen, & Gage, 1989). Recently, the characterization of brain-derived neurotrophic factor (BDNF) and neurotrophin 3 (NT3), both with approximately 50% amino acid sequence identity to NGF, has indicated that NGF is a member of a family of structurally related trophic factors that are produced by differing populations of forebrain neurons which exhibit differences in cellular specificity of trophic action (Ernfors, Wetmore, Olson, & Persson, 1990; Hohn, Leibrock, Bailey, & Barde, 1990; Leibrock et al., 1989; Maisonpierre, Belluscio, Squinto, et al., 1990). While NGF appears specific for the cholinergic basal forebrain neurons, BDNF supports these cells (Alderson, Alterman, Barde, & Lindsay, 1990) as well as dopaminergic neurons of the ventral tegmentum (Knüsel et al., 1991) and retinal neurons (Johnson, Barde, Schwab, & Thoenen, 1986). The central actions of NT3 are not known but the distributions of NT3 and BDNF synthesis in brain (Ernfors et al., 1990) indicates that further responsive neuronal populations will be identified.

Until recently, very little was known about factors that regulate the expression of NGF in brain. Although it had been anticipated that NGF production might be stimulated in instances of neuronal degeneration, and thereby might be mobilized to direct compensatory growth processes, lesions have not been found to stimulate increased NGF synthesis in the adult brain (Lärkfors, Strömberg, Ebendal, & Olson, 1987). Rather, as originally demonstrated by studies from this laboratory, the effects of seizures on NGF mRNA levels indicate that neuronal activity regulates the expression

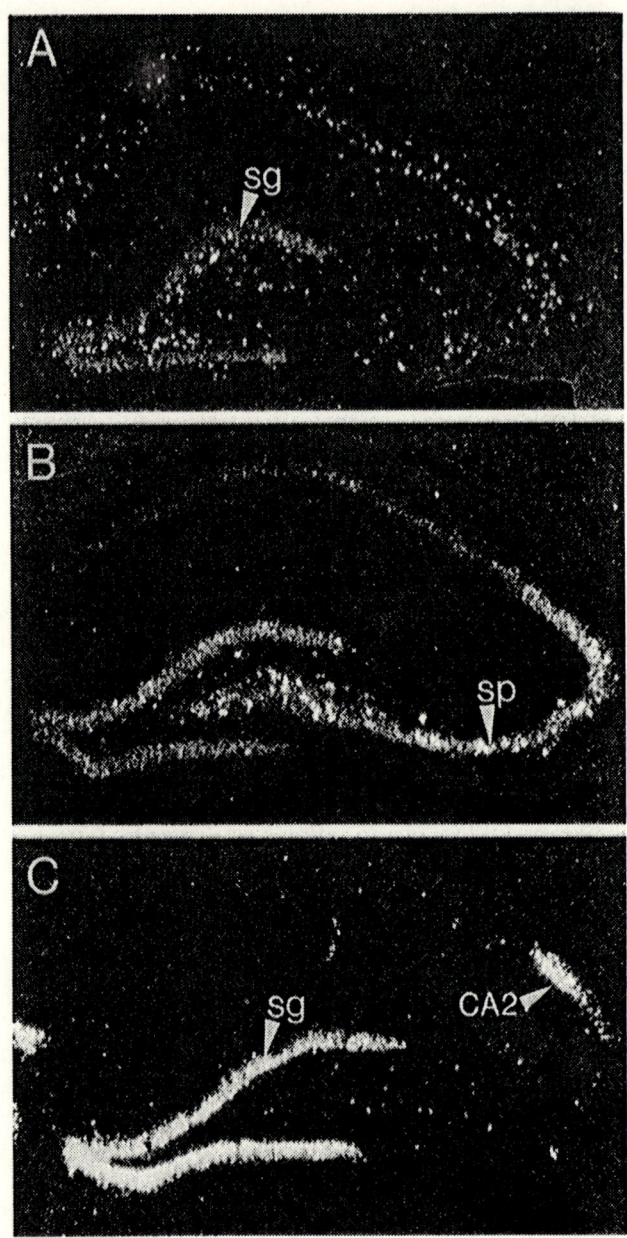

FIGURE 13.5. Dark-field photomicrographs showing the different patterns of in situ hybridization to mRNAs for NGF (A,D), BDNF (B,E), and NT3 (C,F) within coronal sections through rostral hippocampus of a control rat (A,B,C) and experimental seizure rats sacrificed 6 h (D,E) and 24 h (F) following a contralateral hilus lesion. Abbreviations: sg, stratum granulosum; sp, stratum pyramidale.

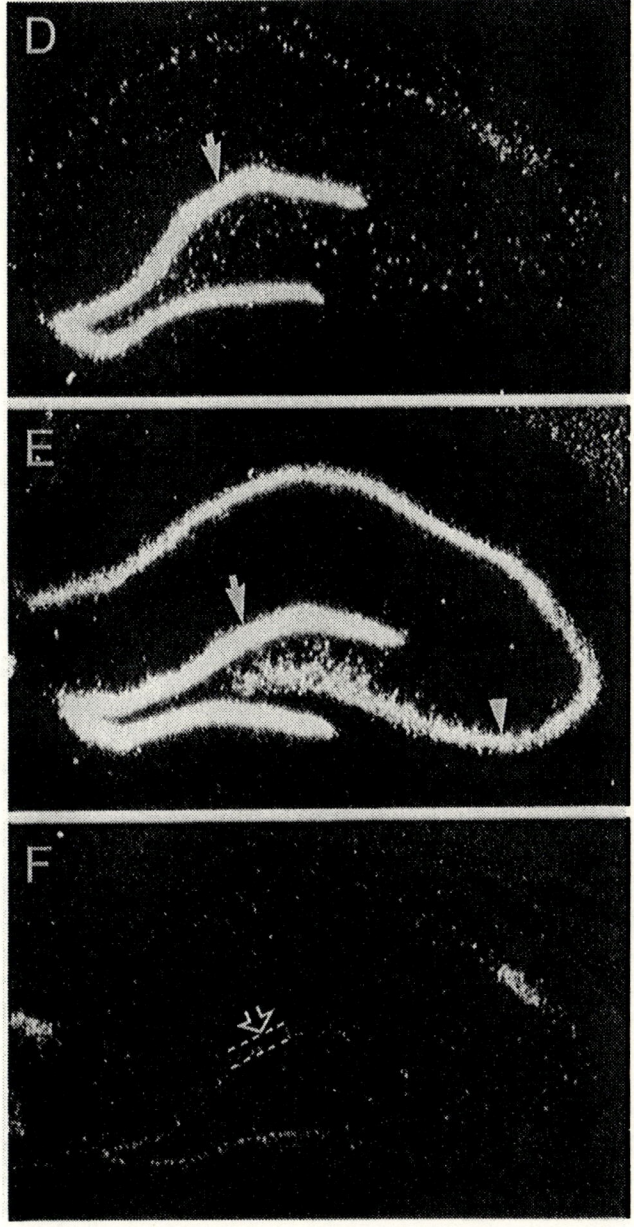

of NGF in brain (Gall & Isackson, 1989). We have now extended our analyses to studies of BDNF and NT3 and find that seizures markedly alter the expression of mRNAs for all three of the NGF-like trophic factors in many different populations of forebrain neurons, but in very different ways.

As can be seen in Figure 13.5, in the untreated rat hippocampus, hybridization to mRNAs for NGF, BDNF, and NT3 exhibit different but overlapping patterns of labeling. Nerve growth factor mRNA is present at low levels within the granule cells but is much more abundant in probable local circuit neurons scattered within the hilus and the pyramidal cell fields. Messenger RNA for BDNF is present at moderate density within both the granule and pyramidal cell layers, whereas neurons in the molecular layers are not labeled. Hybridization to NT3 labels the granule cells and pyramidal cells of region CA2, as well as scattered cells in the pyramidal cell molecular layers.

Recurrent seizure activity induced by either a hilus lesion (Gall & Isackson, 1989; Isackson, Huntsman, Murray, & Gall, 1991), kainic acid (Gall, Murray, & Isackson, 1991; Zafra, Hengerer, Leibrock, Thoenen, & Lindholm, 1990), or electrical stimulation (unpublished observations) stimulates large and rapid increases in levels of mRNAs for NGF and BDNF in hippocampus and other very broadly distributed forebrain structures (Figure 13.5D, E). The change in BDNF mRNA content is the least complex. In hilus lesion rats, hybridization to BDNF mRNA increases rapidly *during* the period of seizures in all affected brain areas to reach maximal levels in hippocampus (stratum pyramidale and stratum granulosum), amygdala, neocortex, olfactory cortex, and other rostral olfactory structures by 6 h postlesion (Figure 13.6). Hybridization to BDNF mRNA begins to decline with the termination of seizure activity to approach control levels in most areas by 24 h postlesion (Isackson et al., 1991). In contrast, in analysis of tissue from the same experimental rats we find the increase in NGF mRNA in hippocampus is biphasic and occurs *after* the period of seizure activity in extrahippocampal loci (Figure 13.7). Specifically, during the period of seizures, NGF mRNA levels increase rapidly, but exclusively, in the dentate gyrus granule cells to reach maximal levels by 3–6 h postlesion and then decline sharply to control levels by 10–12 h postlesion. This is followed by a second increase in the granule cells and increases in hybridization neocortex, olfactory cortex, and amygdala that appear maximal at 24 h postlesion. In contrast to NGF and BDNF, recurrent seizures cause a delayed *decrease* in NT3 mRNA content (Figure 13.5F). Hybridization to NT3 mRNA remains normal through the early period of seizure activity then drops to 20% of control levels in the dentate gyrus granule cells and becomes markedly reduced in cortical fields (caudal neocortex, entorhinal cortex) by 12–24 h after a contralateral hilus lesion (Figure 13.7).

Studies of the effects of electrical stimulation indicate that only very brief periods of activation are necessary to alter the expression of the BDNF and NGF mRNAs. One brief (25–40 s) afterdischarge of hippocampal neurons is sufficient to induce a bilateral 6- to 10-fold increase in the abundance of

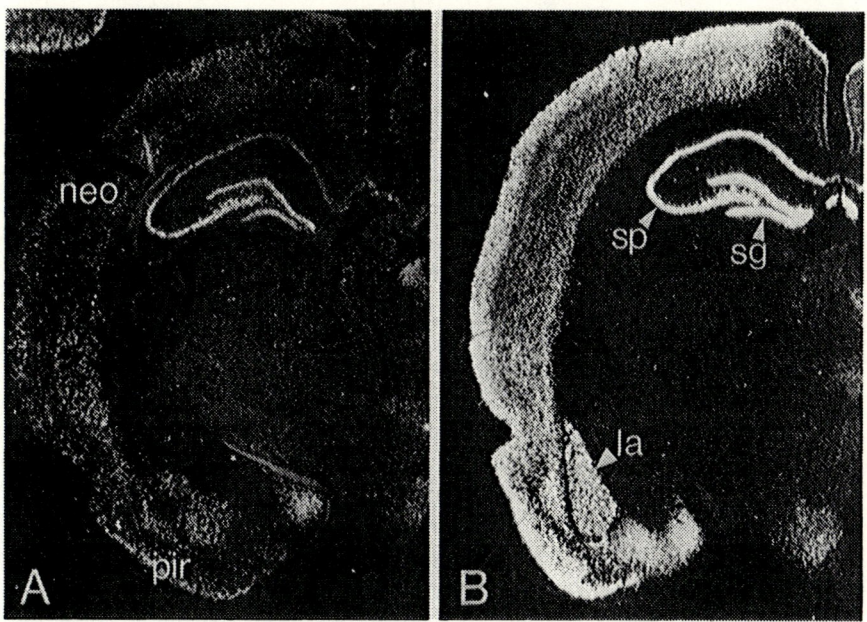

FIGURE 13.6.   Low-magnification dark-field photomicrographs of full coronal hemisections through the plane of rostral hippocampus showing autoradiographic labeling (seen as white) of in situ hybridization localization to BDNF mRNA in tissue from an untreated rat (A) and a paired experimental rat (B) sacrificed 6 h following a seizure-producing hilus lesion. In the experimental case, hybridization is clearly increased in stratum granulosum (sg) and stratum pyramidale (sp) of the hippocampus, neocortex (neo), piriform cortex (pir), and the lateral nucleus of the amygdala (la).

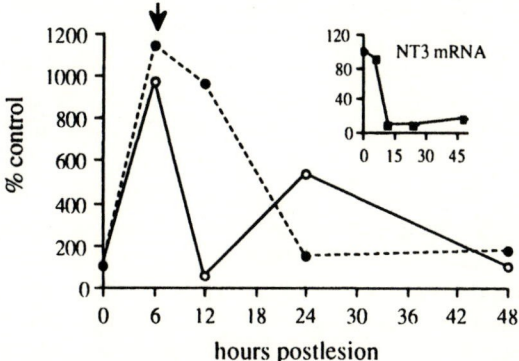

FIGURE 13.7.   Graph showing the relative change in hybridization to mRNAs for BDNF (dashed line), NGF (solid line), and NT3 (insert) in dentate gyrus stratum granulosum at various times following the hilus lesion as determined by calibrated film densitometery (mean values plotted, $n \geq 3$ at each time point).

mRNAs for both NGF and BDNF in the dentate gyrus granule cells (Gall, Lauterborn, & Isackson, 1990; Isackson et al., 1991). This is an extremely rapid response. Both trophic factor mRNAs are elevated by 30 min and reach maximal levels by 2–3 h after the discharge. This growth factor response follows very closely behind stimulated increase in the immediate-early gene mRNAs, which can be detected 10 min, and are maximal at 30 min, following stimulation.

We have yet to determine the threshold stimulation conditions necessary to influence neurotrophic factor synthesis but have reason to believe that subseizure levels of activity will prove effective. In studies of the effects of perforant path stimulation on NGF mRNA levels within the granule cells, we have observed in a small minority of subseizure-stimulation cases, including those receiving either theta burst or 10 Hz stimulation, a marked (greater than seven-fold) increase in hybridization in the granule cell layer ipsilateral to stimulation. In these cases, epileptiform afterdischarges were not recorded; the unilateral induction further reinforces the conclusion that a seizure discharge did not occur. However, the absence of increases in NGF mRNA content in the majority of similarly treated rats suggests that these data should not be overinterpreted. It remains possible that damaged-induced afterdischarges, occurring during electrode placement, may have played a role.

These results demonstrate that the three members of the NGF family of neurotrophic factors are differentially regulated by activity and, in some instances, differentially regulated in the same populations of neurons. As mentioned above, on the basis of data on NGF action it is expected that each of these factors influence the morphological elaboration, synthetic activities, and quite probably the survival of responsive afferent neurons both during development and in the adult. The demonstration that at least extreme levels of activity can influence the synthesis of these neurotrophic factors in adult brain therefore suggests the possibility that, through modulation of NGF production, levels of activity within the targets of the cholinergic neurons might regulate the synthetic activities and influence morphological adjustments by the cholinergic neurons throughout life. Similarly, activity-dependent changes in the expression of BDNF and NT3 would be expected to influence their separate populations of responsive neurons.

The opposing changes in levels of BDNF mRNA and NT3 mRNA in some cell groups (e.g., the granule cells) in response to seizures is particularly intriguing. It is of course possible that this is a pathophysiological response, not truly representative of the influence of normal levels of activity on these trophic substances. However, reciprocal regulation of BDNF and NT3 has been suggested on the basis of changes in levels of expression during development. In some brain areas, early in development, NT3 mRNA levels are high whereas BDNF mRNA levels are low; at later stages NT3 mRNA levels decline while BDNF mRNA expression increases (Maisonpierre, Belluscio, Freidman et al., 1990). If these two factors do indeed influence distinct populations of neurons, one might imagine that, with reciprocal regulation, activity-induced increases in BDNF expression might result in a preferential stabilization of innervation by particular (responsive) afferents and might during the same period leave NT3 responsive afferents without sufficient trophic support. Taking this idea even further, at the cellular level, neurons with higher levels of activity might, over time, receive proportionately greater innervation by BDNF responsive afferents.

It is not difficult to imagine how activity-dependent changes in trophic factor expression might play a role in the morphological adjustments reported to be associated with environmental enrichment effects or with longer periods of training (Greenough & Bailey, 1988). Chronic or intermittent stimulation over days and weeks could effect chronic changes in trophic factor production that might either directly influence the dendritic aborizations of responsive cortical neurons or indirectly induce these changes through stimulating the growth of afferent systems. However, as will be considered below, it is not likely that more rapid morphological adjustments, such as changes in synapse number and spine morphology found to be associated with LTP (Greenough & Bailey, 1988), involve activity-mediated changes in trophic interactions.

Summary of Seizure Studies

The results described above demonstrate that physiological activity, or at least the bursts of intense neuronal activity associated with seizures, influences the expression of four functional classes of genes: the immediate-early genes and genes that encode neuromodulatory peptides, neurotrophic factors, and at least one major neurotransmitter receptor. In each instance, changes in expression were observed in many different neuronal populations and brain areas—changes in gene expression in response to activity were not found to be a specialized property of any particular cell type or types. However, there was a sort of cellular "specificity" as to the particular mRNA species influenced in a given neuronal group. As seen most clearly for the neuroactive peptides and NGF-like neurotrophic factors, seizures induced the expression of a particular gene product in limited subsets of the neurons activated. As such, NGF mRNA expression was only increased in neurons that normally express this neurotrophic factor. Although other cell groups (such as the CA1 pyramidal cells) exhibit changes in gene expression in response to seizure, phenotypic constraints on trophic factor expression appeared to remain in force.

As illustrated most dramatically by the complex pattern of seizure-induced changes in mRNA content in the dentate gyrus granule cells summarized in Table 13.1, these results provide ample evidence for differential regulation of different mRNA species within individual neurons. Moreover, the marked differences in the time courses for these effects and, in some instances, in the threshold to induction, suggest that fundamentally different intracellular regulatory mechanisms are involved. For example, in reviewing the temporal

TABLE 13.1 Latencies to Onset and Maximal Alterations in Levels of mRNAs for Immediate-Early Genes, Neurotrophic Factors, Neuropeptides, and the Glutamate Receptor GluR1

	Onset	Maximal
Immediate-early genes		
c-*fos*	~10 min	30 min
NGFI-A (a.k.a. Tis 8, *zif* 268)	~10 min	30 min
c-*jun*		
Neurotrophic factors		
Brain-derived neurotrophic factor (BDNF)	~30 min	2–3–h
Nerve growth factor (NGF), phase 1	~30 min	2–3 h
Nerve growth factor, phase 2	>12 h	24 h
Neurotrophin 3 (NT3)	>10 h	12–24 h
Neuropeptides		
Enkephalin	~1.5 h	18–24 h
Dynorphin (increase)	~1.5 h	12 h
Dynorphin (decrease)	>12 h	48 h
Neuropeptide Y (NPY), stratum granulosum	~10 h	18–24 h
Neuropeptide Y (stratum pyramidale)	>10 h	18–24 h
Glutamate receptor GluR1		
	20 h	24–30 h

Note: Values derived from densitometric analysis of in situ hybridization in dentate gyrus stratum granulosum (or hippocampal stratum pyramidale where noted) and represent an integration of data from hilus lesion- and electrical stimulation-induced seizure activity.

characteristics of these responses one can see three major tiers in the cascade of gene expression induced by seizure. First, there is the rapid alteration in IEG expression. This is followed closely by changes in NGF and BDNF mRNA content. Finally, one sees the delayed and much more prolonged changes in the expression of the neuropeptide and glutamate receptor genes. In comparing the three, the change in neurotrophic factor expression is much more similar to the IEG response in regard to time course and to the relatively low threshold for induction.

In considering the potential involvement of activity-induced alterations in gene expression in mnemonic processes, it is important to note that all activity-induced changes in expression described here, and reported by others, are transient. With recurrent seizure activity lasting a period of hours, neuropeptide mRNA levels are altered for a period of days, and protein levels are altered for up to a couple of weeks. There is to our knowledge no well characterized example of permanent changes in mRNA or protein synthesis following an individual episode of specialized physiological activity.

MODIFICATIONS OF GENE EXPRESSION BY NORMAL ACTIVITY

Clearly, for activity-dependent changes in gene expression to play a role in memory formation, gene expression must be responsive to normal levels of physiological activity. Although studies in this area are only beginning, there is evidence from a number of groups that normal neuronal activity can indeed influence gene expression. In fact, studies of the expression of c-*fos* indicate that natural patterns of activity are actually more effective than various forms of electrical stimulation in influencing the expression of these genes. Although, as described above, subseizure electrical stimulation of forebrain pathways can increase c-*fos* mRNA expression, this has proven to be more difficult to obtain than originally anticipated. In our own work, we have examined the effects of subseizure stimulation of the perforant path using a number of paradigms and only rarely have seen changes in hybridization to c-*fos* mRNA in hippocampus even though hippocampal neuronal firing was driven by stimulation and LTP was frequently induced. In contrast, natural patterns of activity seem to readily induce c-*fos* mRNA expression in the appropriate neurons. There are now many examples of this. In particular, Fos expression is increased in retinal (Sagar & Sharp, 1990) and suprachiasmatic (Rusak, Robertson, Wisden, & Hunt, 1990) neurons in response to light. We have found that odor-stimulation increased c-*fos* mRNA in "activated" regions of the olfactory bulb, including the stimulation of expression both in periglomerular neurons, which receive direct innervation from the olfactory receptor cells, and in higher order olfactory neurons in the deeper layers of the main olfactory bulb (K. Guthrie & C. Gall, unpublished observations); in these cases the sensitivity of detecting activated neurons is actually greater using c-*fos* mRNA hybridization than using 2-deoxyglucose autoradiography. Even the very subtle stimulation of stress associated with handling and placement in a novel environment will induce an increase in Fos expression in forebrain (Gubits, Smith, Fairhurst, & Yu, 1989). Thus, expression is clearly not directly related to high intensities of stimulation. Rather, it seems that other characteristics, possibly the pattern and duration of stimulation, might be more critical.

Ultimately, one would like to determine if heightened or specialized patterns of gene expression are required for learning. The analysis of IEG induction should be extremely valuable to studies of the involvement of protein synthesis in memory formation. The induction of IEG expression is of relatively low threshold, follows a predictable poststimulus time course, and is seemingly less subject to phenotypic constraints than other changes in gene expression thus far described. Therefore, without having to make predictions as to what particular transcriptional activities might be important to learning, one can screen for changes in IEG expression to determine if transcriptional activities have been stimulated in a given situation.

Recent studies provide evidence that IEG expression is stimulated during particular forms of training but leave the particular association of gene expression with learning open to interpretation. Anokhin and Rose (1991) have studied the effects of food discrimination training in chicks on total brain levels of c-*fos* and c-*jun* mRNA. Their study examined mRNA levels in four groups: (a) quiet control chicks, (b) chicks familiarized with the test chamber and placed in the test chamber prior to sacrifice, (c) chicks pretrained for food discrimination and provided food during the test period prior to sacrifice, and (d) chicks familiarized with the test chamber but only provided food for learning of the food discrimination task during the test period prior to sacrifice. Briefly, all groups handled (placed in the test chamber) prior to sacrifice had higher levels of the c-*fos* and c-*jun* mRNAs than quiet control chicks, and in the feeding groups (c and d) levels of mRNA were higher still. Moreover, the recent learning group (d) exhibited significantly higher levels of c-*jun* mRNA expression than the active but previously overtrained group (c). As indicated by these authors, these results would be consistent with higher levels of IEG induction during learning or, possibly, induction as a part of a less specific arousal-type response to the novel experience.

Studies conducted in this laboratory with U. Hess and G. Lynch have used in situ hybridization to examine the expression of mRNAs for the IEGs c-*fos* and Tis-8 in rats trained for olfactory discrimination. Levels of expression have been examined in (a) untrained/naive rats, (b) previously untrained rats placed in the test chamber prior to sacrifice, (c) previously trained rats placed in the test chamber but not engaged in olfactory discrimination learning immediately prior to sacrifice, and (d) trained rats engaged in olfactory discrimination learning prior to sacrifice. As in the study described above, in all handled rats the levels of c-*fos* mRNA were increased in many forebrain areas, including superficial and deep layers of visual cortex, superficial piriform cortex, hippocampal stratum granulosum and stratum pyramidale, and dorsolateral caudate. These increases were greatest in the previously untrained rat merely placed in the test chamber; hybridization was elevated to a similar extent in both trained groups. Although analysis of this material continues, we have as yet identified no difference in hybridization related to whether rats were involved in olfactory discrimination prior to sacrifice. Thus, neither the magnitude nor distribution of changes in hybridization to c-*fos* mRNA were found to reflect recent olfactory learning but, rather, seemed to reflect the novelty of treatment prior to sacrifice.

CONCLUDING COMMENTS: POTENTIAL ROLES OF ACTIVITY-DEPENDENT GENE EXPRESSION IN MEMORY FORMATION

Studies demonstrating that protein synthesis inhibition disrupts particular types of learning (Davis & Squire, 1984; Staubli et al., 1985) suggest that specialized or heightened patterns of neuronal activity might induce changes in protein synthesis that are critical to memory formation. As described here, studies of seizures have demonstrated that bursts of intense neuronal activity can influence the synthesis of proteins that are likely to play fundamentally important roles in both synaptic and trophic communication between forebrain neurons. Moreover, we have seen that even very subtle and naturalistic forms of stimulation can activate the expression of immediate-early genes that act as intracellular regulators of the expression of other, phenotype specific, genes. However, the spatiotemporal parameters of these responses place limitations on the probable involvement of activity-regulated protein synthesis in learning.

The most rapid physiologically induced changes in gene expression thus far described (e.g., immediate-early genes) require several minutes before their initial appearance and still more time to reach their peaks. Some of the most interesting effects (e.g., altered glutamate receptor expression) did not appear until several hours after intense physiological activity was over. Presumably then, altered genomic activity cannot directly contribute to the *acquisition* of new information. It is informative in this regard to compare the time course of these effects to those for the development and stabilization of LTP, a type of plasticity induced by intense synaptic activity that has been linked to some forms of memory (Morris, Anderson, Lynch, & Baudry, 1986; Staubli, Thibault, DiLorenzo, & Lynch, 1989). Work by Gustaffson, Asztely, Hanse, and Wigstrom (1989) shows that LTP develops within 20–30 s while Arai and colleagues (Arai, Kessler, Lee, & Lynch, 1990; Arai, Larson, & Lynch, 1990) find that synaptic potentiation is converted from a vulnerable to a very stable condition within at most 5–10 min after its induction. These time frames are too short to involve any of the effects described in the present review. Accordingly, it seems unlikely that altered gene expression can play a role in the formation and initial steps of consolidating the stable synaptic modifications likely to be associated with the encoding of specific memories.

A second point that bears emphasis is that physiologically driven modifications in gene activity are transient. Given the wide variety of mRNAs that have been sampled, it is likely that this will be generally true for altered expression. Studies on the LTP effect again provide for a useful comparison. Once induced, LTP in the hippocampus can persist without evident change for weeks (Staubli & Lynch, 1987), a time period over which even the most long-lived of the effects described here will have dissipated. It seems reasonable to conclude then that up- or down-regulation of genes is not likely to contribute products that in any direct way contribute to the consolidation of individual memories.

A third limitation on the role of gene expression in memory formation is that its consequences are not likely to be synapse-specific. In a few cases it was possible to follow the disposition of the proteins synthesized by genes whose activity had been profoundly influenced by seizures. Enkephalin, for example, was found to increase markedly following activity-induced elevations of preproenkephalin mRNA; this effect occurred in most, if not all, terminals formed by the axons projecting from the affected neurons (Gall & White, 1989). There is no reason to assume that down-regulation of GluR1 (glutamate receptor) gene expression would result in decreases in this receptor subunit at subpopulations of synapses. These are important considerations because there are good theoretical reasons for assuming that the encoding of individual memories involves changes in small collections of synapses associated with the processing of the to-be-learned information. The synapse specificity of the LTP effect (Bliss & Lømo, 1973; Dunwiddie & Lynch, 1978) is one of the reasons why this form of plasticity is so attractive as a potential substrate for memory. The more global consequences of altered gene expression again point to the conclusion that this phenomenon is not likely to be a mechanism *encoding* individual memories.

Three points, among others, suggest that effects of the kind described in this chapter could, if they occurred during learning, contribute to memory. First, altered gene expression was prominent in brain regions thought to be critical to formation, storage, and utilization of memory. Second, different genes (e.g., those associated with neuroactive peptides or transmitter receptors) were affected by the same physiological events in different brain regions, something which would be expected if altered expression were to contribute to specialized memory functions of these regions. Third, several of the activity-driven changes in gene expression should have profound effects on the functional properties of the neurons and networks in which they occur. Given the limitations outlined in the preceding paragraphs, how might the various regulatory changes manifest themselves in behavior? Three speculative hypotheses are summarized below:

- *Activity-regulated gene products provide a generalized background against which selective plasticity will (or will not) occur.* According to this idea, events occurring *prior to* a learning episode produce genomic changes that determine the ease with which synapse specific effects such as LTP can be induced. As an example, placing an animal in a familiar testing environment might induce an increase in the activity of trophic factor genes and thus a greater likelihood that growth-related enzymes will be activated by local synaptic events.
- *Tonic activity within individual neurons over days determines via gene regulation their thresholds for plasticity.* Theorists have argued that learning involves not only synapse-specific changes of the type represented by LTP but also generalized changes in the ease with which such effects can be elicited by synaptic activity. Mechanisms of this kind are, for example, needed to explain how experience produces ocular dominance effects in visual cortex (Bear, Cooper, & Ebner, 1987). It is thus possible that mean activity over days, acting through gene regulation, differentiates neurons in terms of their plasticity or other properties and thereby defines where information becomes encoded. Levels of glutamate receptors, trophic factors, or the balance of neuroactive peptides could all be critical to such effects.

- *Activity-dependent gene expression contributes to the decay of learning-induced changes in neuronal properties.* Behavioral studies have produced evidence for a relatively short-lasting type of memory sometimes referred to as "working memory." The hippocampus appears to be critically involved in this effect (Olton, Becker, & Handelman, 1979) as do neuroactive peptides (Jiang, Owyang, Hong, & Gallagher, 1989). Interestingly enough, in vitro it was recently discovered that the mossy fibers exhibit an unusual form of LTP that is qualitatively different from CA1-LTP, raising the possibility that it may serve a specialized function such as working memory (Staubli, Larson, & Lynch, 1990). Other work has shown that the LTP found in the perforant path, unlike that in field CA1, decreases steadily with normal synaptic responses, being recovered in 1–2 weeks (Castro, Silbert, McNaughton, & Barnes, 1989). These observations indicate that hippocampus, and perhaps other regions of the brain, possess plasticities with various durations, thus providing the basis for memories of different durations. While a not unlikely explanation for such effects is that the substrates of potentiation decay with time, it is also conceivable that they reflect an active reversal process. One possibility is that in some systems potentiation reflects a depletion of a protein that normally suppresses transmission and that the same activity responsible for this depletion also up-regulates the gene for this protein. Certain of the neuropeptide effects observed in the mossy fibers would satisfy this scenario.

Evaluation of the above three hypotheses and similar ideas will require tests of the extent to which expression is influenced by naturalistic stimulation and ultimately behavior. Work with brief limbic seizure has identified candidate genes, time courses, and regions, and thus has served as a prelude to the search for the subtle changes that might be expected with less-intense physiological activation. Further studies with the seizure paradigm are needed to test for underlying themes that might explain the diversity of changes so far observed. The complex of up- and down-regulatory events, often occurring within individual cells, reviewed here may reflect the many facets of definable syndromes, the end-points of which are to shift neurons between modes of functioning. Answers to how gene expression affects learning and memory may ultimately be found at this level of analysis.

Acknowledgments: This work was supported by NINDS award NS26748, NIA award AG00538, and NICHD award HD 24236. The authors thank Gary Lynch for helpful discussions of learning mechanisms.

REFERENCES

Alderson, R. F., Alterman, A. L., Barde, Y. A., & Lindsay, R. M. (1990). Brain-derived neurotrophic factor increases survival and differentiated functions of rat septal cholinergic neurons in culture. *Neuron, 5*, 297–306.

Anokhin, K. V., & Rose, S. P. R. (1991). Learning-induced increase of immediate early gene messenger RNA in the chick forebrain. *European Journal of Neuroscience, 3*, 162–167.

Arai, A., Kessler, M., Lee, K., & Lynch, G. (1990). Calpain inhibitors improve the recovery of synaptic transmission from hypoxia in hippocampal slices. *Brain Research, 532*, 63–68.

Arai, A., Larson, J., & Lynch, G. (1990). Anoxia reveals a vulnerable period in the development of long-term potentiation. *Brain Research, 511*, 353–357.

Bear, M. F., Cooper, L. N., & Ebner, F. F. (1987). A physiological basis for a theory of synapse modification. *Science, 237*, 42–48.

Bliss, T. V. P., & Lømo, T. (1973). Long-lasting potentiation of synaptic transmission in the dentate area of the anaesthetized rabbit following stimulation of the perforant path. *Journal of Physiology (London), 233*, 334–356.

Boulter, J., Hollmann, M., O'Shea-Greenfield, A., Hartley, M., Deneris, E., Maron, C., & Heinemann, S. (1990). Molecular closing and functional expression of glutamate receptor subunit genes. *Science, 249*, 1033–1037.

Campbell, K. A., Bank, B., & Milgram, N. W. (1984). Epileptogenic effects of electrolytic lesions in the hippocampus: role of iron deposition. *Experimental Neurology, 85*, 506–514.

Castro, C. A., Silbert, L., McNaughton, B. L., & Barnes, C. A. (1989). Recovery of spatial learning deficits after decay of electrically-induced synaptic enhancement in the hippocampus. *Nature, 342*, 545–548.

Cole, A. J., Saffen, D. W., Baraban, J. M., & Worley, P. F. (1989). Rapid increase of an immediate early gene messenger RNA in hippocampal neurons by synaptic NMDA receptor activation. *Nature, 340*, 474–476.

Curran, T., & Morgan, J. I. (1987). Memories of fos. *Bioessays, 7*, 255–258.

Daval, J.-L., Nakajima, T., Gleiter, C. H., Post, R. M., & Marangos, P. J. (1989). Mouse brain c-*fos* mRNA distribution following a single electroconvulsive shock. *Journal of Neurochemistry, 52*, 1954–1957.

Davis, H. P., & Squires, L. R. (1984). Protein synthesis and memory: A review. *Psychological Bulletin, 96*, 518–559.

Douglass, J., Grimes, L., Shook, J., Lee, P. H. K., & Hong, J.-S. (1991). Systemic administration of kainic acid differentially regulates the levels of prodynorphin and proenkephalin mRNA and peptides in the rat hippocampus. *Molecular Brain Research, 9*, 79–86.

Dragunow, M., Abraham, W. C., Goulding, M., Mason, S. E., Robertson, H. A., & Faull, R. L. M. (1989). Long-term potentiation and the induction of c-*fos* mRNA and proteins in the dentate gyrus of unanesthetized rats. *Neuroscience Letters, 101*, 274–280.

Dragunow, M., & Robertson, H. A. (1987). Kindling stimulation induces c-*fos* protein(s) in granule cells of the rat dentate gyrus. *Nature, 329*, 441–442.

Dunwiddie, T., & Lynch, G. (1978). Long-term potentiation and depression of synaptic responses in the rat hippocampus: Localization and frequency dependency. *Journal of Physiology, 276*, 353–367.

Ernfors, P., Wetmore, C., Olson, L., & Persson, H. (1990). Identification of cells in rat brain and peripheral tissues expressing mRNAs for members of the nerve growth factor family. *Neuron, 5*, 511–526.

Gall, C. (1988). Seizures induce dramatic and distinctly different changes in enkephalin, dynorphin, and cholecystokinin immunoreactivities in mouse hippocampal mossy fibers. *Journal of Neuroscience, 8*, 1852–1862.

Gall, C., Brecha, N., Karten, H. J., & Chang, J.-J. (1981). Localization of enkephalin immunoreactivity in identified axonal and neuronal populations in the rat hippocampus. *Journal of Comparative Neurology, 198*, 335–350.

Gall, C., & Isackson, P. (1989). Limbic seizures increase neuronal production of mRNA for nerve growth factor. *Science, 245*, 758–761.

Gall, C., Lauterborn, J., & Isackson, P. (1990). One paroxysmal discharge stimulates temporally distinct changes in neuronal NGF and immediate-early gene expression. *Journal of Cellular Biochemistry, 14F* (Suppl.), 67.

Gall, C., Lauterborn, J., Isackson, P., & White, J. (1990). Seizures, neuropeptide regulation, and mRNA expression in the hippocampus. In J. Storm-Mathisen, J. Zimmer, & O. P. Ottersen (Eds.), *Understanding the brain through the hippocampus. Progress in brain research* (Vol. 83) (pp. 371–390). Amsterdam: Elsevier.

Gall, C., Murray, K., & Isackson, P. J. (1991). Kainic acid-induced seizures stimulate increased expression of nerve growth factor in adult rat hippocampus. *Molecular Brain Research, 9*, 113–123.

Gall, C., Pico, R., & Lauterborn, J. (1988). Seizures induce distinct long-lasting changes in mossy fiber peptide immunoreactivity. *Peptides, 9*, 79–84.

Gall, C., Sumikawa, K., & Lynch, G. (1990). Levels of mRNA for a putative kainate receptor are affected by seizures. *Proceedings of the National Academy of Sciences, U.S.A., 87*, 7643–7647.

Gall, C., & White, J. (1989). Studies on the expression of opioid peptides and their respective mRNAs in hippocampal seizure. In V. Chan-Palay & C. Köhler (Eds.), *The hippocampus: New vistas* (pp. 153–170). New York: Alan Liss.

Greenberg, M. E., Ziff, E. B., & Greene, L. A. (1986). Stimulation of neuronal acetylcholine receptors induces rapid gene transcription. *Science, 234*, 80–83.

Greenough, W. T., & Bailey, C. H. (1988). The anatomy of a memory: Convergence of results across a diversity of tests. *TINS, 11*, 142–143.

Gubits, R. M., Smith, T. M., Fairhurst, J. L., & Yu, H. (1989). Adrenergic receptors mediate changes in c-*fos* mRNA levels in brain. *Molecular Brain Research, 6*, 39–45.

Gustafsson, B., Asztely, F., Hanse, F., & Wigstom, H. (1989). Onset characteristics of long-term potentiation in the guinea pig hippocampal CA1 region in vitro. *European Journal of Neuroscience, 1*, 382–394.

Hefti, F. (1986). Nerve growth factor (NGF) promotes survival of septal cholinergic neurons after fimbrial transection. *Journal of Neuroscience, 6*, 2155–2162.

Hengerer, B., Lindholm, D., Heumann, R., Rüther, U., Wagner, E. F., & Thoenen, H. (1990). Lesion-induced increase in nerve growth factor mRNA is mediated by c-*fos*. *Proceedings of the National Academy of Sciences, U.S.A., 87*, 3899–3903.

Higgins, G. A., Sookyong, K., Chen, K. S., & Gage, F. H. (1989). NGF induction of NGF receptor gene expression and cholinergic neuronal hypertrophy in the basal forebrain of the adult rat. *Neuron, 3*, 247–256.

Hohn, A., Leibrock, J., Bailey, K., & Barde, Y.-A. (1990). Identification and characterization of a novel member of the nerve growth factor/brain derived neurotrophic factor family. *Nature, 344*, 339–341.

Hollmann, M., O'Shead-Greenfield, A., Rogers, S. W., & Heinemann, S. (1989). Cloning by functional expression of a member of the glutamate receptor family. *Nature, 342*, 643–648.

Isackson, P. J., Huntsman, M. M., Murray, K. D., & Gall, C. M. (1991). BDNF mRNA expression is increased in adult rat forebrain after limbic seizures: temporal patterns of induction distinct from NGF. *Neuron, 6*, 937–948.

Jiang, H. K., Owyang, V. V., Hong, J. S., & Gallagher, M. (1989). Elevated dynorphin in the hippocampal formation of aged rats: Relation to cognitive impairment on a spatial learning task. *Proceedings of the National Academy of Sciences, U.S.A., 86*, 2948–2951.

Johnson, J. E., Barde, Y.-A., Schwab, M., & Thoenen, H. (1986). Brain-derived neurotrophic factor supports the survival of cultured rat retinal ganglion cells. *Journal of Neuroscience, 6*, 3031–3038.

Kanamatsu, T., Obie, J., Grimes, L., McGinty, J. F., Yoshikawa, K., Sabol, S., & Hong, J. S. (1986). Kainic acid alters the metabolism of Met^5-enkephalin and the levels of dynorphin A in the rat hippocampus. *Journal of Neuroscience, 6*, 3094–3102.

Knüsel, B., Winslow, J. W., Rosenthal, A., Burton, L. E., Seid, D. P., Nikolics, K., & Hefti, F. (1991). Promotion of central cholinergic and dopaminergic neuron differentiation by brain-derived neurotrophic factor but not neurotrophin 3. *Proceedings of the National Academcy of Sciences, U.S.A., 88*, 961–965.

Köhler, C., Eriksson, L., Davies, S., & Chan-Palay, V. (1986). Neuropeptide Y innervation of the hippocampal region in the rat and monkey brain. *Journal of Comparative Neurology, 244*, 384–400.

Lärkfors, L., Strömberg, I., Ebendal, T., & Olson, L. (1987). Nerve growth factor protein level increases in the adult rat hippocampus after a specific cholinergic lesion. *Journal of Neuroscience Research, 18*, 525–531.

Leibrock, J., Lottspeich, F., Hohn, A., Hofer, M., Hengerer, B., Masiakowski, P., Thoenen, H., & Barde, Y.-A. (1989). Molecular cloning and expression of brain-derived neurotrophic factor. *Nature, 341*, 149–152.

Macgregor, P.F., Abate, C., & Curran, T. (1990). Direct cloning of leucine zipper proteins—Jun binds cooperatively in the CRE with CRE-BPI. *Oncogene, 5*, 451–458.

Maisonpierre, P. C., Belluscio, L., Friedman, B., Alderson, R. F., Wiegand, S. J., Furth, M. E., Lindsay, R. M., & Yancopoulos, G. D. (1990). NT-3, BDNF and NGF in the developing rat nervous system: Parallel as well as reciprocal patterns of expression. *Neuron, 5*, 501–509.

Maisonpierre, P. C., Belluscio, L., Squinto, S., Ip, N. Y., Furth, M. E., Lindsay, R. M., & Yancopoulos, G. D. (1990). Neurotrophin-3: A neurotrophic factor related to NGF and BDNF. *Science, 247*, 1446–1451.

Marksteiner, J., Ortler, M., Bellmann, R., & Sperk, G. (1990). Neuropeptide Y biosynthesis is markedly induced in mossy fibers during temporal lobe epilepsy of the rat. *Neuroscience Letters, 112*, 143–148.

McGinty, J. F., Henriksen, S. J., Goldstein, A., Terenius, L., & Bloom, F. E. (1983). Dynorphin is contained within hippocampal mossy fibers: Immunohistochemical alterations after kainic acid administration and cholchicine-induced cytotoxicity. *Proceedings of the National Academy of Sciences, U.S.A., 80*, 589–593.

McGinty, J. F., Kanamatsu, T., Obie, J., Dyer, R. S., Mitchell, C. L., & Hong, J. S. (1986). Amygdaloid kindling increases enkephalin-like immunoreactivity but decreases dynorphin A-like immunoreactivity in rat hippocampus. *Neuroscience Letters, 71*, 31–36.

Morgan, J. I., Cohen, D. R., Hempstead, J. L., & Curran, T. (1987). Mapping patterns of c-*fos* expression in the central nervous system after seizure. *Science, 237*, 192–197.

Morgan, J. I., & Curran, T. (1986). Role of ion flux in the control of c-*fos* expression. *Nature, 322*, 552–555.

Morgan, J. I., & Curran, T. (1989). Stimulus-transcription coupling in neurons: Role of cellular immediate early genes. *Trends in Neuroscience, 12*, 459–462.

Morris, B. J., Feasely, K. J., Bruggencate, G. ten, Herz, A., & Höllt, V. (1988). Electrical stimulation in vivo increases the expression of proenkephalin mRNA and decreases the expression of prodynorphin mRNA in rat hippocampal granule cells. *Proceedings of the National Academy of Sciences, U.S.A., 85*, 3226–3230.

Morris, R. G. M., Anderson, E., Lynch, G. S., & Baudry, M. (1986) Selective impairment of learning and blockade of long term potentiation by an N-methyl-D-aspartate receptor antagonist, AP-5. *Nature, 319*, 774–776.

Muller, D., Joly, M., & Lynch, G. (1988). Contributions of quisqualate and NMDA receptors to the induction and expression of LTP. *Science, 242*, 1694–1697.

Olton, D. S., Becker, J. T., & Handelman, G. E. (1979). Hippocampus, spaces and memory. *Behavioral and Brain Sciences, 2*, 313–365.

Rusak, B., Robertson, H. A., Wisden, W., & Hunt, S. P. (1990). Light pulses that shift rhythms induce gene expression in the suprachiasmatic nucleus. *Science, 248*, 1237–1240.

Saffen, D. W., Cole, A. J., Worley, P. F., Christy, B. A., Ryder, K., & Baraban, J. M. (1988). Convulsant-induced increase in transcription factor messenger RNAs in rat brain. *Proceedings of the National Academy of Sciences, U.S.A., 85* 7795–7799.

Sugar, S. M., & Sharp, F. R. (1990). Light induces a Fos-like nuclear antigen in retinal neurons. *Molecular Brain Research, 7*, 17–21.

Sheng, M., & Greenberg, M. E. (1990). The regulation and function of c-*fos* and other immediate early genes in the nervous system. *Neuron, 4*, 477–485.

Shin, C., McNamara, J. O., Morgan, J. I., Curran, T., & Cohen, D. R. (1990). Induction of c-*fos* mRNA expression by afterdischarge in the hippocampus of naive and kindled rats. *Journal of Neurochemistry, 55*, 1050–1055.

Sonnenberg, J. L., Macgregor-Leon, P. F., Curran, T., & Morgan, J. I. (1989). Dynamic alterations occur in the levels and composition of transcription factor AP-1 complexes after seizure. *Neuron, 3*, 359–365.

Staubli, U., Faraday, R., & Lynch, G. (1985). Pharmacological dissociation of memory: Anisomycin, a protein synthesis inhibitor and leupeptin, a protease inhibitor, block different learning tasks. *Behavioral and Neural Biology, 43*, 387–297.

Staubli, U., Larson, J., & Lynch, G. (1990). Mossy fiber potentiation and long-term potentiation involve different expression mechanisms. *Synapse, 5*, 333–335.

Staubli, U., & Lynch, G. (1987). Stable hippocampal long term potentiation elicited by "theta" pattern stimulation. *Brain Research, 435*, 227–234.

Staubli, U., Thibault, O., DiLorenzo, M., & Lynch, G. (1989). Antagonism of NMDa receptors impairs acquisition but not retention of olfactory memory. *Behavioral Neuroscience, 103*, 54–60.

Van Nguyen, T., Kobierski, L., Comb, M., & Hyman, S. E. (1990). The effect of depolarization on expression of the human proenkephalin gene is synergistic with cAMP and dependent upon a cAMP-inducible enhancer. *Journal of Neuroscience, 10*, 2825–2833.

White, J. D., Gall, C. M. (1987). Differential regulation of neuropeptide and proto-oncogene mRNA content in the hippocampus following recurrent seizures. *Molecular Brain Research, 3*, 21–29.

White, J. D., Gall, C. M., & McKelvy, J. F. (1987). Enkephalin biosynthesis and enkephalin gene expression are increased in hippocampal mossy fibers following a unilateral lesion of the hilus. *Journal of Neuroscience, 7*, 753–759.

Whittemore, S. R., & Seiger, A. (1987). The expression, localization, and functional significance of β-nerve growth factor in the central nervous system. *Brain Research Reviews, 12*, 439–464.

Wisden, W., Errington, M. L., Williams, S., Dunnett, S. B., Waters, C., Hitchcock, D., Evan, G., Bliss, T. V. P., & Hunt, S. P. (1990). Differential expression of immediate early genes in the hippocampus and spinal cord. *Neuron, 4*, 603–614.

Zafra, F., Hengerer, B., Leibrock, J., Thoenen, H., & Lindholm, D. (1990). Activity dependent regulation of BNDF and NGF mRNAs in the rat hippocampus is mediated by non-NMDA glutamate receptors. *EMBO Journal, 9*, 3545–3550.

14

Variants of Synaptic Potentiation and Different Types of Memory Operations in Hippocampus and Related Structures

GARY LYNCH
JOHN LARSON
URSULA STAUBLI
RICHARD GRANGER

Recent work indicates that high-frequency stimulation of afferent fibers causes a long-lasting potentiation of synaptic responses in each of the links of a sequence beginning with the olfactory cortex and continuing through the subfields of hippocampus. Taken together, these studies also established the important point that the characteristics of the potentiation vary across different connections and in some cases dramatically so. There are at least two ways in which these variations are potentially useful in developing hypotheses about the types of memory operations carried out by the regions in which they are found. First, the characteristics of the fully expressed potentiation could be directly related to the properties of memory. Duration and specificity provide obvious examples; synaptic changes lasting for hours are suggestive of different types of behavioral phenomena than changes persisting for months, and modifications that affect specific subpopulations of contacts on a fiber or dendrite can be expected to have very different effects than more general changes. Second, it may be possible to convert the physiological rules (e.g., specific patterns or sequences of activity governing the induction of potentiation) into a set of computational operations. Tests could then be made for regional variations in the rules and computations, and hence for regionally specific memory processes. Placing these points in a more psychological context one might assume that variations in expression should relate to types and organization of memory while variations in induction should govern what is (or can be) learned.

The present chapter is concerned with both these points. It begins with a review of the characteristics of synaptic potentiation found in four different links of the olfactory–hippocampal circuit. The point will be made that variants of the long-term potentiation (LTP) effect are found in three of these links while the fourth exhibits a very different type of plasticity. The second section of the chapter describes experiments that define the relationship between spatial and temporal patterns of input activity and the induction of LTP. The argument is made that these data constitute the ingredients needed to construct synaptic learning rules based on LTP. Efforts to define the properties of memory resulting from the characteristics of expressed LTP are described in the third part of the chapter. Some preliminary studies on the computational significance of the LTP-based synaptic learning rules are also discussed. The last section takes up the question of how variations in potentiation might interact with different anatomical architectures (circuit designs) and in particular those found in hippocampus. The hypothesis is advanced that these interactions generate a sequence of memory operations that involves periods of time ranging from several milliseconds to many weeks.

EXPRESSION CHARACTERISTICS OF SYNAPTIC POTENTIATION IN A SEQUENCE OF NETWORKS

LTP in Field CA1: A Postsynaptic Phenomenon?

There is general agreement that the initial induction steps involve (a) stimulation of NMDA receptors (Collingridge, Kehl, & McLennan, 1983), during (b) postsynaptic depolarization of unusual degree and duration (Kelso, Ganong, & Brown, 1986; Malinow & Miller, 1986; Wigstrom, Gustafsson, Huang, & Abraham, 1986), and (c) a change in calcium levels in the postsynaptic cell (Lynch, Larson, Kelso, Barrionuevo, & Schottler, 1983). While it is clear that the triggers for LTP are postsynaptic, the nature and locus of the changes that express it in field CA1 are controversial. Figure 14.1a illustrates four widely discussed possibilities; (a) increased influx of calcium and greater probability of release, (b) greater release resulting from any of a variety of possible mechanisms (Bliss & Lynch, 1988), (c) modification of postsynaptic receptors (Lynch & Baundry, 1984), or (d) enhanced synaptic current because of biophysical changes in spines (Rall, 1978). Figure 14.1b shows what could be a more accurate representation in which individual axons form multiple contacts of unequal strength with individual dendrites. Note that LTP could be a selective strengthening of weaker contacts; any of the mechanisms shown in Figure 14.1a could be used for this purpose. The possibility that new junctions subserve the potentiation effect must also be considered.

Efforts to test the first idea (increased influx of calcium, increased probability of release) have taken advantage of the observation that treatments which augment release are not multiplicative (Rahamimoff,

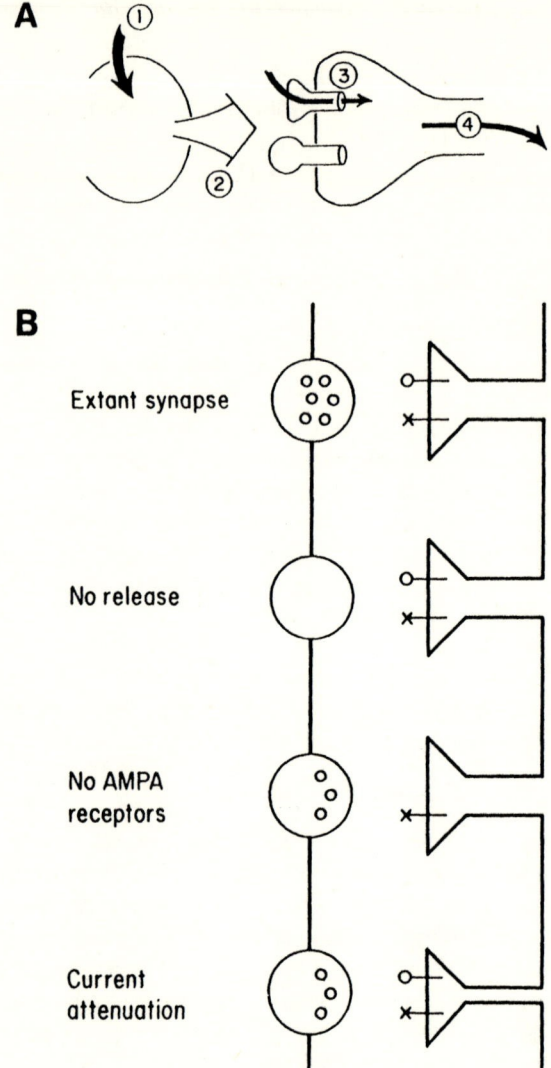

FIGURE 14.1. Possible loci and mechanisms for expression of LTP in field CA1 of hippocampus. (A) Mechanisms involving changes in transmission at existing synapses. Potentiation of transmission could be due to increased presynaptic calcium influx (1), increased transmitter release (2), changes in postsynaptic receptors (3), or changes in spine shape (4). (B) Strengthening of weak or "silent" synapses as a mechanism for LTP. Diagram shows a single presynaptic axon making four synapses on a single postsynaptic dendrite (circles and crosses denote AMPA and NMDA receptors, respectively). Prior to LTP, only one synapse (extant synapse) produces measurable postsynaptic responses; the others are silent because they either do not release transmitter, have no functional AMPA receptors, or the postsynaptic spine greatly attenuates synaptic current. After LTP, the weak synapses could become functional by mechanisms that ameliorate their deficiencies. (Panel B adapted from Larson, Ambros-Ingerson, & Lynch, in press)

1968). Muller and Lynch (1989) confirmed this for CA3–CA1 connections by demonstrating interactions between increased extracellular calcium, 4-aminopyridine, and paired-pulse facilitation, all manipulations thought to affect calcium levels in terminals. If LTP expression involves such effects, then it would be expected that it would show similar interactions. This result was not obtained. Thus, potentiation did not reduce paired-pulse facilitation (see McNaughton, 1982, for a similar result using perforant path) and changes in extracellular calcium levels did not affect the degree of LTP expressed (Muller & Lynch, 1989). Haas and Greene (1985) have also reported that the actions of 4-aminopyridine are not reduced by LTP.

The idea (hypothesis 2 in Figure 14.1) that LTP expression involves increased release because of some change in the release process beyond calcium influx and simple probability (e.g., number of vesicles, amount of transmitter per vesicle, etc.) was tested using preparations in which both NMDA (NMDA-R) and AMPA (AMPA-R) receptors make significant contributions to the postsynaptic response (Muller & Lynch, 1988). The relative size of each component could then be measured using drugs that selectively block either NMDA-Rs or AMPA-Rs (see Figure 14.2). It would be expected that an increased number of transmitter molecules in the synaptic cleft would stimulate more AMPA-Rs and NMDA-Rs and hence increase the size of both components of the composite response. This was confirmed using paired-pulse facilitation; that is, facilitated release increases AMPA-R dependent responses by ~50% and NMDA-R mediated potentials by 70–80%. If LTP were due to increased release, then it follows that it should produce similar results. This was not obtained. Using three different experimental paradigms, it was found that the potentiation effect enhanced AMPA-R responses by 40–60% and NMDA-R responses by 0–15% (Muller & Lynch, 1988; Muller, Joly, & Lynch, 1988; Muller, Larson & Lynch, 1989). Kauer, Malenka, & Nicoll (1988) have reported similar results.

Studies using quantal analysis techniques have led to the conclusion that LTP is accompanied by increased release (Bekkers & Stevens, 1990; Malinow & Tsien, 1990; Voronin, 1988). These results are controversial (see Foster & McNaughton, 1991) and, in any event, could reflect postsynaptic changes in a multisynapse system of the type shown in Figure 14.1b (Larson, Ambros-Ingerson, & Lynch, 1991).

Hypothesis 3 is that LTP alters the properties of postsynaptic receptors. Reasoning as above, evidence for this could be obtained by testing for interactions between LTP and treatments that are known to alter receptor functioning. Ito, Tanabe, Kohda, & Sugiyama (1990) recently described a manipulation of this type. Specifically, they found that aniracetam (a nootropic drug) enhances currents mediated by AMPA-Rs but not those associated with NMDA-Rs or GABA-Rs expressed in frog oocytes. They also showed that the drug enhanced synaptic responses in hippocampus (Ito et al., 1990). We confirmed that aniracetam increases AMPA-R mediated responses in hippocampus (Staubli, Kessler, & Lynch, 1990) and showed that it has no effects on NMDA-R dependent potentials, (Xiao, Staubli,

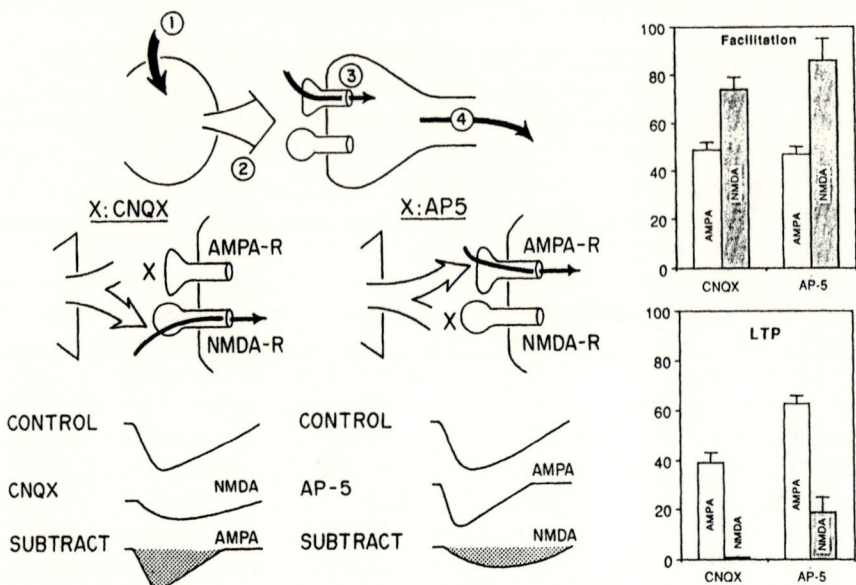

FIGURE 14.2.   Differential expression of LTP by AMPA and NMDA receptors. Two strategies for isolating AMPA-R and NMDA-R responses from composite responses are illustrated: one (X: CNQX) uses the selective AMPA-R antagonist, CNQX, to directly measure NMDA-R responses and estimate AMPA-R responses by subtraction of NMDA-R components; the other (X: AP5) uses the selective NMDA-R antagonist, AP5, to directly measure AMPA-R responses and estimate NMDA-R responses by subtraction of AMPA-R components. Graph at top right shows that NMDA-R dependent responses exhibit greater paired-pulse facilitation than AMPA-R responses using either pharmacological technique; graph at bottom right shows that AMPA-R responses exhibit much greater LTP than NMDA-R responses; y-axis in both graphs is percentage increase from control. (Data from Muller, Joly, & Lynch, 1988; Muller & Lynch, 1988)

Kessler, & Lynch, submitted). Thus the drug has the specificity expected from the oocyte experiments. We then asked if it interacts with LTP and obtained positive results; aniracetam produced percentage increases in the amplitude of control inputs that were nearly double those found in potentiated inputs to the same dendritic targets. Conversely, its actions were unaffected by paired-pulse facilitation, a manipulation that, as noted above, increases release (Staubli, Kessler, & Lynch, 1990; Xiao et al., in press). These results provide direct evidence that LTP expression involves a change in AMPA receptors.

Hypothesis 4 holds that spine shape changes have biophysical consequences that enhance postsynaptic currents. Under certain conditions changes in spine neck resistance can significantly affect the nonlinear relationship between synaptic conductance and synaptic current (Brown, Chang, Ganong, Keenan, & Kelso, 1988; Koch & Poggio, 1983; Rall, 1978; Wilson, 1984) and hence alter the synaptic current driven by a constant conductance. Such an effect could, in principle, account for LTP. A potential problem for the spine resistance hypothesis is the differential expression of LTP by AMPA-R and NMDA-R mediated responses. However, some models indicate that slow currents (e.g., NMDA-R currents) are less affected by spine resistance than fast currents (e.g., AMPA-R currents; Wilson, 1984), thus possibly explaining differential expression. If this were the case, then altering the time course of AMPA-R responses such that they match NMDA-R responses should render them incapable of expressing LTP. However, achieving this by manipulating temperature failed to confirm this prediction (Larson & Lynch, 1991). A second prediction is that control and potentiated synaptic currents should be differentially affected by experimental manipulations of synaptic conductance. Tests of this idea involved measuring relative effects of large reductions in synaptic conductance (by decreasing transmitter release, or partially blocking postsynaptic receptors) on control and potentiated synapses. No differences were observed, again failing to support the spine resistance hypothesis (Jung, Larson, & Lynch, 1991).

In summary, it appears unlikely that expression of LTP in hippocampal field CA1 is mediated by either a simple increase in transmitter release or by biophysical changes resulting from spine shape modifications. A change in postsynaptic receptors is left as a likely alternative, and experimental evidence supports the idea that LTP results from a selective modification of AMPA-R conductance.

Expression Characteristics of LTP

Once induced, LTP in field CA1 has a number of characteristics that are suggestive of the type of memory it might encode. First, the effect is remarkably stable. Experiments using chronically implanted electrodes (Staubli & Lynch, 1987) indicate that LTP can persist without evident change for as long as stable stimulating and recording arrangements can be maintained (weeks in some cases). Explaining this stability is probably the single most difficult problem for hypotheses regarding the substrates of LTP (see Lynch, Kessler, Arai, & Larson, 1990, for a discussion). In any event, the extreme persistence of LTP raises the possibility that hippocampus encodes some equivalently long-lasting forms of memory. Second, LTP is synapse-specific. This was shown using two separate collections of Schaffer-commissural efferents terminating on the same apical dendrites (Andersen, Sundberg, Sveen, Swann, & Wigstrom, 1980; Dunwiddie & Lynch, 1978). Third, fractional degrees of LTP can be produced; that is, the effect is not all-or-none (Douglas & Goddard, 1975; Larson, Wong, & Lynch, 1986). Whether this reflects the number of synapses generated by an input that became potentiated in a single, high-frequency episode as opposed to the degree to which individual synapses become potentiated is not known. As discussed later, fractional LTP can be of considerable computational significance. Fourth, LTP saturates at about a 50–100% increase in synaptic strength. Fifth, LTP does not affect paired-pulse facilitation (see page 335). Repetitive afferent activity causes a transient facilitation of synaptic responses owing to enhanced release. This is likely to be of considerable importance for network operations since it means that high-frequency discharges by neurons will momentarily increase the strength of their connections with other cells and perhaps provide for a kind of frequency filtering whereby target neurons are more likely to discharge in response to some patterns of inputs than others. The observation that LTP does not affect one variant of this type of frequency-dependent synaptic facilitation (i.e., paired pulse facilitation) could be of importance in interpreting its effects on network operations.

Mossy Fiber Potentiation: A Presynaptic Phenomenon

The granule cells of the dentate gyrus and the mossy fibers they send to the pyramidal cells of field CA3 have some of the most unusual features found in mammalian telencephalon. Explaining why this system has so many peculiar aspects constitutes an immediate challenge to any attempt to develop a theory of memory encoding and processing in the olfactory–hippocampal circuit. Several studies have shown that high-frequency stimulation of the mossy fibers produces a long-lasting potentiation effect (Barrionuevo, Kelso, Johnston, & Brown, 1986; Hopkins & Johnston, 1984; Misgeld, Sarvey, & Klee, 1979; Yamamoto & Chujo, 1978). Despite the observation that induction of the effect does not depend on NMDA receptors (Harris & Cotman, 1986), it has been assumed that the potentiation is LTP. However, we have obtained evidence that this is not the case. As discussed, work in our laboratory (Müller & Lynch, 1989) and elswhere (Haas & Green, 1985; Lee, Anwyl, & Rowan, 1986; McNaughton, 1982; Mulkeen, Anwyl, & Rowan, 1988) has established that manipulations which increase transmitter release are unaffected by prior induction of LTP. Paired-pulse facilitation is an example. When two pulses are given in rapid succession (separated by <100 ms) to the same axons, then the synaptic response to the second pulse is greater than that to the first. Extensive work at the neuromuscular junction has shown that the facilitation results from increased release in response to the second pulse, probably because of residual calcium from the influx triggered by the first pulse (Katz & Miledi, 1968). Paired-pulse facilitation is unaffected by LTP, but it is drastically reduced by induction of mossy fiber potentiation (MFP) (see Figure 14.3; Staubli, Larson, & Lynch, 1990; this result has been replicated and extended by Zalutsky & Nicoll, 1990). The finding that paired-pulse facilitation is related to MFP strongly suggests that the latter effect is expressed by an increase in transmitter release and hence is a presynaptic phenomenon. It is noteworthy that the mossy fiber boutons have an enormous surface area and are densely packed with vesicles of different types; it is possible that repetitive stimulation produces an accumulation of calcium in the terminals far beyond that found in more typical endings and that this provides the substrate of MFP.

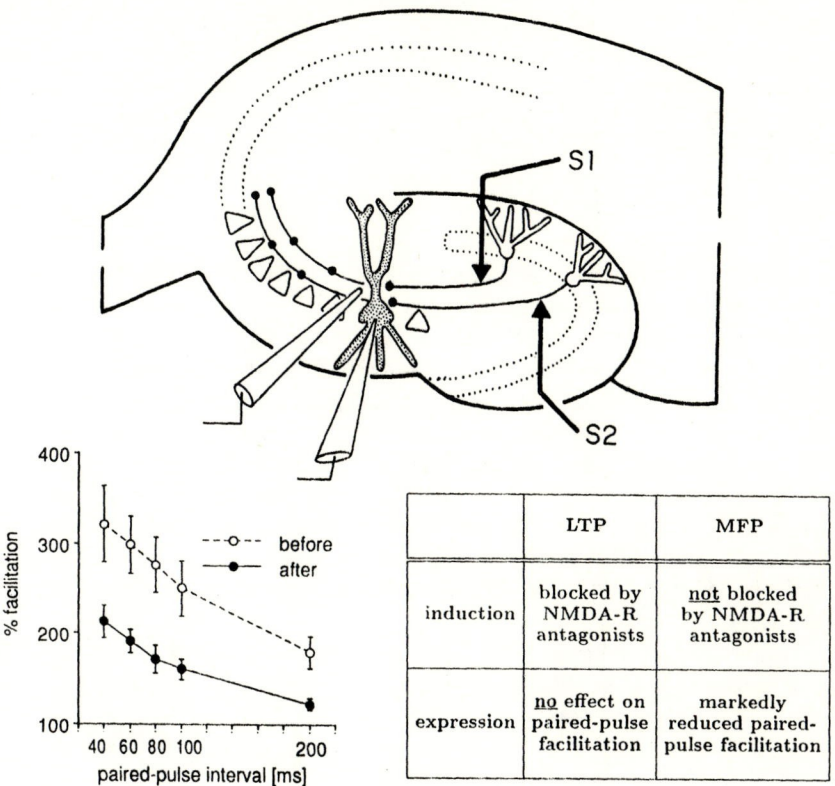

FIGURE 14.3.   Mossy fiber potentiation (MFP) differs from LTP. Diagram shows a hippocampal slice with separate populations of mossy fibers (S1,S2) activated by two stimulating electrodes placed over stratum granulosum and two recording electrodes positioned extracellularly in stratum lucidum and inside a pyramidal cell in field CA3b, respectively. Graph shows the degree of paired-pulse facilitation of mossy fiber field responses obtained before and 15 min after high-frequency stimulation in a group of six slices with stable potentiation. The *y* axis shows facilitation as a percentage of control. The table compares induction and expression mechanisms for LTP versus MFP. (Adapted from Staubli, Larson, & Lynch, 1990)

Two additional aspects of MFP are likely to play a major role in its contributions to the operation of the olfactory–hippocampal circuit. First, the stimulation trains needed to produce the effect appear to be quite different from those required for induction of LTP. In the latter case, very short (30 ms) bursts of four pulses delivered at 5 bursts per second (i.e., theta burst stimulation) have been shown to be optimal (Larson et al., 1986); MFP requires much longer trains (100 Hz for 500–1000 ms). It is indeed interesting that the granule cells alone of the principal components of the olfactory–hippocampal circuit fire in long trains during behavior. Studies on the olfactory cortex showed that layer II cells discharge in very short bursts (see McCollum et al., 1991) and numerous papers have reported a short burst pattern for CA3 and CA1 (Eichenbaum, Kuperstein, Fagan, & Nagode, 1987; Fox & Ranck, 1981; Hill, 1978; Muller, Kubie, & Ranck, 1987, Ranck, 1973). The granule cells, on the other hand, fire in long trains of high-frequency discharges, both in response to learned cues and while the animal is carrying out learned responses to the cue; the discharge pattern in the latter case is modulated by the theta rhythm (Deadwyler, West, & Lynch, 1979; Rose, Diamond, & Lynch, 1983). The possibility thus exists that different forms of potentiation (LTP and MFP) found in the hippocampus have induction requirements that are matched by the firing characteristics of the cells that produce the synapses in which they are found.

Second, the presynaptic nature of MFP suggests that the effect is not synapse specific. That is, paired-pulse facilitation will occur in any terminal on an axon that receives two action potentials in rapid succession and hence can be assumed to occur all along the length of the fiber. Given the close relationship between MFP and paired-pulse facilitation (Staubli, Larson, & Lynch, 1990), it is likely that this argument applies to the former effect as well. If so, then MFP in situ would quickly saturate (i.e., all the terminals would become potentiated) unless the effect was much shorter in duration than LTP.

To summarize, LTP in field CA1 appears to be induced and expressed postsynaptically while MFP is induced and expressed presynaptically. The following section will make the argument that LTP-like effects are found throughout the circuitries leading into and through the hippocampus.

Potentiation in Other Links of the Olfactory–Hippocampal Circuit

The initial stage of hippocampus (dentate gyrus) is only three synapses removed from the odor receptors in the nasal mucosa. It is reasonable then to think of hippocampus as a higher order olfactory structure (although it is of course more than this) and to consider the anatomical steps leading from the receptors through the hippocampus as a circuit (Figure 14.4). Doing so allows one to ask how plasticity of synaptic physiology varies across the links of a well defined corticohippocampal serial network that processes sensory information of a very specific type. Work in our laboratory and elsewhere indicates that LTP is found in all connections in the circuit so far tested with the above described exception of the mossy fibers. However, while the essential features of LTP appear to be present in several instances, variations suggestive of different memory operations are in evidence.

Studies on the connections between the olfactory bulb and olfactory cortex (i.e., the lateral olfactory tract (LOT) projections to piriform and entorhinal cortex) initially led to the conclusion that these synapses do not exhibit LTP (Racine, Milgram, & Hafner, 1983; Stripling, Patneau, & Gramlich, 1988). However, recent work showed that an LTP-like effect was obtained when the stimulation was used as a discriminative cue in a two-odor learning

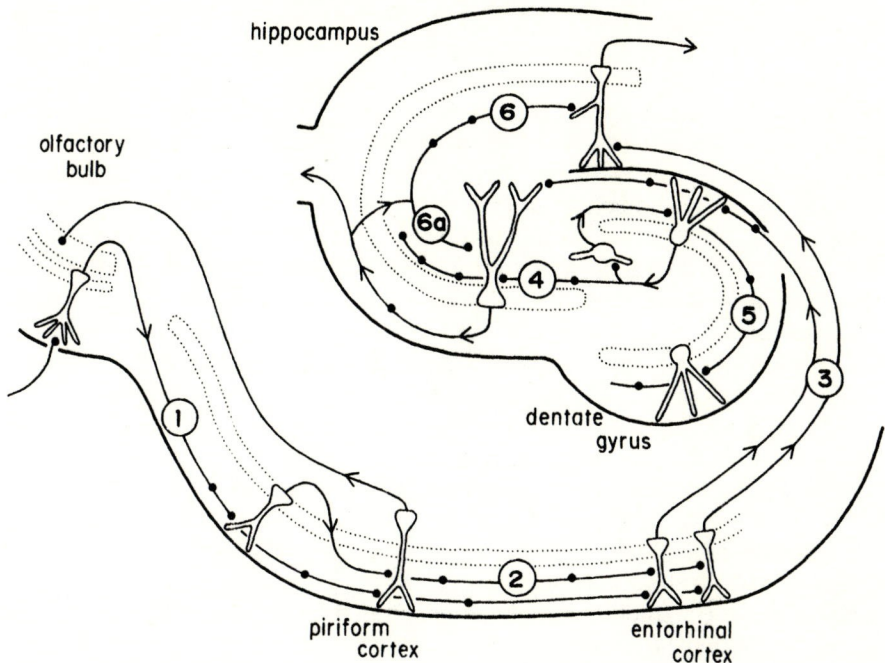

FIGURE 14.4. Main excitatory connections of the olfactory–hippocampal circuit. Olfactory bulb axons form the lateral olfactory tract (1), which innervates superficial layers of piriform and lateral entorhinal cortices. Piriform axons generate an associational system (2) that contacts within piriform and extends to lateral entorhinal cortex. Entorhinal cortex generates the perforant path (3) that innervates dentate gyrus, hippocampal fields CA3 and CA1. Granule cells of the dentate gyrus send mossy fibers (4) to CA3 and polymorph neurons that provide an associational projection (5) for the granule cells. CA3 axons project Schaffer collaterals to CA1 (6) and associational fibers back to CA3 (6a).

problem but not otherwise (Roman, Staubli, & Lynch, 1987). This led us to use in vitro slices to study if the observed potentiation was in fact LTP and to explore why it was more difficult to induce than LTP in hippocampus.

A first set of experiments established that both the LOT and associational synapses in piriform cortex possessed the same receptor pharmacology found in hippocampus. That is, transmission under normal conditions was completely blocked by DNQX, a selective antagonist of the AMPA receptor subclass of glutamate receptors. A second type of response became evident under conditions of unusual depolarization or in low magnesium medium; this potential was blocked by AP-5, an antagonist of the NMDA receptor. In these regards, LOT and associational synapses were indistinguishable from those in hippocampus (Jung, Larson, & Lynch, 1990b). LTP was readily elicited in the associational connections by the same stimulation patterns used to analyze the potentiation effect in hippocampus (Jung, Larson, & Lynch, 1990a; see also Kanter & Haberly, 1990). It was unusual in that it developed over a period of about 1 min; in hippocampus, high-frequency bursts trigger a potentiation effect that appears within 5–10 s (Larson et al., 1986). We had previously reached the conclusion that hippocampal synapses exhibit both short-term and long-term potentiation phenomena (see Larson et al., 1986); it appears that the former effect is not present in piriform (Jung et al., 1990a). LTP was much more difficult to induce in the lateral olfactory tract connections than in the associational system; in fact, only 8% of the slices showed the effect. However, pairing LOT stimulation with associational stimulation dramatically increased this percentage as did lowering the magnesium concentration of the medium. The potentiation found in both associational and LOT synapses was induced by NMDA receptors and expressed by AMPA receptors (Jung et al., 1990a), as is the case for hippocampus (see above).

The above studies point to the following conclusions:

1. Stable LTP is found in both classes excitatory synapses in the superficial layers of piriform cortex.
2. A short-term potentiation phenomenon that is prominent in hippocampus is lacking in the cortex.
3. LTP is difficult to induce in the lateral olfactory tract synapses probably because, by themselves, these connections do not produce sufficient depolarization to trigger the NMDA receptors.
4. LTP in vivo is thus likely to occur only when inhibition has been relaxed so that the LOT inputs discharge enough piriform cells to generate a substantial associational response.
5. These observations provide a basis for understanding how ascending systems (e.g., cholinergic projections) could serve as attentional devices that determine whether or not synaptic changes will occur. This would accord with the finding that LOT stimulation in chronic rats produces LTP only when it is used as a discriminative cue (Roman et al., 1987).

The next link in the olfactory–hippocampal circuit is that which connects lateral entorhinal cortex to the dentate gyrus (i.e., the lateral perforant path). LTP was discovered in the perforant path (Bliss & Lomo, 1973) as was the convergence requirement for induction (Levy & Steward, 1979; McNaughton, Douglas, & Goddard, 1978). It is clear that induction at these synapses also involves NMDA receptors (Morris, Anderson, Lynch, & Baudry, 1986) and that expression does not change paired-pulse facilitation (McNaughton, 1982). LTP in the perforant path is unusual in that it dissipates over a period of 1–2 weeks (Barnes, 1979; Castro, Silbert, McNaughton, & Barnes, 1989); this type of decay is not seen in the CA3-CA1 connections (Staubli & Lynch, 1987) and is probably not present in the LOT–piriform synapses (Roman et al., 1987). A summary of these points is given in Figure 14.5.

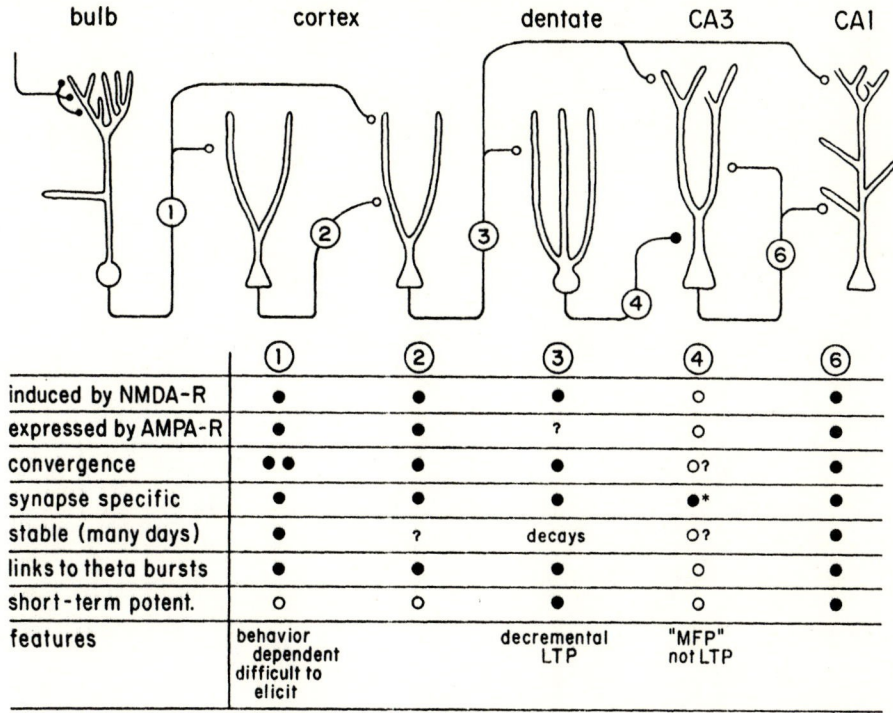

	bulb	cortex	dentate	CA3	CA1
	①	②	③	④	⑥
induced by NMDA-R	●	●	●	○	●
expressed by AMPA-R	●	●	?	○	●
convergence	● ●	●	●	○?	●
synapse specific	●	●	●	●*	●
stable (many days)	●	?	decays	○?	●
links to theta bursts	●	●	●	○	●
short-term potent.	○	○	●	○	●
features	behavior dependent difficult to elicit		decremental LTP	"MFP" not LTP	

FIGURE 14.5. Characteristics of synaptic potentiation at different stages of the olfactory–hippocampal circuit. Projections are numbered as in Figure 14.4. Solid circles represent cases where available data are positive for the relevant characteristic; open circles indicate negative data. Question marks indicate that the issue is unresolved. See text for details.

SYNAPTIC LEARNING RULES AND LTP INDUCTION

LTP appears to be a simple increase in synaptic strength that does not affect paired-pulse facilitation; as such, it is not likely to affect any computations carried out at the level of individual synapses (e.g., frequency filtering effects). The variations across regions for LTP described earlier could have major consequences for the types of information encoded by these regions but in terms of moment-to-moment synaptic operations, the chief effect of LTP would be simply to increase the level of depolarization produced by a subset of contacts. The rules describing the relationship of LTP induction to spatiotemporal patterns of activity involving diverse inputs could, however, carry with them specific types of computational operations. This is the case for learning rules in neural networks; that is, in such models computation arises from rules that dictate changes in synaptic strength based on the degree of correlation between pre- and postsynaptic activity (Hebb rule;

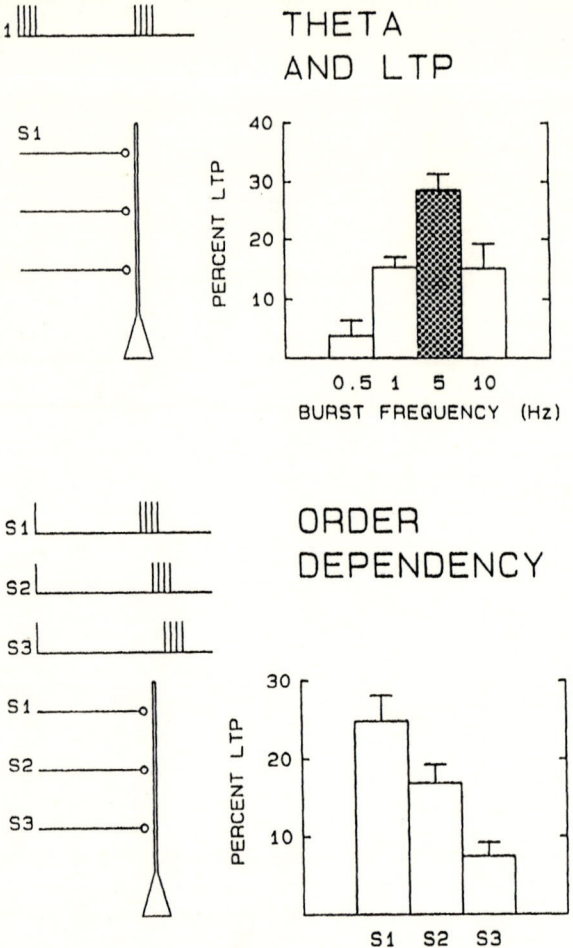

FIGURE 14.6. Some features of CA1 field LTP relevant to derivation of synaptic learning rules for neural networks. Theta and LTP: Short high-frequency bursts to a single set of fibers produce optimal LTP when repeated at 5 Hz, the theta frequency. Graph shows magnitude of LTP 20 min after burst stimulation. (Adapted from Larson, Wong, & Lynch, 1986.) Two input case: When two inputs are stimulated sequentially with bursts separated by 200 ms, only the second (S2) input exhibits LTP. Graph shows measurements of EPSPs before and after burst stimulation. (Adapted from Larson & Lynch, 1986.) Order dependency: Asynchronous stimulation of multiple inputs during the time of one theta peak results in potentiation related to the order of stimulation. Graph shows percentage LTP measured for the three inputs 20 min after burst stimulation. (Adapted from Larson & Lynch, 1989). Reversal of LTP: LTP can be reversed by low-frequency stimulation shortly after its induction in rats with chronic stimulation and recording electrodes. HFS consisted of theta burst stimulation; downward arrow indicates a 1-min period of 1 or 5 Hz stimulation. Solid circles show measurements for the experimental input (stimulated); open circles show measurements for a control pathway in the same animals. The *x*-axis shows time in minutes with the exception of numbers marked "d" for days. (Adapted from Staubli & Lynch, 1990)

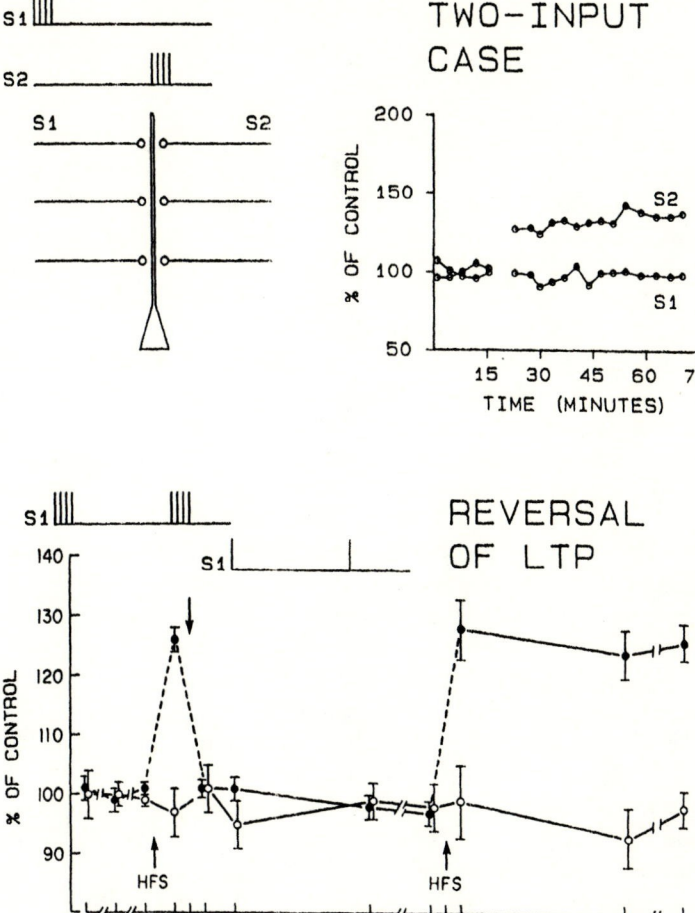

FIGURE 14.6 (*cont'd.*).

Ballard, Hinton, & Sejnowski, 1983; Kelso et al., 1986). While it is commonly said that LTP induction follows such formulations, this is not really the case. Thus, invariant association of presynaptic discharges with postsynaptic spikes does not produce LTP and negative correlations between input and output do not cause synaptic weakening. Experimental work has led to the discovery of a set of more complex rules and these are described below.

Theta Bursting and LTP

The theta rhythm is a characteristic feature of hippocampus in freely moving animals. It is an intriguing observation that theta corresponds in frequency to the sniffing rhythm known to be exhibited by a variety of small mammals when engaged in sampling an odor (Welker, 1964); moreover, the entire olfactory–hippocampal circuit exhibits theta-like activity that is phase locked to the sniffing pattern (Komisaruk, 1970; Macrides, 1975; Macrides, Eichenbaum, & Forbes, 1982). This is highly suggestive of a relationship between theta and network operations associated with the processing of sensory cues. This is not likely to be the whole of the story since theta is also present in rats carrying out well learned locomotor acts (Vanderwolf, 1969). In any event, the very prominence of theta in the hippocampal EEG during behaviors (cue sampling, exploration) raises the question of whether it is somehow linked to learning and LTP.

To test this last idea, it is necessary to first ask what types of spiking activity occur in individual neurons during theta. Numerous studies have shown that pyramidal neurons in CA1 and CA3 fire in short bursts (complex spikes); these bursts appear to be separated by the period of the theta wave ($\sim$150–300 ms) in rats exploring new environments (Hill, 1978) and learning odors (Eichenbaum et al., 1987; Otto, Eichenbaum, Wiener, & Wible, 1991). An explicit relationship between theta and burst discharges has been established in the latter case.

By themselves, short bursts (four pulses in 30 ms) do not produce potentiation but are extremely effective in this regard when given as a series with a between burst interval of 200 ms (see Figure 14.6). Moreover, it was found that longer or shorter intervals produced progressively lesser degrees of LTP (Larson et al., 1986); thus, the naturally occurring theta burst pattern is ideally suited for inducing LTP (the link between theta and LTP has been confirmed and extended by several laboratories; see Diamond, Dunwiddie, & Rose, 1988; Greenstein, Pavlides, & Winson, 1988, Pavlides, Greenstein, Grudman, & Winson, 1988). Having established this point it became possible to search for interactions between different collections of afferents arriving at a common dendritic target at different, theta-related time points. A first study of this type asked what happens when two independent Schaffer-commissural inputs are paired such that a burst to one precedes a burst to the second by 200 ms. When 5 to 10 pairs were given over a period of 1 min, it was found that LTP was induced only in the second (delayed) member of the pair (see Figure 14.6). Moreover, as in the experiments using single inputs, the optimal delay between the two inputs fell within the period of the theta rhythm (Larson & Lynch, 1986). Taken together, the results of these studies provided one aspect of an LTP-based synaptic learning rule describing how interactions over time between inputs can lead to strengthening of specific populations of synapses.

The two-input paradigm also proved to be an excellent tool with which to investigate the connection between the period of the theta wave and the events that induce LTP. Experiments of several kinds revealed that the first input elicited inhibitory postsynaptic potentials (IPSPs) in the target zone (presumably because of contacts on feedforward inhibitory interneurons), which, after their decay ($\sim$50 ms), entered a transient refractory period.

This refractory episode was at its maximum between 100–200 ms after the first input; a second input arriving during this time elicited only very weak IPSPs and hence its excitatory responses were not antagonized by hyperpolarizing currents and conductances (Larson & Lynch, 1986; McCarren & Alger, 1985; Pacelli, Su, & Kelso, 1991). Given that enough synapses were activated by the second input, it was thus able to cause a depolarization of sufficient degree and duration to unblock the voltage sensitive NMDA receptor channels (Larson & Lynch, 1988, 1989). In all, the peculiar efficiency of the theta bust pattern in triggering LTP can be traced to a transient suppression of IPSPs and hence enhanced NMDA receptor function.

Timing Rules for LTP Induction for Inputs Arriving During One Peak of Theta

The theta burst experiments described immediately above used synchronous stimulation of large collections of axons and it can be assumed that different inputs in situ arrive at their targets in a staggered fashion during a single peak of theta. To study this, separate and small populations of Schaffer-commissural axons converging on a common dendritic locus in CA1 were used. Theta bursts were given to each electrode in a staggered sequence; that is, a four-pulse burst (100 Hz) to S1 began 20 ms before that to S2, which in turn began 20 ms before that to S3. The experimental question was simply which input would show the greatest degree of LTP (Figure 14.6). The results were surprising; the amount of LTP corresponded to the order in which the inputs were activated (i.e., S1 >S2 >S3) (Larson & Lynch, 1989). The likeliest explanation for this effect is that the NMDA channels opened by the first input remain open the longest because the subsequent inputs maintain the target cell in a depolarized state.

It will be noted that the "within peak" rule is non-Hebbian in that the greatest degree of convergence and depolarization occurs during the middle input (see Larson & Lynch, 1989) and thus, according to the Hebb correlation rule, this input should show more synaptic change than the first input. Instead the opposite is the case, a result that raises the question of what computational significance, if any, might emerge from the timing rule. This will be discussed below.

Reversal of LTP

Work undertaken several years ago in our laboratory indicated that LTP could be reversed in anesthetized rats by low-frequency stimulation (1–5 Hz) applied within minutes of the induction of the potentiation effect (Barrionuevo, Schottler, & Lynch, 1980). The same stimulation applied to unpotentiated synapses produced only a transient depression. We were unsure if the loss of LTP was a true reversal or an unusually long depression and thus if the potentiation might not reappear after several hours. Subsequent studies addressed this question using rats with chronically implanted electrodes. The results of Barrionuevo et al. (1980) were replicated (i.e., low-frequency stimulation depressed potentiated but not control inputs) and it was found that the LTP did not reappear on testing 24 h later. Moreover, the degree of LTP that could be induced by a second episode of theta burst stimulation given 24 h later in the synapses that had received the high-frequency/low-frequency sequence was the same as that obtained in connections that had only been given high-frequency stimulation (Figure 14.6). These points indicate that the low-frequency trains did in fact reverse LTP (Staubli & Lynch, 1990). It is of interest that a reversal effect has been found in slices of hippocampus (unpublished data).

Little is known of the mechanisms of the reversal effect. Two questions of particular importance for modeling studies are as follows: First, is there a fixed time period following theta burst stimulation during which LTP can be reversed? Recent work in our laboratory indicates that LTP passes through a vulnerable period of less than 5 min during which it can be selectively reversed by hypoxia (Arai, Larson, & Lynch, 1990) or adenosine (Arai, Kessler, & Lynch, 1990). Repetitive low-frequency stimulation might operate by disrupting events needed to consolidate LTP and thus be effective only during a short period of time. Alternatively, synapses could have two states (naive and potentiated) with different patterns of activity causing them to switch back and forth. Second, what are the optimal patterns of stimulation for reversing LTP? It would indeed be intriguing if theta stimulation without bursts proved optimal for reversing LTP just as theta bursts were found to be ideal for inducing it. Studies are also needed to determine the duration of stimulation needed to reverse potentiation and, in particular, if a series of short trains (4–5 s) is as effective as a single long train.

Answers to these questions will provide material needed to evaluate the computational significance of the LTP reversal effect. Minimally it would seem that it could be used to refine or sharpen the representation of a cue in a network, this can only be addressed with computer simulations after the questions raised immediately above have been answered.

INCORPORATING THE EXPRESSION CHARACTERISTICS OF LTP INTO NETWORK MODELS

Simulations of the Initial Stages of the Olfactory–Hippocampal Circuit

Initial simulations of the superficial layers of the olfactory cortex incorporated rhythmic activation (at the olfactory–hippocampal theta rhythm), generating sequences of responses to repeated samples of an input stimulus. These response sequences exhibited the tendency initially to form categories of similar input stimuli and subsequently distinguish among individual category members (Granger, Ambros-Ingerson, Whitson, Staubli, & Lynch, 1989; Lynch & Granger, 1989). Implementation of feedback from the cortex to its primary input structure, the olfactory bulb, provided cue-specific inhibition targeting the glomeruli of the bulb, enabling a process of "masking" or subtracting circumscribed components of the input from bulb activity.

In the first tests of this masking operation, an effect was found in which complex odors consisting of prelearned components could be decomposed into their constituents. Bulbar activity corresponding to the combination of, for example, two components (A and B) gives rise to a cortical response corresponding to one (the largest) such component (e.g., A). Inhibitory corticobulbar feedback arises from that cortical response, and thus it subtracts selectively the bulbar origins of that component. Remaining bulb activity then generates the next cortical response, which will correspond to the remaining component of the mixture (e.g, B). In this fashion the constituents of mixtures are sequentially "read out" in order of their intensity by the repetitive activity of the corticobulbar system (Granger, Ambros-Ingerson, Staubli, & Lynch, 1990).

When trained on unitary cues, that is, those not containing any isolatable components to which pretraining has occurred, there are no specific stimuli to give rise to cortical responses whose bulbar origins can be subtracted. When such a system is trained on populations of cues, the similarities among subsets of these cues corresponds to overlaps in their input structure, for example, the shared elements that cause them to seem similar. These shared elements tend to give rise to "category" responses in cortex, as previously found; the masking operation accomplished by corticobulbar inhibitory feedback subtracts these category responses in the bulb and leaves a remainder that corresponds to the differences among elements in the category. Repetitive operation sequentially extracts categories of stimuli, then subcategories, sub-subcategories, etc., approaching responses that correspond to individual stimuli; this corresponds to the operation of hierarchical clustering of the cues (Ambros-Ingerson, Granger, & Lynch, 1990). Mathematical abstraction of the hierarchical clustering operation led to expression of a novel computational algorithm for performing this task; the algorithm had several properties that rendered it novel and efficient enough to compete against existing such algorithms in the computational literature.

Operation of the bulb–cortex simulation led to testable behavioral predictions, most notably, that animals should spontaneously form similarity based categories during learning. This prediction was tested behaviorally using rats in an olfactory discrimination learning task, with positive results (Granger, Staubli, Powers, Ambros-Ingerson, & Lynch, 1991). In addition, testable physiological predictions arise from the simulation, including sparseness of cell-firing response, relative odor-specificity, and time-locked firing. The presence of these predicted features was supported by single-unit recordings with chronically implanted electrodes in freely moving animals actively engaged in learning olfactory discriminations (McCollum, Larson, Otto, Schottler, Granger, & Lynch, 1991).

Relating Induction and Expression Characteristics to the Properties of Network Memory

It is to be expected that specific phenomena constituting a substrate of some particular behavior will give rise to identifiable features of that behavior. In particular, properties of the induction of LTP should relate to observable properties of learning, whereas expression characteristics of LTP will play out as features of memory: its organization and retrieval. A number of specific properties of induction and expression have been noted here, yet none directly suggests its correlate in overt learning behavior. Here we outline a number of specific ways in which such physiological features of induction and expression may be mirrored in learning and memory, respectively.

Theta Bursting and LTP Induction and Expression

The point has been made that the only naturally occurring physiological activity known to produce LTP is that of brief high-frequency bursts of activity repeated about every 200 ms (i.e., at the theta rhythm). The biophysical reasons why this activity pattern is optimal for LTP induction have been discussed, but the question is raised: what computational characteristics emerge from repeated activation? The combination of relatively long-lasting inhibition (100–500 ms in duration) in cortex and inhibitory feedback from cortex to bulb cause quite different spatial patterns of cell spiking response on successive peaks of theta; as mentioned, analysis of these different responses showed that they were clustering and successively subclustering collections of learned inputs into increasingly finer-grained categories (e.g., food, cheese, cheddar). Thus LTP induction over discrete successive samples has the effect of organizing learned responses into hierarchies of categories; in turn, expression of LTP over these successive repetitive samples sequentially "reads out" the memorial hierarchy, traversing it from general to specific information (Ambros-Ingerson et al., 1990).

Timing Rules for LTP Induction for Inputs Arriving During One Peak of Theta

The unlikelihood of complete synchrony of afferents requires extension of LTP induction rules to account for somewhat asynchronous inputs occurring within the envelope of a single peak of the theta rhythm, that is, brief (<100 ms) sequences of inputs. In terms of synaptic change, a Hebbian coactivity rule would predict that as asynchronous afferents arrive, increased depolarization of the target neuron over the staggered arrival times will cause later inputs to be strengthened more than earlier inputs. However, the experiments described earlier found the opposite effect: earliest-arriving afferents potentiate the most, with subsequently arriving afferents causing successively less potentiation. Networks using this biophysical induction rule and a predicted corresponding expression rule were tested for their abilities to learn brief sequences of the sort that might occur within a single theta peak. Such sequences might be expected to correspond to unitary perceptual events, such as the rapid sequence of phonemes constituting a word. Initial results have suggested that such networks are able to store and recognize sequences of this type with great specificity (i.e., very low error rates). Moreover, these networks exhibit large capacity: in one experiment, a 1,000-cell network was trained on 10,000 dictionary words, and was able to correctly "accept" (recognize) these words and reject others as not recognized, with an error rate of 0.1% (Granger et al., in press).

Reversal of LTP Induced by Theta Spiking

Physiological activity in response to the presence of an olfactory cue is typically characterized by theta rhythm EEG and cell firing activity; only burst activity at theta, not single spikes, induces LTP. Studies of olfactory receptor and bulb representations of olfactory cues have not identified conditions under which burst activity might emerge during perceptual sampling; it is anticipated that burst activity will emerge predominantly when the animal is learning, and evidence to this effect has been found (Otto et al., 1991). Studies to date of the LTP-reversal phenomenon have characterized single spikes at the theta rhythm as a firing pattern that reverses previously induced LTP, and suggest that LTP may remain reversible for a significant time after induction (Staubli & Lynch, 1990). An odor occurs against a background of other environmental odors, and naturally will typically be learned in a "noisy" condition of this kind; this can lead to inaccuracies in the resulting representations formed. A possible computational effect of the LTP-reversal rule may be the selective "erasure" of those synaptic portions of a trace that correspond to portions of a cue that are only weakly present. For example, if strong odor A is learned in the presence of weak spurious background odors B and C, repetitive training trials could initially occur in the presence of cortical response thresholds purposely lowered (e.g., via dampened inhibitory activity) to elicit burst responses to the entire input pattern (ABC). Further sampling with an intermediate threshold (slightly enhanced inhibition) would then elicit burst firing only in the pathways active as a result of the strong component A, and single-spike activity in the B and C afferents. This would effectively erase potentiation of the B and C components of the mixture via the reversal rule. Such a process could have the effect of allowing the B and C background activity to participate in the selection of appropriate cells to respond to the stimulus (via rules for competitive cell selection in cortical local-circuit patches; see Coultrip, Granger, & Lynch, in press), and yet not allow these participants to become potentiated as part of the learned trace of the cue. The computational significance of such an effect may be the ability to learn complex cues in the presence of noise, and the enhancement of the ability to extract individual components from complex cue mixtures (cf. Granger et al., 1989).

Stable Expression of LTP

LTP is expressed only as an increase in efficacy of a synapse, not as a decrease, and once induced, LTP is not decremented or otherwise altered by induction of LTP at other synapses. If this were not the case, it might be expected that subsequent learning could affect prior learning in ways that could be predicted by the interaction. As it stands, the unidirectional nature of LTP and its stability, synapse-specificity, and independence suggest that memories, once formed via this mechanism, will be relatively unaffected by subsequent learning. This property of LTP contrasts with mechanisms that allow decrements to synaptic weights for purposes of normalization of dendritic vectors (see, for example, Grossberg, 1987) or due to learning via "Hebbian" or error correction rules, which allow nonspecific decreases of synaptic weights (cf. Rumelhart & McCelland, 1986).

Fractional Degrees of Induction and LTP Saturation

LTP is not an all-or-none phenomenon; rather, each LTP induction episode increases synaptic strength by a small amount which incrementally brings the synapse to a fixed saturation or ceiling level. Specifically, it has been found (Larson & Lynch, 1986) that each induction episode increases the response by about one-tenth the distance between naive synaptic strength and full or ceiling potentiation. In our studies of the categorization properties conferred on networks by LTP learning rules, it has been noted that these incremental steps correspond to the learning of individual members of a putative category; it is not until a sufficient number are learned and the synapse is at or near saturation that categorization behavior in the network is robust; thus the number of incremental induction steps is a factor in determining the minimum size of categories: the number of similar items that must be learned before a category is created. Empirically, roughly 7–10 induction steps appear to be required in in vitro experiments, and this may imply that about that many items must be learned to constitute a learned category. Empirical findings suggest that learning of similarity-based categories does not occur with a single instance of the category, but requires multiple category members (Granger et al., in press).

LTP is Induced via NMDA Receptors, but Expressed via AMPA Receptors

The observation that expression and induction are accomplished by distinct receptors (Muller et al., 1988) has notable computational consequences. Intuitively it means that the prior learning history has little or no effect on subsequent learning: the NMDA receptor channels that induce new LTP are relatively unaffected by prior LTP induction episodes. Computationally, clustering by the network is improved by this "no-history" rule. Without this property (i.e., if synaptic weights in "learning mode" are increased by learning episodes) then learning tends to generate "attractor cells," which, because of their increased synaptic weights, bias subsequent learning by increasing their own probability of being recruited to become part of the representation of other inputs than the ones they were initially trained on. In experiments with the simulation (Granger et al., 1989), the absence of the "no history" rule tended to give rise to three undesirable properties:

- The ability of the network to subcategorize is diminished, because of the tendency of cells with many potentiated synapses to be recruited for other, similar input vectors.
- Distinction between multiple learned categories is lessened, again because of the appearance of "attractor cells" which generate overlap among representations of multiple categories.
- Learned representations exhibit a strong "order effect": that is, what categories are learned depends on the order in which cues are presented, and initial bias in the cue order can skew the categorization learned by the network.

EFFECTS OF VARIATIONS IN SYNAPTIC POTENTIATION AND NETWORK PROPERTIES ON MEMORY OPERATIONS

The above-described simulation studies led to specific hypotheses regarding the types of memory operations that might emerge from LTP in terms of its characteristics as a form of potentiation and as a set of synaptic learning rules. As discussed in the first section, however, variations in LTP exist in the olfactory–hippocampal circuit and indeed a completely different form of potentiation is found in one link. The question thus arises as to the features of memory promoted by these variations. The separate networks that comprise the individual links of the circuit have quite different anatomical designs accompanied in some cases by different physiological properties. These features presumably contribute to their memory-related functions. The present section takes up these points and begins with a discussion of hippocampus.

An Informal Model of Hippocampus

The contributions of hippocampus to learning and memory have been the object of intense, oftentimes ingenious experimentation and theorizing since the report that patients with temporal lobe damage exhibit a profound anterograde anmesia (Scoville & Milner, 1957). There have not, however, been many attempts to incorporate the specific anatomical characteristics that define hippocampus into hypotheses about its functions as in the manner done for the cerebellum (Albus, 1971; Brindley, 1964; Eccles, 1977; Gluck, Reifsnider, & Thompson, 1990; Ito, 1974; Marr, 1969; Pellionisz & Llinas, 1979). This is surprising since the hippocampus has many unusual features that seemingly should provide clues about how it operates; moreover, these features are such as to have caused the hippocampus to become a kind of standard preparation for neuroscientists and hence much more is known about its anatomy, physiology, etc., than is true for other telencephalic structures. The relative absence of ideas linking neurobiology to hippocampal memory functions also explains why biologically based computer simulations directed at this question have not been developed for dentate gyrus, CA3, etc., as they have for piriform cortex (Ambros-Ingerson et al., 1990; Granger et al., 1989; Haberly & Bower, 1989) and cerebellum (Gluck et al., 1990; Pellionisz & Llinas, 1979). Models are necessarily restricted with regard to the detail they incorporate and thus require a selection of features prior to their construction; they therefore need to be preceded by more qualitative arguments regarding the relative significance of neurobiological character-istics. The following discussion is an effort in this direction with an emphasis on material pertinent to the theme of variations in synaptic potentiation.

The hippocampus, like Gaul, is divided into three parts: dentate gyrus, field CA3 (regio inferior), and field CA1 (regio superior). The by far dominant extrinsic input to the structure arises in the medial and lateral entorhinal cortices and is distributed as projections to each of the three subdivisions; the largest component and the only one that dominates its target cells (in terms of providing the majority of all synapses on the neuron) is that to the dentate gyrus; CA3 and CA1 receive massive intrinsic projections that numerically are much larger than the entorhinal input. Hippocampus also receives a significant input from the medial septum/dia-gonal bands complex, much of which is cholinergic (Lewis & Shute, 1967; Mosko, Lynch, & Cotman, 1973) and directed, at least in part, to interneurons (Lynch, Rose, & Gall, 1978). This basal forebrain projection is much heavier in dentate gyrus and CA3 than in CA1, and via its interactions with interneurons plays a major role in the genesis of theta (see Bland, 1986, for a review).

The superficial layers of lateral entorhinal cortex that generate hippocampal afferents constitute the posterior extension of the olfactory cortex (e.g., they receive most of their input from the olfactory bulb and anterior olfactory cortex). The hippocampus thus receives highly processed sensory information; this is also true for modalities other than olfaction (see Deadwyler et al., 1979; Foster, Christian, Hampson, Campbell, & Deadwyler, 1987). The medial septum/diagonal bands complex is sometimes thought of as a rostral extension of brain stem reticular systems (Lewis & Shute, 1967) and thus relays to hippocampus activity associated with arousal and movement. It is thus reasonable to assume that the hippocampus receives refined sensory input followed in rapid succession by activity associated with the responses generated by that input. It is of interest that both types of inputs are focused on the dentate gyrus. To say more than this it is necessary to consider the physiological activity and anatomical organizations of the three components of hippocampus.

The granule cells of the dentate gyrus, unusual in so many respects, do not generate a collateral associational system like the neurons that precede (layer II piriform cortex, II entorhinal cortex) and follow (CA3 pyramidal neurons) them in the circuit. Instead, they contact a very sparse population of polymorph neurons in the subjacent hilus, which in turn produce an excitatory (see Deadwyler et al., 1975a) projection which distributes to the dendrites of granule cells throughout the ipsilateral and contralateral dentate gyrus. This convergent-divergent associational system is a highly specialized feature and one that seems designed to produce prolonged bursts of firing by many granule cells in response to a temporally discrete input (Lynch, 1986). In accord with this, are studies showing that the granule cells emit a long burst of activity to a brief, previously learned auditory input arriving via the perforant path (Deadwyler, West, Cotman, & Lynch, 1979). These experiments also demonstrated that if the rat performed a learned response, then large numbers of granule cells would discharge at high frequencies in a manner that waxed and waned with theta during the period of movement. A logical interpretation of this latter effect is that the movement activates the cholinergic inputs from basal forebrain and that these suppress interneuron activity (either directly or via interneuron to interneuron contacts), thereby allowing associational inputs to drive the granule cells. Thus sensory information from the perforant path activates a subset of granule cells while septal input associated with movement permits the feedback systems to maintain a level of firing in a still broader population of neurons.

The important question now arises as to whether the firing patterns generated by the granule cells in the above circumstances would be sufficient to produce MFP. While we know that the induction of MFP requires much longer trains than the short bursts used to elicit LTP, there have been no studies to define the optimal parameters for production of the former effect. Nevertheless, experience suggests that the firing patterns described in Deadwyler et al. (1979) and Rose et al. (1983) *could* be sufficient to produce potentiation. This leads to our first postulate:

1. The combination of sensory evoked burst discharges in a subset of granule cells followed by movement related activity in that subset will produce MFP lasting for minutes to hours.

If correct, this postulate would mean that an appropiate behavioral response to a previously learned cue would potentiate a subset of mossy fiber boutons. This in turn could mean that the cue on its first presentation would drive only a small population of CA3 pyramidal cells but a much larger population on later presentations. The CA3 response would thus denote whether or not the animal had sampled *and* responded to the cue earlier. Such memory would last only so long as MFP itself.

Field CA3 projects densely to the lateral septum (Swanson & Cowan, 1977), which in turn innervates the hypothalamus, among other targets. There is evidence that the lateral septal neurons are inhibitory (Stevens, Gallagher, & Shinnick-Gallagher, 1987), resulting in a situation in which a substantial CA3 output could block hypothalamic input to the midbrain locomotor regions delineated by Grillner (1975). Combining these points, MFP would serve to connect a sensory cue to a "stop-response" signal or in other words predispose the animal to avoid a cue sampled and responded to earlier in the day. There is an extensive literature suggesting that hippocampus suppresses learned or prepotent responses. The hypothesis formulated here is that this is accomplished by circuitry involving dentate gyrus–CA3–lateral septum–hypothalamus and that MFP "closes" the circuit by strengthening the connection from dentate gyrus to field CA3.

Field CA3 is dominated by its dense commissural-associational system. The large basal dendritic field and as much as 70% of the apical dendrites are innervated by fibers arising from ipsilateral and contralateral CA3 neurons. Since axons from individual cells project across much of the septotemporal axis, though with a preference for local cells (Swanson, Wyss, & Cowan, 1978), CA3 comes reasonably close to a combinatorial neural network in which activity cycles between its constituent elements: Indeed, network models by Traub, Miles, and Wong (1989) suggest that regenerative patterns of activity can propagate throughout CA3. Our second postulate concerns the possible relationship of the perforant path, mossy fiber, and septal afferents of CA3 to this cycling activity.

2. (a) Perforant path inputs previously strengthened by LTP and briefly activated by an arriving sensory input predispose the CA3 cells toward a particular regenerative spatial pattern of firing that is sustained by the dense associational system; that is, the perforant path "channels" CA3 into a particular cycle by "selecting" a subpopulation of CA3 neurons that initiates the first cycle. (b) Mossy fiber activity related to a movement provides a "forcing" stimulus that helps sustain regenerative patterns of activity. (c) Septal inputs serve to shape the temporal parameters of the pattern by regulating interneuron activity.

LTP in CA3–CA3 would, in this version of events, further define the spatial pattern of cell activity that recurs during cycling activity. Postulate (2) argues that CA3 is designed to generate recurrent patterns of activity with specific spatial features (i.e., which cells fire on an individual cycle) being determined by an initial set of conditions specified by the perforant path and perhaps mossy fiber responses to a transient input.

The above argument treats the granule cell response to movement as being rather nonspecific; that is, large numbers of neurons being brought to activity by the positive feedback loop. As discussed elsewhere, there may be more structure to this response in that subpopulations of granule cells could be affected more by some movements than others. (The anatomical basis of this argument is described in Lynch & Baudry, 1988). If so, then the possibility exists that the recurrent activity pattern in CA3 could reflect the initial input *and* movement-specific mossy fiber activity. In any event, the design of the CA3 system is suggestive of a device that produces a response to a cue that is maintained after the cue is gone and while behavior continues. If the response is seen as a dynamic representation of the cue, then CA3 could provide for associations between cues that are separated in space and time, a short-term memory function that must be vital to behavior.

Field CA1 is perhaps the simplest of the three hippocampal components. The apical and basal dendritic trees of the pyramidal cells are occupied by massive Schaffer-commissural projections (collaterals of the ipsi- and contralateral CA3 associational axons) except for a relatively small region at the tips of the apical dendrites innervated by the entorhinal projections. Alone among the links in the olfactory hippocampal circuit, CA1 lacks a collateral associational system. The efferents of CA1 for the most part are directed to the subiculum and deep layers of the entorhinal cortex, from which projections to regions outside hippocampus originate. Electrophysiological studies also suggest that the deep layers communicate with the superficial layers that give rise to the entorhinal–hippocampal projections (see Deadwyler, West, Cotman, & Lynch, 1975b).

Given that so much of its input comes from CA3, it is reasonable to suppose that field CA1 performs some type of operation on the output from the earlier stage of hippocampal circuitry. One possibility is that it "compares" the recurrent activity pattern in CA3 set in motion by a first cue and maintained during movement with the activity elicited following an encounter with a second cue. The direct entorhinal projections to CA1 could also play a role in this, particularly in the ventral hippocampus where this input is somewhat larger than in the more septal aspects of the structure (Witter, Griffioen, Jorritsma-Byham, & Krijnen, 1988). The idea that CA1 cells match a now present cue with one expected for a given context has been proposed on the basis of physiological recording studies (Muller et al., 1987; O'Keefe & Nadel, 1978) but the details of how this might be achieved with CA1 circuitry needs to be elaborated.

Serial Networks, Sequential Memory Operations

The structures beginning with the olfactory bulb and running through the olfactory cortex and hippocampus and retrohippocampal areas can reasonably be viewed as a sequence of brain networks. Presumably this provides for succession of different computational operations. The presence of physiological plasticity at each step implies that these operations involve memory; the variations that exist across steps, coupled with differences in anatomical designs, suggest that the nature of the memory used also varies along the circuit. Relationships between plasticity and memory proposed above can be summarized as follows (see also Lynch & Granger, in press):

- Olfactory cortex: LTP is present in both the lateral olfactory tract and associational system and results in a recognition memory that is hierarchically organized. The characteristics of LTP can be directly related to the characteristics of the hierarchy; for example, the percentage potentiation defines the width of categories, and the number of LTP increments before saturation is reached affects the number of items that must be learned before a category forms. The theta rhythm also proved to be an essential ingredient both in the formation and use of the hierarchy. The major variation in LTP in the lateral olfactory tract concerned its dependency on the past experience of the animal. It seems only reasonable to suggest that this unique feature provides a point at which attention can determine whether or not learning will occur.

- LTP is known to be present in the synapses formed by the entorhinal cortex to hippocampus; the most striking variation seen in this link is the decremental nature of the potentiation found in the dentate gyrus. The suggestion has been made that this provides for a memory of how much time has elapsed since last exposure to a cue (recency: see Lynch & Granger, in press). Studies on the stability of the LTP in the entorhinal projections to CA3 and CA1 have not been carried out; the model of hippocampus described above assumes that it does not decay over days as reported for the dentate gyrus.
- LTP is not present in the mossy fibers and the nature of potentiation found there is poorly understood. The proposal was made that MFP is a transient (hours) whole axon effect (i.e., not synapse specific) and is a specialized feature that provides a memory of what cues were responded to earlier in a test session.
- The CA3 collateral system (CA3 commissural-associational system, Schaffer-commissural projections) exhibits an extremely stable LTP effect, at least in field CA1. The proposal made here is that in CA3 the potentiation (in conjunction with LTP in the entorhinal–CA3 connections) serves to define recurrent patterns of activity that are initiated by an input and maintained over the several seconds needed to perform a learned response to that input. LTP in the synapses formed by the collaterals in CA1, coupled again with potentiation of the entorhinal inputs, is hypothesized to provide a device that links an activity pattern in CA3 with a second, delayed input; that is, that it connects cue 1 with cue 2 when the two inputs are physically and temporally separated. In the absence of further work, this idea is little more than a suggestion.

Analysis of the computational significance of the LTP-based synaptic learning rules is still in its earliest stages. Preliminary work indicates that the order dependency rule allows a network to encode the temporal structure of cues and, related to this, to have a remarkable capacity. The first property is undoubtedly of great significance given the nature of environmental stimuli such as odors or words, while the second is an essential and evident property of memory. If these early observations are confirmed in more extensive studies, an explicit proposal can be made for how critical aspects of memory emerge directly from the rules for producing synaptic plasticity.

The significance of the other LTP rules for network level operations has not been investigated. The between-peaks rule (i.e., S1 "primes" target cells so that S2 becomes potentiated) seems to provide for a kind of associativity that captures the order in which *separate* cues occur. In this sense, it can be seen as a counterpoint to the order dependency (or within peak) rule that encodes information about the temporal structure of unitary cues. The rule might, for example, provide the basis for the types of operations suggested to occur in the CA3 to CA1 system of hippocampus. The LTP reversal effect cannot be simulated in the absence of further experimental data (i.e., how long after LTP has been induced can it be reversed; is theta an optimal pattern for reversal, etc.).

The above discussion relating specific neurobiological features to particular memory operations points to some general conclusions. Memory, according to these formulations, emerges as a series of operations involving (a) matching an environmental stimulus to a position in a recognition hierarchy, (b) establishing the time from last encounter, (c) deciding if the cue has already been sampled, and (d) determining if it is followed by other, appropriate environmental stimuli. This sequence does not fall naturally into any of the widely discussed categories of memory and, indeed, calls into question the extent to which such categories correspond to any feature of brain. Instead, it would seem that brain networks and perhaps especially those in hippocampus have evolved features that allow animals to deal with the very different time scales required for interacting with the environment. Individual stimuli are composites that occur in rapid succession; different cues can occur reliably in rapid sequence with no intervening behavior, or can be expected to follow one another only after a specific behavioral response. Animals need to recognize cues that have not been sampled for weeks and yet at the same time decide whether they have already dealt with more commonly encountered stimuli at some point earlier in a test session. The neurobiological and modeling studies described here suggest that the brain deals with this diversity of possibilities by using sequential networks possessing specialized features, including several variants of synaptic potentiation.

Acknowledgments: This work is supported by grants from the Office of Naval Research (N 00014–89–J–1255), the Air Force Office of Scientific Research (89–0383), and a Research Scientist Award (G.L.) from the National Institutes of Health (MH00358). We thank Jackie Porter for excellent secretarial assistance.

REFERENCES

Albus, J. S. (1971). A theory of cerebellar function. *Mathematical Biosciences, 10*, 25–61.

Ambros-Ingerson, J., Granger, R., & Lynch, G. (1990). Simulation of paleocortex performs hierarchical clustering. *Science, 247*, 1344–1348.

Andersen, P., Sundberg, S. H., Sveen, O., Swann, J. W., & Wigstrom, H. (1980). Possible mechanisms for long-lasting potentiation of synaptic transmission in hippocampal slices from guinea pigs. *Journal of Physiology (London)*, *302*, 463–482.

Arai, A., Kessler, M., & Lynch, G. (1990). The effects of adenosine on the development of long-term potentiation. *Neuroscience Letters*, *119*, 41–44.

Arai, A., Larson, J., & Lynch, G. (1990). Anoxia reveals a vulnerable period in the development of long-term potentiation. *Brain Research*, *511*, 353–357.

Ballard, D. H., Hinton, G. E., & Sejnowski, T. J. (1983). Parallel visual computation. *Nature*, *306*, 21–26.

Barnes, C. A. (1979). Memory deficits associated with senescence: A neurophysiological and behavioral study in the rat. *Journal of Comparative and Physiological Psychology*, *93*, 74–104.

Barrionuevo, G., Kelso, S. R., Johnston, D., & Brown, T. H. (1986). Conductance mechanism responsible for long-term potentiation in monosynaptic and isolated excitatory synaptic inputs to hippocampus. *Journal of Neurophysiology*, *55*, 540–550.

Barrionuevo, G., Schottler, F., & Lynch, G. (1980). The effects of repetitive low frequency stimulation on control and "potentiated" synaptic responses in the hippocampus. *Life Sciences*, *27*, 2385–2391.

Bekkers, J. M., & Stevens, C. F. (1990). Presynaptic mechanism for long-term potentiation in the hippocampus. *Nature*, *346*, 724–729.

Bland, B. H. (1986). The physiology and pharmacology of hippocampal formation theta rhythms. *Progress in Neurobiology*, *26*, 1–54.

Bliss, T. V. P., & Lomo, T. (1973). Long-lasting potentiation of synaptic transmission in the dentate area of the anaesthetized rabbit following stimulation of the perforant path. *Journal of Physiology (London)*, *232*, 334–356.

Bliss, T. V. P., & Lynch, M. A. (1988). Long-term potentiation of synaptic transmission in the hippocampus: Properties and mechanisms. In P. W. Landfield & S. A. Deadwyler (Eds.), *Long-term potentiation: From biophysics to behavior* (pp. 3–72). New York: Alan R. Liss.

Brindley, G. S. (1964). The use made by the cerebellum of the information that it receives from sense organs. *International Brain Research Organization Bulletin*, *3*, 80.

Brown, T. H., Chang, V. C., Ganong, A. H., Keenan, C. L., & Kelso, S. R. (1988). Biophysical properties of dendrites and spines that may control the induction and expression of long-term synaptic potentiation. In P. W. Landfield & S. A. Deadwyler (Eds.), *Long-term potentiation: From biophysics to behavior* (pp. 201–264). New York: Alan R. Liss.

Castro, C. A., Silbert, L. H., McNaughton, B. L., & Barnes, C. A. (1989). Recovery of spatial learning deficits after decay of electrically induced synaptic enhancement in the hippocampus. *Nature*, *342*, 545–548.

Collingridge, G. L., Kehl, S. J., & McLennan, H. (1983). Excitatory amino acids in synaptic transmission in the Schaffer-commissural pathway of the rat hippocampus. *Journal of Physiology (London)*, *334*, 33–46.

Coultrip, R., Granger, R., & Lynch, G. (in press). A cortical model of winner-take-all competition via lateral inhibition. *Neural Networks*.

Deadwyler, S. A., West, J. R., Cotman, C. W., & Lynch, G. (1975a). A neurophysiological analysis of the commissural projections to the dentate gyrus of the rat. *Journal of Neurophysiology*, *38*, 167–184.

Deadwyler, S., West, J., Cotman, C., & Lynch, G. (1975b). Physiological studies of the reciprocal connection between the hippocampus and entorhinal cortex. *Experimental Neurology*, *49*, 35–37.

Deadwyler, S. A., West, M., & Lynch, G. (1979). Activity of dentate granule cells during learning: Differentiation of perforant path input. *Brain Research*, *169*, 29–43.

Diamond, D. M., Dunwiddie, T. V., & Rose, G. M. (1988). Chracteristics of hippocampal primed burst potentiation in vitro and in the awake rat. *Journal of Neuroscience, 8,* 4079–4088.

Douglas, R. M., & Goddard, G. V. (1975). Long-term potentiation of the perforant path-granule cell synapse in the rat hippocampus. *Brain Research, 86,* 205–215.

Dunwiddie, T., & Lynch, G. (1978). Long-term potentiation and depression of synaptic responses in the rat hippocampus: Localization and frequency dependency. *Journal of Physiology (London), 276,* 353–367.

Eccles, J. C. (1977). An instruction-selection theory of learning in the cerebellar cortex. *Brain Research, 127,* 327–352.

Eichenbaum, H., Kuperstein, M., Fagan, A., & Nagode, J. (1987). Cue-sampling and goal-approach correlates of hippocampal unit activity in rats performing an odor-discrimination task. *Journal of Neuroscience, 7,* 716–732.

Foster, T. C., Christian, E. P., Hampson, R. E., Campbell, K. A., & Deadwyler, S. A. (1987). Sequential dependencies regulate sensory evoked responses of single units in the rat hippocampus. *Brain Research, 408,* 86–96.

Foster, T. C., & McNaughton, B. L. (1991). Long-term enhancement of CA1 synaptic transmission is due to increased quantal size, not quantal content. *Hippocampus, 1,* 79–91.

Fox, S. E., & Ranck, Jr, J. B. (1981). Electrophysiological characteristics of hippocampal complex-spike cells and theta cells. *Experimental Brain Research, 41,* 399–410.

Gluck, M., Reifsnider, E., & Thompson, R. F. (1990). Adaptive signal processing and the cerebellum: Models of classical conditioning and VOR adaptation. In M. Gluck & D. Rumelhart (Eds.), *Neuroscience and connectionist theory* (pp. 131–185). Hillsdale, New Jersey: Lawrence Erlbaum Associates.

Granger, R., Ambros-Ingerson, J., Staubli, U., & Lynch, G. (1990). Memorial operation of multiple, interacting stimulated brain structures. In M. Gluck & D. Rumelhard (Eds.), *Neuroscience and connectionist theory* (pp. 95–129). Hillsdale, New Jersey: Lawrence Erlbaum Associates.

Granger, R., Ambros-Ingerson, J., Whitson, J. W., Staubli, U., & Lynch, G. (1989). Clustering computations of brain network simulations. In R. Pfeifer, Z. Schreter, F. Fogelman-Soulie, & L. Steels (Eds.), *Connectionism in perspective* (pp. 199–212). Amsterdam: Elsevier.

Granger, R., Staubli, U., Powers, H., Ambros-Ingerson, J., & Lynch, G. (1991). Behavioral tests of a prediction from a cortical network simulation. *Psychological Science. 2,* 116–118.

Granger, R., Whitson, J., Larson, J., & Lynch, G. (in press). Non-Hebbian features of LTP enable high-capacity encoding of temporal sequences. Proceedings of the National Academy of Sciences, U.S.A.

Greenstein, Y. J., Pavlides, C., & Winson, J. (1988). Long-term potentiation in the dentate gyrus is preferentially induced at theta rhythm periodicity. *Brain Research, 438,* 331–334.

Grillner, S. (1975). Locomotion in vertebrates: Central mechanisms and reflex interaction. *Physiological Review, 55,* 247–304.

Grossberg, S. (1987). *The Adaptive Brain* (Vol. 2). Amsterdam: North-Holland.

Haas, H. L., & Greene, R. W. (1985). Long-term potentiation and 4-aminopyridine. *Cellular & Molecular Neurobiology, 5,* 297–301.

Haberly, L. B., & Bower, J. M. (1989). Olfactory cortex: Model circuit for study of associative memory? *Trends in Neuroscience, 12,* 258–264.

Harris, E. W., & Cotman, C. W. (1986). Long-term potentiation of guinea pig mossy fiber responses is not blocked by N-methyl-D-aspartate antagonists. *Neuroscience Letters, 70,* 132–137.

Hill, A. J. (1978). First occurrence of hippocampal spatial firing in a new environment. *Experimental Neurology, 62,* 282–297.

Hopkins, W. F., & Johnston, D. (1984). Frequency-dependent noradrenergic modulation of long-term potentiation in the hippocampus. *Science, 226,* 350–352.

Ito, M. (1974). The control mechanisms of the cerebellar motor system. In F. O. Schmitt & R. G. Worden (Eds.), *The neurosciences, third study program.* Cambridge: MIT Press.

Ito, I., Tanabe, S., Kohda, A., & Sugiyama, H. (1990). Allosteric potentiation of quisqualate receptors by a nootropic drug aniracetam. *Journal of Physiology (London), 424,* 533–543.

Jung, M. W., Larson, J., & Lynch, G. (1990a). Long-term potentiation of monosynaptic EPSP's in rat piriform cortex in vitro. *Synapse, 6,* 279–283.

Jung, M. W., Larson, J., & Lynch, G. (1990b). Role of NMDA and non-NMDA receptors in synaptic transmission in rat piriform cortex. *Experimental Brain Research, 82,* 451–455.

Jung, M. W., Larson, J., & Lynch, G. (1991). Evidence that changes in spine neck resistance are not responsible for expression of LTP. *Synapse, 7,* 216–220.

Kanter, E. D., & Haberly, L. B. (1990). NMDA-dependent induction of long-term potentiation in afferent and association fiber systems of piriform cortex in vitro. *Brain Research, 525,* 175–179.

Katz, B., & Miledi, R. (1968). The role of calcium in neuromuscular facilitation. *Journal of Physiology (London), 195,* 481–492.

Kauer, J. A., Malenka, R. C., & Nicoll, R. A. (1988). A persistent postsynaptic modification mediates long-term potentiation in the hippocampus. *Neuron, 1,* 911–917.

Kelso, S. R., Ganong, A. H., & Brown, T. H. (1986). Hebbian synapses in hippocampus. *Proceedings of the National Academy of Sciences, U.S.A., 83,* 5326–5330.

Koch, C., & Poggio, T. (1983). A theoretical analysis of electrical properties of spines. *Proceedings of the Royal Society, London, B218,* 455–477.

Komisaruk, B. R. (1970). Synchrony between limbic system theta activity and rhythmical behavior in rats. *Journal of Comparative and Physiological Psychology, 70,* 482–492.

Larson, J., Ambros-Ingerson, J., & Lynch, G. (1991). Sites and mechanisms for expression of LTP. In M. Baudry & J. Davis (Eds.), *Long-term potentiation: A debate of current issues.* (pp. 121–139) Cambridge: MIT Press.

Larson, J., & Lynch, G. (1986). Induction of synaptic potentiation in hippocampus by patterned stimulation involves two events. *Science, 232,* 985–988.

Larson, J., & Lynch, G. (1988). Role of N-methyl-D-aspartate receptors in the induction of synaptic potentiation by burst stimulation patterned after the hippocampal theta rhythm. *Brain Research, 441,* 111–118.

Larson, J., & Lynch, G. (1989). Theta pattern stimulation and the induction of LTP: The sequence in which synapses are stimulated determines the degree to which they potentiate. *Brain Research, 489,* 49–58.

Larson, J., & Lynch, G. (1991). A test of the spine resistance hypothesis for LTP expression. *Brain Research, 538,* 347–350.

Larson, J., Wong, D., & Lynch, G. (1986). Patterned stimulation at the theta frequency is optimal for the induction of hippocampal long-term potentiation. *Brain Research, 368,* 347–350.

Lee, W. -L., Anwyl, R., & Rowan, M. (1986). 4-Aminopyridine-mediated increase in long-term potentiation in CA1 of the rat hippocampus. *Neuroscience Letters, 70,* 106–109.

Levy, W. B., & Steward, O. (1979). Synapses as associative memory elements in the hippocampus. *Brain Research, 175,* 233–245.

Lewis, P. R., & Shute, C. C. D. (1967). The cholinergic limbic system: Projection to hippocampal formation, medial cortex, nuclei of the ascending cholinergic reticular system, and the subfornical organ and supraoptic crest. *Brain, 90,* 521–540.

Lynch, G. (1986). *Synapses, circuits, and the beginnings of memory.* Cambridge: MIT Press.

Lynch, G., & Baudry, M. (1984). The biochemistry of memory: A new and specific hypothesis. *Science, 224,* 1057–1063.

Lynch, G., & Baudry, M. (1988). Structure-function relationships in the organization of memory. In M. Gazzaniga (Ed.), *Perspectives in memory research* (pp. 23–91). Cambridge: MIT Press.

Lynch, G., & Granger, R. (1989). Simulation and analysis of a simple cortical network. In R. G. Hawkins & G. H. Bower (Eds.), *The psychology of learning and motivation* (Vol. 23) (pp. 205–241). San Diego: Academic Press.

Lynch, G., & Granger, R. (in press). Serial steps in memory processing: Possible clues from studies of plasticity in the olfactory-hippocampal circuit. In H. Eichenbaum & J. Davis (Eds.), *Olfaction as a model system for computational neuroscience.* Cambridge, Mass: MIT Press (1991).

Lynch, G., Kessler, M., Arai, A., & Larson, J. (1990). The nature of causes of hippocampal long-term potentiation. In J. Storm-Mathisen, J. Zimmer, & O. P. Ottersen (Eds.), Understanding the brain through the hippocampus: The hippocampal region as a model for studying brain structure and function [Special issue]. *Progress in Brain Research, 83,* 233–249.

Lynch, G., Larson, J., Kelso, S., Barrionuevo, G., & Schottler, F. (1983). Intracellular injections of EGTA block induction of hippocampal long-term potentiation. *Nature, 305,* 719–721.

Lynch, G., Rose, G., & Gall, C. (1978). Anatomical and function aspects of the septo-hippocampal projections. In L. Weiskrantz & J. Gray (Eds.), *Functions of the septo-hippocampal system.* Ciba Foundation Symposium 58 (pp. 5–24). London: Elsevier/Excerpt Medica/No-Holland.

Macrides, F. (1975). Temporal relationships between hippocampal slow waves and exploratory sniffing in hamsters. *Behavioral Biology, 14,* 295–308.

Macrides, F., Eichenbaum, H. B., & Forbes, W. B. (1982). Temporal relationship between sniffing and the limbic theta rhythm during odor discrimination reversal learning. *Journal of Neuroscience, 2,* 1705–1717.

Malinow, R., & Miller, J. P. (1986). Postsynaptic hyperpolarization during conditioning reversibly blocks induction of long-term potentiation. *Nature, 320,* 529–530.

Malinow, R., & Tsien, R. W. (1990). Presynaptic enhancement shown by whole-cell recordings of long-term potentiation in hippocampal slices. *Nature, 346,* 177–180.

Marr, D. (1969). A theory of cerebellar cortex. *Journal of Physiology, 202,* 437–470.

McCarren, M., & Alger, B. E. (1985). Use-dependent depression of IPSPs in rat hippocampal pyramidal cells in vitro. *Journal of Neurophysiology, 53,* 557–571.

McCollum, J., Larson, J., Otto, T., Schottler, F., Granger, R., & Lynch, G. (1991). Short-latency single unit processing in olfactory cortex. *Journal of Cognitive Neuroscience. 3,* 293–299.

McNaughton, B. L. (1982). Long-term synaptic enhancement and short-term potentiation in rat fascia dentata act through different mechanisms. *Journal of Physiology (London), 324,* 249–262.

McNaughton, B. L., Douglas, R. M., & Goddard, G. V. (1978). Synaptic enhancement in fascia dentata: Co-operativity among coactive afferents. *Brain Research, 157,* 277–293.

Misgeld, U., Sarvey, J. M., & Klee, M. R. (1979). Heterosynaptic postactivation potentiation in hippocampal CA3 neurons: Long-term changes in the postsynaptic potentials. *Experimental Brain Research, 37*, 217–229.

Morris, R. G. M., Anderson, E., Lynch, G. S., & Baudry, M. (1986). Selective impairment of learning and blockade of long-term potentiation by an N-methyl-D-aspartate receptor antagonist, AP-5. *Nature, 319*, 774–776.

Mosko, S., Lynch, G., & Cotman, C. (1973). The distribution of the septal projections to the hippocampus of the rat. *Journal of Comparative Neurology, 152*, 163–174.

Mulkeen, D., Anwyl, R., & Rowan, M. (1988). The effects of external calcium on long-term potentiation in the rat hippocampal slice. *Brain Research, 447*, 234–238.

Muller, D., Joly, M., & Lynch, G. (1988). Contributions of quisqualate and NMDA receptors to the induction and expression of LTP. *Science, 242*, 1694–1697.

Muller, D., Larson, J., & Lynch, G. (1989). The NMDA receptor mediated components of responses evoked by patterned stimulation are not increased by long-term potentiation. *Brain Research, 477*, 396–399.

Muller, D., & Lynch, G. (1988). Long-term potentiation differentially affects two components of synaptic responses in hippocampus. *Proceedings of the National Academy of Sciences, U.S.A., 85*, 9346–9350.

Muller, D., & Lynch, G. (1989). Evidence that changes in presynaptic calcium currents are not responsible for long-term potentiation in the hippocampus. *Brain Research, 479*, 290–299.

Muller, R. U., Kubie, J. L., & Ranck, J. B. (1987). Spatial firing patterns of hippocampal complex-spike cells in a fixed environment. *Journal of Neuroscience, 7*, 1935–1950.

O'Keefe, J., & Nadel, L. (1978). *The hippocampus as a cognitive map*. Oxford: Oxford University Press.

Otto, T., Eichenbaum, H., Wiener, S. I., & Wible, C. G. (1991). Learning-related patterns of CA1 spike trains parallel stimulation parameters optimal for inducing hippocampal long-term potentiation. *Hippocampus. 1*, 181–192.

Pacelli, G. J., Su, W., & Kelso, S. R. (1991). Activity-induced decrease in early and late inhibitory synaptic conductances in hippocampus. *Synapse, 7*, 1–13.

Pavlides, C., Greenstein, Y. J., Grudman, M., & Winson, J. (1988). Long-term potentiation in the dentate gyrus is induced preferentially on the positive phase of theta rhythm. *Brain Research, 439*, 383–387.

Pellionisz, A., & Llinas, R. (1979). Brain modeling by tensor network theory and computer simulation. The cerebellum: Parallel processor for predictive coordination. *Neuroscience, 4*, 323–348.

Racine, R. J., Milgram, N. W., & Hafner, S. (1983). Long-term potentiation phenomena in the rat limbic forebrain. *Brain Research, 260*, 217–231.

Rahamimoff, R. (1968). A dual effect of calcium ions on neuromuscular facilitation. *Journal of Physiology (London), 195*, 471–480.

Rall, W. (1978). Dendritic spines and synaptic potency. In R. Porter (Ed.), *Studies in neurophysiology* (pp. 203–209). Cambridge: Cambridge University Press.

Ranck, J. B., Jr. (1973). Studies on single neurons in dorsal hippocampal formation and septum in unrestrained rats. Part I. Behavioral correlates and firing repertoires. *Experimental Neurology, 41*, 462–531.

Roman, F., Staubli, U., & Lynch, G. (1987). Evidence for synaptic potentiation in a cortical network during learning. *Brain Research, 418*, 221–226.

Rose, G., Diamond, D., & Lynch, G. (1983). Dentate granule cells in the rat hippocampal formation have the behavioral characteristics of theta neurons. *Brain Research, 266*, 29–37.

Rumelhart, D., & McCelland, J. (1986). *Parallel distributed processing*. Cambridge: MIT Press.

Scoville, W. B., & Milner, B. (1957). Loss of recent memory after bilateral hippocampal lesions. *Journal of Neurological and Neurosurgical Psychiatry, 201,* 11–21.

Staubli, U., Kessler, M., & Lynch, G. (1990). Aniracetam has proportionately smaller effects on synapses expressing long-term potentiation: Evidence that receptor changes subserve LTP. *Psychobiology, 18,* 377–381.

Staubli, U., Larson, J., & Lynch, G. (1990) Mossy fiber potentiation and long-term potentiation involve different expression mechanisms. *Synapse, 5,* 333–335.

Staubli, U., & Lynch, G. (1987). Stable hippocampal long-term potentiation elicited by 'theta' pattern stimulation. *Brain Research, 435,* 227–234.

Staubli, U., & Lynch, G. (1990). Stable depression of potentiated synaptic responses in the hippocampus with 1–5 Hz stimulation. *Brain Research, 513,* 113–118.

Stevens, D. R., Gallagher, J. P., & Shinnick-Gallagher, P. (1987). In vitro studies of the role of gamma-aminobutyric acid in inhibition in the lateral septum of the rat. *Synapse, 1,* 184–190.

Stripling, J. S., Patneau, D. K., & Gramlich, C. A. (1989). Selective long-term potentiation in the pyriform cortex. *Brain Research, 441,* 281–291.

Swanson, L. W., & Cowan, W. M. (1977). An autoradiographic study of the organization of the efferent connections of the hippocampal formation of the rat. *Journal of Comparative Neurology, 172,* 49–84.

Swanson, L. W., Wyss, J. M., & Cowan, W. M. (1978). An autoradiographic study of the organization of intrahippocampal association pathways in the rat. *Journal of Comparative Neurology, 181,* 681–716.

Traub, R. D., Miles, R., & Wong, R. K. S. (1989). Model of the origin of rhythmic population oscillations in the hippocampal slice. *Science, 243,* 1319–1325.

Vanderwolf, C. H. (1969). Hippocampal electrical activity and voluntary movement in the rat. *Electroencephalography and Clinical Neurophysiology, 26,* 407–418.

Voronin, L. L. (1988). Quantal analysis of long-term potentiation. In H. L. Haas & G. Buzsaki (Eds.), *Synaptic plasticity in the hippocampus* (pp. 27–40). Berlin: Springer-Verlag.

Welker, W. I. (1964). Analysis of sniffing in the albino rat. *Behaviour, 22,* 223–244.

Wigstrom, H., Gustafsson, B., Huang, Y.-Y., & Abraham, W. C. (1986). Hippocampal long-term potentiation is induced by pairing single afferent volleys with intracellularly injected depolarizing current pulses. *Acta Physiologica Scandinavica, 126,* 317–319.

Wilson, C. J. (1984). Passive cable properties of dendritic spines and spiny neurons. *Journal of Neuroscience, 4,* 281–297.

Witter, M. P., Griffioen, A. W., Jorritsma-Byham, B., & Krijnen, J. L. (1988). Entorhinal projections to the hippocampal CA1 region in the rat: An underestimated pathway. *Neuroscience Letters, 85,* 193–198.

Xiao, P., Staubli, U., Kessler, M., & Lynch, G. (in press). Selective effects of aniracetam across receptor types and forms of synaptic facilitation in hippocampus. *Hippocampus.*

Yamamoto, C., & Chujo, T. (1978). Long-term potentiation in thin hippocampal sections studied by intracellular and extracellular recordings. *Experimental Neurology, 58,* 242–250.

Zalutsky, R. A., & Nicoll, R. A. (1990). Comparison of two forms of long-term potentiation in single hippocampal neurons. *Science, 248,* 1619–1624.

15

Local Plasticity in Neuronal Learning

E. N. SOKOLOV

Two main types of learning processes can be distinguished: stimulus dependent (habituation and sensitization) and effect dependent (classical and instrumental conditioning). The basic characteristic of stimulus-dependent learning is its specificity with respect to the presented stimulus. Effect-dependent learning is selective both with respect to the conditioned stimulus and to the unconditioned response. The major question addressed to stimulus-dependent and effect-dependent learning refers to the neuronal basis of stimulus selectivity. To approach this problem one should explain how external and internal stimuli are represented in the central nervous system. The basic question with respect to effect-dependent learning is concerned with the specificity of the conditioned reflex that is highly similar to the unconditioned reflex. To solve the problem of conditioned reflex specificity, one should explain mechanisms that are responsible for elicitation of unconditioned reflexes.

The associative stimulus–response selectivity involved in the evocation of a conditioned reflex can be elucidated using the strategy of a step-by-step approximation from the behavioral level towards identifiable neurons and identifiable synapses participating in the transfer of information by conditioning. The injection of dyes through the microelectrode into the neuron under recording enables one to reconstruct the distribution of its dendrites and axons. Two synaptically linked neurons injected with dyes demonstrate the structural basis of the identified synapses. The integration of single-unit recording and behavioral manifestation can be achieved in semi-intact preparations.

The plastic changes in identifiable synapses can be studied further with respect to the contribution of pre- and postsynaptic mechanisms. Differentiation of postsynaptic from presynaptic plasticity is achieved by a local iontophoretic application of the transmitter on the membrane of a completely isolated, identified neuron taking part in the conditioned reflex. The identified isolated neuron preparation opens a new stage in the study of plasticity devoted to intracellular signaling.

This chapter concerns the integration of data obtained in *Helix* semi-intact preparations, preparations of isolated nervous systems, and completely isolated neurons.

CONCEPTUAL REFLEX ARC

The results of the study of information processing in snails can be summarized in a scheme that includes the following types of neurons: feature-detectors, command neurons, modulatory neurons, and motor neurons. The feature-detectors are afferent neurons selectively tuned to a particular aspect of the stimulus, its intensity or location on the receptive surface. The command neurons are responsible for generating specific behavioral acts or their fragments. The modulatory neurons, triggering no behavioral acts, modify the synaptic links between detectors and command neurons, which elicit a particular type of behavior under specified conditions. The motor neurons generating local motor responses are stimulated either directly by feature-detectors or indirectly via command neurons (Figure 15.1). The pattern of activated motor neurons in space and time determines the behavior of animals (Sokolov, 1977).

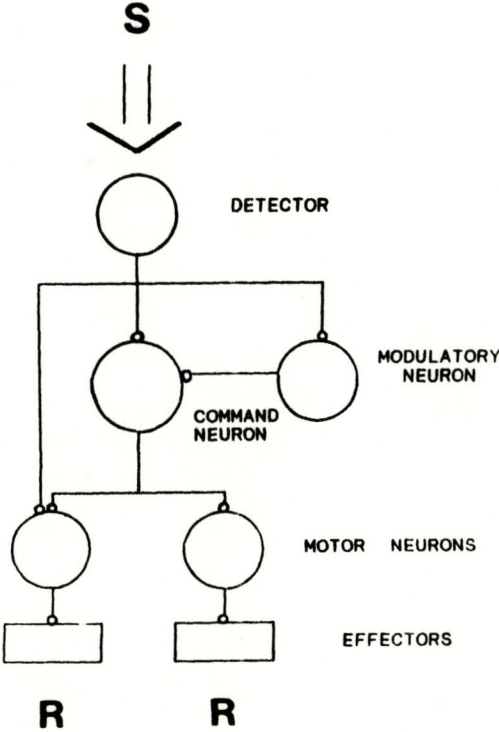

FIGURE 15.1. Conceptual reflex arc. The stimulus stimulating a feature detector reaches the motor neuron either directly evoking a local motor response or indirectly via a command neuron triggering a complex response R in a set of motor neurons. The parallel pathway leads to a modulatory neuron, which in turn modifies the activity of the command neuron.

THE COMMAND NEURON AS A NERVOUS CENTER

Different behavioral acts are triggered by specific sets of command neurons. Avoidance behavior in Helix is characterized by closure of the pneumostome, contraction of the body musculature, and general withdrawal, which is elicited by giant neurons located in the parietal ganglia. The avoidance command neurons have different thresholds of spike generation, which provide overlapping output signals. They constitute the basis for the various subtypes of avoidance behavior. Representatives of avoidance command neurons are giant cells LPa3 and RPa3 located in the left and right parietal ganglia, respectively. The injection of cobalt or nickel in these neurons demonstrates their complex morphology (Figure 15.2). The extensions of the soma constitute the basis of local processes: axons and dendrites widely distributed in different ganglia. The axons incorporated into the left and right pallial anal and skin nerves reach muscles of the mantle directly. The axons that project the pedal ganglia synapse on motor neurons, influence the response of the foot (Arakelov & Sakharova, 1982). Thus, the avoidance command neuron possess the features of both premotor and motor neurons (Arakelov & Palikhova, 1985).

The avoidance command neuron is a latent pacemaker cell. The intracellular injection of depolarizing current results in a sequence of sine-like waves that generate spikes on reaching the firing threshold. The pacemaker potentials are present not only in the cell body but also in local patches of the extensions of the cytoplasm (Arakelov, 1974) or in the axonal branches (Palikhova, 1985). Such local pacemaker mechanisms can be observed in the soma as axonal spikes. The amplitudes of axonal spikes are different depending on the distance and conditions of their passive transduction from axonal branches to the soma (Palikhova, 1985). The axonal spikes recorded in the soma that result from passive electrotonic antidromic effects can reach the firing threshold and generate a somatic spike, resulting in a duplication of frequency in the axon. The somatic spike reaching the distinct pacemaker locus can activate the pacemaker wave as a result of afterdepolarization. If the pacemaker wave reaches the firing threshold, then the local spike is generated, reaching the soma electrotonically where it can trigger the next somatic spike (Figure 15.3). Such a shuttle-like passage of nerve impulses between the soma and a local branch constitutes an intracellular reverberation that is not abolished by synaptic blockade (Palikhova, 1985, in press). The presence of several pacemaker loci in different axonal branches with local dendrites makes the command neuron a complex nervous center.

PLASTICITY OF THE PACEMAKER MECHANISM

The pacemaker potentials of the command neuron are a result of currents passing via ionic channels. The activation of low-threshold voltage-dependent

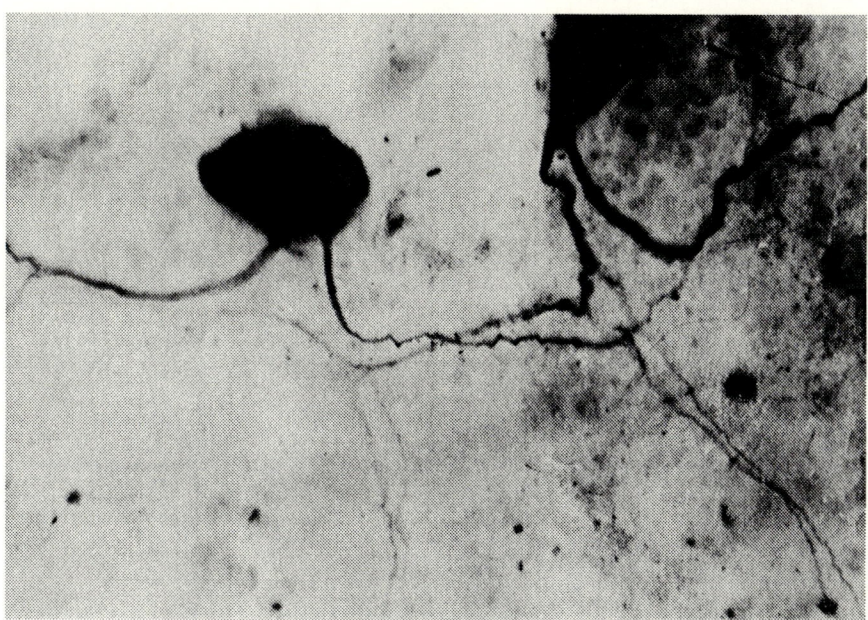

(A)

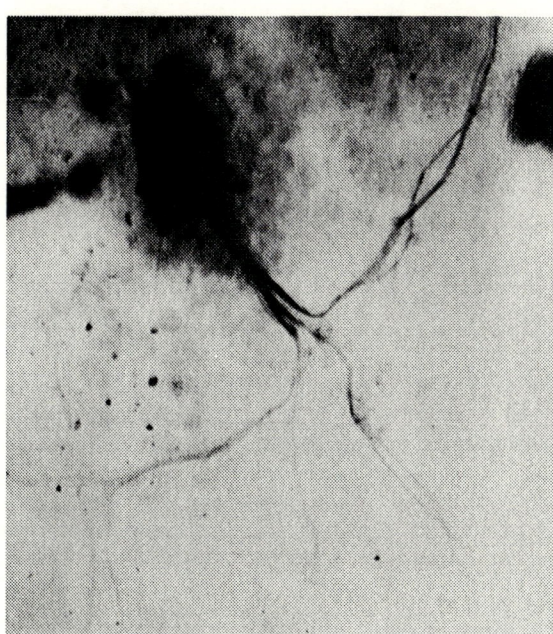

(B)

FIGURE 15.2. (A,B) Morphology of the avoidance command neuron. Example of avoidance command neurons, with typical morphology. The cell body is extended in left and right directions. Fine descending processes represent axons drectly linked with mantel musculature. Some other axons are converging on motor neurons. The dendrites located along the cytoplasmatic extensions collect the input signals from different parts of the ganglia.

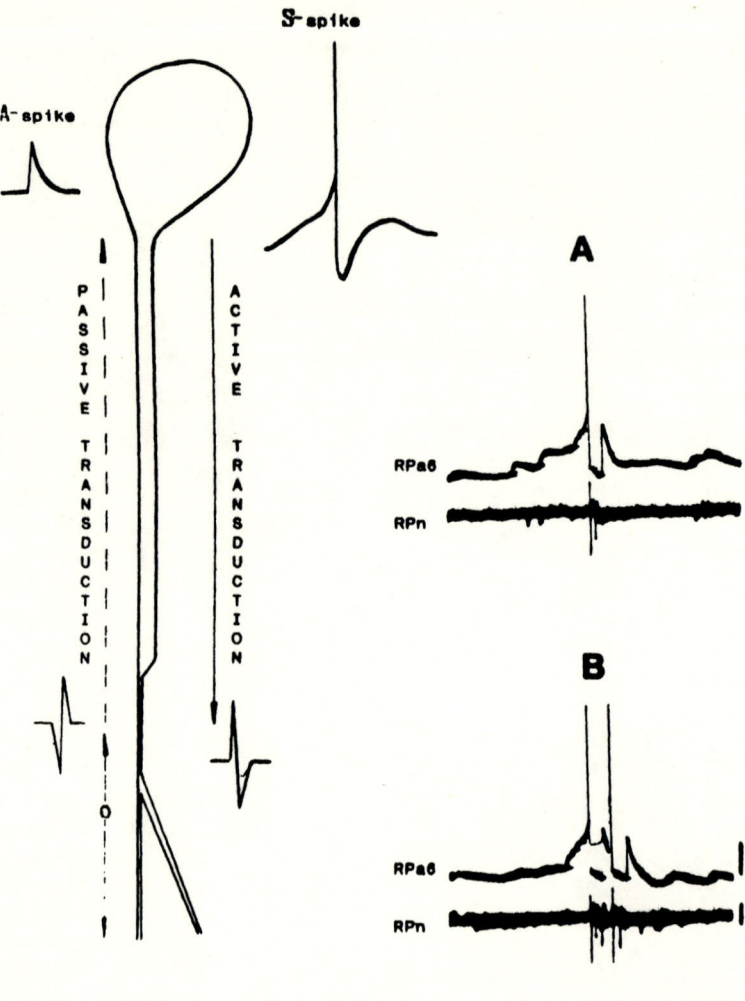

FIGURE 15.3. Intracellular reverberation. The somatic spike (S-spike) can be generated owing to a pacemaker wave or synaptic input. Reaching the axonal pacemaker the somatic spike activates a local pacemaker wave by an afterdepolariz- ation, which triggers a local spike. The locally triggered spike is conducted passively to the soma as an axonal spike (A-spike((A). If the axonal spike activates a new somatic spike, intracellular reverberation occurs (B). (A,B) Simultaneous recording of neuron RPa6 activity in its soma and axon in the right pallial nerve (RPn). Calibration: 10 mV, 50 mkV, 1 s.

calcium channels results in a progressive depolarization of the membrane. The calcium ions entering the cell body in turn activate calcium-dependent potassium channels. The outward potassium current results in a hyperpolarization of the membrane and the closure of calcium channels. The decrease of calcium influx reduces the calcium-dependent potassium current, initiating a new cycle of activity.

The role of calcium in the pacemaker oscillations can be demonstrated in experiments with sodium-free and calcium-free solutions (Figure 15.4). The sodium-free solution does not eliminate the pacemaker oscillations. The calcium-free solution or cobalt blockade of calcium channels usually eliminate the pacemaker waves, demonstrating the basic role of calcium channels in the generation of pacemaker potentials (Khludova & Sokolov, 1982). The calcium pacemaker potentials are habituated by repeated intracellular injection of a depolarizing current. The amplitude of the pacemaker wave decreases progressively and the train of pacemaker waves becomes shorter. The process of habituation can be interrupted by a strong depolarizing current producing a dishabituation effect. If pacemaker waves trigger a train of spikes, the habituation process can be separated into two stages: elimination of spikes and progressive decrease of pacemaker oscillations (Figure 15.5). The decrease in pacemaker activity is due to depolarization of calcium channels resulting in their "sleepy," closed, non-responsive state. A strong depolarization has an opposite effect: owing to the phosphorylation of "sleepy" channels, they become responsive to subsequent depolarizing currents.

THE MOTOR FIELD OF THE COMMAND NEURON

The distributed network of comman neuron axons is the basis of the motor field, constituting complex motor responses generated by intracellular depolarization. The testing of the motor field of the avoidance command neuron is performed by a mechanical sensor measuring local body displacements that are evoked by intracellular stimulation of an avoidance command neuron. The motor field can be divided into a focus and a periphery. The focus of a motor field is concentrated around the pneumostome, which is innervated directly by command neuron axons. The periphery of the motor field occupying the foot is supplied by motor neurons controlled by the command neuron. Cobalt or cadmium blockade of central synapses eliminates the motor responses of the periphery of the motor field while responses in its focus are intact. The mantel muscles are innervated both directly and via motor neurons. The motor response in this area has two components: tonic and short phasic contractions. The late, phasic, component is abolished by the blockade of central synapses. The initial tonic component is not eliminated by such a procedure (Figure 15.6).

The synapses between the command neuron and motor neurons are plastic. Repeated stimulation of the command neuron by depolarizing current

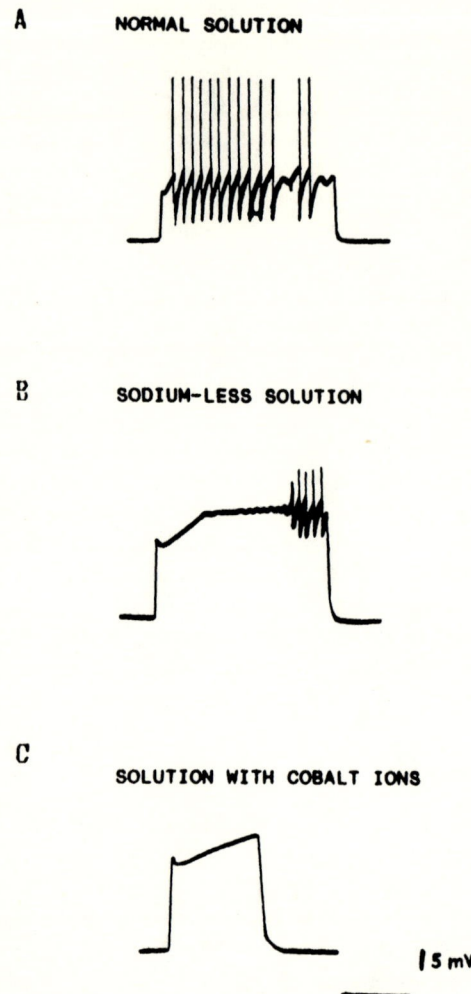

FIGURE 15.4. Ionic mechanisms of pacemaker waves. A sodium-free solution does not prevent the pacemaker waves and spikes (B). The calcium-free solution or cobalt blockade of voltage-dependent calcium usually eliminates both the calcium pacemaker and calcium spikes (C).

pulses (with constant frequency and duration when spike discharge is not changed) results in only a habituation of the late component of the mantel response.

The recording of spikes from nerves that contain axons of a command neuron and motor neurons demonstrates two spike discharges: an initial and late discharge only. The late spike discharge is habituated during repeated intracellular stimulation of the command neuron (Figure 15.7). This effect

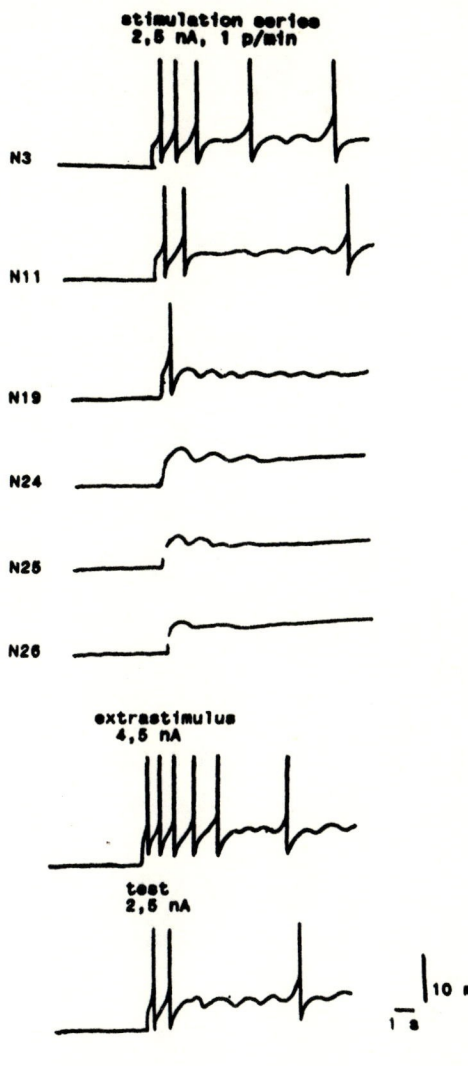

FIGURE 15.5.
Habituation of pacemaker waves and pacemaker spikes. Repeated intracellular depolarization results in a progressive diminution of pacemaker waves and abolishes the generation of pacemaker-dependent spikes. A strong stimulation produces a re-establishment of the response, demonstrating that the habituation cannot be explained by loss of sensitivity.

suggests two neuronal pathways from the command neuron to the mantel: a direct axonal route via unplastic synapses and an indirect route passing via plastic synapses between motor neurons and the command neuron (Arakelov & Palikhova, 1985).

RECEPTIVE FIELD OF THE COMMAND NEURON

The receptive field of the avoidance command neuron occupies the total receptive surface, including intestinal organs. The giant receptive field consists of a focus and a periphery. The focus of the receptive field represents

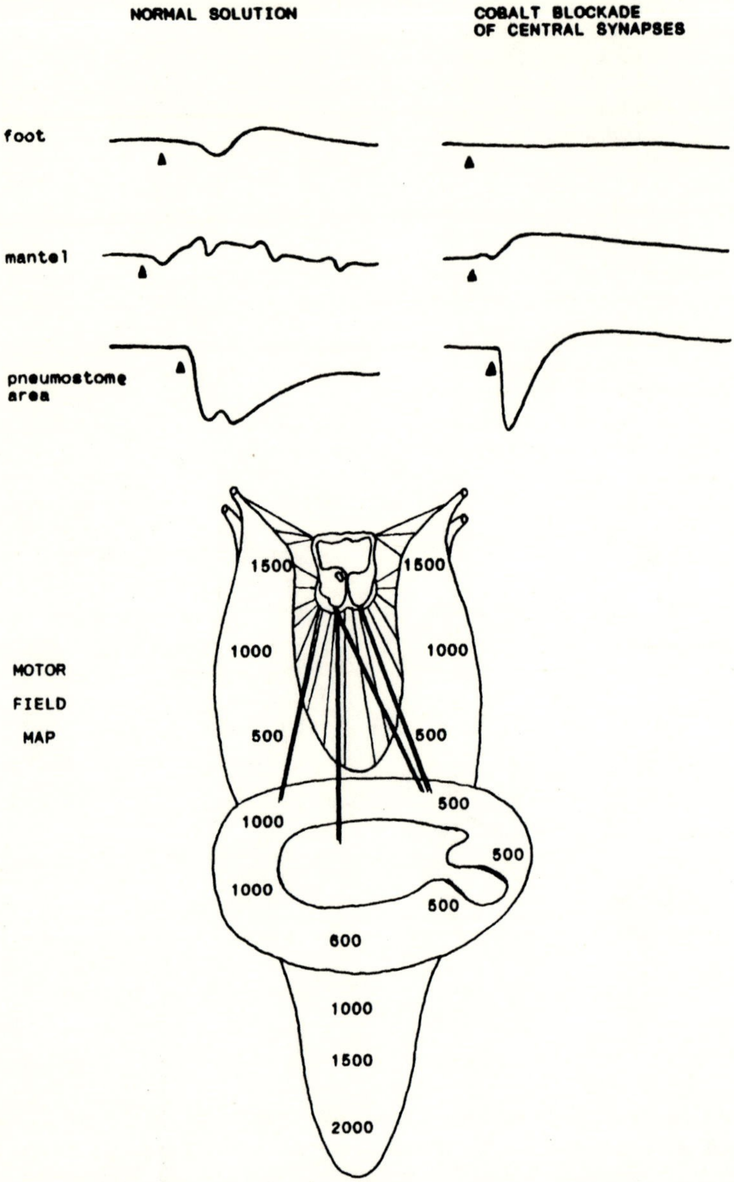

NORMAL SOLUTION

**COBALT BLOCKADE
OF CENTRAL SYNAPSES**

foot

mantel

pneumostome
area

MOTOR

FIELD

MAP

FIGURE 15.6.   Structure of avoidance command neuron motor field. Intracellular depolarizing stimulation of the defensive command neuron results in body displacement of foot, mantel, and pneumostoma areas of the mantel. Cobalt blockade of central synapses results in elimination of response of the foot and phasic mantel component leaving intact its tonic component. Cobalt blocks the late component of the response in the pneumostoma area while the initial response is not affected. The map of latencies of motor responses on the surface of the snail body is given milliseconds.

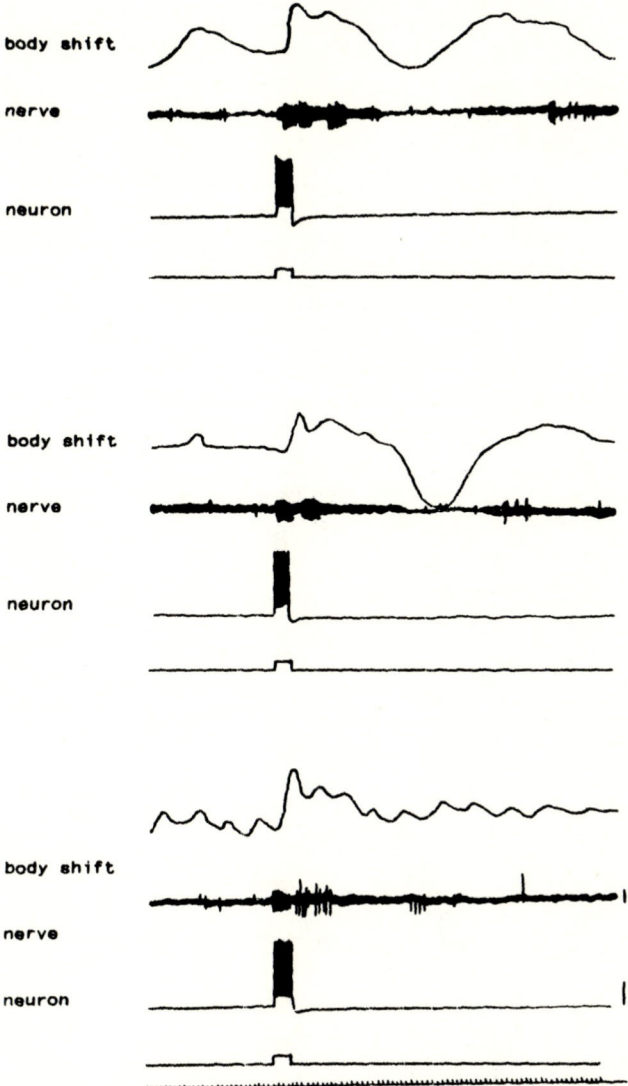

FIGURE 15.7. Plastic synapses between the command neuron and motor neurons. Intracellular depolarization triggers spikes in the command neuron and generates early and late bursts of spike in nerves corresponding to initial and postponed motor responses of the mantel. Repeated intracellular depolarization results in a habituation of the late burst of spikes and late motor component, demonstrating plastic changes of the synapses between the command neuron and motor neuron and stable synapses linking the command neuron with the muscles.

the area around the pneumostome linked with the command neuron through plastic synapses. There are two independent pathways from the pneumostome area evident by two excitatory post synaptic potentials (EPSPs). The repeated tactile stimulation of the receptive field focus results in no habituation of either of these EPSPs.

The mantel is linked with the giant neuron through two independent plastic pathways. The initial EPSP is generated on the periphery and is not abolished after blockade of central synapses. The late EPSP is due to central synapses and is eliminated by their blockade (Figure 15.8). Both components are habituated by repeated tactile stimulation of the mantel.

The foot is linked with the giant neuron through plastic central synapses with participation of skin nerve and pedal nerves (Figure 15.9). Tactile stimulation of the foot produces a late EPSP only. Repeated presentation of stimuli result in habituation of the EPSP (Figure 15.10) (Shehter, Arakelov, 1985).

Strong electrical stimulation of the mantel has elucidated the third late EPSP. Repeated strong electrical stimulation demonstrating habituation of

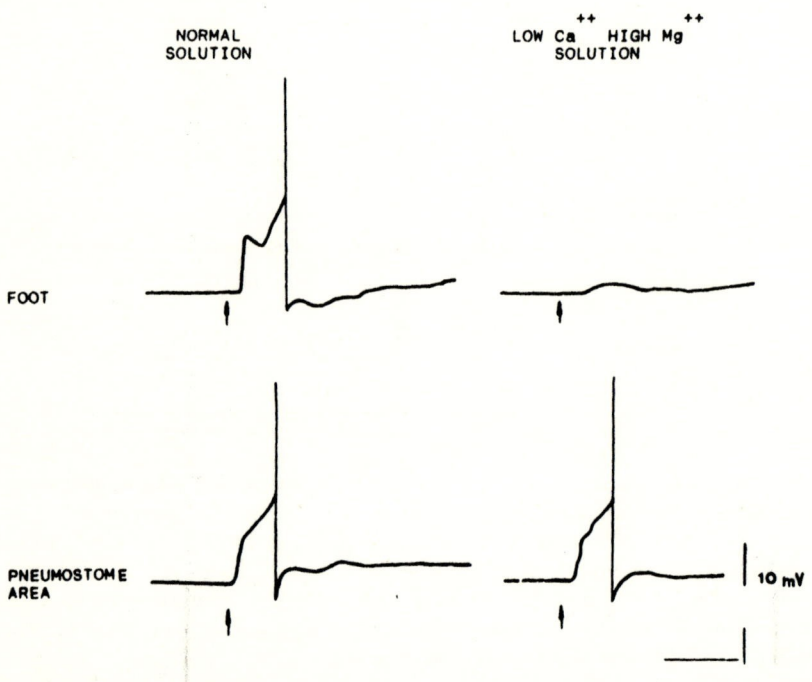

FIGURE 15.8. Structure of the receptive field of the command neuron. The blockade of central synapses by a low Ca^{2+}, high Mg^{2+} solution eliminates the late EPSP evoked from the foot. The initial EPSP from the mantel and the response of the pneumostom are not eliminated.

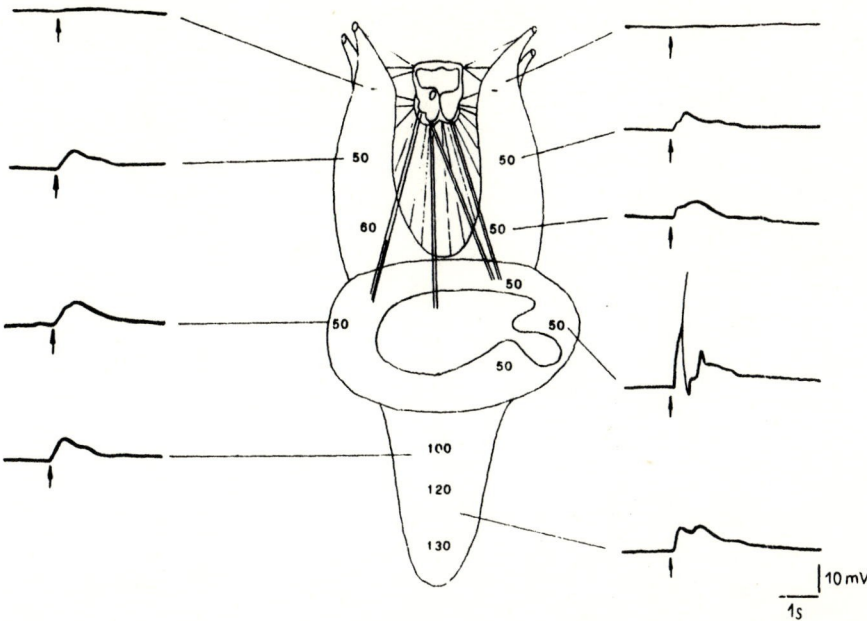

FIGURE 15.9. Receptive field map. The map of EPSP latencies in milliseconds demonstrates late responses from the foot and early responses from the mantel

the first and second EPSP did not abolish the third EPSP, representing a nonplastic nociceptive input to the avoidance command neuron (Figure 15.11) (Shehter, 1988).

Thus, in the receptive field one can identify plastic and nonplastic synapses. The nonplastic synapses are characteristic of the receptive field focus and nociceptive channels. The plastic synapses represent the nonnociceptive periphery of the receptive field (Shehter & Arakelov, 1985). The process of habituation of EPSPs is selective with respect to stimulus location. A minimal shift of the tactile stimulus with respect to the skin evokes an EPSP (Figure 15.12). This means that local areas of the receptive surface send signals to the command neuron through independent parallel channels. It can be assumed that habituation is occurring within separate synaptic contacts.

LOCAL DETECTORS AS PARALLEL CHANNELS

The study of receptive fields of afferent neurons has revealed a population of cells with point-like receptive field areas. Such a population of cells also represents the local areas of intestinal organs (Figure 15.13) (Palikhova & Arakelov, in press). Tactile stimulation of the point-like receptive field generates spikes in the cell body. The tactile stimuli outside the point-like

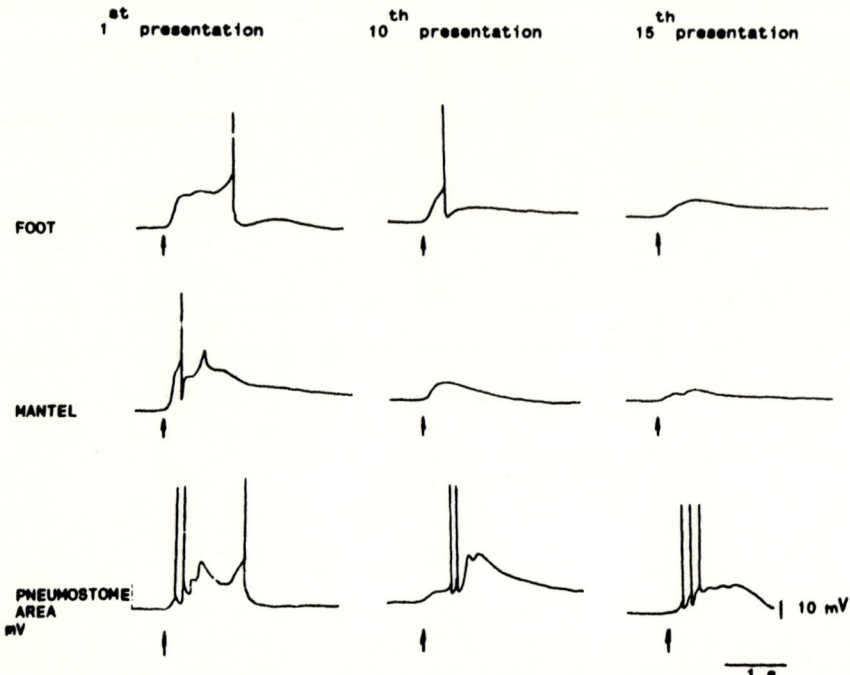

FIGURE 15.10. Plastic and nonplastic synapse of the receptive field. Repeated tactile stimuli do not eliminate the EPSPs from the pneumostoma area representing the focus of the receptive field. In contrast, the late EPSPs evoked by foot and mantel stimulations are habituated.

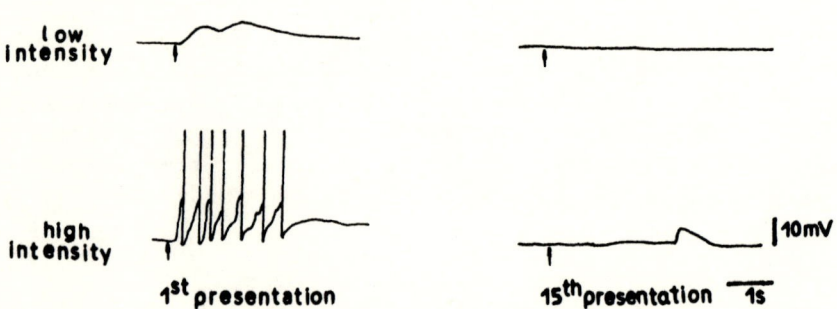

FIGURE 15.11. The nonplastic nociceptive input to the command neuron. Repeated slight electrical stimulation of the skin results in a habituation of two early EPSPs. A repeated strong stimulation parallels the habituation of two initial EPSPs. However, the late nociceptive component is not extinguished.

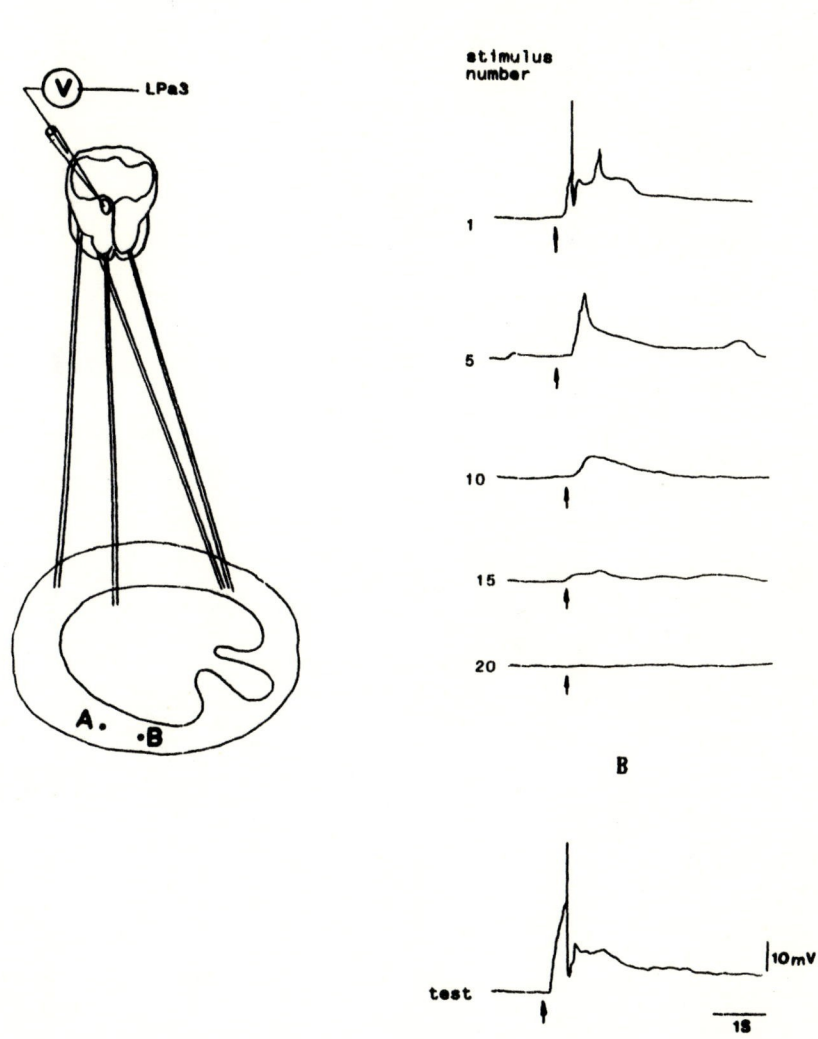

FIGURE 15.12. Selective stimulation of the skin results in an EPSP that is diminished and completely habituated during repeated presentation on the same point (A). A shift of the stimulation locus 1 mm away evokes an EPSP of the initial amplitude (B).

area result in an inhibition that is expressed in long-lasting hyperpolarization. Such an inhibitory surrounding emphasizes the excitation evoked by stimulation of the receptive field center. The receptive field of local detectors demonstrates no habituation effect (Figure 15.13c).

The spikes in the detectors are accompanied by a sequence of EPSPs in the command neuron. The intracellular depolarization of the local detector

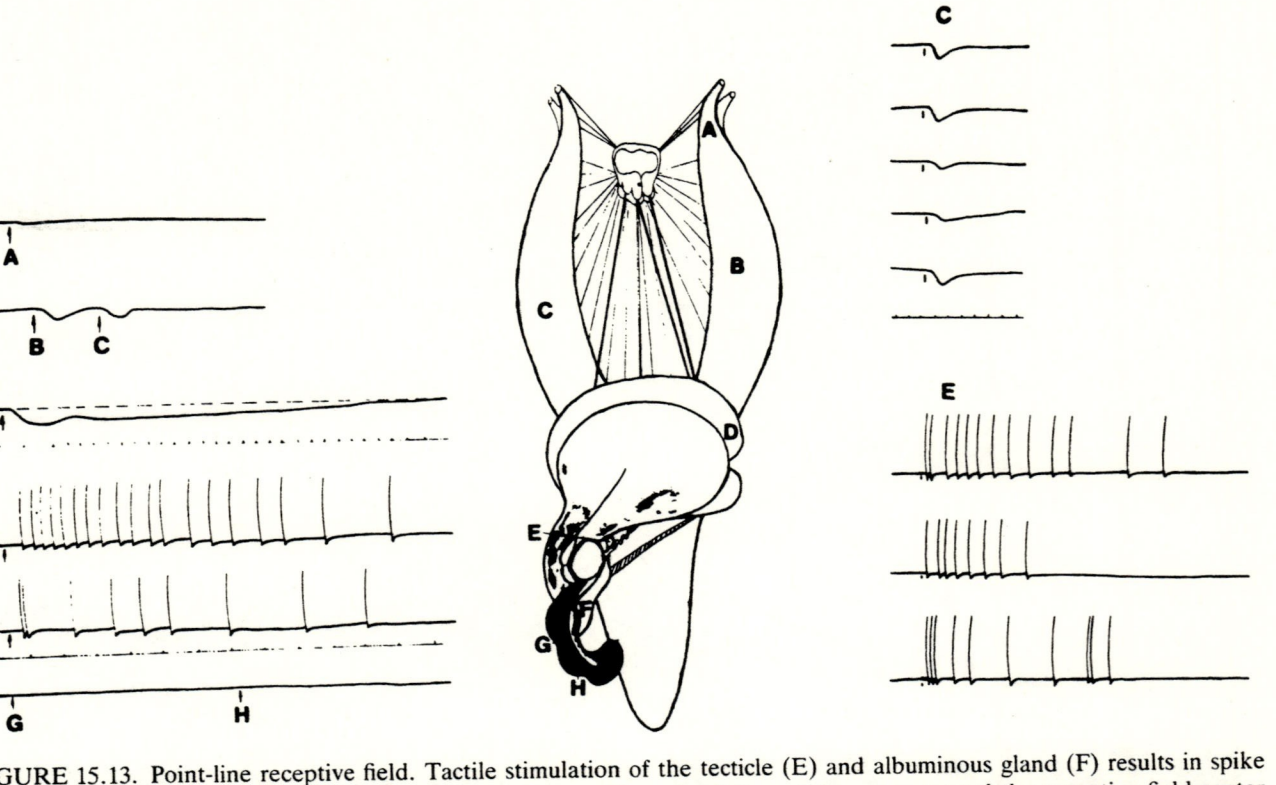

FIGURE 15.13. Point-line receptive field. Tactile stimulation of the tecticle (E) and albuminous gland (F) results in spike generation in a small sensory neuron LPa7. In contrast, tactilke stimulation of the areas around the receptive field center [foot (A,B,C); mantel (D), and liver (G,H)] results in hyperpolarizing potentials or lack of responses. The repeated stimulation of the center (E) and periphery (C) demonstrates no habituation phenomena.

triggers spikes that generate EPSPs in the command neuron (Figure 15.14). Thus the local detectors constitute a set of parallel channels converging on the command neuron via plastic inputs.

IDENTIFIABLE SYNAPSES ON THE COMMAND NEURON

The identification of the avoidance command neuron and local detector synapsing on the command neurons enables an identification of such a synapse. The physiological identification is based on the observation of the EPSPs evoked in the identified command neuron by intracellular depolarization of the identified local detector. the morphological identification of the synapse is based on the injection of cobalt and nickel in respective neurons to identify the areas of localization of synaptic contacts.

The light microscopic data reveal a complex synapse with five boutons located on the processes of the command neuron. The axonal terminals of the local detector are characterized by very fine fibres of different length (Figure 15.15). Thus the spikes reaching the boutons pass various distances through such fine branches. Because of the low speed of the spike travelling in such fine terminals, their time of arrival at each bouton will be different. Such structural organization of the synapse suggests a sequence of EPSPs peaks in accordance with respective spike delay (Marakujeva, Trepakov, Palikhova, & Sokolov, in press).

Detailed study of the shape of the EPSPs evoked by intracellular stimulation of the local detector has demonstrated their complex structure. Recorded superimposed components correlate with different synaptic

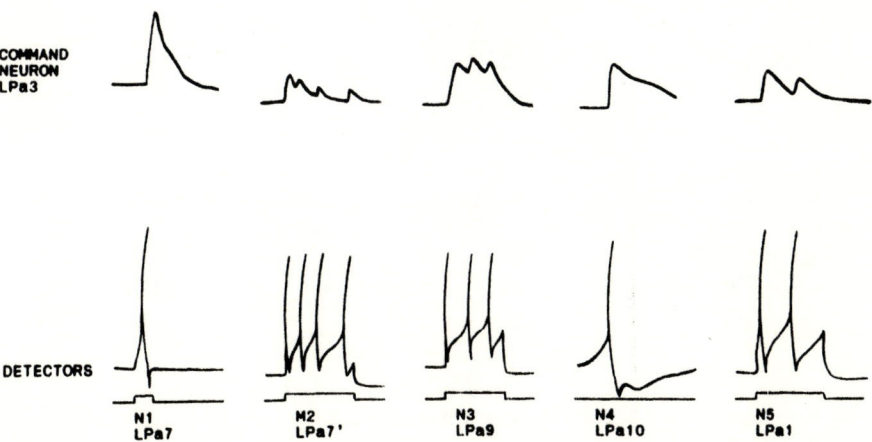

FIGURE 15.14. EPSPs in the command neuron evoked by stimulation of different detectors. Intracellular depolarizatin produces trains of spikes in a local-detector accompanied in the command neuron by sequences of EPSPs.

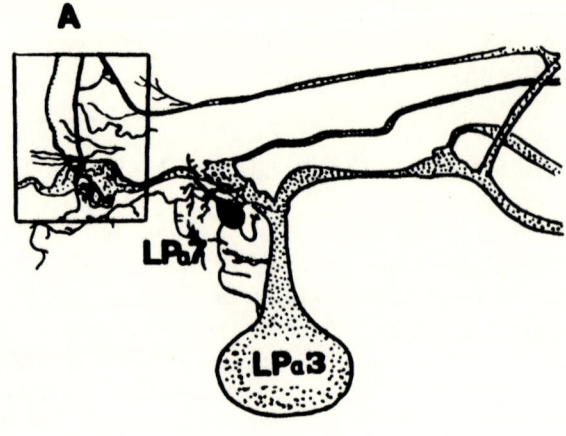

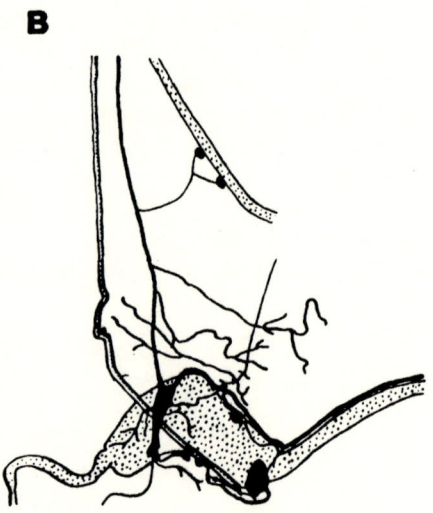

FIGURE 15.15. Identifiable synapse between detector and command neuron. Reconstruction of detector-command neuron preparation (A,B). Injection of nickel in detector LPa7 and mixed cobalt and nickel in command neuron Lpa3 shows the synapses. The boutons are characterized by fine axonal terminals of different length.

boutons. Separated EPSPs during low-frequency, repeated intracellular stimulation of the local detector have shown different habituation effects. The late high-amplitude components were habituated. The initial component is more stable. A high-frequency train of spikes evoked in the local detector results in a sensitization effect expressed as the increase of EPSP amplitude to the subsequent low-frequency (test) stimulation (Figure 15.16) (Arakelov, Marakujeva, & Palikhova, 1990).

MODULATORY NEURONS IN CONTROL OF SYNAPTIC TRANSMISSION

The efficiency of the identified synapse between a local detector and the avoidance command neuron depends on the participation of calcium channels. The decrease of calcium concentration results in a reduction of EPSP amplitude (Figure 15.17). The increase of calcium ions in the solution augments the magnitude of the EPSP. With constant calcium concentration, the EPSP depends on the density of functionally active calcium channels, which is increased by addition of serotonin to the solution (Figure 15.18A) (Balaban, Vehovszky, Maximova, & Zakharov, 1987).

The action of serotonin on calcium channels is controlled by phosphorylation of the channel protein through the following sequence of events: (a) activation of adenylatecyclase, (b) increase of cAMP concentration, and (c) activation of protein kinase. Under natural conditions, serotonin is released from the terminals of avoidance modulatory neurons synapsing on the

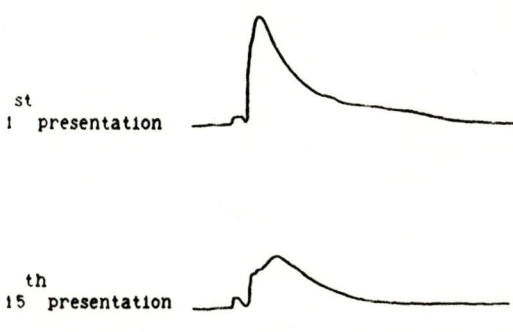

1st presentation

15th presentation

High frequency stimulation

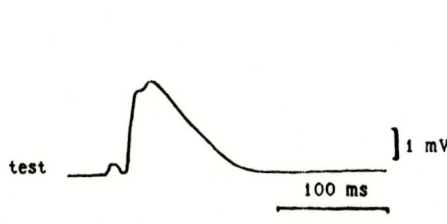

test

1 mV

100 ms

FIGURE 15.16.
Monosynaptic EPSPs in the command neuron. Intracellular stimulation of a detector results in a monosynaptic EPSP in the command neuron. Repeated stimulation shows its complex structure.

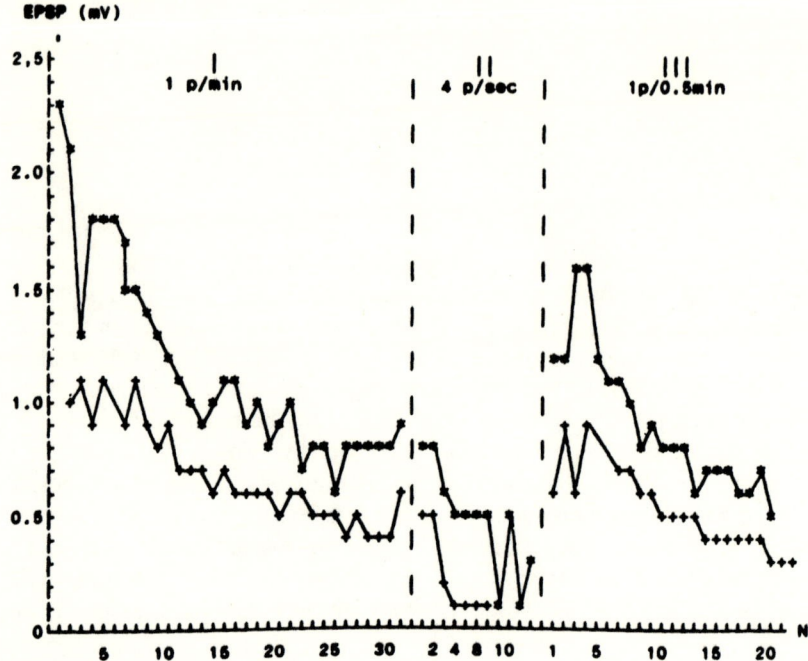

FIGURE 15.17. Habituation and sensitization in an identified synapse. A different rate of habituation due to low-frequency (1 p/min) stimulation demonstrates that different boutons of the synapse are characterized by different plasticity. A high-frequency train of spikes re-establishes the habituated responses, indicating that the direction of plastic changes is frequency-dependent. Decrease of calcium concentration reduces EPSP amplitude, but does not change response dynamics (lower curves, +).

presynaptic branches of detectors that are converging on the avoidance command neuron. The avoidance modulatory neurons are organized as a group of spontaneously active cells in the pedal ganglion (Balaban, Zakharov, & Chistyakova, 1987). Their direct electrical stimulation, increasing spike frequency, results in a release of serotonin and transformation of the "sleepy" calcium channels into responsive ones (Figure 15.18B).

The avoidance modulatory neurons are also responsive to strong stimulation of the skin. Thus the avoidance modulatory neurons emphasize or reduce the responsiveness of the avoidance command neurons to sensory stimulation.

NEURONAL MECHANISMS OF ADVERSIVE CONDITIONING

The food presented to the lip in the semi-intact preparation evokes no response or only rare EPSPs in the avoidance command neuron. No response is seen in avoidance modulatory neurons either. In methacerebral giant

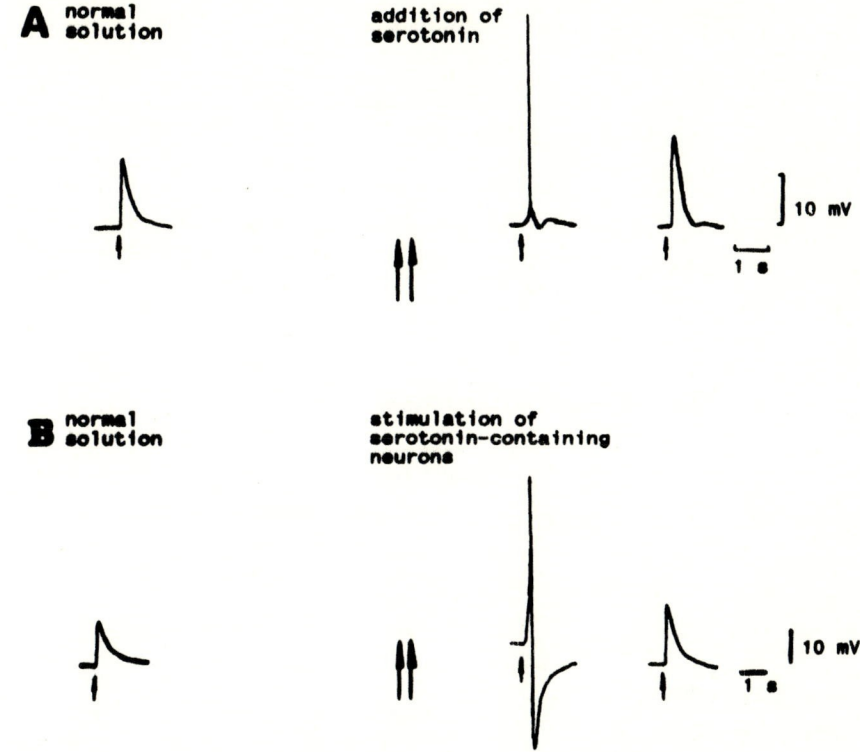

FIGURE 15.18. Serotonin-dependent increase of postsynaptic potential in the avoidance command neuron. The addition of serotonin to the normal physiological solution results in an augmentation of EPSP (A). Similar effects are obtained by intracellular electrical stimulation of avoidance modulatory neurons (B).

cells, known as feeding behavior modulatory neurons, food evokes depolarization and intensive spiking. If, however, application of food is regularly combined with electric shock on the skin, then the response pattern changes radically. The presentation of food now evokes a sequence of EPSPs and spikes in the avoidance command neuron, triggering a withdrawal reaction and the closure of pneumostoma (Figure 15.19). The aversive conditioned reflex established during food-shock association is extinguished when the food is not reinforced by electric shock (Maximova & Balaban, 1982, 1984).

The aversive conditioned reflex at the neuronal level can be explained differently. The first explanation suggests that electric shock stimulating avoidance modulatory neurons increases the efficiency of synapses of chemosensitive detectors present on the defensive command neuron. The other explanation is based on the assumption that the efficiency of plastic synapses of chemosensitive detectors on the command neuron are increased because of a combination of their activation with excitation of the command neuron by shock through nonplastic nociceptive inputs.

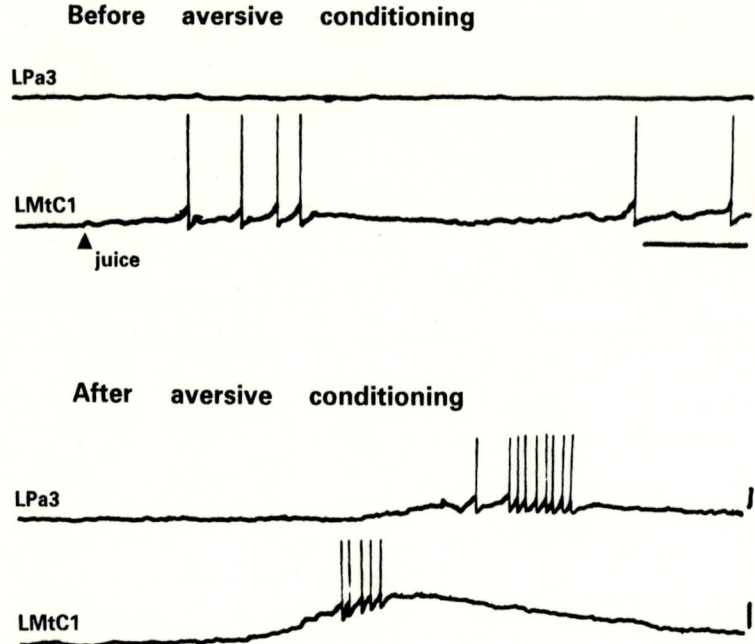

FIGURE 15.19. Intracellular events during aversive conditioning. Food given before aversive conditioning activates modulatory neurons of feeding behavior (LMtC1). The avoidance command neuron (LPa3) is not activated. No avoidacne behavior occurs. After repeated presentation of food in combination with electric shock, the same food generates spiking in avoidance command neurons and releases avoidance behavior.

The suggestion concerning the role of modulatory neurons in selective conditioning represents a presynaptic version of the effect-dependent theory of learning. It implies a long-lasting enhancement of activated feature-detector synapses resulting from shock stimulation of modulatory neurons.

The hypothesis concerned with enhancement of activated plastic synapses due to the contribution of the nonplastic inputs of the command neuron represents a Hebbian type of postsynaptic plasticity based on intracellular signaling.

ASSOCIATIVE LEARNING IN THE COMPLETELY ISOLATED COMMAND NEURON

The hypothesis concerning intracellular signaling as a basis of effect-dependent associative learning can be tested on the completely isolated identifiable avoidance command neuron. The conditioned stimulus reaching the command neuron under natural conditions through the feature-detector synapses is replaced with a micropipette and acetylcholine. The nociceptive stimulation used as a reinforcement for elaboration of the avoidance conditioned reflex in a semi-intact preparation is simulated by depolarizing current injected through an intracellular microelectrode.

The iontophoretic application of acetylcholine results in an excitatory transmitter potential without spike generation. The depolarizing current used as reinforcement triggers a sequence of spikes. The repeated association of the excitatory transmitter potential with a superimposed intracellular depolarization demonstrates a gradual augmentation of the amplitude of the transmitter potential, best seen when a test application of acetylcholine is not followed by intracellular depolarization. In the process of such intracellular conditioning, the transmitter potential can reach firing threshold resulting in spike generation. This intracellular conditioning is gradually extinguished when the transmitter potential is not reinforced by intracellular depolarization (Figure 15.20) (Grechenko & Sokolov, 1987).

Is this augmentation of transmitter potential a distributed or a local

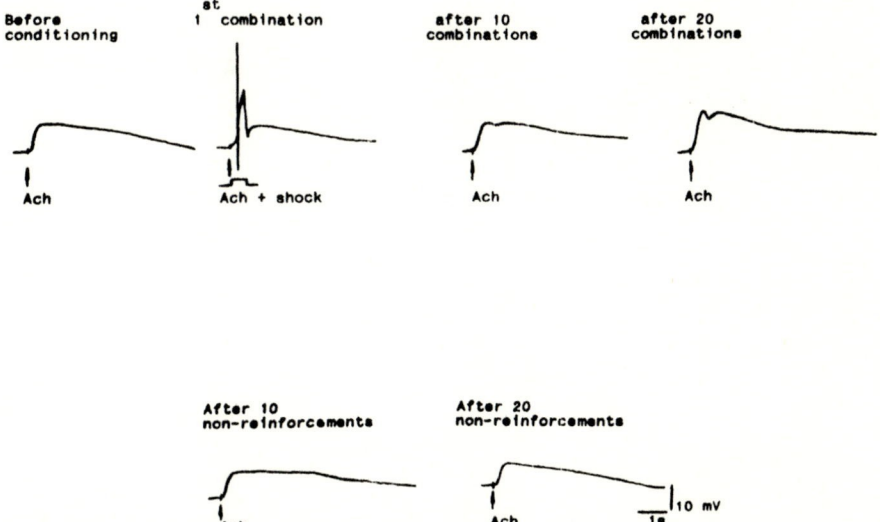

FIGURE 15.20. Intracellular conditioning and extinction in an isolated soma of the avoidance command neuron. The transmitter potential increases after its combination with intracellularly evoked spiking. Non-reinforcment results in a reduction of the transmitter potential.

process? To test this problem two micropipettes were used in experiments. The transmitter iontophoretic application from one pipette simulating the conditioned stimulus was associated with spiking evoked by the intracellular microelectrode. The other pipette simulating a differential stimulus was not reinforced by spiking. It was shown that the increase of the amplitude of the transmitter potential is a *local* event, occurring only with the pipette that was reinforced by intracellular depolarization (Figure 15.21) (Grechenko & Sokolov, 1987).

Local modification of the responsiveness of acetylcholine receptors due to immediately subsequent spike generation of the cell body suggests similar mechanisms of local plasticity of synapses in the process of association of sensory signals with biologically important reinforcement.

INTRACELLULAR SIGNALING IN THE CONDITIONED REFLEX

There are two states of the receptor proteins incorporated into the neuronal membrane and representing ionic channels: open and closed. The category of closed channels is divided into two groups: responsive with respect to a transmitter molecule and nonresponsive or "sleepy." The local application

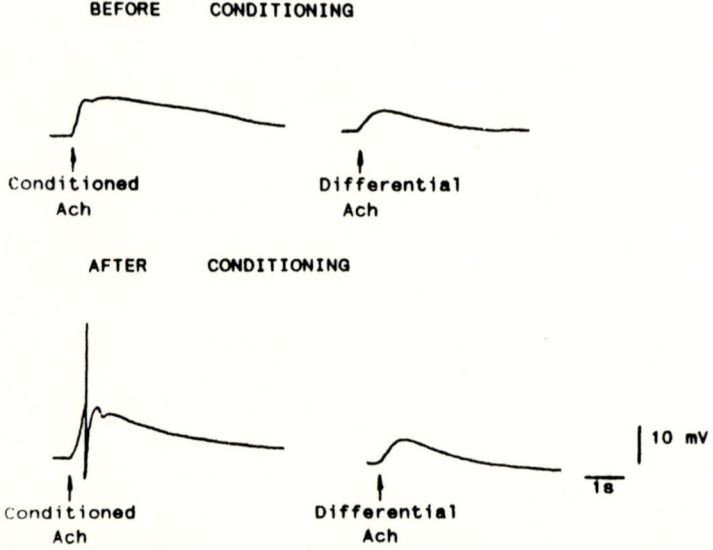

FIGURE 15.21. Differential conditioning in an isolated soma of the avoidance command neuron. Local applications of acetylcholine (Ach) as conditioned and differential stimuli result in a local augmentation of response to the conditioned transmitter only. The differential Ach stimulus evokes a transmitter potential of the initial amplitude. Thus, the conditioning is a local process in an area being stimulated before the intracellular spiking.

of the transmitter on the membrane results in the opening of the responsive channels. The sleepy channels are not opened.

The opening of responsive channels can modify some of them, inducing their sleepy state. The transformation of responsive channels into sleepy ones decreases the number of responsive channels and reduces the effect of the next presentation of the transmitter, constituting the basis of response habituation.

The spiking superimposed on the transmitter potential transforms some of the sleepy channels activated by a transmitter into a responsive state. Thus, the number of responsive channels due to pairing with spiking results in an enhancement of the response to the next presentation of the transmitter. Such an effect of the transmitter-spiking association constitutes the basis of intracellular conditioning.

Short-term and long-term mechanisms of such a modification of channels can be suggested. The short-term transformation might depend on phosphorylation–dephosphorylation of the receptor protein. The responsive channel being activated and opened by the transmitter can be affected by phosphatase and be transformed into a sleepy state owing to dephosphorylation. The spiking opens voltage-dependent calcium channels of the cell body. Calcium entering the cell stimulates calcium calmodulin-dependent protein kinase and results in the phosphorylation of sleepy channels pre-excited by transmitter molecules. This transforms sleepy channels into the responsive state.

The action of the transmitter on the sleepy receptor cannot open it but is a precondition for subsequent phosphorylation of the channel under the influence of the spikes that follow. This means that sleepy channels can be transformed into responsive channels only at the locus of transmitter application after attachment of transmitter molecules. Thus, the conditioned stimulus represented by local application of transmitter should precede the unconditioned stimulus, which is active in the form of calcium influx during cell body spiking (Figure 15.22). The long-term mechanism suggests a more complex sequence of events. The local stimulation of a receptor followed by intracellular depolarization results in the phosphorylation of the channel. This is the initial step.

The phosphorylated receptor protein is transported to the nucleus where it operates in the enhancer for transcription of genes responsible for coding of the specific receptor protein. The selective translocation of the synthesized receptor protein might depend on specific translocation proteins bringing the receptor protein to a predetermined locus on the membrane. The selective synthesis of specific translocation proteins is triggered by a locus-specific protein activated in parallel by the transmitter. Thus, the membrane of the neuron is mapped on the DNA molecule in such a way that each locus of the membrane corresponds to a specific translocation protein, which can be activated by a locus-specific protein operating as an enhancer (Figure 15.23).

To summarize, the map of the membrane is coded by locus-specific

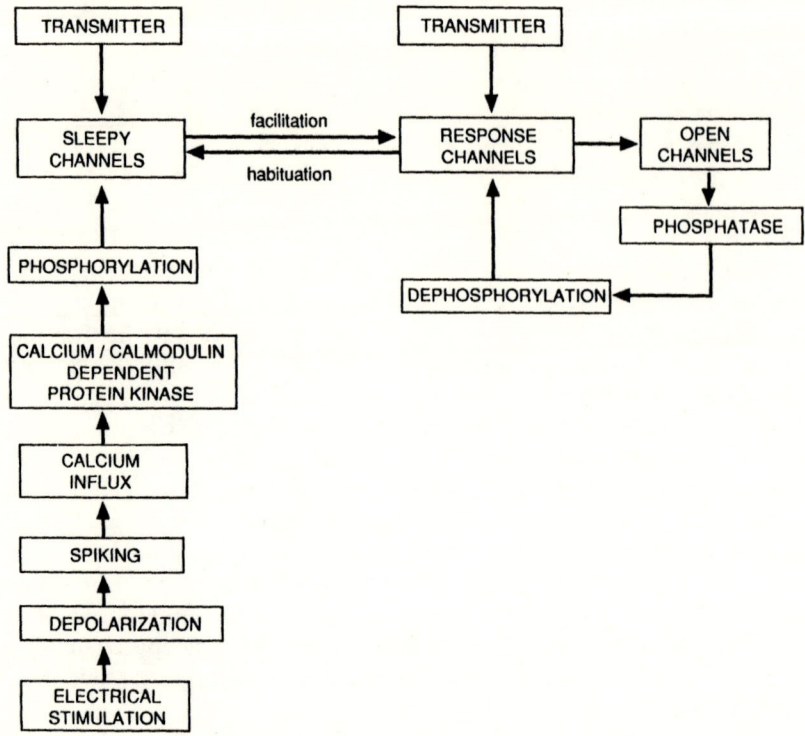

FIGURE 15.22.   Postsynaptic short-term plasticity. Transmitter can influence the state of the ionic channel. Acting on the responsive channel, transmitter opens it and produces an activation of phosphatase, dephosphorylation of the responsive channel makes it "sleepy." This means that the channel is not opening by transmitter. The sleepy channel activated by transmitter can be transformed into a responsive state by being phosphorylated by calcium/calmodulin-dependent protein kinase owing to calcium infux induced by calcium spikes during depolarization of the somatic membrane.

proteins. Different loci of the membrane are represented on the DNA molecule by operons for locus-specific translocating proteins. These operons are expressed with respect to the stimulated loci by locus-specific proteins on the neuronal membrane. The synthesized locus-specific proteins fulfil the function of transportation of receptor proteins to the stimulated locus on the neuronal membrane.

SUMMARY

The processes of habituation, sensitization, and conditioning are localized at specific plastic synapses. At the presynaptic level, the conditioned response is due to a selective increase of efficiency of synapses activated before a

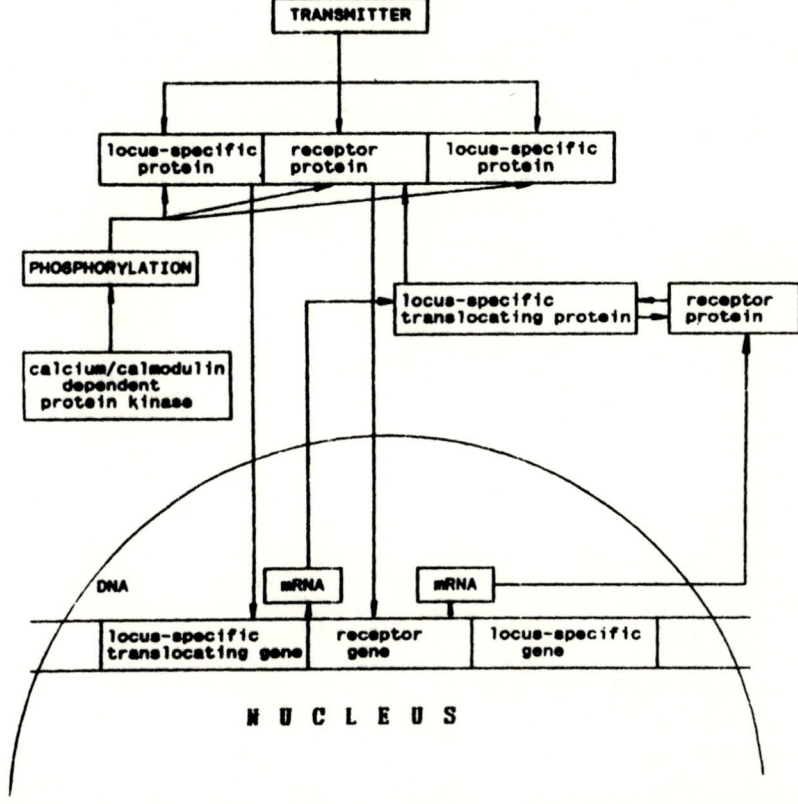

FIGURE 15.23. Postsynaptic long-term plasticity. The loci of the membrane are specified by locus-specific proteins with receptor proteins between them. The transmitter activates both receptor protein and locus-specific protein. Being transported to the nucleus of the cell body these proteins enhance respective gene transcription. The synthesized locus-specific protein functioning as a translocation protein transports the receptor protein to a specific locus of the membrane increasing local density of receptor molecules. The particpation of gene expression makes local increase of receptor density long-lasting.

modulatory neuron is activated. At the postsynaptic level, conditioning is an intracellular process selective with respect to the stimulated locus, which is followed by spiking. Short-term intracellular plasticity is due to phosphorylation–dephosphorylation of receptor protein. Long-term plasticity suggests an enhancement of expression of receptor genes transported to the locus of stimulation with participation of specific translocating proteins expressed by locus-specific proteins on the neuronal membrane.

Acknowledgments: The author wishes to thank all colleagues whose participation made this work possible: Drs G. G. Arakelov, L. K. Khludova, A. L. Krylova, T.

A. Palikhova, and E. D. Shehter from the section of Psychophysiology, Faculty of
Psychology, Moscow State University; scientists from the Institute of Higher Nervous
Activity and Neurophysiology of the Academy of Science, USSR: Drs P. M. Balaban,
O. A. Maksimova, and I. S. Zakharov; Dr T. N. Grechenko from the Institute of
Psychology of the Academy of Science, USSR; and all others who helped me in my
work.

REFERENCES

Arakelov, G. G. (1974). Endogeneus potentials of nerve cells as a result of neuron
    functional and metabolic heterogeneity. *Uspekhi Physiologicheskikh Nauk,
    5*, 52–77 (in Russian).
Arakelov, G. G., Marakujeva, I. V., & Palikhova, T. A. (1990). Monosynaptical
    connection: Identified synapses in CNS of *Helix pomatia. Zhurnal Visshey
    Nervnoy Deyatelnosty, 39*, 737–745 (in Russian).
Arakelov, G. G., & Palikhova, T. A. (1985). Central mechanisms of movement
    organization. In E. N. Sokolov & L. A. Shmelev (Eds.), *Neurocybernetic
    analysis of the mechanisms of behavior* (pp. 84–101). Moscow: Nauka (in
    Russian).
Arakelov, G. G., Palikhova, T. A., & Marakujeva, I. V. (in press). Structural and
    functional analysis of monosynaptical connections between identified
    neurones in snail, *Helix lucorum*. In D. A. Sakharov & B. Winlow (Eds.),
    Simpler nervous systems. Manchester: Manchester University Press.
Arakelov, G. G., & Sakharova, T. A. (1982). Structural-functional analysis of
    identified neurons in the snail. *Neuroscience and Behavior Physiology, 12*,
    75–81.
Balaban, P. M., Vehovszky, A., Maximova, O. A., and Zakharov, I. S. (1987).
    Effect of 5,7-DHT on food-aversive conditioning in the snail *Helix lucorum
    L. Brain Research, 404*, 201–210.
Balaban, P. M., Zakharov, I. S., & Chistyakova, M. V. (1987). Localization of
    plastic changes evoked by aversive learning in the nervous system of the
    snail *Helix lucorum L. Neuroscience, 22*, 659P.
Balaban, P. M., Zakharov, I. S., & Chistyakova, M. V. (1988). Role of serotonergic
    cells in aversive learning in *Helix*. In J. Salanki & K. S.-Rozsa (Eds.),
    Neurobiology of invertebrates. Transmitters, modulators and receptors (pp.
    519–531). Budapest: Akademia Kiado.
Grechenko, T. N., & Sokolov, E. N. (1987). Neurophysiology of learning and
    memory. In P. G. Kostyuk (Ed.), *Handbook of physiology. Mechanisms
    of memory* (pp. 132–172). Leningrad: Nauka (in Russian).
Khludova, L. K., & Sokolov, E. N. (1983). Ion channels in electric sensibility of
    command neuron. *Vestnik Moskovskogo Universiteta: seria 14, Psychology,
    2*, 14–19.
Marakujeva, I. V., Trepakov, V., Palikhova, T. A., & Sokolov, E. N. (in press).
    Complex pattern of monosynaptical EPSP in the *Helix* neuron: Some
    proposition about its nature. *Zhurnal Visshey Nervnoy Deyatelnosty, 41* (in
    Russian).
Maximova, O. A., & Balaban, P. M. (1982). Neural correlates of associative learning
    in vitro. *Neuroscience, 7* (Suppl.), S142.
Maximova, O. A., & Balaban, P. M. (1984). Neuronal correlates of aversive learning
    in command neurons for avoidance behavior of *Helix lucorum L. Brain
    Research, 292*, 139–149.
Palikhova, T. A. (1985). Trigger zones on axonal branches of *Helix* identified
    neurons. In E. N. Sokolov & L. A. Shmelev (Eds.), *Neurocybernetic

analysis of the mechanisms of behaviour (pp. 101–119). Moscow: Nauka (in Russian).

Palikhova, T. A. (in press). Intracellular circulation of spikes in central neurones of snail. In D. A. Sakharov & B. Winlow (Eds.), *Simpler nervous systems*. Manchester: Manchester University Press.

Palikhova, T. A., & Arakelov, G. G. (in press). Monosynaptic connections in *Helix* central nervous system: Receptive fields of the presynaptic neurons. *Zhurnal Visshey Nervnoy Deyatelnosty, 40* (in Russian).

Shehter, E. D. (1988). Sensitivity of the command neuron to the electrical stimulation of its receptive field. In D. A. Sakharov (Ed.), *Simpler nervous systems* (pp. 324–327). Leningrad: Nauka (in Russian).

Shehter, E. D., & Arakelov, G. G. (1985). Receptive field of command neuron. In E. N. Sokolov & L. A. Shmelev (Eds.), *Neurocybernetic analysis of the mechanisms of behavior* (pp. 64–84). Moscow: Nauka (in Russian).

Sokolov, E. N. (1977). Brain functions: neuronal mechanisms of learning and memory. *Annual Review of Psychology, 28*, 85–112.

Sokolov, E. N., & Yarmizina, A. L. (1970). Habituation of molluscan giant neuron to repeating electrical stimulation. In *Neuronal mechanisms of orienting reflex* (pp. 111–117). Moscow: Moscow University Press (in Russian).

Yarmizina, A. L. (1975). Neuronal plasticity. In E. N. Sokolov & N. N. Tavkheladze, *Pacemaker potential of neuron* (pp. 87–103). Tbilisi: Mentsiereba (in Russian).

16

What the Chick Can Tell Us About the Process and Structure of Memory

STEVEN P. R. ROSE

LEVELS OF MEANING AND LEVELS OF ANALYSIS

Being the final chapter in this book has some advantages; the position enables one to try to extract some common themes and to set one's own interests in the context of, or even in contention with, ideas and issues that have been raised earlier. I will try to identify some of these issues and to show how experiments from my own lab, using the young chick as a model for the study of memory mechanisms, may perhaps cast light on them. The overarching problem seems to be whether it is possible to build a general theory that can unify—or at least put into a common context—the disparate approaches and findings concerning the cellular processes of memory formation. As earlier chapters have perhaps inadvertently revealed, we are still far from that point. We do not even yet know how many different theories of memory might be required by the multiplicity of phenomena embraced within that term. Let me try to tease apart some of the paradoxes and dichotomies that, depending on one's viewpoint, either enrich or impede our progress.

One of the terms used most glibly by neurobiologists and neurophilosophers alike is the little word "level," and I have become increasingly concerned at the assumption that the concept is unproblematic, and means no more than the sort of scalar quantity suggested by Churchland and Sejnowski (1988), when they propose the sequence:

CNS (1 m). → System (10 cm) → Map (1 cm) → Network → (1 mm) → Neuron (100 μm) → Synapse (1 m) → Molecule (1 Å)

This is of course neither the only nor yet the most relevant use of the concept of level; organized complexity is more than merely a matter of scale. True, Churchland and Sejnowski (1988) offer an alternative based on

Marr's computer-derived definitions of different classes of analytical question (computational, algorithmic, and implementation), but the neurobiological literature is replete with other uses, for instance:

1. To define different central nervous system (CNS) structures (cortex → midbrain → brain stem).
2. To define phylogeny (human → primate → mammal → vertebrate → invertebrate).
3. To define epistemology (psychology → physiology → biochemistry → molecular biology).
4. To define neural function (motor, verbal; conscious, unconscious, etc.).

In the context of theories of memory, however, we are—or should be—concerned with yet another sense of level; on the one hand, levels of meaning, and on the other, levels of analysis. *Level of meaning* is reflected in Freeman's claim that learning and memory should not be conceived of in information processing terms but in terms rather of meaning and representation—which I understand to imply that the biological significance of the change in behavior that results from learning, occurs during recall, and whose intervening variable we infer to be memory. *Level of analysis* reflects the search for the appropriate level of organized complexity of matter at which to seek for an "explanation" of memory mechanisms. It is the level of analysis that mainly concerns me here. Should we be talking the language of single synapses and their biochemistry and biophysics (cellular alphabets), of small ensembles of synapses and their modified connectivity (connectionism), or global field properties (chaos models)? Protagonists of each of these approaches are present among the authors of the chapters in this volume. Is it presumptious of me to suggest that they cannot all be right and that unification is not simply a question of letting a hundred flowers bloom?

DICHOTOMIES AND PARADOXES

The unresolved question of level has not been the only ghost at our banquet. Brooding over our feast I have observed the shades of Lashley and Penfield, whose modern avatars are still confronting the paradoxes of distributed versus local changes. Other absent presences, I suggest, are Edelman, whose critique (Edelman, 1987) of information processing models of memory, if one disregards the pseudoevolutionary jargon in which it is couched, ought to be obligatory reading, and Garcia, for reasons I will return to later. Thus the physiologists and brain imagers present us with models of memory that are essentially fluid and dynamic: memory as process, the fluctuating records from shifting ensembles of neurons either measured directly or by way of the surrogates given by blood flow or radioactive accumulation following ^{14}C-2-deoxyglucose (DG) injection. By contrast the biochemists and morphologists seem to offer linear sequences of processes in single synapses or cells that fix memories as rigidly as the blackened images of an autoradiogram. Are memories local or global, or, as I shall argue below, mobile?

In our search for appropriate levels of analysis of memory, how are we to interpret the many taxonomies that we have been offered: procedural and declarative, semantic and episodic, recognition and recall? One feature that these dichotomies share is that they all seem to be time-independent; there is no space within them for the stage theories of memory, the transitions between long and short term, that the multitudinous pharmacological studies with animals seem empirically to indicate, that the progenitor of the present volume, McGaugh, has so effectively theorized, and which underly the molecular and cellular models presented here by Lynch, Bailey, and Sokolov. How do conclusions as to the time course of memory formation based on the painstaking delineation of phases of memory pharmacologically dissected in rats, chicks, and mollusks map on to the taxonomy of procedural and declarative memories in humans?

This leads to another rather fundamental question, implicit in the earlier discussions: Is "memory" an omnibus term at the behavioral/psychological level (by which I mean here epistemological level), embracing a multitude of different mechanisms at the analytical level, or can we identify general cellular processes that subserve all, or most forms of memory, the only distinction being the addresses of the cells whose connectivity is being modulated during the learning? Does Hebb universally rule? Is what is true for *H. ermissenda* also the case for *H. sapiens*? Does localism conflict with globalism, or is it embraced within it? Aesthetically I favor such a universalism, but we lack the evidential base for or against at present. The ubiquity of the phenomena of habituation, sensitization, and association at least at the behavioral level speaks to unity theories. So does the apparently near universality of the requirements of protein synthesis for long-term memory. (The only exceptions I know to this rule are some forms of odor discrimination in *Drosophila* and in honey-bees; see discussion in Squire and Lindenlaub, 1990.) I shall describe evidence that even nonassociative learning requires macromolecular synthesis. Does the passionate debate about pre versus postsynaptic mechanisms, of which again more below, reflect real differences in the mechanics of memory, or is it merely methodological and interpretative arm-wrestling among afficionados? Is memory a special case of neural plasticity, in which case seizures, enriched experience, environmental deprivation during development, even transplant technology, all have something to say as to mechanism, or is it *sui generis*? Does not the richness of human experience suggest multiplicity rather than unity?

THE CHICK MODEL

So much for the generalities; let me try to address some of these questions more precisely by way of work from our own laboratory, based on studies of early learning in that most amenable of laboratory vertebrates, the domestic chick. Show a young chick a small bright object, and it will quickly peck at it. If the object is a colored bead dipped in a bitter-tasting liquid, the chick will subsequently avoid pecking at even a dry bead of that color and shape, although its general pecking activity is unimpaired. This behavior forms the basis of the one-trial passive avoidance learning task introduced by Cherkin more than 2 decades ago (Cherkin 1969). It is but one of the large repertoire of forms of early learning about key features of its environment, such as mother (imprinting, see Horn, 1985) and edible food, which the naive but precocial young chick, hatched with a large brain and considerable behavioral competence, must achieve rapidly if it is to survive. Avian learning, from canary song to marsh-tit food catching, is becoming increasingly popular as possible model systems in which to study vertebrate memory formation (e.g., Horn & Krebs, 1990), and the chick, with its repertoire of strongly ontogenetically driven learning, is particularly atttractive (Andrew, 1991). Chicks are, after all, vertebrates (if not even honorary mammals), and there are merits in working with "natural" learning in intact animals rather than the cellular models thereof which long-term potentiation (LTP) represents.

Learning to suppress pecking at the bitter bead initiates an intracellular cascade of cellular processes, which, beginning with pre- and postsynaptic membrane transients and proceeding by way of genomic activation to the lasting structural modification of these membranes, occurs in identified regions of the chick forebrain. I believe that these synaptic modifications form in some way the neural representations of the aversive bead-pecking experience and encode the instructions for the changed behavior (avoid pecking a bead of these characteristics) that follows. I will summarize the key steps that we have identified as occurring in this cascade, emphasizing commonalities and distinctions between these and the data presented in earlier chapters, and then ask what these processes can reveal about the mechanisms and nature of memory storage in vertebrates.

THE LOCI OF CHANGE

In the basic experimental design (e.g., Lossner & Rose, 1983) day-old chicks are placed in small pens under controlled illumination and, after a period of equilibration, may be injected intracerebrally with appropriate precursors or potentially amnestic agents. The procedure is made very simple, without the need for anesthesia, because of the chick's soft, unossified skull (Davis, Masouka, Gerbrandt, & Cherkin, 1979). The birds are then presented with a small chrome bead dipped either in water (W) or the bitter aversant methylanthranilate (M). Chicks pecking at the bead are tested at times ranging from 30 min to 24 h subsequently before their brains are taken for analysis. More than 80% of W birds peck on testing, and more than 75% of M birds avoid; the percentage avoidance amongst the M birds, by comparison with W birds, is taken as a measure of recall.

Because we had no initial preconceptions about which areas of the brain might be involved in the response to pecking at the bitter bead, in an early series of experiments we gave chicks a 30 min pulse of ^{14}C-2-DG just prior to or after training on the bead and compared autoradiograms of forebrains from M and W birds (Kossut & Rose, 1984). Two regions, in particular, showed enhanced accumulation of radioactivity in the 30 min after training, the intermediate medial hyperstriatum ventrale (IMHV) and lobus parolfactorius (LPO), with some evidence for a third, the paleostriatum augmentatum (PA) (Figure 16.1). Interestingly, and of considerable relevance to our subsequent studies, there was also evidence of lateralization, with the greatest changes being seen in the left hemisphere regions (Rose & Csillag, 1985). For those more familiar with mammalian than avian brain structures, IMHV has been regarded as homologous with striate cortex, the LPO with basal ganglia; the hyperstriatum ventrale in general seems to be a type of association area, receiving inputs from many different sensory systems, while the LPO, as part of the paleostriatal complex, lies on the

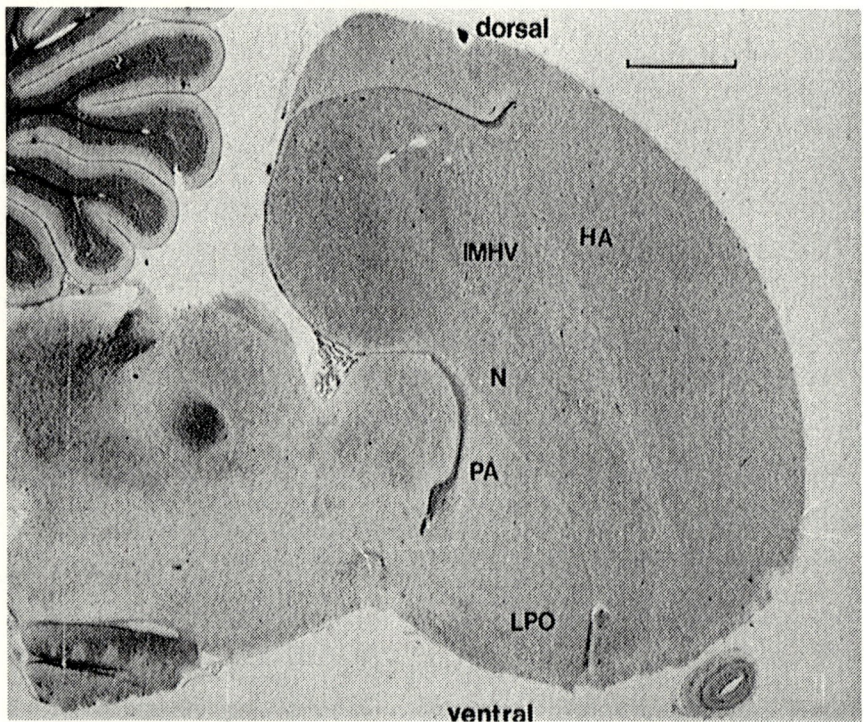

FIGURE 16.1. Saggital section through day-old chick brain; Nissl staining. Hp, hippocampus; HA, hyperstriatum accessorium; IMHV; intermediate medial hyperstriatum ventrale; N, neostriatum; LPO, lobus parolfactorius; PA, paleostriatum augmentatum. (Photograph courtesy of Dr. Mike Stewart)

output side and is concerned with the integration of motor responses, although there are no known direct connections from IMHV to LPO. Even more relevantly, perhaps, the IMHV is an area that has also been implicated as showing cellular plasticity during visual imprinting (Horn, 1985; see also Andrew, 1991).

SYNAPTIC PHOSPHORYLATIONS

Having identified IMHV and LPO as sites of enhanced neural activity in the minutes following training on the passive avoidance task, in subsequent experiments we have followed biochemical, physiological, and morphological changes in these regions (Table 16.1). Because it seemed probable, by analogy with LTP and other models of neural plasticity, that early events following training would include membrane phosphorylations, we isolated synaptic plasma membranes (SPMs) and post-synaptic densities (PSDs) from IMHV-enriched tissue and phosphorylated them in vitro with ^{32}P-ATP. The phosphorylation patterns showed the presence of an exclusively presynaptic, 52 kD component immunologically identical to the phosphoprotein variously called B50, GAP 43, or F1 (Ali, Bullock, & Rose, 1988; Benowitz & Routtenberg, 1985; Bullock, de Graan, Oestreicher, Gispen, & Rose, 1990). Thirty minutes after training, M chicks showed a specific, transient in vitro reduction in the phosphorylation of this component. (There is a somewhat tortuous debate in the literature about whether in vitro reductions in phosphorylation imply an increase in in vivo occupancy of phosphorylable sites, which I will not enter into here. For discussion see, for example, Gispen & Routtenberg, 1986.)

B50 is a protein kinase C (PKC) substrate, and PKC inhibitors such as melittin, staurosporine, or H7 prevent its phosphorylation. If the phosphorylation step is essential for memory formation, it should follow that intracerebral injection of PKC inhibitors should result in amnesia for the passive avoidance; that is, on test M birds should peck rather than avoid the bead. This indeed turns out to be the case; unilateral injection of, for instance, melittin or H7 into left but not right IMHV, just before or just after training, results in amnesia on test 6–24 h subsequently (Burchuladze, Potter & Rose, 1990). PKC exists in a number of isoforms, partially membrane-bound and partially cytosolic, and one widely canvassed model for the regulation of phosphorylation of its membrane substrates is by way of translocation from cytosol to membrane (Akers, Lovinger, Colley, Linden, & Routtenberg, 1986). We have found a small but significant increase in the membrane-bound PKC, assayed using a specific antibody to the α/β (translocatable) forms of the enzyme, in synaptic membranes of the left IMHV 30 min after passive avoidance training.

These processes are analogous to those occurring in LTP, where PKC inhibitors have been reported to affect the maintenance, although not the initiation of the effect (Reymann, Schulzeck, Dase, & Matthies, 1988). This

TABLE 16.1 Cellular Cascade During Memory Formation for Passive Avoidance

Time scale	Process		Location	Inhibited By (Amnesia)
Seconds–minutes	Glucose uptake	↑	IHMV, LPO (L and R)	—
	Receptor binding (muscarinic, NMDA)	↑	IMHV?	APV, MK801
Minutes–hours	PKC translocation	↑	L IMHV	—
	Presynaptic B50 phosphorylation	↑	L IMHV	Polymixin B, Melittin, H7, Staurosporine
	c-fos, c-jun expression	↑	L IMHV	—
1–6 hours	Protein synthesis ↑ (tubulin)		IMHV	Cycloheximide, anisomycin, etc.
	Glycoprotein synthesis (pre- and postsynaptic)	↑	L and K IMHV	
			L and R LPO	2-D-galactose, electroshock
	Fucokinase	↑	R LPO	—
	Neuronal bursting	↑	L and R IMHV L and R LPO	Electroshock
12–24 hours	Dendritic branching	↑	L IMHV	Electroshock
	Spine head diameter	↑	L IMHV	—
	Synapse number	↑	L and R LPO	—
	Vesicle number	↑	L IMHV L LPO	—
	PSD length	↑	L IMHV L LPO	—

L: left; R: right.

claim, it is true, has been challenged by Lynch (Muller, Buchs, Dunant & Lynch, 1990) although supported by others (Loveringer, Colley, Akers, Nelson, & Routtenberg, 1989). By contrast with the presynaptic effect of PKC inhibitors on our B50 phosphorylation, Malinow and others (e.g., Malinow, Schulman, & Tsien, 1989) have reported that the postsynaptic injection of specific PKC pseudosubstrates blocks LTP. However, until workers with LTP are able to show that presynaptic application of PKC inhibitors is *without* effect, or we demonstrate that the *only* phosphorylation step blocked by the inhibitors in the chick is that of presynaptic B50, the contradiction (along with other aspects of the somewhat heated dispute amongst workers with LTP on pre- versus postsynaptic loci of effects, see, for example, Bliss, 1990) may be more apparent than real. However, it is worth emphasizing that, at least in our hands, the B50 phosphorylation does seem to be exclusively presynaptic. This may just be a developmental phenomenon; there is some evidence that postsynaptic B50 is present in older animals. It is also worth mentioning that we do find a 45 kD phosphorylable component that is postsynaptic; we do not yet know whether, at later times after training, this component also shows learning-associated changes (Ali et al., 1988). Nor do these data eliminate the possibility of the additional involvement of a cAMP-dependent protein kinase of the type proposed by Lynch and Kandel in their chapters.

FROM SYNAPSE TO NUCLEUS

In any event, conversion of such transient modifications of membrane properties into more lasting pre- or postsynaptic modulations of connectivity must depend on the synthesis of new membrane constituents. The molecular biological mechanisms involved in triggering the synthesis of such membrane proteins are assumed to involve the initial activation of members of the family of immediate early genes of which the protein oncogenes c-*fos* and c-*jun* are amongst the best-known, as described by Gall. C-*fos* and c-*jun* expression is believed to be initiated by signals emanating from the membrane, especially the opening of calcium channels and the activation of the phosphoinositide (PI) cycle mediated by the phosphorylation steps described above (see, for example, Chiarugi, Ruggiero & Corradetti, 1989 and references therein). We (Anokhin, Mileusnic, Shamakina, & Rose, 1991) have recently been able to show that, 30 min after M-training, c-*fos* and c-*jun* mRNAs are induced in IMHV and LPO. However, as Gall's paper makes clear, the induction of these genes is notoriously sensitive to many types of sensory stimulation (including, as we also observed, pecking at a water-coated bead), and it was important to test whether the large increases we found in M-training were directly associated with memory formation.

To do this, we altered the training task from an aversive to an appetitive one. If chicks are placed on a floor on which food grains are scattered amongst immobile inedible objects of similar size and colour (small pebbles, glued to the floor surface) they soon learn to distinguish food from nonfood particles, pecking at the former but not the latter—an observation first made by Andrew and Rogers (1972). We took three groups of birds (as well as a quiet control group that remained undisturbed in their pens for the duration of the experiment). All three groups were exposed to the "pebble floor" during training trials on Day 1, and a final trial on Day 2, after which forebrain c-*jun* expression was measured by Northern blotting. On Day 1, Groups 1 and 2 were placed on the floor with no food grains; Group 3 had food on all trials. On Day 2, Groups 1 and 3 repeated their experience of

Day 1; Group 2, however, also had food grains for the first time on Day 2, and was thus learning the discrimination at the time c-*jun* was measured, while Group 3 was overtrained with respect to Group 2. All birds pecked during the third trial (Group 3 most of all) and showed some increase in c-*jun* expression over that in the quiet controls. However, much the greatest c-*jun* expression occurred in Group 2, the "learning" rather than the merely "behaving" Group (Figure 16.2), and seems therefore to be specifically learning-related (Anokhin & Rose, 1991).

FROM NUCLEUS TO SYNAPSE

Whatever the intervening intracellular signals and genomic mechanisms, within an hour after training there is enhanced synthesis of a variety of

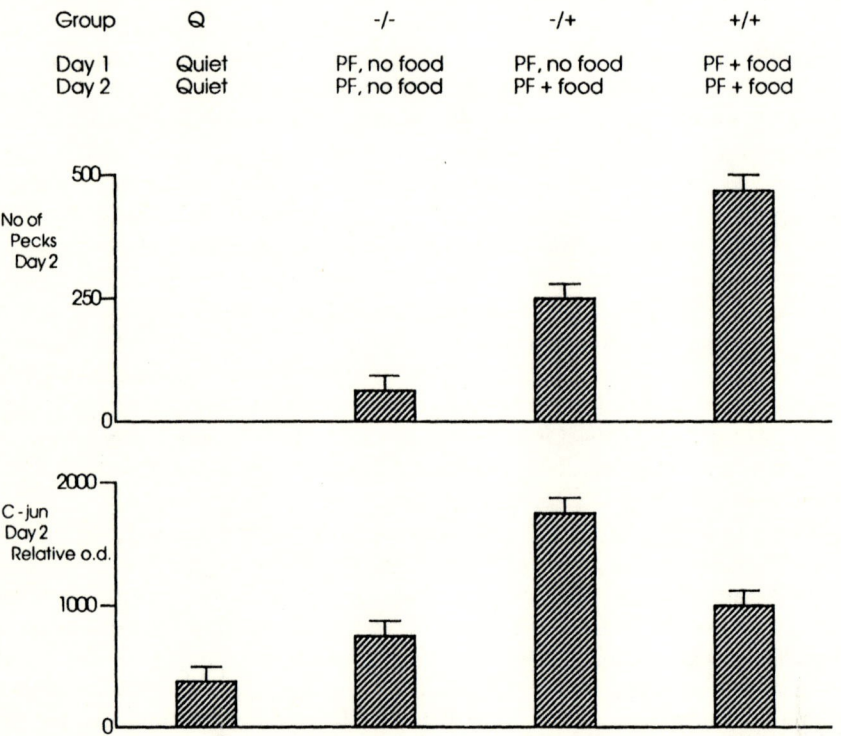

FIGURE 16.2. C-*jun* expression during pebble floor learning. Three groups of chicks and a Quiet control were trained over 2 days as indicated in the top two rows (PF = pebble floor) and number of pecks at the pebbles and/or scattered food recorded during an 8-min trial on Day 2, following which c-*jun* was estimated by Northern blotting. (Data redrawn from Anokhin & Rose, 1991)

proteins intended for export from the cell body. Although in our early work we observed increases in the synthesis of cell proteins, notably the microtubular protein tubulin (Mileusnic, Rose, & Tillson, 1980), most of our attention has been directed towards the glycoproteins of the synaptic membrane (Rose, 1989), because of the major role that several glycoprotein families (for instance, the N-CAMs and integrins discussed by Lynch and Kandel in this volume, and see also (Edelman, 1987) play as cell recognition and adhesion molecules in stabilizing intercellular connections. There is enhanced incorporation of radioactively labeled fucose into pre- and postsynaptic membrane glycoproteins for many hours following training (Sukumar, Rose, & Burgoyne, 1980) regulated by increased activity of the rate-limiting enzyme fucokinase (Lossner & Rose, 1983). Using double-labeling techniques, we have separated the glycoproteins on SDS gels and identified a number of fractions of interest. In particular, in IMHV and LPO, a presynaptic component of molecular weight around 50 kD and postsynaptic components of molecular weight 100–120 and 150–180 kD seem particularly training-sensitive (Bullock, Potter, & Rose, 1991; Bullock, Zamani, & Rose, unpublished results).

As with the phosphorylation and protein synthesis steps of this series of reactions, we would expect to find that, if the synthesis of glycoproteins was a necessary step in the formation of long-term memory, then inhibiting this synthesis should produce amnesia. Jork, in Magdeburg, has used a specific inhibitor of fucoglycoprotein synthesis, 2-deoxygalactose (2-dgal), a competitive inhibitor to galactose, which, incorporated into the nascent glycoprotein chain, prevents terminal fucosylation. Intracerebral administration of 2-dgal produces amnesia for a number of tasks in rodents (Jork, Grecksch, & Matthies, 1986). In collaborative experiments we have found that it has a similar effect in chicks when injected within a time window of an hour before to an hour after training (Rose & Jork, 1987). However, I have recently observed a curious additional aspect of 2-dgal amnesia; although not amnestic when given between 2 and 4+ h after training, if injected between 5 and 8 h after training, animals were amnesic when tested 24 h subsequently (Figure 16.3). Thus, there appears to be a "second wave" of memory-related glycoprotein synthesis occurring some hours downstream of the first, a phenomenon that has also been observed during memory formation in rats by the Magdeburg group (Pohle, Rüthrich, Popov, & Matthies, 1979). I return below to the possible relevance of this "second wave" in the context of the models suggested by Lynch (this volume).

How does this intracellular biochemical cascade "translate" into altered pre- and postsynaptic morphology? Working on the hypothesis that changes in synaptic connectivity might be expressed by changes in the numbers or dimensions of axo-dendritic synapses, a series of studies by my colleague Stewart has quantitatively examined morphological parameters, at light and electron microscope level, in IMHV and LPO of chicks 24 h after training on the passive avoidance task (reviewed in Stewart, 1991). At this time, there is a large (60%) increase in the density of dendritic spines on the

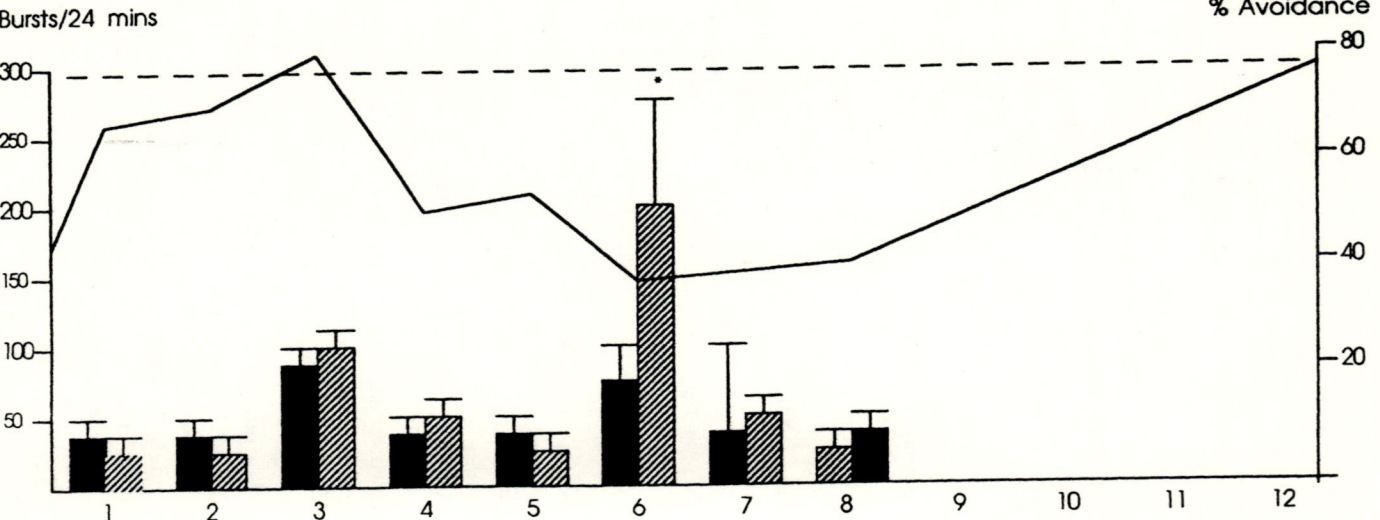

FIGURE 16.3. Bursting and the second wave of glycoprotein synthesis. Histograms show frequency of neuronal bursting recorded from left and right IMHV of anesthetized chicks at various times after training (Filled bars, left; hatched bars, right, IMHV) (data from Gigg, Patterson, & Rose, 1990). Superimposed graphs show percentage avoidance (retention score) tested 24 h after training in birds injected bilaterally into IMHV with either saline (dotted line) or 20 μM 2-deoxygalactose at the times shown.

large multipolar neurons of the left IMHV in the M-trained compared with W-trained chicks. This lateralized change is superimposed on a left–right assymmetry that already exists in control chicks (and that we also observe using monoclonal antibody markers for synaptic membrane constituents; Bullock, Csillag, & Rose, 1987), and is accompanied by a significant increase in the spine head diameter (Patel & Stewart, 1988). There is also increased dendritic growth in these neurons (Lowndes, Stanford, & Stewart, 1989).

Stereological analysis of the synapses of the IMHV and LPO has also shown training-related changes, the most striking of which include increases in synapse number in both left and right LPO and a 60% increase in the numbers of synaptic vesicles per synapse in the left IMHV and left LPO. Changes in synapse numbers in the LPO can be detected as soon as 12 h after training. These changes are reminiscent of those found by Greenough following exposure of rats to enriched versus impoverished environments, and Chen and Bailey in the synapses involved in the gill withdrawal reflex in *Aplysia* (see the references in Bailey's chapter in this volume). Bailey argues—and this would certainly be compatible with the data from the chick—that changes in vesicle number are relatively transient, whilst those in synapse number are longer lasting.

PHYSIOLOGICAL CORRELATES

What might these biochemical and structural changes to the synapse "mean" in terms of changed physiology? The IMHV of the young chick shows a number of interesting neurophysiological properties, the most relevant of which is perhaps its capacity to express LTP-like phenomena in vitro (Bradley, Burns, & Webb, 1988, 1990). Extracellular recordings from the IMHV and LPO of anesthetized chicks in the hours after training with the bitter bead show dramatic, several-fold increases in the incidence of bouts of high-frequency neuronal firing—bursting activity (Gigg, Patterson, & Rose, in preparation; Mason & Rose, 1987)—increases that, in the IMHV, show two peaks of intensity, one at 3–4 h after training, the second at 6–7 h after training. Whilst the first peak occurs in both left and right IMHV, the second is confined to the right IMHV (Figure 16.3). At the same time, John Gigg in our lab has found increased bursting in both left and right LPO.

It is of course essential to show that these substantial biochemical, morphological, and physiological changes are no mere epiphenomena, perhaps the sequelae of the combination of sensory, motor, and aversive experiences associated with pecking a bitter bead, but rather are directly associated with memory formation. The experimental design we have used to check for this possibility exploits the fact that a brief subconvulsive transcranial electroshock given in the minutes after training on the passive avoidance task results in subsequent amnesia; birds peck on test (a phenomenon first described by Benowitz & Magnus, 1973). If the electroshock is delayed however, until around 10 min after training, birds show recall on test. This phenomenon is presumably a consequence of the fact that the very earliest phases of memory formation are dependent on transient ionic fluxes at the synapse that the electroshock disrupts. In any event this effect makes it possible for us to dissociate the sequelae of the experience of pecking the bead from those of memory for the avoidance, by simply comparing our presumed biochemical, morphological, or physiological markers in birds that have all pecked the bead and been shocked, but, because of the time of administering the shock, some of which show recall whilst others do not. Using this paradigm we have shown that enhanced fucosylation, increased spine density, and neuronal bursting all occur only in birds showing recall; the mere tasting of the bead is without effect on these markers (Mason & Rose, 1988; Patel, Rose, & Stewart, 1989; Rose & Harding, 1984).

LESIONS AND THE LOCI OF MEMORY

The story I have told of the chick so far shows strong similarities with the picture of cellular processes mediating synaptic connectivity told for hippocampal processes by Lynch and for the serotonin-induced plasticity of the *Aplysia* synapse demonstrated by Kandel to be associated with long-term facilitation. It is also in accord with relatively straightforward cellular-association models of memory formation best summarized as Hebb rules. One could argue that, in an association region of the chick brain like the IMHV, convergent inputs from pathways associated on the one hand with visual signals from the bead and on the other its bitter and aversive taste resulted in modifying an output pathway (perhaps directly or indirectly via LPO) so that the original Peck response was switched to a No Peck one. Within individual IMHV cells a linear set of processes passes smoothly through the molecular steps associated with short-to-intermediate and long-term stages of memory (see chapters by Gibbs and by Rosenzweig in Andrew, 1991, for discussion of such stage theories).

However, it turns out that things are not so simple. The complexity has been revealed by a series of lesion experiments recently made by Gilbert, Patterson, and myself. We started from the premise that if IMHV, and particularly left IMHV, is the locus of memory for the passive avoidance task, then bilateral lesions of IMHV made prior to training should produce amnesia for the task. And indeed, if bilateral or unilateral left IMHV lesions are made on the day of hatch, and the chicks trained on the following day, they show amnesia for the avoidance when tested several hours later; equivalent right hemisphere IMHV lesions are, however, without effect. This would imply that left IMHV is necessary for memory formation, in accord with the biochemical and structural observations (Figure 16.4).

Doubts as to this simple interpretation arise from the next observation, that if the IMHV lesions (unilateral or bilateral) are made 1 or 6 h posttraining and the chicks tested 24 h later, they show full recall; thus once

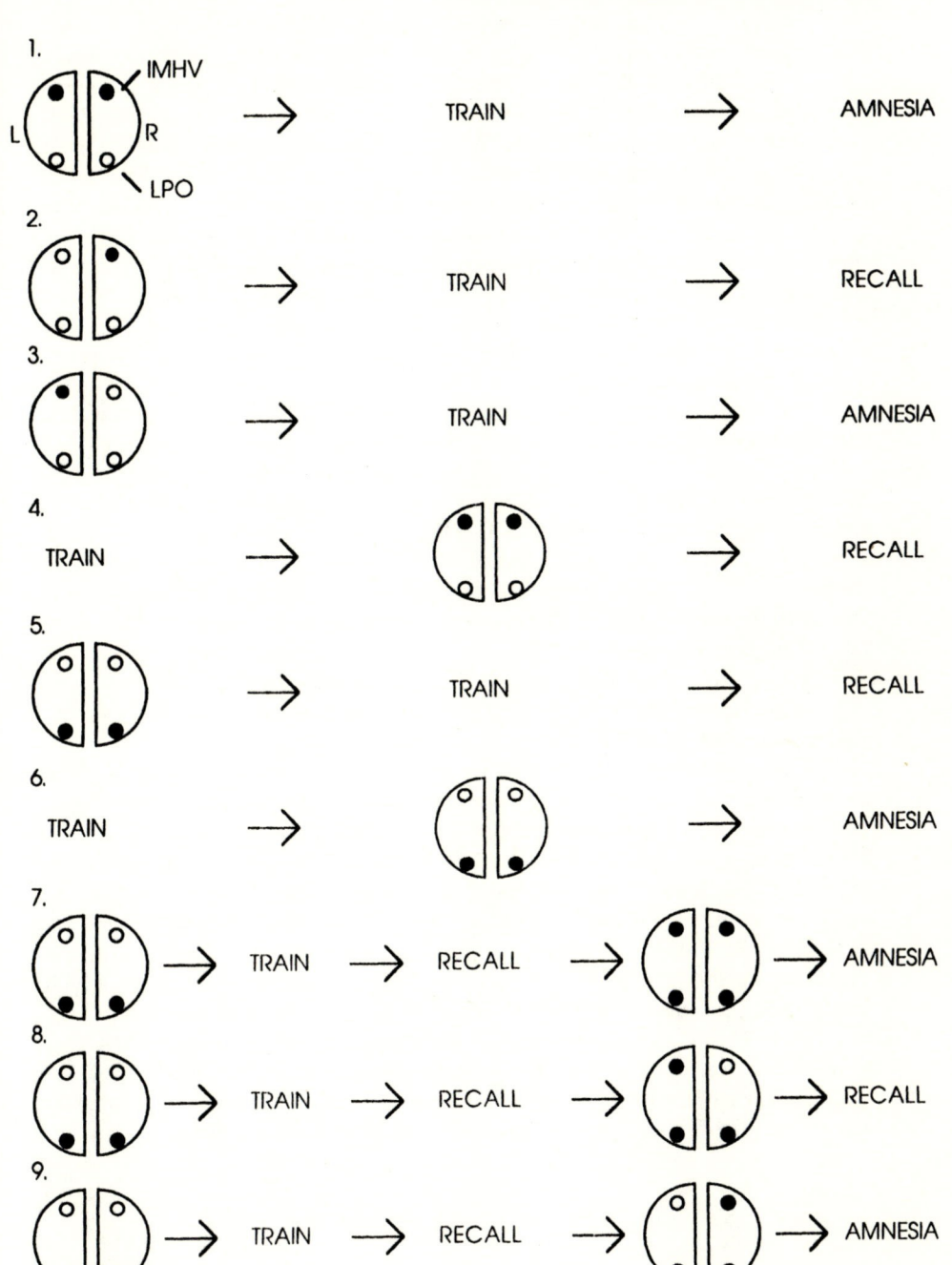

FIGURE 16.4. Effects of IMHV and LPO lesions on recall for passive avoidance (unilateral LPO lesions are without effect).

the animals have learned the task, left IMHV is no longer necessary (Patterson, Gilbert, & Rose, 1990). This observation resembles a finding first made in the context of imprinting by Horn and his colleagues (Cipolla-Neto, Horn, & McCabe, 1982). Horn, in the context of imprinting, suggested that the memory trace had in some way migrated out of the IMHV to a further, unspecified store. In the context of passive avoidance, an obvious question to ask was whether this could be the LPO? In accord with this possibility, we found that while even bilateral LPO lesions made prior to training are without effect, posttraining (bilateral but not unilateral) lesions are amnestic. In the presence of the LPO at training then, the memory seems in some way to end up there, whilst if the LPO is absent at training, some other structure must take over from it.

If this argument, of the migrating trace, is valid, then in the absence of the LPO, one possible argument is that the trace simply "backs up" and becomes "stranded" in the IMHV. Accordingly, we made pretraining lesions of the LPO (which were, of course, not amnestic) and then, after training, right or left hemisphere lesions of IMHV, neither of which *would* have been amnestic had the LPO been present. In the absence of the LPO, however, posttraining *right* IMHV lesions now resulted in amnesia. This sequence is shown in Figure 16.4. The simplest interpretation is shown in the "memory flow" diagram of Figure 16.5, in which a migratory trace, beginning in the left IMHV, flows first to right IMHV and then on into LPO. If the flow is interrupted at any point, however, the trace simply stays permanently stored in the structure preceding the interruption.

If this somewhat mechanical interpretation is correct, then with a pretraining right IMHV lesion, which is not itself amnestic, posttraining LPO lesions, which *would* be amnestic in the intact animal, would no longer be so, as the "memory flow" would no longer be able to pass through the right IMHV. Figure 16.6 shows that this experiment indeed gives the predicted results. However, a further prediction of this simple model is that, with a right IMHV lesioned pretraining, the memory should become "stranded" in the left IMHV, so that a posttraining left IMHV lesion, which would not be amnestic with an intact right IMHV, should now become so. As Figure 16.6 shows, however, this does *not* happen; the result of this set of dissociations is still that the chick shows recall. In the absence of the right IMHV, there must be yet another route out of the IMHV to some as yet unspecified locus (Figure 16.7) (Gilbert, Patterson, & Rose, 1991).

MEMORY STORAGE: LOCALIZED OR DISTRIBUTED?

What do these data have to say about how memories are stored in the brain? The biochemical and cellular cascade that I have described implies, as do most cellular models of memory formation, that a linear sequence of processes in a pair of neurons, or more realistically, in a small ensemble of such neurons, results in lasting modification of synaptic connectivity within

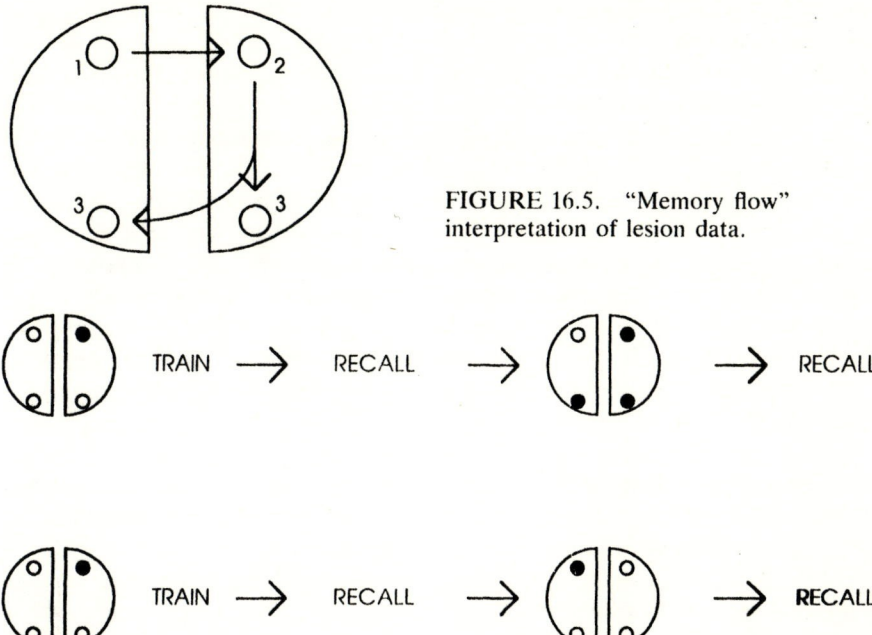

FIGURE 16.5. "Memory flow" interpretation of lesion data.

FIGURE 16.6. Lesions to test predictions from Figure 16.5.

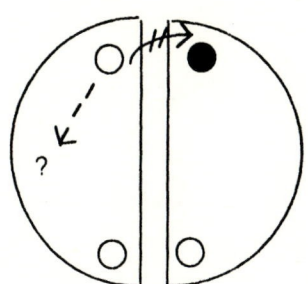

FIGURE 16.7. "Modified memory flow" interpretation. (From Gilbert, Patterson, & Rose, 1991.)

the ensemble, a modulation that is the brain representation of some association of events and experiences whose consequences are changed behaviors. The lesion studies, however, cast doubt on such a simplistic sequential model. Memory traces are not, it would appear, stably located within a single neuronal ensemble but are dynamic and fluid, moving from site to site within the brain. Representations are multiple, a result more in accord with Freeman's views than with the "frozen" cell ensemble biochemistry and morphology with which they have been contrasted.

Let me return to the phenomenon of the "double wave" of glycoprotein synthesis already described and consider its implications for this model. I said at the beginning of this chapter that another brooding presence at our feast was that of Garcia, whose observation of conditioned taste aversion (e.g., Garcia, Ervin, & Keolling, 1966) has presented a difficult theoretical challenge for the "temporal-contiguity" models of learning that dominate both association psychology and its cellular manifestation, the famous Hebb rules. It turns out that one can obtain a strong Garcia-type effect in the chick by simply offering it a dry green bead to peck, and 30 min to an hour later making it mildly sick by injecting lithium chloride intraperitoneally. The chick will avoid the green bead on presentation 3 h later (Figure 16.8). Thus the chick must form some representation of the bead in its brain even without explicit pairing with a contiguous aversive or appetitive stimulus (unlike early attempts to explain away the Garcia effect when animals were trained on colored or flavored water by claiming that some residual taste was being impaired with the lithium chloride).

This intriguing result in itself presents some challenges to simple cellular memory models, but the point I wish to make here is that inhibition of glycoprotein synthesis at the time of pecking the bead by injecting 2-dgal prevents the subsequent association of the lithium-chloride-induced sickness with the bead peck. As a result, birds that have been made sick with the lithium chloride nevertheless peck the bead when offered it 3 h later (Figure 16.8; Barber, Gilbert, & Rose, 1990). The 2-dgal must be injected at the

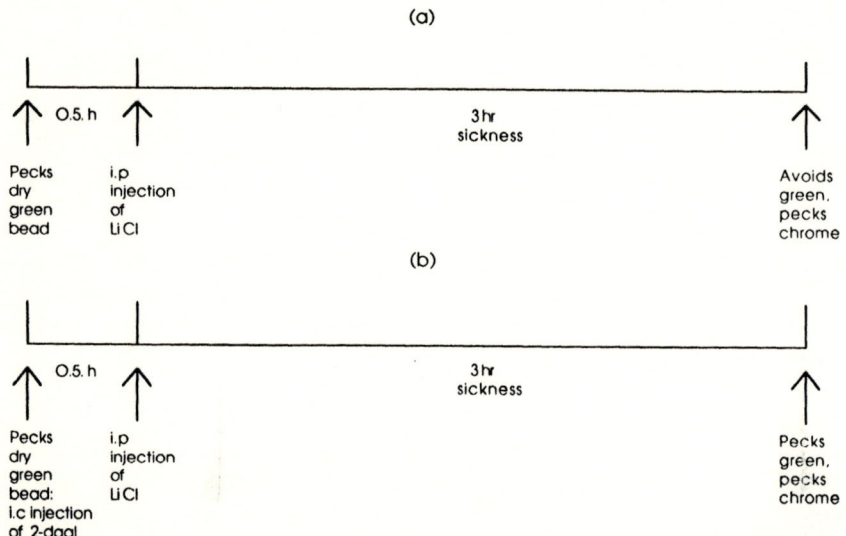

FIGURE 16.8.   2-Deoxygalactose and the Garcia effect in chicks. (See Barber, Gilbert, & Rose, 1990)

time of bead peck; there is no amnesia when it is injected at the time of administering the lithium chloride, nor is the phenomenon a state-dependent effect. Thus the chick not only makes a brain representation of the bead without specifically associating it with either appetitive or aversive consequences, but making that representation requires macromolecular—or at least glycoprotein—synthesis (this could be posttranslational modification of existing proteins).

Unlike the memory for the bitter-tasting bead, however, such simple representations, if unassociated with any strongly aversive or rewarding experience, soon fade; the chick cannot associate bead peck with sickness if the lithium chloride is given more than an hour after the bead. And weak aversive associations, such as pairing bead peck not with methylanthranilate but with the taste of quinine, which is remembered only for a few hours, do not produce any increase in glycoprotein synthesis over and above that found for pecking at the water bead alone (Bourne, Davies, Stewart, & Cooper, 1991). I suggest that in these weak learning cases only a first wave of glycoprotein synthesis is involved, and the memory is thus impermanent. Only if the memory is to be more permanently represented does the "second wave" of glycoprotein synthesis occur. The initial representation, and the first wave of protein synthesis, occurs in the left IMHV. During the processing and stabilizing of the trace, there is a sequential activation of the right IMHV and LPO. This is why, at around 6 h after training, the time of the second wave, the neuronal bursting is no longer found in the left, but only in the right IMHV and in the LPO. It is the second wave, then, that is responsible for producing the glycoproteins that stabilize the changed synaptic connectivities, by creating new synapses or dendritic structures or altering the locations of pre-existing ones. It is there that the various families of N-CAMs and integrins, synaptic recognition molecules, may play their part. This would explain why Lynch and his colleagues find that the integrins are essential for stabilizing but not initiating LTP. A related observation by Regan (personal communication) is also highly relevant here. Working with a step-down passive avoidance task in rats, he has found that a polyclonal antibody against N-CAM produces amnesia if injected at around 6 h after training but not if injected at around the time of training. The anti-N-CAM in this experiment would, in my interpretation, be disrupting the vital second wave of insertion of synapse recognition glycoproteins into the membrane and hence blocking permanent memory. If this turns out to be a generalizable mechanism—from LTP and rats to chicks and even *Aplysia*—perhaps we will have identified a further universal molecular step in memory formation.

Meantime, it is a global functional system, and not simply Hebb, who rules—O.K.?

Acknowledgments: The experiments described in this paper have been based on collaborative work by many members of the Brain and Behaviour Research Group over the past decade; I thank all who are cited, and those whose work forms part of the essential background to the results foregrounded here. An additional special thanks to Steve Walters and Dawn Sadler for consistently efficient animal care. The work described has been funded through the Open University, the UK Medical, and Science and Engineering, Research Councils, the Royal Society, the Wellcome Foundation, and the UK Department of Health.

REFERENCES

Akers, R. F., Lovinger, D. M., Colley, D., Linden, D., & Routtenberg, A. (1986). Translocation of protein kinase C activity after LTP may mediate hippocampal synaptic plasticity. *Science, 231*, 587–589.

Ali, S., Bullock, S., & Rose, S. P. R. (1988). Phosphorylation of synaptic proteins in chick forebrain: Changes with development and passive avoidance training. *Journal of Neurochemistry, 50*, 1579–1587.

Andrew, R. J. (Ed.). (1991). *Neural and behavioural plasticity; The use of the domestic chick as a model.* Oxford: Oxford University Press.

Andrew, R. J., & Rogers, L. J. (1972). Testosterone, search behaviour and persistence. *Nature, 237*, 343–346.

Anokhin, K. V., Mileusnic, R., Shamakina, I. Y., & Rose, S. P. R. (1991). Effects of early experience on c-*fos* gene expression in the chick forebrain. *Brain Research. 544*, 101–107.

Anokhin, K., & Rose, S. P. R. (1991). Learning-induced increase of immediate early gene messenger RNA in the chick forebrain. *European Journal of Neuroscience. 3*, 162–167.

Barber, A. J., Gilbert, D. B., & Rose, S. P. R. (1990). Glycoprotein synthesis is necessary for memory of sickness-induced learning in chicks. *European Journal of Neuroscience, 1*, 673–677.

Benowitz, L. I., & Magnus, J. G. (1973). Memory storage processes following one-trial aversive conditioning in the chick. *Behavioural Biology, 8*, 367–380.

Benowitz, L. I., & Routtenberg, A. (1985). A membrane phosphoprotein associated with neuronal development, axonal regeneration, phospholipid metabolism and synaptic plasticity. *Trends in Neuroscience, 10*, 527–532.

Bliss, T. V. P. (1990). Memory: Maintenance is presynaptic. *Nature, 346*, 698–699.

Bourne, R. C., Davies, D. C., Stewart, M. G., & Cooper, W. (1990). Cerebral glycoprotein synthesis and long term memory formation in the chick, follows passive avoidance training, depends on the nature of the aversive stimulus. *European Journal of Neuroscience. 3*, 243–248.

Bradley, P. M., Burns, B. D., & Webb, A. C. (1988). Response characteristics of neurons in chick forebrain slices. *Proceedings of the Royal Society of London B234*, 145–157.

Bradley, P. M., Burns, B. D., & Webb, A. C. (1991). Potential of synaptic responses in slices from the chick forebrain. *Proceedings of the Royal Society of London, B243*, 19–29.

Bullock, S., Csillag, A., & Rose, S. P. R. (1987). Synaptic vesicle proteins and acetylcholine levels in chick forebrain nuclei are altered by avoidance training. *Journal of Neurochemistry, 49*, 812–820.

Bullock, S., de Graan, P. N. E., Oestreicher, A. B., Gispen, W.-H., & Rose, S. P. R. (1990). Identification of a 52 kD chick brain membrane protein showing changed phosphorylation after passive avoidance training as B50 (GAP 43). *Neuroscience Research Communications, 6*, 181–186.

Bullock, S., Potter, J., & Rose, S. P. R. (1990). Effects of the amnestic agent 2-deoxygalactose on incorporation of fucose into chick brain glycoproteins. *Journal of Neurochemistry, 54*, 135–142.

Burchuladze, R., Potter, J., & Rose, S. P. R. (1990). Memory formation for passive avoidance in the chick depends on membrane-bound protein kinase C. *Brain Research, 535*, 131–138.

Cherkin, A. (1969). Kinetics of memory consolidation: Role of amnestic treatment parameters. *Proceedings of the National Academy of Sciences, U.S.A., 63*, 1094–1100.

Chiarugi, V. P., Ruggiero, M., & Corradetti, R. (1989). Oncogenes, protein kinase C, neuronal differentiation and memory. *Neurochemistry International, 14*, 1–9.

Churchland, P. S., & Sejnowski, T. J. (1988). Perspectives on cognitive neuroscience. *Science, 242*, 741–745.

Cipolla-Neto, J., Horn, G. & McCabe, B. J. (1982). Hemispheric asymmetry and imprinting: The effect of sequential lesions to the hyperstriatum ventrale. *Experimental Brain Research, 48*, 22–27.

Davis, H. P., & Squire, L. R. (1984). Protein synthesis and memory: A review *Psychological Bulletin, 96*, 518–559.

Davis, J. L., Masouka, D. T., Gerbrandt, L. K., and Cherkin, A. (1979). Autoradiographic distribution of L-proline in chicks after intracerebral injection. *Physiology and Behavior, 22*, 177–184.

Edelman, G. (1987). *Neural Darwinism.* New York: Basic Books.

Garcia, J., Ervin, F. R., & Keolling, R. (1966). Learning with prolonged delay of reinforcement, *Psychonomic Science, 5*, 121–122.

Gilbert, D. B., Patterson, T. A., & Rose, S. P. R. (1991). Dissociates of brain sites necessary for registration – storage of memory for a one-trail passive avoidance task in the chick. *Behaviour Neuroscience, 105*, 553–561.

Gispen, W.-H., & Routtenberg, A. (Eds.) (1986). Phosphoproteins in neuronal function. *Progress in Brain Research* (book series), *69*. Amsterdam: Elsevier.

Horn, G. (1985). *Memory, imprinting and the brain.* Oxford: Oxford University Press.

Horn, G., & Krebs, J. R. (Eds.). (1990). *Proceedings of the Royal Society of London, B329*, No. 1253.

Jork, R., Grecksch, G., & Matthies, H. (1986). Impairment of hippocampal glycoprotein fucosylation—consequences on memory formation. In H. J. Matthies (Ed.), *Learning and memory: Mechanisms of information storage in the central nervous system* (pp. 223–228). Oxford: Pergamon Press.

Kossut, M., & Rose, S. P. R. (1984). Differential 2-deoxyglucose uptake into chick brain structures during passive avoidance learning. *Neuroscience, 12*, 971–977.

Linden, D. J., & Routtenberg, A. (1989). The role of protein kinase C in long term potentiation: A testable model *Brain and Behavior Review, 14*, 1357–1363.

Lossner, B., & Rose, S. P. R. (1983). Passive avoidance training increases fucokinase activity in right forebrain tissue of day-old chicks. *Journal of Neurochemistry, 48*, 1357–1363.

Lovinger, D. M., Colley, P. A., Akers, R. F., Nelson, R. B., & Routtenberg, A. (1989). Direct relationship of long-term synaptic potentiation to phosphorylation of membrane protein F1, a substrate for membrane PKC. *Brain Research, 536*, 177–183.

Lowndes, M., Stanford, D., & Stewart, M. G. (1989). A system for the reconstruction and analysis of dendritic fields, *Neuroscience Letters, 38* (Suppl.), S87.

Malinow, R., Schulman, H., & Tsien, R. W. (1989). Inhibition of postsynaptic PKC or Cam K II blocks induction but not expression of LTP. *Science, 245*, 862–866.

Mason, R. J., & Rose, S. P. R. (1987). Lasting changes in spontaneous multi-unit activity in the chick brain following passive avoidance training. *Neuroscience, 21*, 931–941.

Mason, R. J., & Rose, S. P. R. (1988). Passive avoidance learning produces focal elevation of bursting activity in the chick brain: Amnesia abolishes the increase. *Behavioral and Neural Biology, 49*, 280–292.

Mileusnic, R., Rose, S. P. R., & Tillson, P. (1980). Passive avoidance learning results in region-specific changes in concentration of and incorporation into colchicine-binding proteins in the chick forebrain. *Journal of Neurochemistry, 34*, 1007–1015.

Muller, D., Bucks, P. A., Dunant, Y., & Lynch, G. (1990). Protein kinase C activity is not responsible for the expression of long term potentiation in hippocampus. *Proceedings of the National Academy of Sciences, U.S.A., 87*, 4073–4077.

Patel, S. N., Rose, S. P. R., & Stewart, M. G. (1988). Training-induced dendritic spine density changes are specifically related to memory formation processes in the chick. *Brain Research, 463*, 168–173.

Patel, S. N., & Stewart, M. G. (1989). Changes in the number and structure of dendritic spines, 25 h after passive avoidance training in the chick *Gallus domesticus*. *Brain Research, 449*, 34–46.

Patterson, T. A., Gilbert, D. B., & Rose, S. P. R. (1990). Pre- and post-training lesions of the intermediate medial hyperstriatum ventrale and passive avoidance learning in the chick. *Experimental Brain Research, 80*, 189–195.

Pohle, W., Rüthrich, H.-L., Popov, N., & Matthies, H. (1979). Fucose incorporation into rat hippocampus structures after acquisition of a brightness discrimination. *Acta Biologica et Medica Germanica, 38*, 53–63.

Reymann, K. C., Schulzeck, K., Dase, H., & Matthies, H. (1988). Phorbol ester-induced hippocampal long-term potentiation is counteracted by inhibitors of PKC. *Experimental Brain Research, 71*, 227–230.

Rose, S. P. R. (1989). Glycoprotein synthesis and post-synaptic remodelling in long-term memory. *Neurochemistry International, 14*, 299–307.

Rose, S. P. R., & Csillag, A. (1985). Passive avoidance training results in lasting changes in deoxyglucose metabolism in left hemisphere regions of chick brain. *Behavioral and Neural Biology, 44*, 315–324.

Rose, S. P. R., & Harding, S. (1984). Training increases ^{3}H-fucose incorporation in chick brain only if followed by memory storage. *Behavioral and Neural Biology, 12*, 663–667.

Rose, S. P. R., & Jork, R. (1987). Long term memory formation in chicks is blocked by 2-deoxygalactose, a fucose analogue. *Behavioral and Neural Biology, 48*, 246–258.

Squire, L. R., & Lindenlaub, E. (Eds.). (1990). *The biology of memory*. Symposia Medica Hoechst, 23. Stuttgart: Schattauer Verlag.

Stewart, M. G. (1991). Changes in dendritic and synaptic structure in the chick forebrain consequent on passive avoidance training. In R. J. Andrew (Ed.), *Neural and behavioural plasticity: The use of the domestic chick as a model* (pp. 305–328). Oxford: Oxford University Press.

Sukumar, R., Rose, S. P. R., & Burgoyne, R. (1980). Increased incorporation of ^{3}H-fucose into chick brain glycoprotein following training on a passive avoidance task. *Journal of Neurochemistry, 34*, 1000–1007.

Index

Accessibility of stored information 8
Acetylcholine (ACh) 250, 251, 385, 386
Acquiring rules 165
Activity-dependent gene expression
 301–29
 potential roles of 322–5
Adenylatecyclase 279, 381
Adult callosal connections 148
Adversive conditioning, neuronal
 mechanisms of 382–4
Alpha-amino-3-hydroxy-5-methyl-4-
 isoxazolepropionate. *See* AMPA
Amino acid receptors 210
Amino acids 295
Amino butiric acid 59
Amnesia 20–2, 401, 404
 anterograde 205
 common threads in human and animal
 164–8
 defining feature of 22
 retrograde 239
 types of 18
AMPA 311, 333, 334, 339, 340, 350–1
AMPA-R 333, 335
Amygdala 206–11, 260, 316
Amygdaloid nucleus 208
Anterior ventral temporal cortex 245
Anterograde amnesia 20–2
AP-1 303, 311
AP-5 339
Aplysia 273–300
 central nervous system synapse 273–7
 central synapses 277
 changes in structure of transmitter
 release sites at CNS synapses 293
 gill withdrawal reflex 278, 292, 403
 increases in synapse number following
 long-term sensitization 293
 long-term memory in 281, 292
 mechanoreceptor sensory neurons 293
 memory for long-term sensitization
 278–80

morphological changes at specific
 synaptic loci 292
morphological changes in long-term
 facilitation 293
nonassociative learning 278
presynaptic active zone 273–7
presynaptic specialization 276
short-term memory in 292
siphon-withdrawal reflex 278, 292
structural changes at sensory neuron
 synapses 295
synaptic junction 274
synaptic plasticity in 280–1
transmitter mediated changes in cell
 adhesion molecules 296
Artificial intelligence 46
Association 165
 among memorized objects 243–5
 configural 165
 hyperspecific 168
 stimulus–stimulus 245
 visual–visual 240
Associative learning in command neuron
 384–6
Associative memory 116
Associative stimulus–response selectivity
 364
Associativity 210
ATP 397
Auditory cortex 207, 208
Auditory imprinting
 2-deoxyglucose (2-DG) in 116–18
 of Guinea fowl and domestic chicks
 116–17
 synaptic selection in 114–59
Auditory system 207
Availability of stored information 8

B50 397–9
Basal forebrain cholinergic system
 (BFCS) 250, 260

Basal forebrain cholinergic tissue, intrahippocampal implants of 258–60
Basal ganglia 102, 396
BDNF 313, 316, 318–20
Behavior, brain mechanisms of 206
Behavioral manipulation 218
Behavioral tasks
  and recording of neural activities 241–2
  engaging small skin locus 225–30
Behavioral training 217–38
Benzodiazepines 211
Beta-endorphin 263
BFCS. *See* Basal forebrain cholinergic system (BFCS)
Bicuculline 59, 220
Binding problem 36
Biological determinancy 8
Blood flow changes, location of 89, 90
Blood vessels artifacts apparent in functional maps 69
Brain
  /behavior/cognition systems 25
  blood flow, changes in 86
  cells 51
  functional mapping of neuronal activity in 87
  information processing in 86–94
  lesions 205
    of anatomical structures 95
  mechanisms of behavior 206
  networks 355
  optical imaging of architecture and function 49–85
  structures participating in visual learning, tactile learning, and motor learning 95–113
Brain derived neurotrophic factor. *See* BDNF
Bulb–cortex simulation 347
Bulbocavernosus muscle 149

c-*fos* 302–6, 313, 321, 322, 399
c-*jun* 303, 322, 399
Calbindin 134, 136, 138, 140
Calcium
  channels
    depolarization of 369
    participation of 381
    sleepy 382
    voltage-dependent 387
  control, intracellular, in MNH 132–40
  role in pacemaker oscillations 369

Calmodulin 133
Calretinin (CaR) 136–8, 140
  immuno-reactivity 124
cAMP 311, 381
cAMP response element binding proteins (CREBs) 303
Carbachol 252–3
Carrier wave 45
Cat areas 17 and 18, functional architecture of 72–3
Cat visual cortex
  directionality columns in 72
  orientation columns in 72
  orientation preference in 72
  selective visualization of neuronal assemblies in 62–3
CCD camera 67, 69, 75
Cellular cascade during memory formation 398
Center-surround inhibitory interactions 59
Central nervous system (CNS)
  structures 393
  synapses of 273–7
Cerebellum
  changes of rCBF in 101
  role in high-level information processing 91
Cerebral cortex, synaptic mechanism in 221
Chick brain 396
Chick model 394–6
Chicks
  auditory filial imprinting 116–17
  Golgi–Cox analysis 126–32
  imprinted 126–32
  visual imprinting and pecking avoidance related to plasticity in hyperstriatum ventrale 140–6
Choline uptake in hippocampus 256–8
Cholinergic antagonists 263
Cholinergic hypothesis 261
Cholinergic neurons
  and nonspatial recent memory 254–6
  and recent memory in aged rats 253–4
Cholinergic receptors 250
Cholinergic septohippocampal system, mnemonic functions of 250–69
Classificatory concepts 4
CO_2 arterial partial pressure 97
Codetermination of tasks 22–4
Cognitive learning and motor learning, differences between 107–11
Cognitive mapping theory 170
Cognitive memory deficits 95
Cognitive systems 13

Collateral system in field CA3 352–5
Command neuron
  as nervous center 366
  associative learning in 384–6
  identifiable synapses on 379–81
  receptive field of 371–5
Commissural-associational system in field
    CA3 356
Computational modeling 195
Concepts
  central 4
  importance and role of 4
Conceptual reflex arc 365
Conditioned reflex, intracellular signaling
    in 386–8
Conditioned responses (CR) 208, 209
Conditioned stimulus (CS) 207–9
Configural association 165
Configurations 166
Contextual encoding 165
Convergent dissociations 14
Cortical activity
  in the awake monkey, high-resolution
    optical imaging of 77
Cortical anatomy of single-word
    processing 88
Cortical interactions between adjacent
    visual stimuli 71–72
Cortical neurons 217
Cortical neuropil 59
Cortical organization, hypotheses and
    models of 231
Cortical receptive fields 223
Corticocortical interactions 221
Corticocortical projections 46
Corticolimbic circuits in visual learning
    107
Corticostriatal circuits in visual learning
    107
Corticothalamic interactions 221
Coupled cortical neuron groups, acute
    alteration 222–5
Cyclic AMP 279, 295, 296, 303

Declarative information 19
Declarative memory 12, 22, 116, 165–8
Delayed response tasks 189
Dentate gyrus 352–5
  granule cells 318
2-deoxygalactose 401, 408
2-deoxyglucose (2-DG) 51, 72, 142, 145,
    393, 396
  in auditory imprinting 116–18

Depolarization
  intracellular 386
  of calcium channels 369
Diode array
  apparatus 52
  mapping of functional organization in
    cat visual cortex 67
Directionality columns in cat visual cortex
    72
Dishabituation effect 369
Dissociations
  between outcomes of tests 14
  convergent 14
Distributed neural responses 218
Distributed oscillation 44
DNA 303, 387
DNQX 339
Dopamine 125
Dorsomedial thalamic nuclei
    (DMP/DMA) 120, 122, 124, 144
Drosophila 394
Dye-signal source 59
Dyes
  optical imaging of neuronal activity
    52–4
  organization and interaction of *in vivo*
    neuronal populations using 55–64
  see also Voltage-sensitive dyes
Dynorphin 306, 309, 320

ECG 56, 77
Ecphoric information 6
Ecphory 6
Ectostriatum 117
EEG 38, 39, 41, 44, 50, 62, 97, 111, 265,
    344
Effect-dependent learning 364, 384
Electrical stimulation 316
Electroencephalogram. *See* EEG
Electromyogram (EMG) 97
Electroshock 403
EMG 97
Emotional disorders 206
Emotional memory, systems and synapses
    of 205–16
Encoding 6
Engram 6
Enhancement phenomenon 186
Enkephalin 306, 309, 320, 323
Ensemble activity 193
Entorhinal cortex 356
Environmental enrichment effects 319

Epigenetic specification of networks by regressive phenomena 146–51
Episodic memory 11–24
Episodic/semantic distinction 20–2
Epistemology 393
Event-related potentials (ERPs) 8–9
Excitatory postsynaptic potentials (EPSPs) 38, 295, 374–5
Explicit memory 12, 17, 165
External context attributes 165
Eye movements recordings 97

Fear
  conditioning
    and synaptic plasticity 209–12
    neuroanatomy of 206–8
  processes, localization of 206
Feature detection by hippocampal neurons 181–90
Field CA1 352–6
  LTP in 331–5, 338
Field CA3 352–5
  collateral system 356
  commissural-associational system 356
Filial imprinting 115
Fixation helmet 97
Fornix transection (FX) 171–9
Fos protein 303
Fos-related antigens (FRAs) 303
FRA/Jun heterodimer 304
Fractal patterns 244
Fucoglycoprotein 401
Fucokinase 401
Functional architecture
  of cat areas 17 and 18 72–73
  of primate visual areas 17 and 18 67–9
Functional cortical reorganization 219–21
Functional domain 169
  of hippocampus 169–79
Functional mapping of neuronal activity in the brain 87
Functional organization 169
  in cat visual cortex
    infrared imaging of 75–7
    through intact dura 75–7
    using diode array 67
  of hippocampus 179–95
    in behaving animals 180–1
  of orientation tuning in monkey striate cortex 74

GABA 125, 138, 211, 212, 220
  agonists 260

receptors 333
GABAergic afferents 251
GABAergic agonists 253, 263
GABAergic inhibition 255
GABAergic neurons 138
GABAergic receptors 250
Galactose 401
GAPS. *See* General Abstract Processing System
Garcia effect 408
Gene expression
  activity-dependent 301–29
  modification by normal activity 321–2
  seizure- and stimulation-induced changes in 302–20
General Abstract Processing System (GAPS) 5–7, 13, 19
  component processes of 7
  structure of 6
Giant cells 366
Globus pallidus 101, 110
GluR1 311, 320
Glutamate 210
  receptors 311–13, 320, 324
Glycoproteins 401, 408, 409
Golgi–Cox analysis of imprinted chicks 126–32
Golgi studies of neurons 126–32
Golgi Type 1 neurons 211
Golgi Type 2 cells 211
Guinea fowl, auditory filial imprinting 116–17

H. ermissenda 394
H. sapiens 394
Habit formation 168
Habituation 12, 278, 279, 369
Hebb rules 404
Hebbian learning 43, 44
High affinity choline uptake (HACU) 251–2
  in hippocampus 256–8
High-density mapping studies 221
High-resolution optical imaging of cortical activity in the awake monkey 77
Hilus lesion (HL) 304, 316
Hippocampal cells, changes in place fields of 187
Hippocampal cellular activity 186, 189
Hippocampal cellular responses 186
Hippocampal formation 95
Hippocampal gyrus cells 189
Hippocampal lesion 239
Hippocampal neural circuits 240

Hippocampal neuronal activity 189
Hippocampal neurons
  feature detection by 181–90
  firing of 189
Hippocampal place cells 186
Hippocampal representation
  characterization 168–9
  in memory 195–7
Hippocampal system
  and mnemonic flexibility 175–9
  and relational representation 171–4
  damage 165
Hippocampal theta 252–6
Hippocampal unit activity 189
Hippocampus 210, 240, 245, 250, 254,
    316, 325
  contributions to learning and memory
    351
  functional domain of 169–79
  functional organization of 179–95
  high affinity choline uptake in 256–8
  informal model 351–5
  memory representation in 163–204
  relating variants of synaptic potentiation
    to memory operations in 330–63
  topographical organization in 190–5
Horseradish peroxidase (HRP) 219,
    280–1, 283, 285
HVc 133, 150, 151
Hyperspecific associations 168
Hyperstriatum dorsale (HAD) 117
Hyperstriatum ventrale (HV) 117, 140–6

ICMS. *See* Intracortical microstimulation
Identifiable synapses on command neuron
    379–81
Imaging techniques 51
IMHV 142–4, 396, 397, 399, 401, 403–6,
    409
Immediate early genes (IEG) 302–6, 320,
    321
Implicit memory 12, 165
Imprinting
  filial 115
  see also Auditory imprinting; Visual
    imprinting
Individual representation 166
Inferior temporal cortex 240
Inferotemporal cells 186
Inferotemporal cortex 194
Information processing
  and storage, in learning 95
  in the brain 86–94
  role of cerebellum in high-level 91

Infrared imaging of functional organization
  through intact dura in cat visual
  cortex 75–7
Inhibitory postsynaptic potentials (IPSPs)
  211, 344–5
Intact dura, in cat visual cortex, infrared
  imaging of functional organization
  through 75
Interaction between storage and retrieval
  8
Intermediate medial hyperstriatum
  ventrale. *See* IMHV
Intertrial inverval (ITI) 255, 256
Intracellular activity of neuronal
  populations 52
Intracellular calcium control in MNH
  132–40
Intracellular depolarization 386
Intracellular signaling 384–6
  in conditioned reflex 386–8
Intracortical microstimulation (ICMS)
  217–38
Intrahippocampal grafts 265
Intrahippocampal implants of basal
  forebrain cholinergic tissue 258–60
Intraseptal infusions 252–6
Intrinsic signals
  determining source and nature of 66
  optical imaging based on 55, 64–77
Ionic channels 386

Jun/Jun homodimer 304
Jun protein 303

Kainic acid 123, 316
Kety autoradiographic technique 87

Lateral entorhinal cortex 352–5
Lateral olfactory tract (LOT) 338–40
Lateral-rostral neostriatum 142
Learned stimuli 241–4
Learning
  along the performance line 165
  anatomical basis for 280–1
  associative, in command neuron 384–6
  cognitive, and motor learning,
    differences between 107–11
  effect-dependent 364, 384
  Hebbian 43, 44
  hippocampal contributions to 351–5
  hippocampal participation in 180
  in mammals 278

Learning (*contd.*)
information processing and storage in 95
motor, and cognitive learning, differences between 107–11
neuronal, local plasticity in 364–91
nonassociative 278
nonspatial 171
semantic 24
somatosensory information 102–6
stimulus-dependent 364
synaptic rules 341–6
see also Motor learning; Tactile learning; Visual learning
Learning-induced changes in neuronal properties, decay of 325
Lesions and loci of memory 404–6
Levels of analysis 392–3
Levels of meaning 392–3
Linkage problem 44
Lithium-choride-induced sickness 407
LMtC1 384
Lobus parolfactorius (LPO) 122, 140, 396–7, 399, 401, 403, 405, 406, 409
Local detectors as parallel channels 375–9
Local field potentials (LFPs) 38, 46, 62
Local plasticity in neuronal learning 364–91
Long-term depression (LTD) 114, 140
Long-term facilitation, morphological changes in 293
Long-term memory
and varicosity number 285
formation of 401
in *Aplysia* 281, 292
labile component 240
morphological perspective 291–6
nature of 291–6
primal 238–49
stages with distinguishable localizations 239–40
Long-term potentiation (LTP) 114, 140, 209–10, 306, 319, 324, 325, 331, 395, 397–9
and theta bursting 343–5, 348
development and stabilization of 323
expression characteristics of 335–6
expression via AMPA receptors 350
in field CA1 331–5, 338
in MNH 132–40
incorporating the expression characteristics into network models 346–51
induction 341–6
and theta bursting 348

fractional degrees of 350
timing rules 345, 348
via NMDA receptors 350
mechanisms 131
reversal of 345–6, 349–50
saturation 350
stable expression of 350
structures reducing 132
Long-term sensitization in *Aplysia* 273–300
LOT–piriform synapses 340
LPa3 366, 384

Machine vision 40
Macroscopic activity in visual perception 45
Magnetic tomographic image 97
Magnocellular nucleus of the neostriatum (MAN) 122
reduction of neurons in lateral nucleus 150
Major systems, ordering of 12
Medial geniculate body (MGB) 207, 209
Medial–lateral axis 59
Medial septal area (MSA) 250–1, 260, 262
Medial temporal lobe 95
Melittin 397
Membrane
properties 399
proteins 399
Memory
anatomical basis for 280–1
classification 9–18
clinical neurological investigations 18
cognitive, deficits 95
concepts of 3–32
disorder and primal long-term memory 246–7
effect of network properties 351–7
emotional, systems and synapses of 205–16
episodic 11–24
explicit 12, 17, 165
flow diagram 406
formation
cellular cascade during 398
cellular processes of 392
potential roles of activity-dependent gene expression in 322–5
storage and utilization of 324
hippocampal contributions to 351–5
hippocampal representation in 195–7
history of research 3

implicit 12, 165
inhibition of MSA neurons impairment
of 252–3
loci of 404–6
mechanisms, model for study of 392
neural basis of 205
neuroanatomical organization of 205
nonassociative 116
nonspatial 180, 254–6
normal 3, 22–4
pathological 3
primary 13
procedural 11–18, 116, 165, 166
propositional 12
reference 165
representation in hippocampus 163–204
semantic 11–24
spatial 180, 193
storage, localized or distributed 406–9
study of 4–5
systems
  components defining 10–11
  concept of 9–11
  five major types 11–18
  functional analysis of 14
  functionally incompatible 11
  proliferation of 11
with record 164
without record 164
working 165
see also Long-term memory; Recent
  memory; Short-term memory;
  Visual memory
Microscopic activity in visual perception
45
MK-801 306
Mnemonic flexibility 169, 175–9
Mnemonic functions of cholinergic
  septohippocampal system 250–69
MNH 143
functional properties and connections
  118–25
Golgi studies of neurons in neostriatal
  part of 126–32
intracellular calcium control in 132–40
LTP in 132–40
regressive changes in 146
storage of new information in 146
Modified memory flow interpretation 407
Modulatory neurons in control of synaptic
  transmission 381–2
Molecular biological techniques 301
Monkey
distributed changes induced by
  behavioral tasks 225–30

high-resolution optical imaging of
  cortical activity in the awake 77
striate cortex 61
functional organization of orientation
  tuning in 74
visual areas 17 and 18, functional
  organization *in vivo* 67–9
Mossy fiber 356
Mossy fiber potentiation (MFP) 336–8,
353
presynaptic nature of 338
Motor
arm sectors 102
cortices 102
field of command neuron 369–71
learning 99–102
  and cognitive learning, differences
  between 107–11
  brain regions changing rCBF during
  100
  rCBF in 110–11
program storage 101–2
skills, acquisition of 95
units of skeletal muscle 148–9
MRI 66
mRNA 302, 304, 310, 313, 316, 318–23,
399
synthesis 303
MSA 260, 262
Multiple microelectrode recordings 52
Muscimol 252–3, 256, 260

N-CAM 409
Naloxone 260
Neocortex 316
Neocortical function 217
Neostriatum 117
Nerve growth factor (NGF) 316, 318, 320
Nerve growth factor (NGF)-like
  neurotrophic factors 302
Nervous center, command neuron as 366
Network memory, relating induction and
  expression characteristics to
  properties of 348–51
Network models, incorporating expression
  characteristics into 346–51
Network properties, effects on memory
  operations 351–7
Neural activity, simultaneous multichannel
  recording of 46
Neural discharges, selectivity of 242–3
Neural function 393
Neuroactive peptides 306–11, 324
Neurobiological analysis 206

Neuron coupling in temporal domain
    230–3
Neuronal activity, optical imaging with
    dyes 52–4
Neuronal assemblies 50
    oscillations of ongoing and evoked
        activity in 64
    selective visualization in cat visual
        cortex 62–3
    spatiotemporal patterns of 64
Neuronal gene expression, activity-
    dependent 301–29
Neuronal learning, local plasticity in
    364–91
Neuronal mechanisms of adversive
    conditioning 382–4
Neuronal membrane 386
Neuronal populations
    intracellular activity of 52
    spatiotemporal patterns of activity of
        52
Neuronal tuning alterations 187
Neurons, Golgi studies of 126–32
Neuropeptide Y (NPY) 260, 306–7, 310,
    320
Neuropeptides 320
Neurophysiological properties 403
Neuropil arbor 296
Neurotrophic factor synthesis 318
Neurotrophic factors 320
Neurotrophin 3 (NT3) 313, 320
NGF-like growth factors 311
NGF-like neurotrophic factors 313–19
N-methyl-D-aspartate (NMDA) 145, 212,
    306, 333, 336, 339, 340, 350–1
N-methyl-D-aspartate (NMDA) receptors
    210, 333, 335
Nonassociative learning 278
Nonassociative memory 116
Nonlinear dynamics in studies of olfactory
    perception 37
Non-NMDA glutamate receptors 311–13
Nonspatial learning 171
Nonspatial memory 180, 254–6
Nonspatial recent memory 254–6
Normal memory 22–4
NT3 316, 318, 319
Nucleus basalis magnocellularis (NBM)
    260, 262

Ocular dominance columns in visual
    cortex 147–8
Odor discrimination 171–2, 175–7, 181–2,
    187, 189, 394

Odor-specificity 347
Olfaction and vision 35–6
Olfactory bulb 37, 38, 44
Olfactory cortex 316, 355
Olfactory discriminations 348
Olfactory dynamics model 38–9
Olfactory–hippocampal circuit 331,
    338–40, 351
Olfactory perception
    neurodynamics of 37
    nonlinear dynamics in studies of 37
    physiological bases of 37–8
Olfactory processing 37
Olfactory psychophysiology 36
Olfactory system 35–48
Olfactory tract 39
Opioid agonists 263
Opioid peptides 263
Optical chamber 52
Optical imaging
    based on instrinsic signals 55
    of architecture and function in the living
        brain 49–85
    of mammalian brain *in vivo* 55–64
    of neuronal activity with dyes 52–4
    spatial resolution of 80
    surround inhibition revealed by 59–62
    using intrinsic signals 64–77
    with and without voltage-sensitive dyes
        77–81
Orientation centers
    in cat visual cortex 72
    in monkey striate cortex 74
Orientation columns in cat visual cortex
    72
Orientation preference in cat visual
    cortex 72
Oscillatory spatiotemporal patterns 50
Oxotremorine 254, 260

Pacemaker
    mechanism, plasticity of 366–9
    oscillations, role of calcium in 369
    potentials 366–9
Paleostriatal complex 396
Paleostriatum augmentatum (PA) 396
Parahippocampal cortex 194
Parallel channels, local detectors as 375–9
Parasympathetic system, functions of 261
Parietal cortex 195
Parvalbumin (PV) 133–5, 138, 140
Pattern classification 40–1
Pavlovian defensive conditioning 205–6
Perception 35

Perceptual priming 11–18
Perceptual representation systems (PRS)
 11, 14–18
 neuroanatomical and neurophysiological
 correlates of 18
Performance line storage 13
Perirhinal cortex 247
Phaeochromocytoma PC12 cell 303
Phosphoinositide (PI) 399
Phosphorylation–dephosphorylation of
 receptor protein 387
Phylogeny 393
Physical indeterminancy 8
Picture memorization 245–6
Pinwheels
 in cat visual cortex 72–3
 in monkey striate cortex 74
Place cell
 phenomenon 182, 189
 properties 186
Place cues 170
Place fields 195
Place learning 165, 172–4, 177–9
Place tasks 182–90
Plasticity
 of pacemaker mechanism 366–9
 thresholds 324
Pleural sensory neurons 295
Polymodal neocortical areas 183
Positron emission tomography (PET) 51,
 66, 86–94, 257
Posterior intralaminar nucleus (PIN) 207
Postsynaptic cells 59
Postsynaptic dendrites, subthreshold
 excitation of 59
Postsynaptic density (PSD) 145, 397
Postsynaptic short-term plasticity 388
Preproenkephalin cRNA 307
Preproenkephalin mRNA 307, 309, 311
PreproNPY (ppNPY) mRNA 310
Primal long-term memory 239–49
 and memory disorder 246–7
Primary memory 13
Primary somatosensory cortex 217–38
Primate temporal cortex 239–49
Primate visual areas 17 and 18, functional
 architecture 67–9
Priming effects 16–17
Procedural memory 11–18, 116, 165, 166
Processing concepts 4
Propositional information 19
Propositional memory 12
Prorhinal cortex 247
Protein kinase 381
Protein kinase C (PKC) 397, 398

Protein phosphorylation 221, 280
Protein synthesis 295, 301
Putamen 101, 110

QM (quasi-memory) system 15
Q–Q plots 97
Quantitative tissue autoradiogram 87

Rats
 cholinergic neurons and recent memory
 in 253–4
 learning performance 171
 reaction times in 173
 somatosensory cortex 59
rCBF 96–8
 in motor learning 101, 110–11
 in tactile learning 102–6
 in tactile recognition 106
 in visual learning 106–7, 110–11
Reaction times in FX rats 176
Recent memory
 and cholinergic neurons in aged rats
 253–4
 nonspatial 254–6
 and cholinergic neurons 254–6
Receptive field of command neuron
 371–5
Receptor proteins
 open and closed 386
 phosphorylation–dephosphorylation of
 387
Recognition 165
Recurrent seizure activity 316
Reference memory 165
Regional cerebral blood flow. *See* rCBF
Regional cerebral metabolic rate of oxygen
 (rCMRO$_2$) in tactile learning 102–6
Regional synaptic activity 96
Regressive phenomena, epigenetic
 specification of networks by 146–51
Relational representation 166, 167, 169,
 171–4
Remembering
 act of 5, 6
 processes of 4–9
Representational topography 218
Response perserveration hypothesis 169
Response tolerance under stimulus
 transformation 246
Retinotopic imaging experiments in
 monkey striate cortex 56
RH-795 dye 62
Rhinal cortex 247

Rhinal sulcus   247
RNA synthesis   295, 301
Rostral–caudal axis   59
Rostral neostriatum   117
RPa3   366

Schaffer-commissural projections   356
Scopolamine   252–3
Seizure studies, summary   319–20
Selective plasticity   324
Self-organizing system   43
Semantic learning ability   24
Semantic memory   11–24
Sensitization   12, 278
  long-term, in *Aplysia*   273–300
Sensory-evoked responses, topographical
  mapping of   56–9
Sensory information processing   51
Sensory neuron synapses   283–90
Sensory preprocessing   42
Sensory-to-follower cell connection   280
Septohippocampal cholinergic system   264
Sequential memory operations   355–7
Serial networks   355–7
Serial position number (SPN)   241, 243,
  244
Serotonin   279, 381, 382
Short-term memory   11–18
  in *Aplysia*   292
Simple association   165
Single-word processing, cortical anatomy
  of   88
Skeletal muscle, motor units of   148–9
Skin
  locus, behavioral tasks engaging   225–30
  stimulation, temporal response of
    neurons to   230–3
Somatosensory information, learning of
  102–6
Songbirds
  sex difference in song behavior   149
  vocal repertoire in   149–51
Spatial memory   180, 193
Spatial resolution
  increasing   67
  of optical imaging techniques   80
Spatiotemporal patterns
  of neuronal assemblies   64
  of neuronal populations   52
Specificity   260–3
Staurosporine   397
Stimulus-dependent learning   364
Stimulus onset asynchrony   24
Stimulus–response relationship   115

Stimulus selection, behavioral criteria   115
Stimulus–stimulus association   245
Stimulus transformation, response
  tolerance under   246
Stratum granulosum   316
Stratum pyramidale   316
Striate cortex   396
Structural regression   146–7
Study/test paradigm   4–5
Subseizure afferent stimulation   306
Substance P   260
Subthreshold excitation of postsynaptic
  dendrites   59
Supplementary motor area (SMA)   91
Supramodal perceptual processing   186
Synapsin I   274
Synaptic activity and rCBF   101
Synaptic junctions, visualization of   275–6
Synaptic learning rules   341–6
Synaptic mechanism in the cerebral
  cortex   221
Synaptic phosphorylations   397–9
Synaptic plasma membranes (SPMs)   397
Synaptic plasticity   114
  and fear conditioning   209–12
  in *Aplysia*   280–1
Synaptic potentiation
  expression characteristics of   331–41
  variants, relating to memory operations
    in hippocampus   330–63
  variations, effects on memory
    operations   351–7
Synaptic selection in auditory imprinting
  114–59
Synaptic transmission, modulatory neurons
  in control of   381–2
Synergistic ecphory   7–9

Tactile learning   102–6
  regional cerebral metabolic rate of
    oxygen (rCMRO$_2$) in   102–6
Tactile recognition, rCBF in   106
Taxon learning   165
Taxons   170
Temporal domain, neuron coupling in
  230–3
Temporal response of neurons to skin
  simulation   230–3
Temporal tagging   166
Tetracaine   252–3
Thalamoamygdala projection   210
Thalamocortical afferents   219
Thalamocortical inputs   220
Thalamus   95

Theta bursting and LTP 343–5, 348
Theta spikings 349–50
Threshold stimulation conditions 318
Time-locked firing 347
Timing rules for LTP induction 345, 348
Tis-8 306, 310, 322
Tonic activity within individual neurons 324
Topographical mapping of sensory-evoked responses 56–9
Topographical organization in the hippocampus 190–5
Transmitter iontophoretic application 386
Transmitter potential 385
Trophic factor expression 319
Trophic factor mRNAs 318
Trophic factors 324
Type 1 cells 210
Type 1 neurons 211
Type 2 cells 210
Type I neurons 127–8, 130, 131, 138, 150
Type II neurons 138

Unconditioned responses (UR) 208
Unconditioned stimulus (US) 207, 208

Varicosity number 296
  and long-term memory 285
Ventrolateral thalamus 102
Video monitoring 97
Vision and olfaction 35–6
Visual and association cortex 206
Visual cortex 39, 41, 46
  functional architecture of orientation and ocular dominance columns in 50

functional organization in cat 67
  ocular dominance columns in 147–8
Visual images 36
Visual imprinting, related to plasticity in hyperstriatum ventrale 140–6
Visual learning 106–7
  corticolimbic circuits in 107
  corticostriatal circuits in 107
  rCBF in 106–7, 110–11
Visual memory
  system 240
  task 241
Visual perception 35–48
  macroscopic activity in 45
  microscopic activity in 45
  proposed model for 42–6
Visual physiology 36
Visual processes, verified predictions and extensions for 41–2
Visual psychophysiology 36
Visual stimuli, cortical interactions between adjacent 71–72
Visual–visual association 240
Vocal repertoire in songbirds 149–51
Voltage-sensitive dyes, optical imaging with and without 77–81

Wave packet 44
Working memory 165

Y-maze tests 123

Zebra finches 150
zif/268 306